MICROBES, VIRUSES AND PARASITES IN AIDS PROCESS

Edited by **Vladimír Zajac**

Microbes, Viruses and Parasites in AIDS Process
Edited by Vladimír Zajac

Published by InTech

Janeza Trdine 9, 51000 Rijeka, Croatia

Publishing Process Manager Alenka Urbancic

Technical Editor Teodora Smiljanic

Cover Designer InTech Design Team

Additional hard copies can be obtained from orders@intechopen.com

Microbes, Viruses and Parasites in AIDS Process, Edited by Vladimír Zajac
p. cm.
ISBN 978-953-307-601-0

For EU product safety concerns:
IN TECH d.o.o., Prolaz Marije Krucifikse Kozulić 3, 51000 Rijeka, Croatia, info@intechopen.com or visit our website at intechopen.com.

Meet the editor

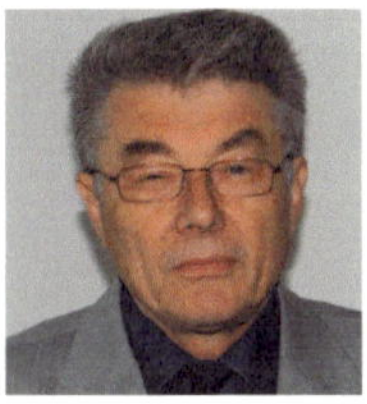

Assoc. Professor Zajac Vladimír, PhD. graduated from Comenius University (Bratislava, Slovakia) in 1973 and ever since has been working at the Cancer Research Institute, SAS (Bratislava), where he obtained his PhD degree in 1981, since then. He joined the Medical Faculty of the Comenius University as Associate Professor in Genetics in 2007. Dr. Zajac began working with bovine leukemia virus (BLV) in 1976., and has been engaged in the study of the role of bacteria in bovine leukosis and AIDS since 1990. The fundamental study was done in Prof. F. Wong-Staal's laboratory (UCSD, San Diego). Since 1994, Dr. Zajac's research is focused on hereditary forms of colon, breast and ovarian cancer. His cancer genetics study culminated in Prof. A. P. Monaco's laboratory (University of Oxford). His particular interest and life-long scientific work concerns the study of horizontal transfer of genetic information between eukaryotic and prokaryotic systems, with focus on retroviruses and the consequences of transmission in induction of cancer and AIDS.

Contents

Preface

A large number of diseases have appeared during the past half century, yet for many of them the reasons have so far remained unexplained. One of the most feared representatives is the acquired immune deficiency syndrome (AIDS). AIDS emerged suddenly, unexpectedly, and in the course of less than two decades it became one of the leading diseases in the world. The majority of scientists and clinicians, except Duesberg and some others, have accepted the data leading to the conclusion that HIV alone is the etiologic agent responsible for this disease, which has been identified as a global pandemic.

Despite the unquestionable success in diagnosis and therapy, there are many unanswered questions which preclude a more successful treatment of the disease. The substantial argument of this predication is the fact that it is still not possible to stop the worldwide pervasion of AIDS, especially in Africa and Asia.

The presented book is predominantly focused on opportunistic diseases of HIV positive patients. The majority of the chapters are from African authors, providing the reader with a fair overview on the prevalence of opportunistic infections of AIDS patients in several African countries. The overall picture of the AIDS situation in Africa is inconsolable, if not apocalyptic. Poverty, parasitosis and AIDS are closely interlinked and co-circulate in many populations. AIDS, parasitic infections and other opportunistic infections are by far the commonest causes of illness and death in the poorest countries of the world, that happen to be in the tropics and temperate countries in Africa, Asia, and South America. Parasitic infections remain an important cause of morbidity and mortality in developing countries, especially among HIV-infected persons.

This alarming situation evokes the question whether opportunistic infections induced by microbes, viruses and parasites are not only the consequence of the immunodeficient condition of the patients, but play a rather more active role in AIDS than acknowledged so far. To date this question could not be answered and its elucidation requires further intensive and target-aimed research.

Africa suffered very markedly from iatrogenic AIDS through dangerous medical interventions, including mass vaccination programs carried out by poorly trained individuals. Recent work by researchers from some laboratories has provided serious evidence that the heterosexual route for transmission of AIDS in Africa has been greatly overstressed and that iatrogenic factors have been very much underestimated.

The book raises the basic question – what is the origin of HIV? The explanation that AIDS arose from a secluded area in Africa, where a virus was transmitted to man from another primate is unacceptable for some researchers. This concept is not able to answer the crucial questions: 1) Why would the immunodeficiency viruses stay put in simians for thousands of years and then suddenly, within a decade atack humans? 2) Was the virus, according to this concept, transferred by several accidental events from apes to humans, resulting in a world- wide pandemics? 3) The diversification of the ancestors of HIV into the HIV-1 and HIV-2 halves of the evolutionary tree would have occurred long before that, perhaps hundreds or even thousands of years ago, and not during the last three-four decades?

In the book an original, for some readers maybe heretical idea, is presented, maintaining that HIV, similarly as other retroviruses, have been an integral part of a particular host organism since the beginning of their existence as species and were passed on from generation to generation. The hosts – including humans - inherited them from their ancestors. In accordance with this idea, it is assumed that transfer of the HIV from apes to humans in Africa, as a consequence of their accidental contact, is not the cause of AIDS pandemics. This hypothesis is confirmed by experimental results, which should be verified by other laboratories. New ideas in this health field are highly needed, as they may open new ways for research and therapy.

Several studies have shown that probiotics could enhance the health and well-being of AIDS patients, but sadly the use of probiotics in Africa has not become popular for several reasons. First, pharmaceutical companies that manufacture probiotics would be forced to lower prices, which would adversely affect their revenues. Secondly, storage and distribution problems make the administration of probiotics difficult. The lack of any probiotic fermented, clinically proven products in Africa at present, with some exceptions, makes it hard to perform studies and provide benefits to the population.

The fight against AIDS is challenging and should be realized in a more complex manner, overcoming all the taboos and dogmas surrounding the disease. As presented by a couple of book authors, it is necessary to consider other potential factors, not only HIV, which may be involved in this disease. They try to offer a new way ahead of our understanding of AIDS and the mechanisms underlying it, which may be very important to future development of research and treatment.

Assoc. Prof. Vladimir Zajac, PhD.
Cancer Research Institute, SAS,
Bratislava,
Slovakia

1

Clinical Manifestations of HIV-Infection in the Era of Highly Active Antiretroviral Therapy

Sara Guillén, Luis Prieto, Marta Ruiz Jiménez and José T. Ramos
Hospital Universitario de Getafe
Spain

1. Introduction

Today, more than 25 years after the description of the first AIDS cases in children, major advances have been made on the prevention and treatment of the infection caused by human immunodeficiency virus (VIH-1), mainly after the availability of highly active antiretroviral therapy (HAART). Despite improved access to antiretroviral treatment and prevention, the HIV-infection epidemic continues to expand. The progression of the disease is much faster in children than in adults as well as the risk of complications. Since most infections occur perinatally, the virus overcomes the capacity of the immature immune system to control the HIV replication and dissemination occurs to all organ systems including the central nervous system (CNS). As a consequence the clinical course is more accelerated in children than in adults, and the immunological dysfunction is greater. Without antiretroviral treatment, HIV-infection in children has a bimodal pattern: a rapidly progressive form (15-20%) characterized by the development of severe opportunistic infections (OI), encephalopathy and death in the first 3 years, and a second form less aggressive and more alike to the presentation seen in adults, that accounts for around 80% of cases. Furthermore as there are no accurate prognostic surrogate markers of disease progression at diagnosis, most children should be treated early. Nevertheless, there is a delay in the development and implementation of antiretroviral treatment in children and adolescents. In addition, the need for a lifelong medication, with complex schedules, frequent high pill burden and lack of suitable paediatric formulation with insufficient data for children makes more difficult to maintain a permanent adherence to medication. Currently, although most children are on a stable situation with high CD4 counts and complete control of viral replication, the long-term consequences of the disease and of the accumulated effects of HAART are unknown and of major concern.

2. Clinical manifestations of HIV-infection in the era of HAART

The mortality and morbidity in HIV-infected children has declined since 1996 with the introduction of HAART. The studies comparing pre-HAART and post-HAART era marked a significant difference with a reduction in rates of mortality and progression to AIDS (Brady et al., 2010, Sánchez Granados J, 2003). The hospitalization has markedly decreased in HIV-infected children who have access to HAART. Frequent causes of hospitalization like bacterial infections and opportunistic infections have diminished after introduction of HAART (Puthanakit et al., 2007). Many children died of *Pneumocystis carinii* pneumonia whereas others succumbed to a variety of opportunistic infections, including disseminated cytomegalovirus, disseminated *Mycobacterium avium complex* (MAC) and recurrent, severe bacterial infections (Abrams, 2000). Opportunistic infections and other related infections are uncommon in children in the HAART era in developed countries (Gina et al., 2006). On the other hand, children with persistently low CD4 percentage are at risk for opportunistic illnesses (Ylitalo et al., 2006). Children who experienced opportunistic infections have higher mortality rates than do those who do not (Nesheim et al., 2007). The incidence of bacterial infections have decreased in the post-HAART era, as well as the time elapsed to the first bacteraemia episode has been prolonged, although children with a decline of CD4 T cells are still more likely to develop bacteraemia (Kapogiannis et al., 2008). Nevertheless, severe bacterial infectious still occurred at considerable high rates, even in the absence of a severe CD4 cell depletion (Chiappini et al., 2007). Antimicrobial prophylaxis has resulted in a successful prevention of several opportunistic infections in children with low CD4 cells. Since the advent of HAART has led to an increase the numbers of CD4 T cells and CD4 percentage to a level of lower risk in children, there is the possibility of safe discontinuation of prophylaxis for opportunistic infections once HIV-infected children demonstrate improvement in CD4 cell counts to levels at which such prophylaxis would not be initiated according to current guidelines (Nachman et al., 2005). Organ-specific diseases such as cardiomyopathy, nephropathy, encephalopathy, and others contribute substantially to the morbidity and mortality associated to with HIV infection. HAART results in a resolution of most of these organ-specific complications (Saulsbury, 2001). Other organ-specific diseases like, thrombocytopenia, wasting syndrome and lymphoid interstitial pneumonia, have dropped dramatically since the introduction of HAART (Guillén et al., 2010) and are also improved with effective antiretroviral therapy. As survival has been prolonged in perinatally HIV-infected children and adolescents in the HAART era and many of them are now reaching adulthood, an increase in the incidence rates over time in pregnancy-related conditions and gynaecological dysplasia is being observed in parallel with a decrease of the incidence of the other non infectious conditions. (Nachman et al., 2009).

Clinical	N	A	B	C
	Asymptomatic	Mild symptoms	Moderated symptoms	Severe Symptoms
Immunological*				
- Not significant immunodeficiency[1]	N1	A1	B1	C1
- Moderate immunodeficiency[2]	N2	A2	B2	C2
- Severe immunodeficiency[3]	N3	A3	B3	C3

Table 1. Clinical and immunological stages (CDC 1993)

In 1994, the CDC proposed a classification of HIV-disease in children into 4 clinical categories (N, A, B, C) and 3 immunological categories (1, 2, 3), according to the degree of immunosuppression (CDC, 1994) (Table 1). In developing countries, WHO classification also considers 4 clinical categories according to severity and 3 immunological categories (WHO, 2007)(Table 2). There are a variety of OI and organ-specific diseases in different clinical classification and AIDS events. Since the CD4 absolute numbers decline physiologically from birth and the CD4 percentage is more preserved across ages, this parameter is preferred in children below 6 years of age, as it is a better predictor of disease progression. The absolute number of CD4 cells does not predict accurately the risk of complications like in adults, although the degree of immunosuppression influences the occurrence of an infection event or development of an organ-specific involvement.

*	< 12 moths	1-5 years	6-12 years
[1]CD4	> 1500/mm^3, > 25%	>1000/mm^3, > 25%	> 500/mm^3, >25%
[2]CD4	750-1499/mm^3, 15-24%	500-999/mm^3, 15-24%	200-499/mm^3, >15-24%
[3]CD4	< 750/mm^3, < 15%	<500/mm^3, < 15%	< 200/mm^3, < 15%

Table 1. Centers for Diseases Control. 1994 revised classification system for HIV infection in children less than 13 years of age. (CDC, 1994)

2.1 Impact of HAART on organ-specific diseases

In developed countries, HAART has dramatically changed the natural history of HIV infection in children. HAART has reduced the morbidity and mortality among HIV-infected children leading to substantial increase in CD4 T-lymphocyte count and a parallel decrease in HIV viral load. Perinatally-acquired HIV-infection has become a chronic disease, in which many infected children in developed countries are entering adolescence and adulthood.

There are a variety of organ-specific diseases in different clinical classification and AIDS events classified in the CDC and WHO classifications (Tables 1 and 2). The most frequent organ-specific diseases in pre HAART era in children were encephalopathy, cardiomyopathy, wasting syndrome, lymphoid interstitial pneumonia, thrombocytopenia and nephropathy. Most of them occur in advanced stages of immunosuppresion, although sometimes they may present as the initial manifestation of the disease, even with relatively preserved CD4 cell count or CD4 percentage. With successful HAART, the weight and height growth curves tend to normalize over time. In addition, the incidence of organ-specific diseases has dramatically decreased with the use of HAART. Most organ-specific diseases improve with HAART, and in many cases the organ-function is completely restored.

2.1.1 Category A organ-specific diseases

Hepatomegaly is a common clinical manifestation of paediatric HIV disease and is likely caused by the replication of HIV within the reticuloendothelial system. In HIV-infected children a variety of factors may be involved in hepatomegaly besides HIV itself, like concomitant hepatitis viruses, opportunistic infections, medications and malnutrition.

Generalized lymphadenopathy is another common clinical finding in HIV-infected children, but a differential diagnosis must be done with other viral infections, opportunistic and mycobacterial infections, and malignancy.

Clinical stage 1
Asymptomatic
Persistent generalized lymphadenoapathy
Clinical stage 2
Unexplained persistent hepatosplenomegaly
Papular pruritic eruptions
Fungal nail infections
Angular cheilitis
Lineal gingival erythema
Extensive wart virus infection
Unexplained persistent parotid enlargement
Extensive molluscum contagiosum
Recurrent oral ulceration
Unexplained persistent parotid enlargement
Herpes zoster
Recurrent of chronic upper respiratory tract infections (otitis media, otorrhoea, sinusitis, tonsillitis)
Clinical stage 3
Unexplained moderate malnutrition or wasting not adequately responding to standard therapy
Unexplained persistent diarrhoea (14 days or more)
Unexplained persistent fever (above 37.6°C, intermittent or constant, for longer than one month)
Persistent oral candidiasis (after 6-8 weeks of life)
Oral hairy leukoplakia
Acute necrotizing ulcerative gingivitis or periodontitis
Lymph node tuberculosis
Pulmonary tuberculosis
Severe recurrent bacterial pneumonia
Symptomatic lymphoid interstitial pneumonitis
Chronic HIV-associated lung disease including bronchiectasis
Unexplained anaemia (<8.0g/dl), neutropaenia ($<0.5x10^9/L^3$) and or chronic thrombocytopenia ($<50 \times 10^9/L^3$)
Clinical stage 4
Unexplained severe wasting, stunting or severe malnutrition not responding to standard therapy
Pneumocystis pneumonia
Recurrent severe bacterial infections (e.g. empyema, pyomyositis, bone or joint infection, meningitis, but excluding pneumonia)
Chronic herpes simplex infection; (orolabial or cutaneous of more than one month's duration, or visceral at any site)
Extrapulmonary TB
Kaposi sarcoma
Oesophageal candidiasis (or candiadisis of trachea, bronchi or lungs)
Central nervous system toxoplasmosis (after the neonatal period)
HIV encephalopathy

Cytomegalovirus (CMV) infection; retinitis or CMV infection affecting another organ, with onset at age more than 1 month
Extrapulmonary cryptococcosis including meningitis
Disseminated endemic mycosis (extrapulmonary histoplasmosis, coccidioidomycosis, penicilliosis)
Chronic cryptosporidiosis (with diarrhoea)
Chronic isosporiasis
Disseminated non-tuberculous mycobacterial infection
Cerebral or B cell non-Hodgkin lymphoma
Progressive multifocal leukoencephalopathy
HIV-associated cardiomyopathy or nephropathy

Table 2. WHO clinical staging of HIV for infants and children with established HIV infection. (WHO, 2007)

Parotid swelling is thought to be caused by the HIV virus itself, although EBV may also play a role. Suppurative bacterial parotiditis is rare in HIV-infected children. Although very inusual, in progressive parotid swelling a malignancy must also be considered in the differential diagnosis.

Dermatitis in children can be secondary to infections or due to medications. The most common non-infectious diseases are atopic dermatitis and seborrheic dermatitis.

These manifestations are still common but less frequently observed since the introduction of HAART. In addition they all tend to improve or even disappear with the use of HAART

2.1.2 Category B organ-specific diseases

Hematologic disorders like anemia, neutropenia and thrombocytopenia more than 30 days of duration are category B manifestations. These manifestations can occur for many reasons like peripheral destruction, the most common cause of the HIV-associated thrombocytopenia, adverse effect of medications (zidovudine) or medications to treat opportunistic infections (ganciclovir), by HIV virus itself, nutritional status and changes in the bone marrow associated with chronic illness. Various studies have demonstrated a reduction in thrombocytopenia and other cytopenias when HAART is started.

Dilated cardiomyopathy has been described in 10%-20% of children with HIV infection. The mean age at diagnosis of cardiomyopathy in children is 18-24 months, but symptomatic cardiomyopathy may occur in children who are as young as 6 months age. Patients with dilated cardiomyopathy have been preceded by myocarditis, due to direct infection of myocardial cells by HIV. The resolution of this cardiomiopathy after introduction HAART has been described, with complete restoration of ventricular ejection fraction. Although cardiomyopathy appears to be rare nowadays in developed countries, it is not uncommon in children coming from high-prevalence areas with advances states of immunosuppression. In these patients a cardiac ultrasound is recommended as baseline evaluation.

Leiomyosarcoma is described in HIV-infected children, but the incidence is very low. The proportion of leiomyosarcoma or leiomyoma in HIV-infected children is 17% of all cancers in these children. Smooth-muscle tumors are reported in the gastrointestinal tract, liver, spleen and lung. In HIV-infected children these tumors are strongly associated to Epstein-Barr virus. In a study of malignancy in HIV-infected children no significant differences were found in the overall rates of soft tissue cancer between HIV-infected children and uninfected children. Leiomyosarcoma was the only soft tissue cancer to occur in HIV-infected children whereas various different soft tissues sarcomas occurred in non-infected children. (Kest et al., 2005).

Lymphocitic interstitial pneumonia (LIP) is common in HIV–infected children non-treated with HAART. The etiology is unknown but it has been suggested that the coinfection with Epstein-Barr virus and HIV may result in a lymphoproliferative response. The patients are initially asymptomatic or have mild symptoms. They may include cough, mild tachypnea and in advanced stages hypoxemia. The course is usually complicated with recurrent episodes of acute lower respiratory tract infections frequently leading to bronchiectasis. The chest radiography usually shows a diffuse reticulonodular pattern more pronounced centrally. High resolution CT may improve the diagnostic accuracy; typical features include micronodules 1-3 mm in diameter, with a perylymphatic distribution, and subpleural nodules. Lung biopsy may show interstitial infiltrate of lymphocytes and lymphoid aggregates surrounding the airways. LIP has been associated with chronic liver disease and bilateral parotid enlargement. Treatment is symptomatic. Oral corticosteroids have been used. HAART has been described to improve the respiratory status in adults and has been reported to be associated with the resolution of radiographic abnormalities in children. LIP is a stage 3 of WHO AIDS defining illness it is an indication to start HAART in children who are not received antiretroviral treatment. (Zar, 2007).

Nephropathy prevalence varies from 2% to 10% in HIV-infected children, and has been reported to be more common in African-American children than Hispanic or white HIV-infected children. The clinical presentation varies from asymptomatic proteinuria to symptomatic renal tubular acidosis, hematuria, proteinuria and acute renal failure. Nephropathy is associated with a higher degree of immunosupresion and a higher mortality. Biopsy diagnosis can reveal the typical histologic features of minimal change nephritic syndrome, mesangioproliferative glomerular lesions, and "lupus-like" renal lesions. Other patients show renal changes consistent with the diagnosis of HIVAN (HIV-associated nephropathy) or HIV-immune complex disease (HIVICK). The introduction of HAART has revolutionized the clinical management of HIV-associated renal disease. The use of HAART is associated with a marked improvement of HIVAN, resulting in slower progression to end-stage renal disease or even in recovery from dialysis-dependent renal failure provided the kidney damage is not too severe (Mc Culloch et al., 2008).

2.1.3 Category C organ-specific diseases

Encephalopathy has been reported between 13-35% of children with HIV infection and in 35-50% of children with AIDS. Studies have demonstrated that HIV enters the central nervous system (CNS) soon after the infection and may persist in this compartment over the entire course of HIV infection. Mechanisms of pediatric HIV neuropathogenesis and factors associated with neurodevelopmental abnormalities in perinatally infected children are not yet fully understood. Neurotropic HIV likely develops distinct genotypic characteristics in response to this unique environment. (Van Rie et al., 2007). Complementary studies are usually non-specific, in fact the isolation of HIV from cerebrospinal fluid does not correlate with clinical symptoms. Neuroimaging has provided the best evaluation showing cortical atrophy with abnormalities in the subcortical white matter and in basal ganglia regions. The use of HAART is highly effective in reducing the incidence of HIV encephalopathy among perinatally infected children. CNS-penetrating antiretroviral regimens are important in affecting survival after diagnosis of HIV encephalopathy (Patel el al., 2009).

Malignancy prevalence in HIV infected children is significantly higher than in the normal population, approximately 2% compared with 1%. The types of malignancy reported show the following proportions of malignancies: 65% non-Hodgkin´s lymphoma, 17% leiomyosarcoma or leiomyoma, 8% leukemia, 5% Kaposi´s sarcoma, 3% Hodgkin´s lymphoma and less than 2% vaginal carcinoma in situ and tracheal neuroendocrine carcinoma. Non-Hodgkin´s lymphoma occurred most commonly in the gastrointestinal tract (37%), followed by the CNS (17%), liver and spleen involvement were common sites too. Although the immunosupresion of HIV disease in cancer pathogenesis is recognized, the etiology of cancer in paediatric HIV infection is not well-understood. In one study, a high viral load of Epstein-Barr virus was associated with the development of malignancy, but only in children with CD4 T cells counts > 200/µl (Pollock et al., 2003). In other study, the incidence of cancer in HIV infected children was highest in patients who received HAART less than 2 years compared to children with more than 2 years of HAART. (Kest et al., 2005)
The wasting syndrome has been described in HIV infected children. The relationship between protein-energy malnutrition and adverse effects on the immune system result in immune deficiency states. Malnutrition may exacerbate the immunological effects. The causes of malnutrition in HIV children include decreased nutrient intake, gastrointestinal malabsorption, increased nutritional requirements or tissue catabolism and psychosocial factors, as well as medications and infections that may also cause malnutrition. HAART has decreased the incidence of wasting syndrome, but new side effects like lipodystrophy has been well defined in children (Miller, 2003). HIV-infected children have experienced significant improvement on growth since the introduction of HAART. An increase in the mean of weight z-scores to normal values was obtained by week 48 and an increase in mean height z-scores approached normal values by 96 week (Verweel et al., 2002; Guillén et al., 2007)

2.2 Impact of HAART on bacterial and opportunistic infections

Bacterial infections and OI infections still occur in the HAART era in children, mostly in those with persistently low CD4 T lymphocyte counts caused by failure of adherence to multiple drugs or drug resistance. By contrast, OI and serious bacterial infections, herpes zoster and tuberculosis (TB) continue to present in children who are not severely immunocompromised. The incidence of OI is higher in developing countries, where the use of HAART is less extended, the follow-up more difficult and the socioeconomic conditions worse.

In contrast with adults, OI in children usually reflect a primary infection by a pathogen, whereas in adults they are often secondary to reactivation from latent infections. Perinatal transmission of hepatitis C virus and cytomegalovirus are more frequent in HIV-infected women than in non-infected women. Children undiagnosed of HIV infection are at risk to suffer an OI because of the lack of HAART and primary prophylaxis. Besides, in children the diagnosis of OI in some situations is difficult. In the first moths of live it is not possible to distinguish between specific antibodies against common pathogens and antibodies belonging to the mother due to transplacental transfer. Furthermore, the diagnostic yield for many OI in children is usually lower than in adults and requires admission or invasive procedures. TB diagnosis requires obtaining smears of induced sputum or gastric lavage, with lower sensitivity than sputum smears in adults, and therefore the diagnosis often rely on an epidemiological history of an adult being diagnosed of TB.

The most frequent bacterial and OI in the pre HAART era in children were severe bacterial infections (bacteraemia and pneumonia), herpes zoster, *Pneumocystis jirovecii* pneumonia, esophageal candidiasis and disseminated *Mycobaterium avium complex* (MAC), less common were cryptosporidiasis, tuberculosis (TB), systemic fungal infections and toxoplasmosis.(Dankner et al., 2001). The widespread use of HAART has decreased the incidence of bacterial infections and OI in children. Some of the opportunistic infections complicating HIV are not curable with available treatments, effective HAART has resulted in improved immune status leading to control the infection. (Gona et al., 2006) Early diagnosis, primary prophylaxis and antiretroviral treatment in vertically infected children are of major importance. The recommendation to start HAART in children has shifted towards an earlier initiation, to include infants less than 2 years in WHO guidelines in developing countries and in less than one year old in American and European guidelines, independently of immunological stage (WHO, 2010; CDC, 2010; PENTA, 2009).

Primary and secondary prophylaxis is important to prevent OI in children. All children below 1 year old must to receive primary prophylaxis for PCP, children aged 1 to 4 years should receive it if they have a CD4 count below 20% of total lymphocyte count. Children aged 5 and above should receive such prophylaxis if they have a CD4 count below 200-250 cells/mm3 or less than 15%. There are few data for recommendations for prophylaxis of other OI. Secondary prophylaxis is used after the treatment of some opportunistic infections to prevent the reactivation or re-infection. Discontinuation of primary prophylaxis for *Pneumocystis jirovecci* and other OI is possible and safe when immune reconstitution is reached.

Vaccines are other important tool to prevent potential severe infections in HIV-infected children, including varicella and human papillomavirus vaccine. Recent evidence shows that children who were already HIV-infected when vaccinated with BCG at birth, and who later developed AIDS, were at increased risk of developing disseminated BCG disease. This has changed the recommendations for not using this vaccine in countries with a high burden of TB, until a diagnosis of HIV-infection has been ruled out. Live attenuated vaccines are not recommended in children with severe immunosuppresion, those with CD4 cells percentage less than 15%.

As patients are living longer, other infections have assumed more importance in the prognosis, as has been well documented with viral hepatitis in co-infected adults. Improvement in the immune system after the introduction of HAART, even in the absence of complete viral suppression, may serve as prevention and therapy for many AIDS-defining OI, particularly those lacking effective therapy. With the immune boost achieved shortly after the initiation of HAART, a new immune reconstitution inflammatory syndrome (IRIS) has emerged. IRIS occurs shortly after the initiation of HAART due to an exaggerated inflammatory response. It is less well characterized in children than adults. The incidence is higher in children with low CD4 count and in developing countries. It is common in infants immunized with Bacille Calmette-Guerin (BCG) vaccine. Typically, IRIS occurs between 2 and 6 weeks after the introduction of HAART, but may occur up to 7 months later. This syndrome consists of an exacerbation of signs and symptoms associated with the underlying disease, of infectious and non-infectious etiology, resulting in an apparent clinical worsening. IRIS result from a rapid rebound in immune function that respond to a variety of clinically occult or latent infections that were present at the time of initiation of HAART, not previously recognized by a severely dysfunctional immune system. IRIS can complicate the management of these children.

It is important to distinguish between failure in HAART, failure in treatment of an OI and antimicrobial resistance or compliance. If an OI becomes apparent in the first 12 weeks of HAART initiation and there is a suspicion, HAART must be continued and treatment for the OI started. When an OI present after 12 weeks on HAART with virologic and immunological responses, it may be either IRIS or manifestations of the OI with partial immune reconstitution that have not controlled the infection. In the last situation HAART should be continued and treated accordingly. If an OI occurred in the setting of a virologic and immunological failure on HAART, this regimen must be revaluated while treatment for the OI given as early as possible.

The time of initiate HAART when an OI is present is unknown. The risk of complications associated with some antiretrovirals, the drug-drug interactions that make more difficult the management and the confusion with IRIS syndrome has led to suggest, in some circumstances, to wait some time before HAART initiation. Some OI improve with the early use of HAART. In other infections, like cryptococcal meningitis, it is recommended to wait a response to therapy to start HAART. In general, HAART should be initiated early after the OI has been diagnosed. Recently, a trial conducted in South Africa showed that the initiation of HAART simultaneously with TB treatment significantly improved survival.

In HIV infected children other difficulty is that the pharmacokinetics data of many commonly used drugs are incompletely known and the potential interactions between the different antiretrovirals and the drugs used to treat the OI may be significant, reducing the number of options available for treatment (CDC, 2009).

2.2.1 Impact of HAART on bacterial infections

During pre-HAART era, serious bacterial infections were the most commonly diagnosed infections in HIV-infected children. Pneumonia was the most common bacterial infection followed by bacteraemia and urinary tract infection. Other serious bacterial infectious including osteomyelitis, meningitis, abscess and septic arthritis occurred as well. HIV-infected children are at risk of serious bacterial infections during the early years of life, and in these patients the risk is magnified by the direct effects of HIV related with T and B cell dysfunction. The most common blood isolate organism among HIV-infected children is *Streptococcus pneumoniae*. A significant decrease in bacteraemia incidence and the time to first bacteraemia incident were seen in the post HAART era. In pre-HAART era children with a decline of CD4 T cells were more likely to develop bacteraemia, and children who experienced bacteraemia had an associated higher mortality (Kapogiannis et al., 2008). In era post-HAART the bacteraemia has decreased but the incidence remains substantially higher than in HIV-uninfected children. There are no data currently on whether initiation of HAART during acute sepsis reduces short-term morbidity or mortality. Paediatric HIV infection is not a homogeneous condition in the era of HAART. Susceptibility to sepsis differs according to stage of disease, access to HAART, and virologic and immunologic response to treatment. HIV-infected children have higher risk of developing pneumonia and of more severe disease than immunocompetent children. Pneumonia remains a major cause of death and hospitalization, particularly in developing countries. HAART has demonstrated to decrease the incidence of pneumonia. The vaccine, early HAART and antibiotic prophylaxis are preventive strategies to prevent pneumonia (Gray & Zar, 2010).

The prophylaxis with vaccination is important in these children and prophylaxis with Trimethoprim-sulphametoxazole (TMP-SMX) produce a benefit to reduce the incidence of these infections. In developing countries where the access to HAART is limited, these children can benefit from prophylaxis with TMP-SMX to avoid bacterial infectious. The WHO recommends prolonged daily prophylaxis for HIV-infected infants and children. Intermittent prophylaxis was associated with more invasive bacterial disease than daily prophylaxis, but the survival was similar (Zar et al., 2010). Opportunistic infections prophylaxis can be withdrawn safely for HIV-infected patients who experience CD4 cell recovery while receiving stable antiretroviral therapy, no increase in the rate of serious bacterial infection was observed. (Nachman et al., 2005).

2.2.2 Impact of HAART on opportunistic infections

Oropharyngeal candidiasis continues to be one of the most frequent opportunistic infection in HIV-infected children and often present as an initial manifestation of the disease. Oesophageal or pulmonary candidiasis has decreased after introduction of HAART. In children who not respond to HAART, candida esophagitis can occur and be concomitant to another opportunistic infection. Disseminated candidiasis is rare among HIV-infected children. There are no data in children to make recommendations for treatment or prevention of oropharyngeal candidiasis. With the available data from adults no conclusion can be made about the effectiveness of what antifungal is better for prophylaxis, although fluconazole is better than placebo. Ketoconazole, fluconazole, itraconazole and clotrimazole improved the treatment outcomes (Pienaar et al., 2010).

Cytomegalovirus infection can be acquired during infancy, early childhood or adolescence. HIV-infected women with CMV infection have a higher rate of CMV shedding from the cervix than do women without HIV infection and the risk for mother to infant transmission of CMV may increased among infants born to women infected by both CMV and HIV. After being born, HIV-infected children have higher risk for CMV infection (Schleiss MR, 2009). In era pre HAART co-infection appear to have faster progression of HIV disease. CMV retinitis is a frequent manifestation in HIV infected children. Viral dissemination can affect multiple organs producing pneumonitis, gastrointestinal disease and involvement of the central nervous system. Disseminated disease and retinitis must be treated with induction therapy and after chronic suppressive therapy. The safety of discontinuation of secondary prophylaxis in children with retinitis has not been well studied, but if the child has completed 6 months of HAART and the CD4 count are >15% in children 1-5 years old or > 100 cells/mm^3 in older than 6 years, secondary prophylaxis is usually withdrawn safely.

HSV-1 (*Herpes simplex virus-1*) causes gingivostomatitis in HIV-infected children when they experiment the primary infection by contact with infected oral secretions. If the patient is severely immunocompromised the HSV-1 may produce severe local lesions or disseminated infection with visceral involvement like esophagus, CNS, lung, spleen, liver and kidney. HAART has decreased the rates of systemic HSV infection. The HIV infected children can also have recurrences of gingivostomatitis. Neonatal transmission occurs with the exposure to maternal genital fluids. Congenital HSV infection is rare but it has cutaneous, ocular and CNS involvement. Caesarean delivery must be considered in women with active genital HSV. HSV-2 is acquired in adolescents by contact with infected genital secretions and the risk of genital HSV reactivation increases with the immunosupresion. HSV infection can increase the risk for mother to child HIV transmission. The treatment is acyclovir orally or intravenously depending on the severity of the infection. Valacyclovir, a prodrug of acyclovir, can also be effective.

The virus *varicella zoster* (VZV) is associated with more severe disease in HIV infected children in pre-HAART era than in uninfected children. After HAART and vaccination the rates of varicella has decreased. In some cases, disseminated varicella can develop in children with severe immunocompromise, but not in children with higher CD4. Retinitis can be a complication of varicella. Herpes zoster after infection of varicella is described like a decline in specific cellular immunity to VZV and can involve various dermatomes. HIV-infected children before HAART with low CD4 percentage at the time of primary varicella were at higher risk to subsequent zoster. In HIV-1 infected children the incidence of herpes zoster was higher in advances stages of immunusuppression. It has been reported an increase of herpes zoster after the introduction of HAART, but the incidence is less than pre-HAART era, possible due to vaccination. (Levin et al., 2009) A VZV-associated IRIS has been described after 1-3 months after the introduction of HAART with mild cutaneous manifestations and with the distribution by dermatomes, responding to acyclovir (Puthanakit et al., 2006). The treatment of choice is acyclovir, other alternatives are valacyclovir or famciclovir. The prevention for varicella in a contact must be the vaccination or varicella zoster immunoglobulin, in some cases acyclovir can be used.

Congenital toxoplasmosis has been rarely reported in HIV-infected children. It may occur when a HIV-mother acquired the primary Toxoplasma infection during the pregnancy, although perinatal transmission has been described in women with chronic Toxoplasma infection because the reactivation of replication in women with severe immunosupresion. The symptoms in congenital infection are generalized lymphadenopathy, hepatosplenomegaly, jaundice, hematologic abnormalities and CNS disease. CNS disease in HIV-infected children acquired after the delivery is very rare, and this occur like in adults when the CD4 were less than 50 cells/mm^3, but in HIV-infected children with neurologic symptoms, it must be considered. Ocular toxoplasmosis often is associated with CNS infection. Mother with acute toxoplasmosis must be treated and empiric therapy in newborn initiated. The treatment in congenital toxoplasmosis is pyrimethamine combined with sulfadiazine with folinic acid with a recommended duration of 12 months. Cerebral toxoplasmosis should be treated during 6 weeks depending of the evolution. Corticosteroids and anticonvulsants may be necessary. Primary prophylaxis must be done with TMP-SMX in children with CD4<15% in children under 6 years old or CD4 < 100 cells/mm^3 or older than 6. Discontinued primary prophylaxis is possible when the immune restoration occurs. Secondary prophylaxis must be used until immune reconstitution with HAART is initiated, then discontinuation of secondary prophylaxis must be considered.

Cryptococcosis occurs less frequent in children than in adults. In era pre-HAART cryptococcosis cases were in older children and with severe immunosuppression. In the HAART era the rate of this infection has decreased, remaining uncommon. The clinical manifestations of this infection are meningoencephlalitis, pulmonary or disseminated infection. The treatment is therapy of induction during 2 weeks with amphotericin B or liposomal amphotericin B and flucytosine in CNS disease and after the consolidation therapy during 8 weeks with fluconazole. When CNS is not affected the flucytosine may not be used. Fluconazole is used to prevent recurrences. If a restoration of immune status is produced by HAART, fluconazole can be discontinued. In some cases IRIS may develop when HAART is initiated simultaneously and therefore it is recommended to delay HAART, but if the patient is on HAART previously, this must be continued.

Cryptosporidiosis/isosporidiosis have declined dramatically after HAART. Before HAART these infections occurred with advanced immunosupresion. Although the incidence of these parasitic infections has declined with HAART, developing countries with less access to HAART have high incidence of these infections. Watery diarrhea is the most common manifestation of *crypstosporidium*, that can migrate into bile duct resulting in inflammation and slerosing cholangitis. Pancreatitis occurs rarely. Effective HAART is the main treatment for these infections. In crypstosporidiosis a 3-day course of nitazoxanide significantly improved the resolution of diarrhoea, parasitological eradication, and mortality in HIV seronegative, but not HIV seropositive, children (Amadi et al., 2002). IRIS has not been described with cryptosporidiosis treatment.

The incidence of tuberculosis depends on the site, and where the incidence of tuberculosis is high, it depends on the age and is increased in HIV co-infected children. So in sub-Saharan countries the incidence rate in HIV-children below 12 months of age is 1595/100.000 compared with 659/100.000 in HIV-uninfected. In older than 12 months-old the incidence rate is 5930/100.000 in HIV-infected children (Verhagen et al., 2010). The resistance of tuberculosis is increasing and it is an obstacle to control the TB worldwide. The diagnosis in children is more difficult than in adults due to the difficulty to obtain a smear of bronchial secretions for a bacteriologic diagnosis. The tuberculin skin test (TST) in HIV-infected children with tuberculosis disease can be negative. Recently, an IFN-γ release assay from lymphocytes after stimulation by highly specific synthetic *Mycobacterium tuberculosis* antigens has been developed, which sensitivity is higher than TST, but is commonly leads to indeterminate results in young and immunocompromised children. To obtain a specimen for microbiologic diagnosis is more combersome in children because of their difficulty in producing sputum, so there is a need to rely on gastric aspirates, although hypertone saline induced sputum induction has shown good results (Zar et al., 2005). The microbiological diagnosis relies on microscopic acid-fast bacilli staining, the isolation the mycobacteria in the culture, and recently nucleic acid amplification can improve the diagnostic yield. Drugs susceptibility testing is important due to increasing resistance. It is recommended a standardization of clinical and radiographic case definition to avoid confusion in the diagnosis. To prevent *M. tuberculosis* infection, BCG vaccine is not currently used due to the risk of disseminated disease in HIV-infected children (WHO, 2007). Treatment of latent tuberculosis infection is indicated in HIV infected children with isoniazide, if resistance to this drug is not suspected in the source case. There are insufficient data to guide isoniazide prophylaxis in HIV-infected children in high-prevalence countries in the absence of TB exposure (Gray et al., 2009). In HIV-infected children with TB disease, initiation of TB treatment is the priority although the optimal timing of HAART initiation is uncertain. Recently, a trial conducted in South Africa in adults showed that the initiation of HAART simultaneous with TB treatment significantly improve survival. (Abdool et al., 2010). Rifampin is a potent induction of the CPY3A that precludes treatment with all protease inhibitors (IP) but may allow the treatment with non-nucleoside reverse transcriptase inhibitors (NNRTIs). In many countries of Africa a PI-based antiretroviral regimen is indicated in HIV-infected children less than 36 months like first line regimen: in children older than 3 years IP can be replaced by efavirenz to avoid interactions with TB treatment; in younger than 3 years efavirenz can be replaced by nevirapine however there is a high percentage of resistance in children exposed to single dose nevirapine used for prevention of mother to child transmission (PMTCT). The management of TB resistance in cases of MDR and XDR TB must be guided by expert based on guidelines (WHO, 2008) (CDC, 2007).

IRIS has been described in children and must be suspected in children with advanced immunosupression who start HAART. TB therapy must not be discontinued and symptomatic treatment can be used including corticosteroids. BCG IRIS has been reported in children initiating HAART.

Mycobacterium avium complex (MAC) disease is caused by multiple species of nontuberculous mycobacteria. The incidence has decreased after introduction of HAART. MAC produces lymphadenitis and a disseminated infection in children with advanced immunologic deterioration. The main treatment is to preserve the immune function with HAART. The specific treatment is combined therapy with a minimum of 2 drugs. IRIS may occur, so antimycobacterial therapy should be started 2 weeks before HAART to minimize the IRIS symptoms. The chronic suppressive therapy may be safely discontinued if immune reconstitution is reached.

Pneumocystis jirovecii pneumonia has decreased in HAART era. Around 80% of immunocompetent children have acquired antibodies for *Pneumocystis* by the age of 2-4 years, and the infection is usually asymptomatic or presenting with mild respiratory symptoms. However, in HIV-infected children the infection frequently is very severe associated with high mortality, being an AIDS event occurring in the first year of life between 3-6 moths. HAART and prophylaxis for *Pneumocystis* has decreased the incidence. *Pneumocystis* pneumonia depends of the grade of immunosupression of the child, so marked decrease in CD4 is a risk factor for this. *Pneumocystis* pneumonia is characterized by fever, tachypnea, cough with hypoxia low arterial oxygen pressure, lactic dehydrogenase is often increased and the radiography can indicate bilateral diffuse parenchymal infiltrates. The microbiologic diagnosis is based on the identification of *Pneumocystis* in respiratory secretions. Bronchoalveolar lavage is the procedure of choice with a high diagnostic yield in HIV-infected children. Coinfection by other microorganisms must be considered. Prophylaxis is recommended in all the children since 4-6 weeks of age during the first year of age independently of CD4 count, with TMP-SMX. Infants with indeterminate HIV infection must received prophylaxis until they are confirmed to be non-infected. In older children prophylaxis is indicated if the CD4 are less than 15%. TMP-SMX is also effective to prevent toxoplasmosis and bacterial infections. The treatment is with TMP-SMX intravenously during 21 days. IRIS is rare to occur with this infection. Adverse reactions are frequent with TMP-SMX so other drugs must be considered. In cases of severe infection corticosteroids must be considered starting in the first 72 hours of diagnosis.

2.2.3 Impact of HAART in other infections

Malaria and HIV infection are two infections with a similar distribution in most countries, mainly in sub-Saharan Africa. An increased susceptibility in HIV-infected patients has been described in adults due to impaired immune response to malaria through cellular immunosuppression resulting in a higher likelihood of increased parasitaemia and severe malarial infections. HIV infection increases the incidence of clinical malaria, inversely correlated with the degree of immunodepression. HIV infection is associated with an increase of cerebral malaria (Imani et al., 2011). The effect of malaria on HIV infection is not as well established. Malaria, when fever and parasitemia are high, may be associated with transient increases in HIV viral load. The effect of subclinical malaria on HIV viral load is uncertain.

TMP-SMX may be effective in the prevention of malaria but the development of resistance is of concern. Severe malaria is clinically similar to other severe febrile illnesses. However, in endemic areas, parasitological confirmation of parasitaemia is often unavailable or unreliable and false positive malaria microscopy is common. The routine use of parenteral antibiotics among children with a positive malaria slide and life-threatening disease is warranted because invasive bacterial infections are likely to be overlooked and are associated with increased mortality. During pregnancy, placental malaria is associated with higher plasma and placental HIV viral loads, independently of the severity of immunodeficiency. Both infections have been associated with maternal and infant morbidity and mortality (Brentlinger et al., 2006)). HIV-1 exposure and HIV-1 infection are associated with increased prevalence of severe malarial anaemia during acute *P. falciparum* infection, independent of parasite density. HIV infection status does not affect the choice of therapy and no recommendations exist for alternative dosing of antimalarial drugs in HIV-infected persons. IRIS caused by malaria has been not reported.

HBV-HIV co-infection in children is less frequent nowadays in developed countries since the universal policy o HBV vaccination to newborns. Nevetheless, HBV is still a major problem in developing countries.

The clearance rates in HBV monoinfected children are 10% in newborns, 70% in children 1-5 years old, and 94% in >5 years. Chronic hepatitis is defined as persistence of HBsAg for more than 6 months. Children can acquire the infection perinatally, parenterally or through sexual transmission. Most children with chronic HBV infection are asymptomatic. They can develop cirrhosis and hepatocellular carcinoma over 2 or 3 decades. The diagnosis is made by detection of HBsAg. HBeAg seroconversion is defined as loss of HBeAg followed by the production of antibodies to HBeAg (anti-HBe) and is defined as an inactive carrier state. HBV DNA is a marker of replication of HBV. Biopsy determines the grade of hepatic inflammation and fibrosis by metavir classification. Percutaneous transient elastography (Fibroscan) is less aggressive than biopsy and useful to determine the grade of inflammation and fibrosis of the liver. The indications for treatment of chronic HBV in HIV co-infected children include evidence of HBV viral replication indicated by detectable serum HBV DNA, with or without HBeAg positivity, for >6 months, persistent elevation of serum transaminase levels or evidence of chronic hepatitis on liver biopsy. Treatment is not recommended for children with immunotolerant chronic HBV infection (i.e., normal serum transaminase levels despite detectable HBV DNA). After initiation of HAART, liver function may worsen due to immune reconstitution syndrome causing an increased immune response to HBV in the liver and subsequently a "flare" of hepatitis. HBV itself, however, has no detrimental effect on the course of the HIV infection.

HCV-HIV co-infection occurs approximately in 30% of adults. Vertical transmission of HCV is 3-5 fold higher in HIV-HCV co-infected mothers. HCV can be accelerate the progression of HIV infection increasing the viral replication, produce a worse immune reconstitution and there is an increase of hepatic toxicity. HIV influences in HCV infection increasing the progression of the liver disease. In HIV-HCV coinfection liver pathology develops more rapidly than in HCV mono-infection. The HCV is usually asymptomatic. Chronic HCV infection is defined as the presence of HCV RNA for > 6 months. In perinatally-acquired HCV-infected children, 20% had apparent clearance of infection, 50% had chronic asymptomatic infection and 30% had chronic active infection. During the infancy there might be an immunotolerance to this infection. The diagnosis is by serologic antibodies but these can be persistently negative in HIV-infected children. Therefore, HCV RNA qualitative or quantitative should be used for diagnosis of infection. HCV viral load does not correlate with the degree of liver damage. There are different genotypes of HCV, genotypes 2 and 3 are more likely than 1 or 4 to achieve sustained virologic response to treatment. The biopsy or fibroscan are used to know the grade of inflammation or fibrosis of the liver. The indications for HCV treatment can be detectable HCV-RNA, persistent elevation of transaminases, evidence of chronic hepatitis on liver biopsy, children >3 years old and no decompensated liver disease. The treatment accepted in children is standard interferon-alfa-2b with ribavirin. Pegilated interferon-alfa administered for 24-48 weeks with ribavirin is recommended in adults. Although, the experience of HCV treatment in coinfected children is scarce, (Navarro et al., 2007) and there is a need of studies. HAART should be initiated. HAART should be initiated earlier than in non-HCV infected children

2.2.4 Immune Reconstitution Inflamatory Syndrome (IRIS)

Antiretroviral therapy improves immune function and CD4 cell count in HIV-infected children within the first few months after starting HAART producing an increase of CD4 cells and decrease in viral load. This changes are associated with an increase in the capacity to develop inflammatory reactions. Some patients develop a paradoxical inflammatory response by their reconstituted immune system to infectious or non-infectious antigens, resulting in apparent clinical worsening. There are two types of IRIS: ¨unmasking¨ IRIS and ¨paradoxical¨ IRIS. The unmasking IRIS is an occult and subclinical opportunistic infection, unmasked by immune recovery following the HAART initiation. Paradoxical IRIS is a clinical recrudescence of a successfully treated infection, symptomatic relapse despite initial clinical improvement and continued microbiologic treatment success; the antigen driving the immune activation often elicits a robust immune response in the setting of few or no detectable organism and the culture may be sterile due to effective opportunistic infection treatment.

The criteria for diagnosis of paediatric IRIS are: a) evidence of clinical response to ART with a virologic response with > 1 log_{10} copies/ml, decrease in HIV RNA; b) clinical deterioration from an infectious or inflammatory condition temporally related to the initiation of ART (unmasking or paradoxical); c) symptoms cannot be explained by an alternative infection or neoplasm, treatment failure of the opportunistic infection, adverse drug reaction or complete non-compliance to ART or TB treatment.

The commonest causes are mostly mycobacterial, including tuberculosis, atypical mycobacteria and BCG-related and herpes zoster.

The incidence of IRIS is between 10-20% in developing countries. IRIS often occurs in older children who start HAART with an advanced stage of immunosupresion, although in young infants it may also occur. Risk factors for IRIS include a high pathogen load and very low CD4 cell count when HAART is initiated. Many children have a marked mortality within the first 90 days of HAART.

The treatment of ¨unmasking¨ IRIS is the treatment of the underlying opportunistic infection, in some cases also anti-inflammatory therapy and rarely discontinuation of HAART. Screening of occult infections before starting HAART can reduce IRIS. The treatment of ¨paradoxical¨ IRIS is observation in mild cases, non-steroidal anti-inflamatory drugs in moderate reactions, and corticosteroids in severe cases, considering the temporary cessation of HAART and surgical debulking (Boulware et al., 2008).

When a child starts HAART, is difficult to distinguish between HAART toxicity, from toxicity due to treatment to the opportunistic infection and IRIS. Opportunistic infections can occur in HIV-infected children experiencing virologic and immunologic failure on HAART. If symptoms appeared within the 12 weeks after initiation HAART, it may indicate ¨unmasking IRIS¨, so HAART must be continued and opportunistic infection treatment initiated. If symptoms occurred after 12 weeks and there is immunologic and virologic response, it may be due to ¨paradoxical IRIS¨ or incomplete immune reconstitution allowing a new opportunistic infection. In both cases HAART must be continued and if the microbiologic evaluation demonstrates a microorganism, it should be treated.

2.2.5 Prophylaxis and vaccines

2.2.5.1 Prophylaxis

TMP-SMX prophylaxis is indicated in HIV-infected children since 4-6 weeks of age until the first year of life and in older children with CD4 less than 15%. TMP-SMX prophylaxis is indicated to prevent *Pneumocystis jirovecci* pneumonia but it has activity against a wide range of pathogens including *Pneumococcus, non-typhoidal Salmonella, Isospora, Cyclospora, Nocardia, Plasmodium falciparum and Toxoplasma gondii.* In developing countries, the CHAP study, a randomized study placebo-controlled trial of cotrimoxazole in Zambia, showed the impact of TMP-SMX on reducing mortality in HIV infected children from 6 months to 14 years (Chintu et al., 2004). WHO guidelines on co-trimoxazole prophylaxis published in 2006, recommend prophylaxis in infants less than 1 year until infection can be excluded or until 6 weeks after the cessation of breastfeeding (WHO, 2006). TMP-SMX prophylaxis has potential risk of resistance and side effects. Currently the number of HIV-infants children infected is decreasing due to the interventions to prevent mother to child transmission and WHO now recommend that breastfeeding women receive HAART or the infants receive nevirapine prophylaxis. Thus, a lower number of children are expected to become HIV-infected and to receive prophylaxis. Breastfeeding decreased the risk of infections such diarrhoea and pneumonia due to the immune protection. These preventive options and the molecular tests are more accessible in these countries, allows limiting the prophylaxis for the uninfected infants (Coutsoudis et al., 2010). WHO guidelines for HIV-infected children of 1-4 years recommend prophylaxis if they are symptomatic or have less than 25%. Similarly, the infants who start prophylaxis before the age of one and who subsequently are asymptomatic and/or have CD4> 25% should remain on co-trimoxazole prophylaxis until they reach five years old. In older than 5 years the recommendations are similar than adults. A randomized controlled trial has compared daily versus intermittent prophylaxis in South Africa, finding that the intermittent prophylaxis was associated with more invasive bacterial disease than daily prophylaxis, but survival was similar (Zar et al., 2010).

TMP-SMX has a range of side effects like skin rashes, gastrointestinal disturbances and marrow suppression which lead to neutropenia and anaemia, in rare cases Stevens-Johnson syndrome may occur. In adults has been studied when there is a hypersensitivity to co-trimoxazole, the management of these adverse reactions has included continuing the drug (treating-through) and reintroducing the drug at a later date, either using dose-escalation (desensitization), or rechallenge at full dose. It observed that cotrimoxazole desensitization resulted in better outcome. Data in children are required (Lin et al., 2007).

Discontinuation of primary and secondary prophylaxis with TMP-SMX in children is possible if a restoration of immune system has occurred (Urchel et al., 2005). Studies have studied the incidence of serious bacterial infections after the withdrawal of prophylaxis (Nachman et al., 2005).

2.2.5.2 Vaccines

HIV-infected children are at increased risk of infections, particularly invasive bacterial infections due to encapsulated bacteria. Cotrimoxazole prophylaxis and associated HAART have shown improvements in morbidity and mortality in HIV-infected children. (Walker et al, 2007). However, even in the ART era, HIV infected children have increased susceptibility to vaccine preventable diseases.

Routine immunizations are generally well tolerated by HIV-infected children but vaccine safety remains an important issue. There have been concerns that vaccination itself could result in immunologic deterioration. Although plasma viral loads could be temporally increased after vaccination, no evidence of HIV disease progression has been observed. Recent evidence shows that children who were already HIV-infected when vaccinated with bacille Calmette-Guérin (BCG) at birth, and who later developed AIDS, were at increased risk of developing disseminated BCG disease. Among HIV-infected infants, the benefits of potentially preventing severe tuberculosis therefore appear to be outweighed by the risks associated with the use of BCG vaccine. In 2007, HIV infection in infants was considered a full contraindication to BCG vaccination in the new revised World Health Organization guidelines (WHO, 2007). Live viral vaccines (eg. varicella, mumps, measles and rubella) are generally not contraindicated in children who have stable CD4 status and not have severe immune suppression.

HIV-infected children in the pre-HAART era had poorer responses to vaccines and more rapid waning of immunity. Lower CD4 cell counts, higher viral load, age or advanced HIV stage at vaccination, have been associated with the immunity response, although these risk factors have not been consistent across the studies. HAART is effective in HIV-infected children by suppressing viral replication and restoring immune function. However, HAART is unlikely to restore memory T cells for vaccine antigens to which children were exposed before treatment. Previously vaccinated children showed low levels of immunity after being started on HAART. No epidemiological, virological or immunological factors consistently predicted immunity after starting HAART in these children. There is increasing evidence of improved immunization responses following effective HAART (Sutcliffe & Moss, 2010).

Once children are commenced on ART, it is generally recommended to initiate vaccination or revaccination 6 months after CD4 cells recovery to the normal range of age. This recommendation is based on the progressive but not immediate immune recovery of HIV-infected children starting HAART (Weinberg, 2008). Nowadays, it is recommended in children who were vaccinated before starting on HAART to measure the immune response to previous vaccines to guide the need for further doses. If non protective antibody levels are demonstrated; booster doses or revaccination should be considered, based on the response after one booster dose. Some benefit may be gained from vaccination even when severe immunosupression, so this should be especially considered for high risk patients. Complete revaccination after immune reconstitution is recommended. Although most children on HAART respond to vaccination, immune reconstitution is not sufficient to ensure long-term immunity for some children. These suggest that children on HAART would benefit from revaccination.

Age of the patient when started on HAART might be important in enhancing vaccine responses. Early administration of HAART preserved the memory B-cell compartment. Children who were started on HAART in infancy, less than 12 months of age, had greater protective immunity that did children who were started on HAART later in childhood, and had similar levels of immunity compared with uninfected children of the same age (Pensieroso, 2009). These findings support recommendations for early administration of HAART among infants.

It is currently recommended to start vaccination of HIV-infected children in infancy with some modifications of the routine immunization schedule:

- Hepatitis B virus (HBV) immunization in a four-dose-schedule starting soon after birth is recommended. Standard doses are advised as the infant should not be immunocompromised at this age. Testing for adequate seroconversion at or after the time of the fourth dose is important. Booster dose o revaccination is recommended accordingly to anti-HBs titre for protection. Newborns of HBV-coinfected mothers also require one dose of anti-HBV immunoglobulin with the first dose of HBV vaccine.
- Diphteria, tetanus and acellular pertussis vaccine (DTPa) is recommended in a five-dose-schedule as in routine vaccination programs. One dose of dTpa adult vaccine (low dose diphtheria and pertussis) is recommended for adolescents who have completed the series of DTPa in childhood. Revaccination with dTpa is recommended every 10 years for adults.
- Four doses of parenteral polio vaccine (IPV) and Haemophilus influenzae type b (Hib) are recommended as in routine immunization programs. Hib vaccine could be considered in HIV-infected children more than 5 years old who did not receive the vaccine before.
- Meningococcal C vaccine is recommended in a three dose scheme in first year of life. It is also advised to vaccinate older HIV infected children with two doses, especially adolescents who have not been vaccinated before.
- A 3 dose primary immunization schedule of conjugate 13-valent pneumococcal vaccine (PCV13) in the first year of life is recommended, with a re-enforcing dose during the second year. The first dose of polysaccharide 23-valent pneumococcal vaccine (PPV23) is recommended after 24 moths old and at least 2 months after the final dose of PCV13. Revaccination with PPV23 every 5 years thereafter should be considered. For children aged 24 months or more, who have not been vaccinated against pneumococcal disease, 2 doses of PCV13 administered at least 2 months apart, and later PPV23 immunization schedule is recommended.
- Hepatitis A virus (HAV) vaccine could be considered in a two dose scheme for all hepatitis A seronegative HIV-infected children over 12 months of age, especially focussing on adolescents or populations with high endemic or epidemic diseases.
- Measles, mumps and rubella (MMR) vaccine is recommended in a two dose schedule unless there is evidence of severe immunocompromise (CD4 cell percentage $< 15\%$).
- Varicella vaccine is indicated in two dose schedule in HIV-infected children more than 12 moths of age, in CDC clinical class N, A or B with CD4 threshold as stated for MMR vaccination and without evidence of varicella immunity.
- Live-attenuated human rotavirus vaccine have been studied in HIV infected infants, in clinical stages I and II according to WHO classification, in a three dose schedule starting on 6 to 10 weeks of age. The vaccine was safe and a satisfactory immune response was mounted without aggravating their immunologic or HIV condition (Steele, 2011). Although the data are limited, this vaccine could be considered in HIV infected infants within the routine age range recommended in HIV healthy infants.
- Human papillomavirus (HPV) vaccine. Data of quadrivalent human papillomavirus vaccine (QHPV) in HIV-infected children (60% female) aged from 7 to 12 years, with a CD4% ≥ 15 and on stable antiretroviral therapy showed that the vaccine is safe and immunogenic for the 4 antigens (Levin, 2010). Although the data are limited, this

vaccine is recommended for girls from 12 years of age (minimum age 9, maximum age 26 years), irrespective of CD4 count in a 3 dose schedule.

- Trivalent inactivated influenza vaccine is recommended yearly from 6 months of age. Vaccination schedule and doses are similar to those recommended for healthy children and adolescents.

3. Conclusion

HAART has dramatically decreased the incidence of opportunistic infections in children and organ-specific diseases in developed countries. Opportunistic infections may complicate the treatment of HIV due to the disease itself, toxicity of the drugs and immune reconstitution inflammatory syndrome. HAART, prophylaxis, vaccines help to reduce the incidence of opportunistic infections. However in developing countries where there is a greater number of new diagnosis of HIV-infected children, less access to antiretroviral drugs and higher prevalence of opportunistic infections like tuberculosis, the prevention and the treatment must to be a priority.

4. Acknowledgment

The Madrid Group of Pediatric HIV Infection: participing hospitals and personnel:
1- Hospital de Getafe: Beatriz Soto, Marta Ruiz, Luis Prieto, Sara Guillén, Bárbara Rubio, JT Ramos. 2- Hospital 12 Octubre: María Isabel González-Tomé, Pablo Rojo, Daniel Blázquez, Luis I. González-Granado, Adriana Navas, Jesús Ruiz Contreras. 3- Hospital La Paz: María Isabel de José. 4- Hospital Carlos III: María José Mellado, Pablo Martín-Fontelos. 5- Hospital Alcalá de Henares: José Beceiro. 6- Hospital Móstoles: Miguel Angel Roa. 7- Hospital de Leganés: Cristina Calvo. 8- Hospital Niño Jesús: Jorge Martínez-Pérez. 9- Hospital Gregorio Marañón: ML Navarro, MD Gurbindo, Jesús Saavedra, José Mª Bellón, Santiago de Ory, MªAngeles Muñoz-Fernández. 10- Hospital Ramón y Cajal: África Holguín, Miguel de Mulder Rougvie.
Proyecto FIS 2007 (PI070236), Proyecto FIPSE 2009 (360829/09) y Proyecto FIS 2009 (PS09/01878).

5. References

Abdool, SS. (2010). Timing of initiation of antiretroviral drugs during tuberculosis therapy. *N Engl J Med,* Vol. 362, No. 8, (February 2010), pp. 697-706.

Abrams, EJ. (2000). Opportunistic infections and other clinical manifestations of HIV disease in children. *Pediatr Clin North Am,* Vol. 47, No.1, (February 2000), pp. 79-108.

Amadi, B. (2002). Effect of nitazoxanide in morbidity and mortality in Zambian children with criptosporidiosis : a randomised controlled trial. *Lancet,* Vol. 360, No. 9343, (November 2002), pp. 1375-1380.

Boulware, DR, et al. (2008). Pediatric HIV Immune Reconstitution Inflammatory Syndrome (IRIS). *Curr Opin HIV AIDS,* Vol. 3. No. 4, (July 2008), pp. 461-467.

Bretlinger, PE, (2006). Challenges in the concurrent management of malaria and HIV in pregnancy in sub-Saharan Africa. *Lancet infect Dis,* Vol. 6, No. 2, (February 2006), pp. 100-111.

CDC. (1994). Revised classification system for human immunodeficiency virus infection in children less than 13 years of age. *MMWR CDC Surveill Summ,* Vol. 43, (1994), pp. 1-10.

CDC. (2007). Managing drug interactions in the treatment of HIV-related tuberculosis. Available from: http://www.cdc.gov/tb/publications/guidelines/TB_HIV_Drugs/PDF/tbhiv.pdf

CDC. (2009). Guidelines for the prevention and treatment of opportunistic infections among HIV-exposed and HIV.infected children. *MMWR Recomm Rep,* Vol. 58. No. RR11, (September 2009), pp. 1-166. Available from : www.cdc.gov/mmwr.

CDC (2010). Guidelines for the use of antiretroviral agents in pediatric HIV infection. (August 2010). Available from: http://aidsinfo.nih.gov/contentfiles/PediatricGuidelines.pdf

Chiapinni, E et al. (2007). Changing patterns of clinical events in perinatally HIV-1-infected children during the era of HAART. *AIDS,* Vol. 21, No.12, (2007), pp. 1607-1615.

Chintu, C et al. (2004). Co-trimoxazole as prophylaxis against opportunistic infections in HIV-infected Zambian children (CHAP) : a double-blind randomised placebo-controlled trial. *Lancet,* Vol. 364, (2004), pp. 1865-1871.

Coutsoudis, A et al. (2010). Time for new recommendations on cotrimoxazole prophylaxis for HIV-exposed infants in developing countries. *Bull World Health Organ,* Vol. 88, (2010), pp. 949-950.

Dankner, WM et al. (2001). Correlates of opportunistic infections in children infected with immunodeficiency virus managed before highly active antiretroviral therapy. *Pediatr Infect Dis J,* Vol. 20, No.1, (January 2001), pp. 40-48.

Gona, P, et al (2006). Incidence of opportunistic and other infections in HIV-infected children in the HAART era. *JAMA,* Vol. 296, No.3, (July 2006), pp. 292-300.

Gray, DM, et al. (2009). Impact of tuberculosis preventive therapy on tuberculosis and mortality in HIV-infected children. *Cochrane Database Syst Rev,* Vol. 21. No.1.

Gray, DM. & Zar, HJ. (2010). Community-acquired pneumonia in HIV-infected children : a global perspective. Curr Opin Pulm Med. Vol. 16, pp. 208-216. ISSN 1070 5287.

Guillén, S, et al. (2007). Impact on growth with the use of HAART. *Pediatr Infect Dis J,* Vol. 26 No.4, (April 2007), pp. 334-338. ISSN 1468 1293

Guillén, S, et al. (2010). Opportunistic infections and organ-specific diseases in HIV-1-infected children : a cohort study (1990-2006). *HIV Medicine,* Vol. 11, No.4, (April 2010), pp. 245-252. ISSN 1468 1293

Imani, PD, et al. (2011). Human immunodeficiency virus infection and cerebral malaria in Uganda : a case-control study. *BMC Pediatrics,* Vol. 11, No. 5, (2011), pp.1-8.

Kapogiannis, BG, et al. (2008). Trends in bacteremia in the Pre and Post Highly Active Antiretroviral Therapy among HIV-infected children in the US Perinatal AIDS Collaborative Transmisssion Study (1986 2004). *Pediatrics,* Vol. 121, No.5, (May 2008), pp. e1229-e1239. ISSN 0031 4005

Kest, H, et al. (2005). Malignancy in perinatally human immunodeficiency virus-infected children in the United States. *Pediatr Infect Dis J,* Vol. 24, No. 3, (March 2005), pp. 237-242. ISSN 0891 3668

Levin, MJ, et al. (2009). Short-term and long-term effects of Highly active antiretroviral therapy on the incidence of herpes zoster in HIV-infected children. *J Acquir Immune Defic Syndr,* Vol. 50. No. 2, (February 2009), pp. 182-191.

Levin MJ, et al. (2010). Safety and immunogenicity of a quadrivalent human papillomavirus (types 6, 11, 16, and 18) vaccine in HIV-infected children 7 to 12 years old. *J Acquir Immune Defic Syndr.* Vol. 55, (2010), pp. 197-204.

Lin, D, et al. (2007). Cotrimoxazole for prophylaxis or treatment of opportunistic infections of HIV/AIDS in patients with a previous history of hipersensitivity to cotrimoxazole. Cochrane Database Syst Rev, Vol.18, No.2.

McCulloch, MI, et al. (2008). Kideney disease in HIV-positive children. *Semin Nephrol,* Vol. 28. No. 6, (November 2008), pp.585-594.

Miller, TL. (2003). Nutritional aspects of HIV-infected children receiving highly active antiretroviral theraphy. *AIDS,* Vol. 17, No.suppl 1, (2003), pp. S130-S140.

Nachman, S, et al. (2005). The rate of serious bacterial infections among HIV-infected children with immune reconstitution who have discontinued opportnistic infection prophylaxis. *Pediatrics,* Vol. 115, No.4, (April 2005), pp. e488-e494. ISSN 0031 4005

Nachman, S, et al. (2009). Incidence of noninfectious conditions in perinatally HIV-infected children and adolescents in the HAART era. *Arch Pediatr Adolesc Med,* Vol. 163, No.2, (February 2009), pp. 164-171

Navarro, ML, et al (2007). Chronic hepatitis C virus infection in a large cohort of HIV-infected children. 14th Conference on retrovirus and opportunistic infections (CROI). Abstract 708. Los Angeles (February 2007).

Nesheim, SR, et al. (2007). Trends in opportunistic infections in the Pre and Post Highly Active Antiretroviral Therapy eras among HIV-infected children in the perinatal AIDS collaborative transmission study, 1986 2004. *Pediatrics,* Vol. 120, No.1, (July 2007), pp. 100-109. ISSN 0031 4005

Patel, K, et al. (2009). Impact of HAART and CNS-penerating antiretroviral regimens on HIV encephalopathy among perinatally infected children and adolescents. *AIDS,* Vol. 23, No.14, (2009), pp. 1893-1901. ISSN 0269 9370

Pensorioso S, et al. (2009). Timing of HAART defines the inegrity of memory B cells and the humoral responses in HIV-1 vertically-infected children. *Proc Natl Acad Sci USA,* Vol 106, (2009), pp. 7739-7344.

PENTA. (2009). PENTA guidelines for the use of antiretroviral therapy in paediatric HIV-1 infection. *HIV Med,* Vol. 10, No. 10, (November 2009), pp. 591-613.

Pienaar, ED, et al. (2010). Interventions for te prevention and management of oropharyngeal candidiasis associated with HIV infection in adults and children. *Cochrane Database Syst Rev,* Vol 11, CD003940, (November 2010).

Puthanakit, T, et al. (2006). Immune reconstitution syndrome after the Highly Active Antiretroviral Therapy in human immunodeficiency virus.infected thai children. Pediatr Infect Dis J, Vol. 25. No. 1, (January 2006), pp. 53-58.

Puthanakit, T, et al. (2007). Hospitalization and mortality among HIV-infected children after receiving Highly Active Antiretroviral therapy. *CID,* Vol. 44, (February 2007), pp. 599-604. ISNN 1058 4838

Sánchez-Granados J, Ramos JT, Rojo P, et al. Impact of HAART on the survival and disease progression in HIV-1 infected children. *Pediatr Infect Dis J,* Vol 22 (October 2003); pp. 863-867.

Saulsbury, FT. (2001). Resolution of organ.specific complications of human immunodeficiency virus infection in children with the use of Highly Active Antiretroviral Therapy. *CID,* Vol. 32, (February 2001), pp. 462-468. ISNN 1058 4838

Schleiss, MR. (2009). HIV and cytomegalovirus co-infection in congenitally infected children: copathogens fanning each other´s flames? *AIDS*, Vol. 23, No. 16, (October 2009), pp. 2215-2217.

Steele, AD. (2011). Safety, Reactogenicity, and Immunogenicity of Human Rotavirus Vaccine RIX4414 in Human Immunodeficiency Virus-positive Infants in South Africa. *Pediatr Infect Dis J*. Vol. 30, No. 2, (February 2011), pp. 125-30.

Sutcliffe, CG, & Moss, WJ. (2010). Do children infected with HIV receiving HAART need to be revaccinated ? *Lancet Infect Dis,* Vol. 10. (September 2010), pp630-642.

Urchel S, et al. (2005). Withdrawal of Pneumocystis jirovecci prophylaxis in HIV-infected children under highly active antiretroviral therapy. *AIDS,* Vol. 19. (2005), pp. 2103-2108.

Van Rie, A, et al. (2007). Neurologic and neurodevelopmental manifestations of pedatric HIV/AIDS : a global perspective. *Eur J Paediatr Neurol,* Vol. 11, No. 1, (November 2006), pp. 1-9.

Verweel, G, et al. (2002). Treatment with highly active antiretroviral therapy in human immunodeficiency virus type 1-infected children is associated with a sustained effect on growth. *Pediatrics,* Vol. 109, No. E25. pp.1-7. ISSN 0031 4005

Verhagen LM, et al. (2010). Human immunodeficiency virus and tuberculosis coinfection in children. *PediatrInfect Dis J,* Vol. 29, No. 10, (October 2010), pp. e63-e70. ISSN 0891 3668

Walker AS, et al. (2007). The impact of daily cotrimoxazole prophylaxis and antiretroviral therapy on mortality and hospital admissions in HIV-infected Zambian children. *Clin Infect Dis,* Vol. 44, (2007), pp. 1361-1367.

Weinberg A, et al. Continuous improvement in the immune system of HIV-infected children on prolonged antiretroviral therapy. *AIDS,* Vol. 22, (2008), pp. 2267-2277.

WHO. (2006). Guidelines on co-trimoxazole prophylaxis for HIV-related infections among children, adolescents and adults. Available from : http://www.who.int/hiv

WHO. (2007). WHO case definitions of HIV for surveillance and revised clinical staging and immunological classification of HIV-related disease in adults and children. Available from: http://www.who.int/hiv

WHO. (2007). Revised BCG vaccination guidelines for infants at risk for HIV infection, Wkly Epidemiol Rec, Vol. 82, (2007), pp. 193-196.

WHO. (2008). Guidelines for the programmatic management of drug-resistan tuberculosis. Available from: http://www.who.int/hiv

WHO. (2010). Antiretroviral therapy for HIV infection in infants and children : towards universal access. Available from: http://www.who.int/hiv

Ylitalo, N, et al. (2006). Risk factors for opportunistic illnesses in children with Human Immunodeficiency Virus in the era of Highly Active Antiretroviral Therapy. *Arch Pediatr Adolesc Med,* Vol. 160, (August 2006), pp. 778-787.

Zar, HJ. (2010). Induced sputum versus gastric lavage for microbiological confirmation of pulmonary tuberculosis in infants and young children : a prospective study. *Lancet,* Vol. 365, No. 9454, (January 2005), pp. 130-134.

Zar, HJ. (2007). Chronic lung disease in human immunodeficiency virus (HIV) infected children. *Pediatr Pulmonol,*Vol. 43, (2008), pp. 1-10.

Zar, HJ, et al. (2010). A rabdomized controlled trial of intermittent compared with daily cotrimoxazole preventive therapy in HIV-infected children. *AIDS,* Vol. 24. No. 14, (September 2010), pp2225-2232. ISSN 0269 9370

2

HIV-1 Super Infection

Maria Pernas and Cecilio López-Galindez
Centro Nacional de Microbiología (CNM). Instituto de Salud Carlos III, Majadahonda, Madrid, Spain

1. Introduction

Human immunodeficiency virus type 1 (HIV-1) infection with more than one strain, termed dual infection (DI), encompasses both co and superinfection (SI). Co-infection is the acquisition of two viral strains during primo-infection, whereas SI is the infection with a second heterologous strains after primary infection or during the course of an established infection.

The first evidence that support HIV-1 DI, is the existence of numerous circulanting recombinant forms, because recombination requires that a single cell is infected by two viruses. Recombination could arise inter-subtype (where viruses differ by ~30% in the viral envelope sequence) and intra–subtype (where viruses differ by only ~10% in the envelope). The first case of a intersubtype SI in a man, infected with a CRF01-AE recombinant form, who became superinfected with a subtype B strain was described by (Jost et al., 2002). Similar inter subtype cases have been reported by (Ramos et al., 2002). Intrasubtype cases, where the first and the second strain belong to the same B subtype, have been described (Altfeld et al., 2002; Pernas et al., 2006).

2. Detection

Different methods have been used to detect DI: restriction fragment length polymorphism (RFLP) (Ramos et al., 2002), multiregion hybridization assay (MHA), heteroduplex tracking assay (HTA), hetroduplex mobility assay (HMA) (Manigart et al., 2004), sequencing of single copy PCR amplifications (Salazar-Gonzalez et al., 2008), clonal sequencing followed by phylogenetic analysis (Pernas et al., 2006). All these methods are expensive, time consuming and require a laborious analysis.

Recently, new approaches to detect SI have been developed. Within population–based sequences multiple nucleotides are possible at a single position, which is called ambiguity codes. The presence of high number of ambiguous codes in the Viro-Seq HIV-RT sequence, vastly used for routine determination of resistance-associated mutations, has been applied to detect DI. In 16 out 37 patients, the existence of more than 34 ambiguous sites (34-99) in the Viro-Seq HIV-RT sequence revealed new cases of dual infections (Cornelissen et al., 2007). However, this method was less sensitive when compared to HMA (Rachinger et al., 2010) since minor variants present below 20-30% in the quasispecies population could not be detected in the sequence chromatogram. Because non synonymous positions are selected by immune response or HAART, a new method focused on mixtures only in the synonymous positions (SM-index) was applied to discriminate between dually and single infection in highly-risk patients. To confirm the cases of DI, ultra-deep sequencing (UDS) was compared to the single genome sequence (SGS) method, considered as the gold standard method. In most of the samples, UDS identified minority variants that were not detected by SGS. Only in samples with very low viral load, SGS could detect minority variants more accurately than the UDS. These results showed that UDS could eventually replace SGS as the method for DI screening (Pacold et al., 2010).

The study of HIV-1 SI is highly dependent on the availability of the appropriate samples. Due to the high recombination rate in HIV (Jost et al., 2002), it is necessary to have samples close to the SI event, because after SI, recombinant strains could arise and mask the phylogenetic segregation of the clades. Serial sampling permits the detection of SI because it allows the identification of the resident strain; detect the appearance of the new strain and the emergence of recombinant strains (Gerhard M. Mloka, 2004; Pernas et al., 2006). Sometimes, soon after SI one of the virus strains overgrow the other which could no longer be detected (Templeton et al., 2009), and also the expression of one strain can vary with time (Kozaczynska et al., 2007; McCutchan et al., 2005).

Analysis of a second region in the HIV genome, that has permitted the detection of new cases of DI (Piantadosi et al., 2008), should be considered a standard approach for HIV SI detection.

We analyzed SI in an HIV-1 infected patient showing high-risk practices (Pernas et al., 2006). Viral quasispecies were analyzed in *pol* and *env* genes in several plasma samples during the patient follow up. Analysis in *env* gene confirmed the existence of 3 different strains in the viral population, one of them a recombinant (Figure 1). The analysis of serial samples as well as the analysis of a second genomic region in *env* gene (Figure 1) has permitted the detection of SI and the identification of recombinant variants.

One important issue is how to discriminate between co-infection and SI. SI implies that the second infection can occur after the development of an immune response, suggesting that natural infection does not provide enough protection against SI; whereas co-infection occurs during primoinfection while the immune response is still not completely functional. To distinguish between these two events, the analysis of sequential samples is necessary. However it is not always possible.

In our group, we developed a method that permits the estimation of the dating time of viruses (Casado et al., 2000). The viral dating time is estimated by the use of a linear-correlation equation, previously developed on the basis of a large set of Spanish samples, that correlates the V3 nucleotide-sequence divergence to the Spanish-epidemic MRCA with the sampling time. Using this approach (Casado et al., 2007) we interpolated the year of the nucleotide sequence of each of the different patient clades (Table 1), were able to discriminate between co-infection and a SI in two LTNPs patients, supporting the usefulness of the viral dating methodology. The years calculated for clades a and b for patient 1 were identical (1992), whereas those obtained for clades a and b for patient 2 was 1987 for clade a, close to the seroconversion time, and 1996 for cluster b (9 years later). The viral dating indicates that a SI had occurred in patient 2, whereas analysis of the first sample from patient 1 showed that he already was coinfected, although a previous SI could not be ruled out.

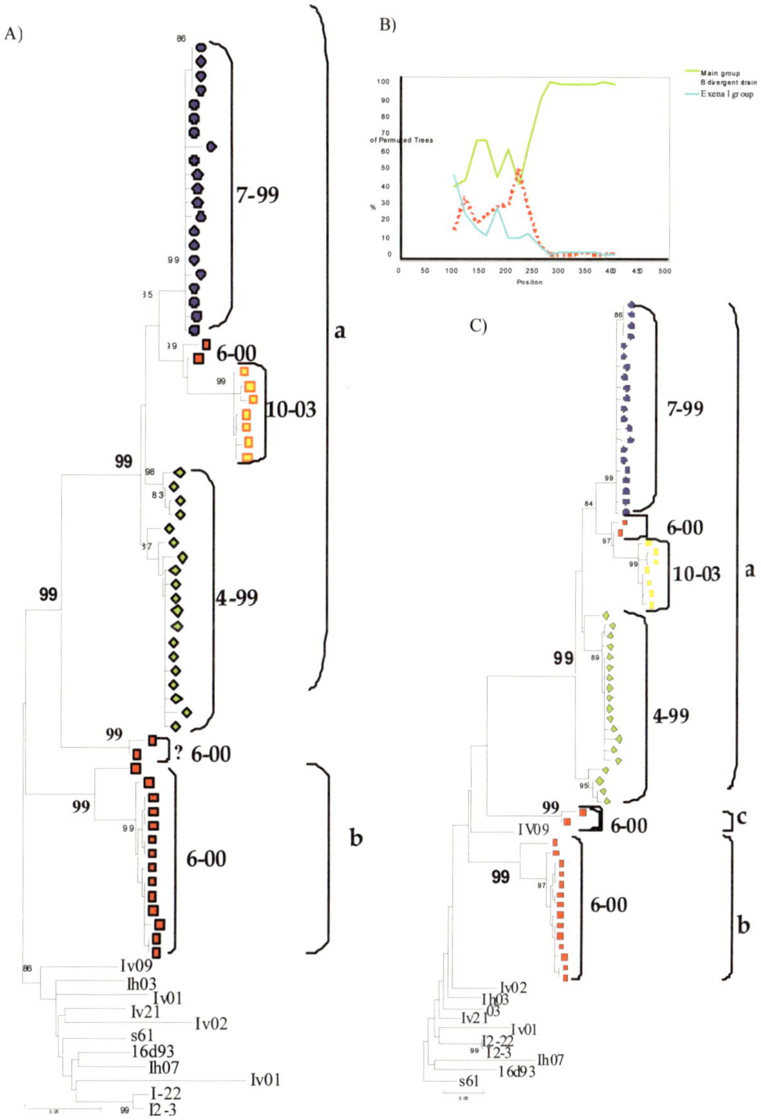

Fig. 1. **A)**. Maximum likehood tree of the sequence quasispecies derived from the C2-C5 region (501 nt) in the *env* gene. Clones were obtained at different time points 4-99♦, 7-99●, 6-00■ and 10-03■. Brackets in the right hand of the phylogenetic tree group the sequences corresponding to a , b and recombinant strain (?). Samples included as external group are designed by letters. **B)** Bootscan plot in the same *env* region of the virus marked with an ? in panel A. Main strain (—) and recombinant strain (···) and external group (—) are included in the analysis. In the first 240 nt the (?) virus showed an homology below 70% with the three compared viruses. C) Maximum likehood tree of the first 240 nt from the C2-C5 region in the *env*. Brackets in the right hand of the phylogenetic tree correspond to a , b and recombinant (c?) virus. Samples designed with letters are reference Spanish strains. Bar represents 10 % genetic distance.

	First HIV-1+Test documented (year)	Genetic Distance to Spanish MRCA	Viral Dating
PATIENT 1	**1986**	**6.9% ± 0.020% (a)** **6.9% ± 0.019% (b)**	**1992 ± 3 (a)** **1992 ± 3 (b)**
PATIENT 2	**1988**	**3.6% ± 1.4% (a)** **9.2% ± 2.3% (b)**	**1987 ± 2 (a)** **1996 ± 4 (b)**

Table 1. Viral dating of dual infected LTNP patients.

3. Incidence

Although it is well establish that SI is frequent in HIV natural history, incidence studies have yielded contradictory results. Several studies found no evidence of HIV-1 SI, in a cohort of 718 HAART treated patients (Gonzales et al., 2003) nor in 37 injecting drug user patients who reported a high risk behaviour (Tsui et al., 2004). In contrast, three population-based studies found SI rates of ~5% which is similar to the primoinfection rate (Chohan et al., 2005). Other authors (Piantadosi et al., 2008) have found higher percentages of 7.7% per year, or even higher (17%) among 36 individuals (Piantadosi et al., 2007).

Super-infection has been reported in every risk group, including men who have sex with men (MSM) (Campbell et al., 2009), heterosexual women (Templeton et al., 2009), and injection drug users (IDU) (Ramos et al., 2002; Yerly et al., 2004). Several cases of SI involving drug-resistant HIV-1 strains have been described (Ramos et al., 2002). Patients, inially infected with a drug-sensitive virus, has been superinfected with a resistant strain (Pernas et al., 2006; Smith et al., 2005) and vice versa (Koelsch et al., 2003). In another case, both viruses were drug-resistant (Brenner et al., 2004).

4. SI and immune response

Study about the role of the immune response in SI is limited. It is still unclear whether only the subset of individuals with a poor immune response are superinfected, or whether immune response during HIV-1 infection is in general inadequate to prevent infection. If SI is a common event, this implies that the immune response generated against HIV infection is not completely protective (Chohan, Piantadosi, and Overbaugh, 2010).

4.1 CTL response

SI has been observed in an individual who showed a cytotoxic acitvity (CTL) against the initial strain, but this response did not protect for SI with a second virus of the same (Altfeld et al., 2002) or different subtype (Ramos et al., 2002). Another case of SI in a patient who developed a high CTL response agaisnt the first virus has been described (Yang et al., 2005). Other authors have suggested that the ability of the SI strain to overcome the preexisting immune response, is related to its ability to rapidly recombine in regions under immune pressure (Streeck et al., 2008).

4.2 Neutralization antibodies response

Unlike CTL response, neutralization antibodies (NAbs) can prevent infection in animal models (Sealy et al., 2009), suggesting that this response might be able to prevent SI in humans. The lack of neutralizing antibody response was related with the predisposition to SI (Smith et al., 2006). On the contrary, a more extensive study showed that at the time of SI, there were not deficits in the Nabs response in the patients who became superinfected compared to the controls, concluding that NAbs elicited during natural infection was not sufficient to block infection (Blish et al., 2008).

5. DI and disease progression

Despite the varying disease progression rates, the majority of untreated HIV-infected individuals progress to AIDS in a period of around 10 years. In some of the HIV-1 dual infected patients, an acelerated disease progression has been observed. In a cohort of 34 patients, in the five individuals with dual infection, the progression to AIDS was very rapid (<3.4 years) (Gottlieb et al., 2004). SI with a dual tropic HIV-1 virus and rapid progression was reported (Gottlieb et al., 2007). In a cohort of HIV-1 subtype C infected female sex workers, DI was associated with an increase viral set point (Grobler et al., 2004). However is not clear whether SI leads allways to clinical progression (Fung et al., 2010).

6. SI in long term non progressor patients

It is very interesting to study SI in a special group of infected patients clasified as long term non progressor (LTNP) -a subset of HIV-positive individuals, who maintain high CD4+ T-cell counts without therapy for more than 15 to 20 years- or in LTNP-Elite controllers (EC) who are LTNPs maintaining undectable viral loads. This group has attracted a lot of interest to disclose the factors contributing to the natural control of the viral replication. Viral control appears to be mediated by multiple mechanism including virological, host genetic and immune response factor:

a. Virological factors

Some studies supported that mutations or deletions in HIV functional proteins or in the accessory genes can lead to viral control like in the virus from the Sidney Cohort (Learmont et al., 1992). Recently, lower replicative capacity and reduced entry capacity in virus obtained from elite controller patients have been reported (Lassen et al., 2009). Other works attribute an important role to the impaired replicative capacity of *gag* (Miura et al., 2009) and *pol* regions obtained from these patients (Brumme et al., 2011). In addition, the presence of viruses with reduced replicative capacity in the initial stages of the infection has been described (Miura et al., 2010). In contrast, other authors did not find relevant deletions or defects after analyzing viral sequences from a large cohort of EC (Miura et al., 2007). Replication competent viruses, which replicated like standard laboratory strains "in vitro", were obtained in 4 out of 10 ES patients, (Blankson et al., 2007). Similar results were obtained by (Lamine et al., 2007) discarding the role of virological factors in the disease control in these patients.

b. Host genetic

Host genetic polymorphisms mapping in the coding and the promoter regions of the co-receptor CCR5 have also been associated with protection against HIV-1 (Gonzalez et al.,

1999). However, the most relevant host factor associated with viral control in HIV infected individuals is the presence of certain major histocompatibility complex class (MHC) I group B HLA I alleles (Deeks and Walker, 2007). HLA B* 57, B* 27 and B* 58 haplotypes are consistently overrepresented in these patients (Fellay et al., 2009; Migueles et al., 2000) .

c. Immune response

One of the most effective mechanisms to control HIV-1 infection is the CD8+T cell response. The effectiveness of the cytotoxic T-lymphocyte (CTL) response does not appear, however, to correlate to the number of the responsive cells but with its functionality (multiple cytokines secretion, degranulation, the ability to proliferate upon to encounter with HIV antigens) which is higher in controllers compared to non controllers (Hersperger et al.,2011). The maintenance of a robust HIV-specific CD4+ T cell response, providing help to CD8+T cells, may also help to the long term control of HIV replication as has been recently described (Blankson, 2010).

Several investigations have studied if ECs have broadly neutralizing antibody (NAb) responses. It appears that this response is not present in most ECs and does not have a major protective role in the early or chronic phase of viral replication (Doria-Rose et al., 2010).

In the majority of the cases described in EC, SI is associated with loss of disease control. In a LTNP female sex worker, an abrupt decline in CD4T cells counts was associated to super-infection (Fang et al., 2004). In two elite controller patients, an accelerated rate of disease progression was observed after a documented super-infection (Clerc et al., 2010). Control of disease after infection by a *nef*-defective strain is lost after SI by a fully competent virus in a B*57 HIV-1 LTNP patient (Braibant et al., 2010). However, other reports have stated SI in patients without apparent clinical consequences. Recovery of viremic control after SI in a long term elite controller patient has been also described although viral load was higher after SI, which implies that the patient did not fulfil the definition of elite controller (Rachinger et al., 2008). For the first time, SI in a long term EC patient able to control both viruses and maintain undetectable viral loads for > 20 years has been reported (Casado et al., 2007). This patient presented strong immune response and viruses with low "in vitro" replicative capacity (Pernas et al, manuscript in preparation).

More studies of SI in people who control infection could be very useful in two ways:

- - Understanding why some EC patients lost viral control after SI while others maintain their EC status.
- - Analysis of SI in this group of patients could help to estimate the real incidence rate of SI in HIV natural infection, because in EC and LTNPS patients there is no or very little viral evolution (Wang et al., 2003), consequently less recombinant forms appear and the detection of SI should be easier than in the patients with typical progression.

7. Conclusion

The study of SI is a very productive topic in HIV research because it provides useful information for different aspects of HIV infection. SI patients constitute an interesting group of patients to investigate the role of the immune response generated against HIV infection and to investigate which factors, including host genes, contribute to protection against new infections. Also, the study of the phenotypic characteristics of the infecting and super-infecting strains will produce very interesting information for HIV pathogenesis. Analysis of SI in LTNPs and EC patients could offer an excellent model for these studies. Moreover, from the clinical perspective, detection of SI, with the potential pathogenic consequences, demonstrate the importance of reducing risky behaviors in HIV-1 infected individuals.

8. Acknowledgements

Work in CNM is supported by grant SAF 2007-61036 and SAF 2010-17226, by Fundacion para la Investigacion y Prevencion del SIDA en España (FIPSE) grants 36558/06, 36641/07, 36779/08, 360766/09 and in part by the Red Temática Cooperativa de Investigación en SIDA (Red de grupos 173) of the Fondo de Investigaciones Sanitarias de la Seguridad Social (FISss).

9. References

Altfeld, M., Allen, T. M., Yu, X. G., Johnston, M. N., Agrawal, D., Korber, B. T., Montefiori, D. C., O'Connor, D. H., Davis, B. T., Lee, P. K., Maier, E. L., Harlow, J., Goulder, P. J., Brander, C., Rosenberg, E. S., and Walker, B. D. (2002). HIV-1 superinfection despite broad CD8+ T-cell responses containing replication of the primary virus. *Nature* 420(6914), 434-9.

Blankson, J. N. (2010). Effector mechanisms in HIV-1 infected elite controllers: highly active immune responses? *Antiviral Res* 85(1), 295-302.

Blankson, J. N., Bailey, J. R., Thayil, S., Yang, H. C., Lassen, K., Lai, J., Gandhi, S. K., Siliciano, J. D., Williams, T. M., and Siliciano, R. F. (2007). Isolation and characterization of replication-competent human immunodeficiency virus type 1 from a subset of elite suppressors. *J Virol* 81(5), 2508-18.

Blish, C. A., Dogan, O. C., Derby, N. R., Nguyen, M.-A., Chohan, B., Richardson, B. A., and Overbaugh, J. (2008). Human Immunodeficiency Virus Type 1 Superinfection Occurs despite Relatively Robust Neutralizing Antibody Responses, Vol. 82, pp. 12094-12103.

Braibant, M., Xie, J., Samri, A., Agut, H., Autran, B., and Barin, F. (2010). Disease progression due to dual infection in an HLA-B57-positive asymptomatic long-term nonprogressor infected with a nef-defective HIV-1 strain. *Virology* 405(1), 81-92.

Brenner, B., Routy, J. P., Quan, Y., Moisi, D., Oliveira, M., Turner, D., and Wainberg, M. A. (2004). Persistence of multidrug-resistant HIV-1 in primary infection leading to superinfection. *Aids* 18(12), 1653-60.

Brumme, Z. L., Li, C., Miura, T., Sela, J., Rosato, P. C., Brumme, C. J., Markle, T. J., Martin, E., Block, B. L., Trocha, A., Kadie, C. M., Allen, T. M., Pereyra, F., Heckerman, D., Walker, B. D., and Brockman, M. A. (2011). Reduced replication capacity of NL4-3 recombinant viruses encoding reverse transcriptase-integrase sequences from HIV-1 elite controllers. *J Acquir Immune Defic Syndr* 56(2), 100-8.

Campbell, M. S., Gottlieb, G. S., Hawes, S. E., Nickle, D. C., Wong, K. G., Deng, W., Lampinen, T. M., Kiviat, N. B., and Mullins, J. I. (2009). HIV-1 superinfection in the antiretroviral therapy era: are seroconcordant sexual partners at risk? *PLoS One* 4(5), e5690.

Casado, C., Pernas, M., Alvaro, T., Sandonis, V., Garcia, S., Rodriguez, C., del Romero, J., Grau, E., Ruiz, L., and Lopez-Galindez, C. (2007). Coinfection and superinfection in patients with long-term, nonprogressive HIV-1 disease. *J Infect Dis* 196(6), 895-9.

Casado, C., Urtasun, I., Martin-Walther, M. V., Garcia, S., Rodriguez, C., del Romero, J., and Lopez-Galindez, C. (2000). Genetic analysis of HIV-1 samples from Spain. *J Acquir Immune Defic Syndr* 23(1), 68-74.

Clerc, O., Colombo, S., Yerly, S., Telenti, A., and Cavassini, M. (2010). HIV-1 elite controllers: Beware of super-infections. *J Clin Virol.*

Cornelissen, M., Jurriaans, S., Kozaczynska, K., Prins, J. M., Hamidjaja, R. A., Zorgdrager, F., Bakker, M., Back, N., and van der Kuyl, A. C. (2007). Routine HIV-1 genotyping as a tool to identify dual infections. *Aids* 21(7), 807-11.

Chohan, B., Lavreys, L., Rainwater, S. M., and Overbaugh, J. (2005). Evidence for frequent reinfection with human immunodeficiency virus type 1 of a different subtype. *J Virol* 79(16), 10701-8.

Chohan, B. H., Piantadosi, A., and Overbaugh, J. (2010). HIV-1 superinfection and its implications for vaccine design. *Curr HIV Res* 8(8), 596-601.

Deeks, S. G., and Walker, B. D. (2007). Human Immunodeficiency Virus Controllers: Mechanisms of Durable Virus Control in the Absence of Antiretroviral Therapy. *Immunity* 27(3), 406-416.

Doria-Rose, N. A., Klein, R. M., Daniels, M. G., O'Dell, S., Nason, M., Lapedes, A., Bhattacharya, T., Migueles, S. A., Wyatt, R. T., Korber, B. T., Mascola, J. R., and Connors, M. (2010). Breadth of human immunodeficiency virus-specific neutralizing activity in sera: clustering analysis and association with clinical variables. *J Virol* 84(3), 1631-6.

Fang, G., Weiser, B., Kuiken, C., Philpott, S. M., Rowland-Jones, S., Plummer, F., Kimani, J., Shi, B., Kaul, R., Bwayo, J., Anzala, O., and Burger, H. (2004). Recombination following superinfection by HIV-1. *Aids* 18(2), 153-9.

Fellay, J., Ge, D., Shianna, K. V., Colombo, S., Ledergerber, B., Cirulli, E. T., Urban, T. J., Zhang, K., Gumbs, C. E., Smith, J. P., Castagna, A., Cozzi-Lepri, A., De Luca, A., Easterbrook, P., Gunthard, H. F., Mallal, S., Mussini, C., Dalmau, J., Martinez-Picado, J., Miro, J. M., Obel, N., Wolinsky, S. M., Martinson, J. J., Detels, R., Margolick, J. B., Jacobson, L. P., Descombes, P., Antonarakis, S. E., Beckmann, J. S., O'Brien, S. J., Letvin, N. L., McMichael, A. J., Haynes, B. F., Carrington, M., Feng, S., Telenti, A., and Goldstein, D. B. (2009). Common genetic variation and the control of HIV-1 in humans. *PLoS Genet* 5(12), e1000791.

Fung, I. C., Gambhir, M., van Sighem, A., de Wolf, F., and Garnett, G. P. (2010). Superinfection with a heterologous HIV strain per se does not lead to faster progression. *Math Biosci* 224(1), 1-9.

Gerhard M. Mloka, T. S. S.-B. E. O. H. M. L. B. D. L. M. H. M. (2004). *HIV dynamics & evolution, UCLA (CA).*

Gonzales, M. J., Delwart, E., Rhee, S. Y., Tsui, R., Zolopa, A. R., Taylor, J., and Shafer, R. W. (2003). Lack of detectable human immunodeficiency virus type 1 superinfection during 1072 person-years of observation. *J Infect Dis* 188(3), 397-405.

Gonzalez, E., Bamshad, M., Sato, N., Mummidi, S., Dhanda, R., Catano, G., Cabrera, S., McBride, M., Cao, X. H., Merrill, G., O'Connell, P., Bowden, D. W., Freedman, B. I.,

Anderson, S. A., Walter, E. A., Evans, J. S., Stephan, K. T., Clark, R. A., Tyagi, S., Ahuja, S. S., Dolan, M. J., and Ahuja, S. K. (1999). Race-specific HIV-1 disease-modifying effects associated with CCR5 haplotypes. *Proc Natl Acad Sci U S A* 96(21), 12004-9.

Gottlieb, G. S., Nickle, D. C., Jensen, M. A., Wong, K. G., Grobler, J., Li, F., Liu, S. L., Rademeyer, C., Learn, G. H., Karim, S. S., Williamson, C., Corey, L., Margolick, J. B., and Mullins, J. I. (2004). Dual HIV-1 infection associated with rapid disease progression. *Lancet* 363(9409), 619-22.

Gottlieb, G. S., Nickle, D. C., Jensen, M. A., Wong, K. G., Kaslow, R. A., Shepherd, J. C., Margolick, J. B., and Mullins, J. I. (2007). HIV type 1 superinfection with a dual-tropic virus and rapid progression to AIDS: a case report. *Clin Infect Dis* 45(4), 501-9.

Grobler, J., Gray, C. M., Rademeyer, C., Seoighe, C., Ramjee, G., Karim, S. A., Morris, L., and Williamson, C. (2004). Incidence of HIV-1 dual infection and its association with increased viral load set point in a cohort of HIV-1 subtype C-infected female sex workers. *J Infect Dis* 190(7), 1355-9.

Hersperger, A. R., Migueles, S. A., Betts, M. R., and Connors, M. (2011). Qualitative features of the HIV-specific CD8+ T-cell response associated with immunologic control. *Curr Opin HIV AIDS*.

Jost, S., Bernard, M. C., Kaiser, L., Yerly, S., Hirschel, B., Samri, A., Autran, B., Goh, L. E., and Perrin, L. (2002). A patient with HIV-1 superinfection. *N Engl J Med* 347(10), 731-6.

Koelsch, K. K., Smith, D. M., Little, S. J., Ignacio, C. C., Macaranas, T. R., Brown, A. J., Petropoulos, C. J., Richman, D. D., and Wong, J. K. (2003). Clade B HIV-1 superinfection with wild-type virus after primary infection with drug-resistant clade B virus. *Aids* 17(7), F11-6.

Kozaczynska, K., Cornelissen, M., Reiss, P., Zorgdrager, F., and van der Kuyl, A. C. (2007). HIV-1 sequence evolution in vivo after superinfection with three viral strains. *Retrovirology* 4, 59.

Lamine, A., Caumont-Sarcos, A., Chaix, M. L., Saez-Cirion, A., Rouzioux, C., Delfraissy, J. F., Pancino, G., and Lambotte, O. (2007). Replication-competent HIV strains infect HIV controllers despite undetectable viremia (ANRS EP36 study). *Aids* 21(8), 1043-5.

Lassen, K. G., Lobritz, M. A., Bailey, J. R., Johnston, S., Nguyen, S., Lee, B., Chou, T., Siliciano, R. F., Markowitz, M., and Arts, E. J. (2009). Elite suppressor-derived HIV-1 envelope glycoproteins exhibit reduced entry efficiency and kinetics. *PLoS Pathog* 5(4), e1000377.

Learmont, J., Tindall, B., Evans, L., Cunningham, A., Cunningham, P., Wells, J., Penny, R., Kaldor, J., and Cooper, D. A. (1992). Long-term symptomless HIV-1 infection in recipients of blood products from a single donor. *Lancet* 340(8824), 863-7.

Manigart, O., Courgnaud, V., Sanou, O., Valea, D., Nagot, N., Meda, N., Delaporte, E., Peeters, M., and Van de Perre, P. (2004). HIV-1 superinfections in a cohort of commercial sex workers in Burkina Faso as assessed by an autologous heteroduplex mobility procedure. *Aids* 18(12), 1645-51.

McCutchan, F. E., Hoelscher, M., Tovanabutra, S., Piyasirisilp, S., Sanders-Buell, E., Ramos, G., Jagodzinski, L., Polonis, V., Maboko, L., Mmbando, D., Hoffmann, O., Riedner, G., von Sonnenburg, F., Robb, M., and Birx, D. L. (2005). In-Depth Analysis of a Heterosexually Acquired Human Immunodeficiency Virus Type 1 Superinfection: Evolution, Temporal Fluctuation, and Intercompartment Dynamics from the Seronegative Window Period through 30 Months Postinfection. *J. Virol.* 79(18), 11693-11704.

Migueles, S. A., Sabbaghian, M. S., Shupert, W. L., Bettinotti, M. P., Marincola, F. M., Martino, L., Hallahan, C. W., Selig, S. M., Schwartz, D., Sullivan, J., and Connors, M. (2000). HLA B*5701 is highly associated with restriction of virus replication in a subgroup of HIV-infected long term nonprogressors. *Proc Natl Acad Sci U S A* 97(6), 2709-14.

Miura, T., Brockman, M., Pereyra, F., Li, B., Sheneidewind, A., Trocha, A., Heckerman, D., Alllen, T., and Walker, B. (2007). Gross viral genetic defects unlikey explain many of spontaneous HIV-1 viremia controllers.

Miura, T., Brockman, M. A., Schneidewind, A., Lobritz, M., Pereyra, F., Rathod, A., Block, B. L., Brumme, Z. L., Brumme, C. J., Baker, B., Rothchild, A. C., Li, B., Trocha, A., Cutrell, E., Frahm, N., Brander, C., Toth, I., Arts, E. J., Allen, T. M., and Walker, B. D. (2009). HLA-B57/B*5801 Human Immunodeficiency Virus Type 1 Elite Controllers Select for Rare Gag Variants Associated with Reduced Viral Replication Capacity and Strong Cytotoxic T-Lymphotye Recognition, Vol. 83, pp. 2743-2755.

Miura, T., Brumme, Z. L., Brockman, M. A., Rosato, P., Sela, J., Brumme, C. J., Pereyra, F., Kaufmann, D. E., Trocha, A., Block, B. L., Daar, E. S., Connick, E., Jessen, H., Kelleher, A. D., Rosenberg, E., Markowitz, M., Schafer, K., Vaida, F., Iwamoto, A., Little, S., and Walker, B. D. (2010). Impaired replication capacity of acute/early viruses in persons who become HIV controllers. *J Virol* 84(15), 7581-91.

Pacold, M., Smith, D., Little, S., Cheng, P. M., Jordan, P., Ignacio, C., Richman, D., and Pond, S. K. (2010). Comparison of methods to detect HIV dual infection. *AIDS Res Hum Retroviruses* 26(12), 1291-8.

Pernas, M., Casado, C., Fuentes, R., Perez-Elias, M. J., and Lopez-Galindez, C. (2006). A dual superinfection and recombination within HIV-1 subtype B 12 years after primoinfection. *J Acquir Immune Defic Syndr* 42(1), 12-8.

Piantadosi, A., Chohan, B., Chohan, V., McClelland, R. S., and Overbaugh, J. (2007). Chronic HIV-1 Infection Frequently Fails to Protect against Superinfection. *PLoS Pathog* 3(11), e177.

Piantadosi, A., Ngayo, M. O., Chohan, B., and Overbaugh, J. (2008). Examination of a second region of the HIV type 1 genome reveals additional cases of superinfection. *AIDS Res Hum Retroviruses* 24(9), 1221.

Rachinger, A., Navis, M., van Assen, S., Groeneveld, P. H., and Schuitemaker, H. (2008). Recovery of viremic control after superinfection with pathogenic HIV type 1 in a long-term elite controller of HIV type 1 infection. *Clin Infect Dis* 47(11), e86-9.

Rachinger, A., van de Ven, T. D., Burger, J. A., Schuitemaker, H., and van 't Wout, A. B. (2010). Evaluation of pre-screening methods for the identification of HIV-1 superinfection. *J Virol Methods* 165(2), 311-7.

Ramos, A., Hu, D. J., Nguyen, L., Phan, K. O., Vanichseni, S., Promadej, N., Choopanya, K., Callahan, M., Young, N. L., McNicholl, J., Mastro, T. D., Folks, T. M., and Subbarao, S. (2002). Intersubtype human immunodeficiency virus type 1 superinfection following seroconversion to primary infection in two injection drug users. *J Virol* 76(15), 7444-52.

Salazar-Gonzalez, J. F., Bailes, E., Pham, K. T., Salazar, M. G., Guffey, M. B., Keele, B. F., Derdeyn, C. A., Farmer, P., Hunter, E., Allen, S., Manigart, O., Mulenga, J., Anderson, J. A., Swanstrom, R., Haynes, B. F., Athreya, G. S., Korber, B. T. M., Sharp, P. M., Shaw, G. M., and Hahn, B. H. (2008). Deciphering Human Immunodeficiency Virus Type 1 Transmission and Early Envelope Diversification by Single-Genome Amplification and Sequencing. *In* "J.Virol", Vol. 82, pp. 3952-3970.

Sealy, R., Zhan, X., Lockey, T. D., Martin, L., Blanchard, J., Traina-Dorge, V., and Hurwitz, J. L. (2009). SHIV infection protects against heterologous pathogenic SHIV challenge in macaques: a gold-standard for HIV-1 vaccine development? *Curr HIV Res* 7(5), 497-503.

Smith, D. M., Strain, M. C., Frost, S. D., Pillai, S. K., Wong, J. K., Wrin, T., Liu, Y., Petropolous, C. J., Daar, E. S., Little, S. J., and Richman, D. D. (2006). Lack of neutralizing antibody response to HIV-1 predisposes to superinfection. *Virology* 355(1), 1-5.

Smith, D. M., Wong, J. K., Hightower, G. K., Ignacio, C. C., Koelsch, K. K., Petropoulos, C. J., Richman, D. D., and Little, S. J. (2005). HIV drug resistance acquired through superinfection. *Aids* 19(12), 1251-6.

Streeck, H., Li, B., Poon, A. F. Y., Schneidewind, A., Gladden, A. D., Power, K. A., Daskalakis, D., Bazner, S., Zuniga, R., Brander, C., Rosenberg, E. S., Frost, S. D. W., Altfeld, M., and Allen, T. M. (2008). Immune-driven recombination and loss of control after HIV superinfection. *In* "J. Exp. Med", Vol. 205, pp. 1789-1796.

Templeton, A. R., Kramer, M. G., Jarvis, J., Kowalski, J., Gange, S., Schneider, M. F., Shao, Q., Zhang, G. W., Yeh, M. F., Tsai, H. L., Zhang, H., and Markham, R. B. (2009). Multiple-infection and recombination in HIV-1 within a longitudinal cohort of women. *Retrovirology* 6, 54.

Tsui, R., Herring, B. L., Barbour, J. D., Grant, R. M., Bacchetti, P., Kral, A., Edlin, B. R., and Delwart, E. L. (2004). Human immunodeficiency virus type 1 superinfection was not detected following 215 years of injection drug user exposure. *J Virol* 78(1), 94-103.

Wang, B., Mikhail, M., Dyer, W. B., Zaunders, J. J., Kelleher, A. D., and Saksena, N. K. (2003). First demonstration of a lack of viral sequence evolution in a nonprogressor, defining replication-incompetent HIV-1 infection. *Virology* 312(1), 135-50.

Yang, O. O., Daar, E. S., Jamieson, B. D., Balamurugan, A., Smith, D. M., Pitt, J. A., Petropoulos, C. J., Richman, D. D., Little, S. J., and Leigh-Brown, A. J. (2005). Human Immunodeficiency Virus Type 1 Clade B Superinfection: Evidence for Differential Immune Containment of Distinct Clade B Strains. *J. Virol.* 79(2), 860-868.

Yerly, S., Jost, S., Monnat, M., Telenti, A., Cavassini, M., Chave, J. P., Kaiser, L., Burgisser, P., and Perrin, L. (2004). HIV-1 co/super-infection in intravenous drug users. *Aids* 18(10), 1413-21.

3

HIV/Aids Fact Sheet – Predisposing Factors the Nigeria Situation

Uju Marie Esther Dibua
Department of Microbiology, Faculty of Biological Sciences, University of Nigeria, Nigeria

1. Introduction

HIV/AIDS has become a global scourge, a devastating challenge to human dignity and a generalized threat to sociocultural and socioeconomic growth. The deadly epidemic has grossly annihilated Millennium Development Goals, reduced life expectancy and heightened poverty levels particularly in the developing and underdeveloped countries of the world. The brunt of the plague is borne chiefly by the sub-Saharan Africa, where it takes its toll mostly on the most productive and sexually active persons of child bearing age.

Co-infection with HIV, TB and STIs has worsened the effect of the epidemic. The World Health Organization (WHO, 2009) declared TB to be a global health emergency, which disproportionately affects people in resource-poor settings, particularly those in Asia and Africa. In 2008, an estimated 11.1 million people were living with (active) TB, including 9.4 million new cases, with an estimated 1.8 million TB deaths including 500,000 deaths that were HIV-positive. TB and HIV are frequently referred to as co- or dual-epidemics as a result of the high morbidity and mortality rates emanating from the co-infection. Resurgence of latent TB in the developing world has largely been attributed to HIV infection.

Sexually transmitted infections (STIs) have similarly been closely associated with HIV as a result of their similar transmission modes, namely, sexual contact. Hence, STIs of different categories: treatable and untreatable, ulcerative and non-ulcerative, etc., have been known to fuel the transmissibility and/or co-infectivity of HIV by a peculiar paradigm: reduction in immunological functions and subsequent progression to the active disease, AIDS.

The future remains bleak as a result of the un-abating HIV prevalence in Nigeria. Estimates by the Federal Ministry of Health (FMOH, 2009), indicated that 2.98 million people were living with HIV/AIDS in Nigeria in 2009 with a total AIDS death of 192,000; the increasing number of orphans and vulnerable children estimated at 2.12million in 2008 and 2.175million in 200; the stigmatization of people living with HIV/AIDS and violation of their rights, their roles and responsibilities; the lack of adherence to the messages on behaviour change and safe sex options especially among young people aged 12-28 years old in secondary and tertiary institutions of learning and the difficulties associated with increased access to treatment options. Far from being an executive summary, this paper merely attempts to provide some useful data/or information on the prevailing situation and the predisposing factors to HIV epidemic in Nigeria and calls for a collaborative and concerted initiative by all and sundry including the already established governmental and non-governmental parastatals in Nigeria towards a wholistic HIV intervention strategies/or programmes.

2.1 HIV situation

Nigeria, the most populous country in Africa, is located on the West Coast of Africa with a land mass of 923,768 square kilometers between 4°16′ and 13°53' north of equator, and between 2°40' and 14°41'east of Greenwich. It is bordered by Niger Republic (north), Chad (north-east), Cameroon (east), Benin Republic (west) and Atlantic Ocean (south). Nigeria had a population of 140million in 2006; an estimation of 152.6 million in mid-2009, making Nigeria the eighth most populous country in the world (Population Reference Bureau 2009 Data Fact Sheet)

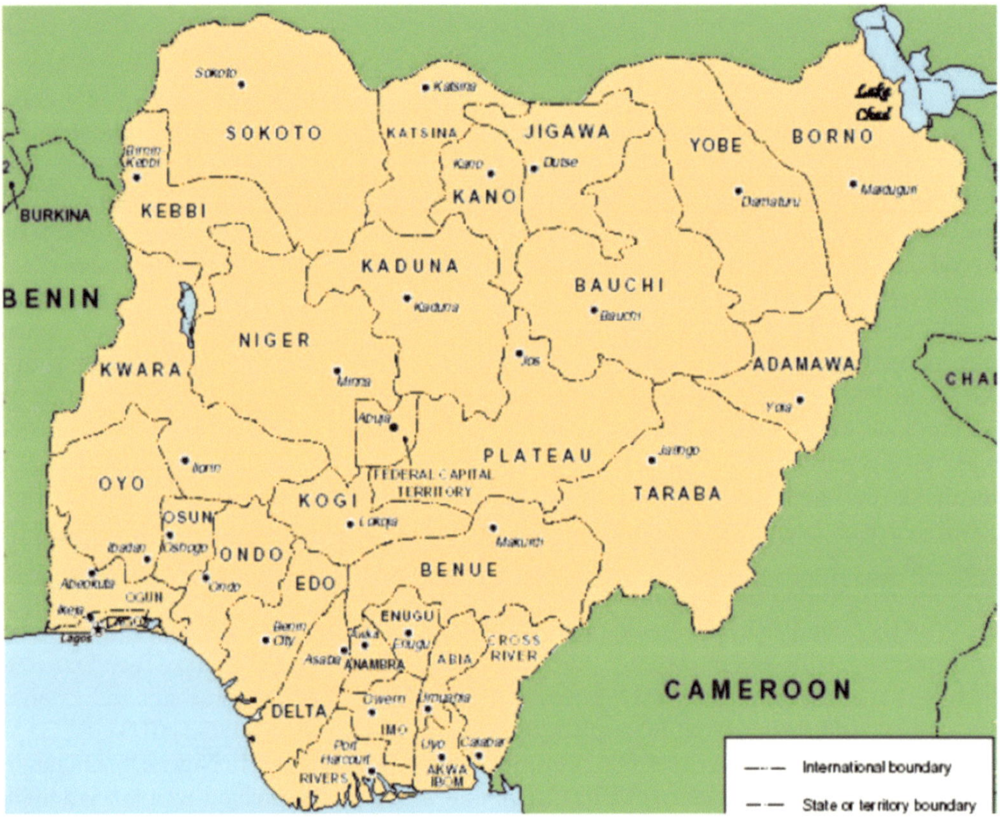

(Population Reference Bureau 2009 Fact Sheet)

Fig. 1. Nigerian Map showing major cities and international boundries

2.2 Global and national HIV/AIDS prevalence

AIDS has become a pandemic. There are 33.3 million people worldwide living with HIV/AIDS, with 2.6 million new infections per year and 1.8 million annual deaths due to AIDS (AVERT, 2009). In 2007, UNAIDS estimated: 33.2 million people worldwide had AIDS that year; AIDS killed 2.1 million people in the course of that year, including 330,000 children, and 76% of those deaths occurred in sub-Saharan Africa (UNAIDS/WHO, 2007). UNAIDS 2009 report indicated that worldwide some 60 million people have been infected, with some 25 million deaths, and 14 million orphaned children in southern Africa alone since the epidemic began (UNAIDS, 2009)

The index reported case of AIDS in Nigeria was in 1986 (Akinsete *et al.,* 1999). Two people were initially identified as sero-positive and by the end of the same year, a total of 6 were reported. By 1989, the figure had escalated to 65, and there is currently a very steady increase. HIV epidemic in Nigeria rose From 1.8% in 1991, the figure rose to 3.8% in 1993; 4.5% in 1995; 5.4% in 1999 and currently 5.8% in 2001 showing an average National HIV prevalence (Federal Ministry of Health 2001). Nevertheless, there was an observed slight increase in HIV from 4.4% in 2005 to 4.6% in 2008, with a state variation in some states and local government areas. From the 2008 ANC survey, a paradigm of variation was observed: at the zonal level, prevalence is lowest in the South West (2.0%) and highest in the South-South (7.0%).

Age specific prevalence is highest among 25-29 years age group (5.6%) and lowest among 40-44 years age group (2.9%) (NASCP Abuja, 2008). In the pattern of HIV transmission and prevalence, women are more affected; with policy implications for prevention of mother to child transmissions, hence, addressing gender inequality which is crucial in the control of the epidemic (Quinn and Overbaugh 2005; Ezumah, 2003).

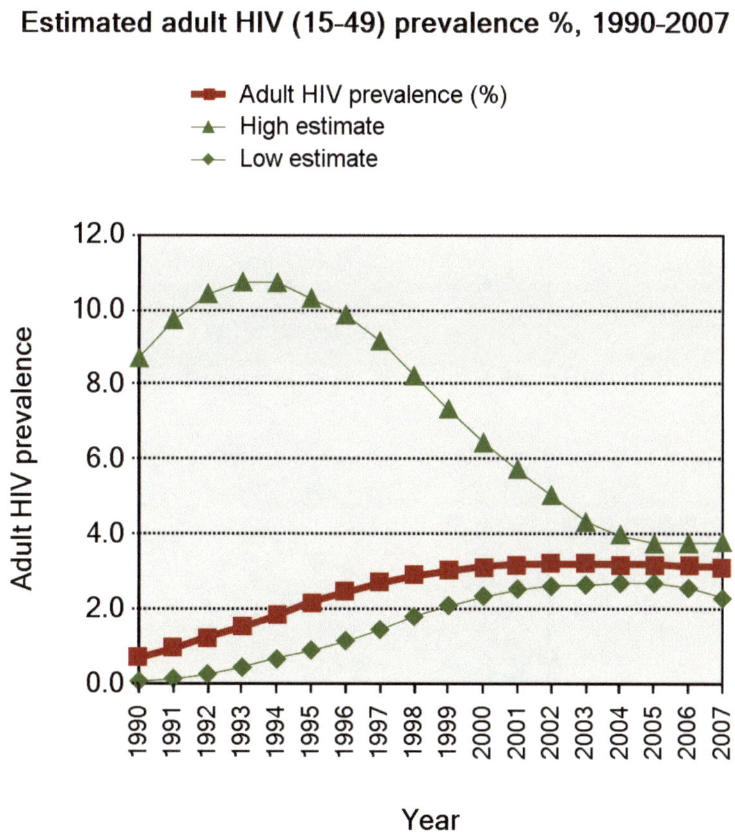

Fig. 2. UNAIDS/WHO estimate giving number of adults living with HIV

With a population of 152.6 million people and estimated HIV prevalence of 3.6 % in the general population, Nigeria has been reported to have the second largest population of people living with HIV/AIDS after South Africa: an 2.98 million people are living with HIV/AIDS by the end of 2009 (Population Reference Bureau 2009 Data Fact Sheet).
The UNAIDS/WHO reports presented below give estimated number of adults and children living with HIV. Figure 1, is an estimated adult HIV (15-49 years) % prevalence. The figure shows a decline in adult HIV prevalence from 1990 to 2007 (UNAIDS/WHO, 2007)
In Figure 2, estimate of people living with HIV is presented with a similar decline in % prevalence from 1990 to 2007. The estimates are based on methods and parameters informed by advice given by the UNAIDS Reference Group on HIV/AIDS Estimates, Modeling and Projections. (The median prevalence rates (in percentages) are given for each of the categories). Several deaths were reported in same year (Figure 3); the death toll does not however seem to be completely on the decline.
The observed decline in HIV epidemics in Nigeria can be attributed to a mirage of factors, including the upsurge in the use of antiretroviral therapy. Estimated number of people receiving and needing antiretroviral therapy at the end of each year has been on the increase (Figure 4). Presented here are coverage estimates based on the estimated unrounded numbers of people - all age groups - receiving antiretroviral therapy and the estimated

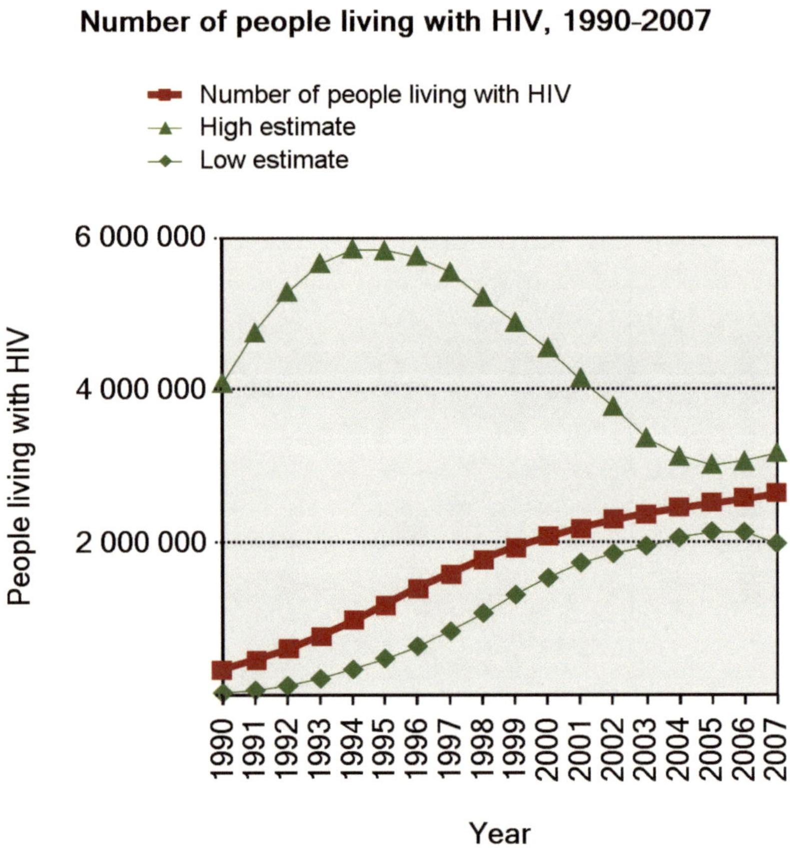

Fig. 3. Estimated HIV/AIDS death 1990-2007

unrounded need for antiretroviral therapy (based on UNAIDS/WHO methodology) (UNAIDS/WHO, 2008).

3.1 HIV transmission dynamics

Heterosexual sex remains the primary mode of transmission for HIV (Dibua, 2009), and accounts for 80-95% of HIV infections in Nigeria. According to the Federal Ministry of Health, high-risk groups significantly contributed to new HIV infections. The high risk groups are about 1% of the general population, and are men that have sex with men, female sex workers and injecting drug users. They contributed almost 23% of new infections. Also, the high risk groups and their partners contributed 40% of new infections. However, people practicing low-risk sex (clandestine sex) in the general population contribute 42% of the infections due to low condom use and high sexual networking (FMH, 2007) Furthermore, long distance truck drivers and traders who spend several days away from their homes and families and who engage the services of commercial sex workers or mistresses (Dibua, 2010), are also identified as important channels in the HIV distribution saga.

Evidence of the enormous contribution of sex working (in its diverse forms) to HIV dissemination abound following the index screening of sex workers in 1988-1989 in Lagos State. Federal Ministry of Health (FMH, 1999), reported an increase from 2 -15% HIV prevalence among this group in 1993. This figure has escalated. Currently, HIV seroprevalence among prostitutes ranges from 18 - 51.8% with a national average of 22.9%.

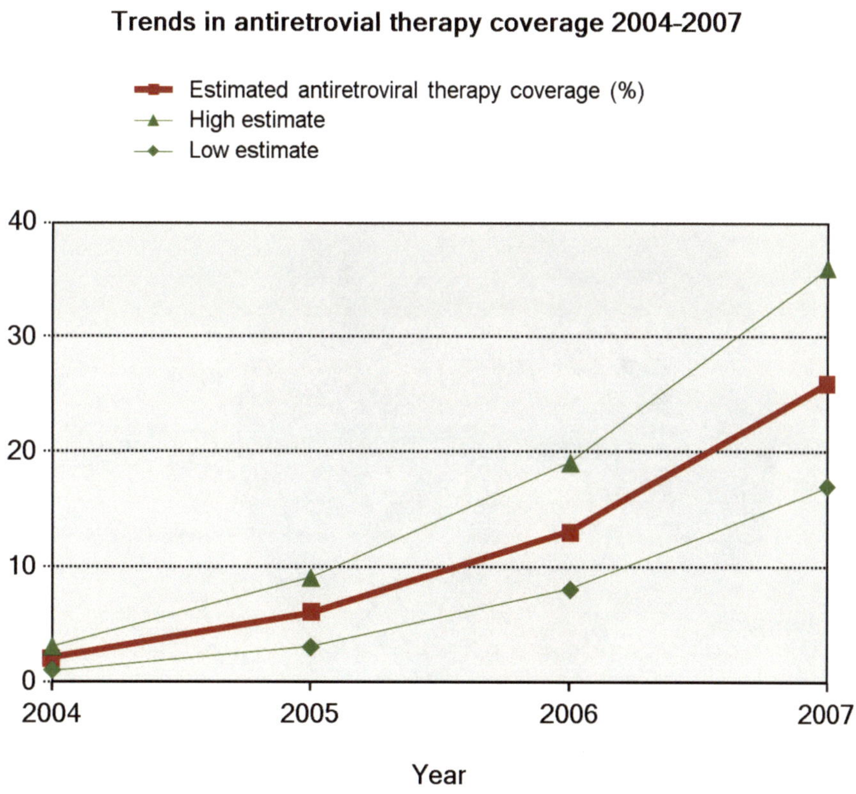

Fig. 4. Trend of Antiretroviral therapy in 2004-2007

Summary of HIV trend

The trend of the HIV epidemic is summarized in Table 1. The estimate of the percentage of adults (aged 15-49) living with HIV/AIDS is reported to be 3.6%. This is calculated by dividing the estimated number of adults living with HIV/AIDS at year-end by the total adult population at year-end.

Year	HIV/AIDS - adult prevalence rate	Rank	Percent Change	Date of Information
2003	5.80 %	26		2001 est.
2004	5.40 %	21	-6.90 %	2003 est.
2005	5.40 %	21	0.00 %	2003 est.
2006	5.40 %	21	0.00 %	2003 est.
2007	5.40 %	21	0.00 %	2003 est.
2008	5.40 %	21	0.00 %	2003 est.
2009	3.10 %	23	-42.59 %	2007 est.
2010	3.10 %	23	0.00 %	2007 est.
2011	3.60 %	17	16.13 %	2009 est.

Source: CIA World Fact-book March 11, 2010

Table 1. Nigeria HIV/AIDS - adult prevalence rate

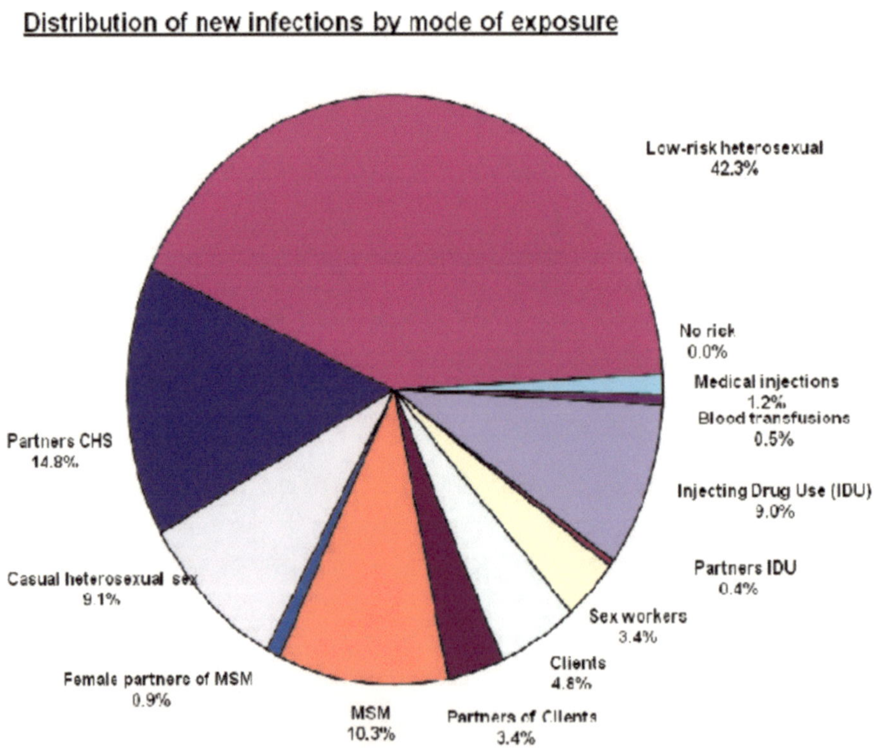

Fig. 5. Modes of HIV Transmission in Nigeria

A similar report on high risk groups and associated high HIV prevalence in the North-East trucking routes of Enugu State, indicated as follows: Commercial sex workers (CSW)(23%) > Students (21.%), Single parents (20%), Long Distance Truck Drivers - LDTD (19%) and Street Children (16%) (Figure 6) (Dibua, 2010)

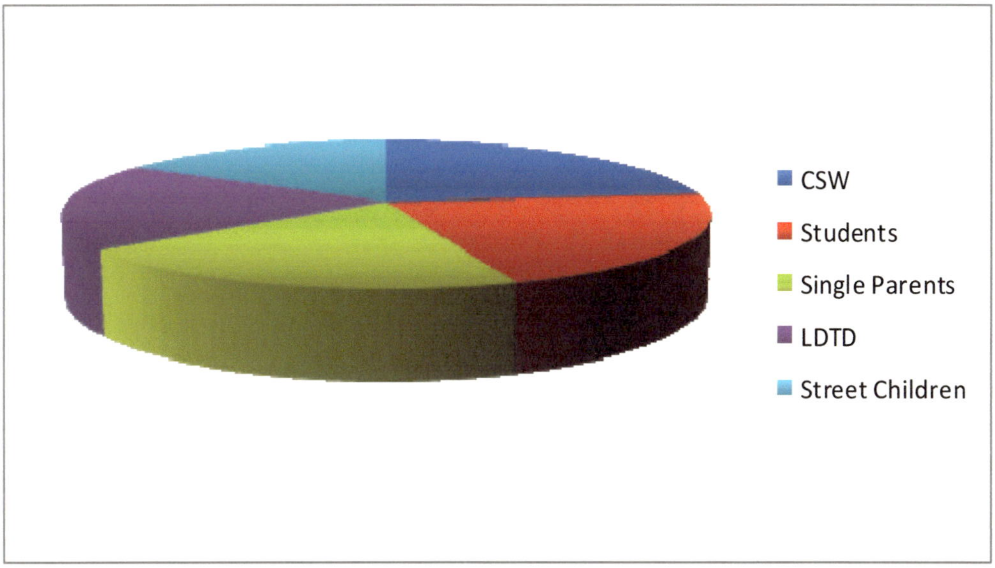

Fig. 6. HIV Transmission and Associated High Risk Groups

According to Dibua (2010), HIV spread in Nigeria is primarily a heterosexual phenomenon (multiple sex partnering): a function of sociocultural and economic predisposition: each filters out and merges into the final outcome: HIV/AIDS (Figure 7). However, there is no strict age or class divide or bias, as young and old are involved in commercial or clandestine sex working (though not resident in hotels), while the ultimate perpetrators are the rich or apparently rich financiers or customers. Anecdotal cases of HIV prevalence were mostly observed in the rural areas where people abscond to elude the social stigma of the disease. To arrest the hideous trend, the Nigeria Government under the auspices of the Federal Ministry of Health, responded by organizing series of surveillance campaigns at the grassroots.

With heterosexual intercourse driving the HIV epidemic, sex with prostitutes or commercial sex workers (identified here as individuals who exchange sex for money, not limited to those in brothels or hotels) has thus been identified as the largest single vector of HIV infection in the country. The steep increase in the rate of prostitution arising from economic recession as well as freedom of sexual expression are major factors responsible for the introduction /dissemination of HIV/AIDS into Nigerian homes. The study further indicated that HIV is a sociocultural and socioeconomic disease in Nigeria, and the paradigm of its infection and spread particularly within the local communities is a reflection of the sociocultural and socioeconomic profile of the people. Incriminated sociocultural predisposing factors to the HIV epidemic include marriage for the dead, surrogate marriage of woman to woman, concubinage, marriage of young girls to older men for favour or economic reasons. The factors have overlapping or interconnected relationships - none excludes the other in importance or in enhancing HIV spread and progression. The precipitating factors of HIV infection as reported by Dibua (2010) is described below.

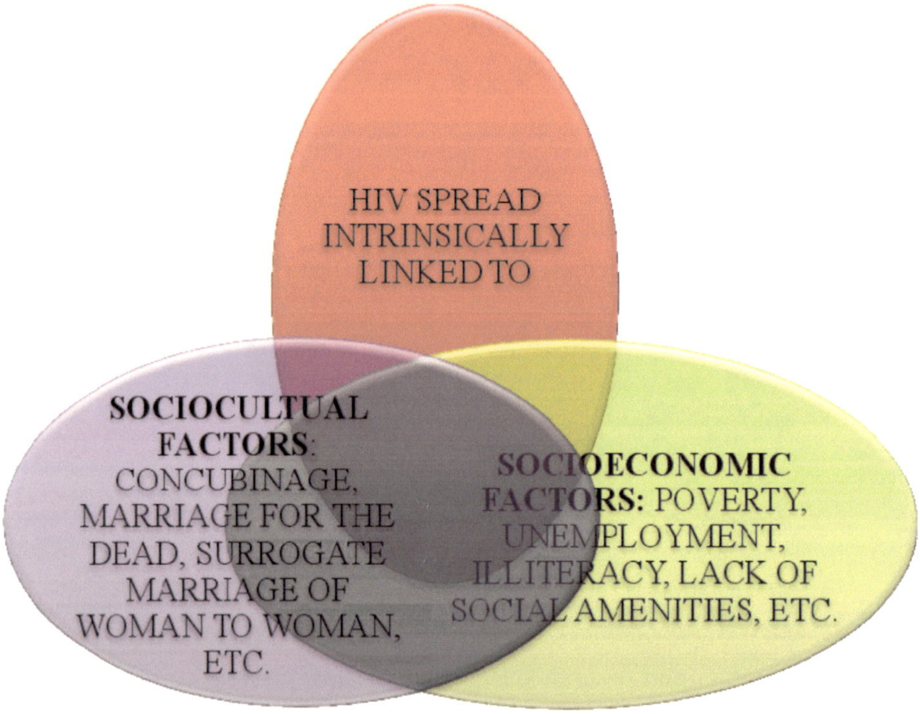

Fig. 7. Interlocking Paradigm Of HIV/AIDS Precipitating Factors

The concentration of the HIV epidemic in Nigeria is observed to be linked inextricably to socio-economic and political factors, which creates particular vulnerability to the agonizing consequences of the infection. Poverty, the incriminated factor, necessitates among others, population movement, thereby exacerbating the dissemination of the disease (Dibua, 2010); ignorance and low perception of risk/risk factors and risk groups in matters of sex and sexual contact among the men-folk, inability of women to negotiate for safe sex for fear of losing friends or finance, migrational activities due to economic repression, social/political conflicts which create avenue for stressful movements, and tend to separate spouses, thereby exposing the partners to sexual escapade, poverty, which makes people tend to be less anxious about risk-taking particularly for a long incubation period and gradual killer disease like AIDS. All these factors fuel the epidemic in significant but variable manner. Other incriminated factors include poor attitude/beliefs about AIDS and people living with HIV/AIDS. The absence of tolerance and involvement of these individuals in intervention programs creates some level of fear and shame/withdrawal that enhances re-infection. Similarly, the unwarranted social stigma and bitter cultural ostracization of the infected persons is on the increase. Furthermore, absence of safe and operational blood banking systems and good transfusion techniques especially in rural areas, where mostly untrained nurses, nursing aids and unqualified laboratory scientists/technicians are allowed to manage hospitals/clinics and medical laboratories are contributing factors in Nigeria.

3.2.1 HIV transmission modes

The risk of HIV infection depends on the amount of the virus in the transmitting fluid as well as the site of inoculation of that fluid. Retrospective studies have shown that there are some fluid-site combinations likely to result to HIV infection and those that are quite unlikely.

3.2.2 Blood transfusion

Blood given intravenously is observed to be the most likely combination with the highest probability of HIV infection (Busch et al, 1991). It is the mode with high risk of transmission of the HIV (CDC, 1982; Ammann et al, 1983). The association of transmissibility with inoculum of virus is most strikingly demonstrated in blood-borne infections. For small inocula, as with a needle prick infection, the risk is rather low, about 1/1000ml (CDC, 1987). On the other extreme, the recipient of a large volume, of instance, the 500ml in a unit of blood, is almost guaranteed to be infected (Busch et al, 1991). In some surgical operations such as heart transplant, HIV can be transmitted too when organs of an infected individual is transplanted into an uninfected person (CDC, 1993; Garner and Simmons 1983). Several cases of HIV transmission through blood transfusion has been reported in Nigeria and this calls for urgent action in personnel training and good blood screening protocols.

3.2.3 Parenteral transmission

In blood-borne transmission, the infectious inoculum transgresses the skin through needle prick, etc., while intact skin proves an effective barrier to HIV (Conley and Holmerg, 1992). Sharp objects such as needles, knives, razors, clippers, cosmetology tools, tattoo, piercing tools etc. can cut or wound the skin of individuals (Heald and Ransohoff, 1990). These objects used on infected individuals in whom cuts are made can, when used on wounded persons, transmit the virus from the objects containing blood particles (Henry and Campbell, 1995). Injection needles used on infected people can also transmit the virus when used on uninfected individuals if the needles are not discarded or sterilized before use (Gilmore, 1996).

Though individual cases of these transmission routes have not been well reported in Nigeria, they are nevertheless considered great possibilities in remote communities where tattooing and circumcision are done and several clinics and maternities are managed by unqualified and illiterate personnel

3.2.4 Perinatal or vertical transmission

Several cases have been reported on transmissions of the infection perenatally. This constitutes greater risk of mother to child (M-T-C) transmission of the virus.

a. Trans-placental infection

Perenatal transmission is common where the prevalence of infection among childbearing women is high (John and Kreiss,1996). Infection also occurs after child delivery through breast milk from HIV-infected mother, or at time of delivery through blood transfusion. The mechanism of placental HIV transfer is as follows: the foetus is developed from the amniotic fluid; the placenta on the other hand surrounds the amniotic fluid, which contains the foetus (Minkoff et al, 1990). The umbilical cord connects the foetus and placenta, which in turn has an attachment on the uterine wall. The placenta thus mediates between the foetus and the uterine wall. The foetus absorbs oxygen and other nutrients from the maternal placenta through diffusion. The umbilical cord, which is connected to the foetus, is also connected to the placenta, while blood vessels or capillaries transverse between the uterine wall and the umbilical cord. The capillaries are formed by the action of the progesterone during the implantation. The placenta receives the nutrients, oxygen etc., from the mothers' uterine wall and sends it to the foetus, then receives the liquid wastes products, carbon dioxide (CO2) from the foetus and transports through the umbilical cord into the system where it is now filtered and is excreted as waste through the urinary tract. HIV can then penetrate by diffusion; as the nutrients are being absorbed, the virus is also absorbed: from the infected mother to the foetus and hence the fetus becomes infected. Therefore, when the child is born it is already infected and so becomes an HIV-positive child (Minkoff et al, 1990).

b. Breastfeeding

The potential for transmission of HIV by breast-feeding is well established although the exact mechanism by which the transmission occurs has not been characterized. Below are two prospective mechanisms reported by researchers. Foremost, secretory Leukocyte protease inhibitor levels are high in both colostrums and breast milk as well as saliva of the new borne. Immediately at postpartum; only the breast milk shows dramatic decrease in the protease inhibitor level few weeks of postpartum (WHO, 1992; Peckman and Gibb, 1995). However if the mother of the child is HIV positive, the breast milk will show high levels of HIV as cell free virus as well as infections within the milk monocytes and macrophages. These high level of HIV present coupled with the relatively low levels of the protease inhibitor in breast milk may facilitate the viral entry in the tonsiliar and intestinal crypts of the new born and the child will be infected thereby leading to the transmission and establishment of the HIV infection (Peckman and Gibb, 1995). Therefore, it appears that the local inhibitory factors that are important in hindering the HIV oral mucosal transmission are not efficient in preventing infection of the new born through breastfeeding. Secondly, it was observed that after the birth of the child, at the early stage of breast-feeding, the milk contains some droplets of blood particles from the infected mother, which could also be infected with HIV (WHO, 1992). When the child consumes this milk, the virus is thus transmitted to the child Southern and Southern (1997).

It is important to understand that finding a small amount of HIV in a body fluid does not necessarily mean that HIV can be transmitted by that body fluid. HIV has not been recovered from the sweat of HIV-infected persons. Contact with saliva; tears, or sweat has never been shown to be a major mode of transmission of HIV in Nigeria. Nevertheless, more research is needed to further unravel the possibilities of HIV infection through these modes.

3.2.5 Sexual contacts

The highest risky means of transmission of the HIV is through sexual contact (Ogbuagu and Charles, 1993; Dibua, 2010). Contaminated vaginal or seminal fluids are very sure sources of HIV transmission through sex by homosexuals, lesbians, bisexual and the heterosexuals (Liuzzi *et al,* 1996). The mechanism is as follow: the walls of the vagina of the female or the anus of the male (lesbians, homosexuals) have mucus membrane which contain the CD4+

cells such as macrophages, dendrites etc (Schwarz *et al* 1995). In the course of the sexual act, there are vaginal and penal secretions; if either the male or female is HIV positive, the secreted fluid, containing the virus now binds to the mucus membrane of the vagina or the opposite sex. In some cases (for those that use stimulants/drugs such as homosexuals, to enhance the pace of the sexual act), this up-thrust and forceful thrust of penis results in the wounding of the anal membrane of the counterpart or the vaginal walls and secretion of fluids from any party of the two individuals enhances the possibility of the virus to easily attach to the blood or the wounded membrane which has the CD4+ cells (Liuzzi *et al,* 1996). Moreover, in some sexual acts, leaking/sucking of the cunnus of the ladies results in sucking of the HIV from the cunnus of the vagina of the infected individual into the saliva, then to the mucus membrane and possibly to the blood stream. Even in the protected sex, there are reported cases of condoms being fake and breaking or slippage in the course of sex, instances which enhance viral entry and replication. Another mechanism is through penal secretions from the HIV positive man during sexual arousal, when he releases the sperm bearing the virus into the female. If fertilization occurs in the female, both the mother and the fetus are infected with the virus.

3.2.6 Saliva

Although transmission of HIV through sexual contact with saliva (oral sex) has not been widely shown (Fox, 1988), oral exposures to HIV infected semen, blood and breast milk can lead to infection in subtle ways. Unprotected orogenital contact, especially receptive oral intercourse are associated with greater risk of HIV transmission than previously thought (Southern and Southern 1997; Fleming and Wasserheit, 1999). The salivary anti- HIV properties, the local and mucosal integrity, and the level of infectious HIV present at the oral mucus site all influence the potential for HIV infection through the oral mucus membrane. WHO statistics has it that oral transmission of HIV does not constitute a great risk but makes 15% of the means of transmission of HIV (WHO, 1986; Fultz 1986).

Casual contact through "closed-mouth" or "Social kissing" has not been well shown to be a risk for transmission of HIV and no case of this has been reported in Nigeria. However, since the month of individuals has mucous membrane, which contains CD4+ receptors, when the virus gets to the mouth, it binds to the CD4 receptors at the oral mucosa and then replicates and spread to the other parts of the body (Ho *and* Byington, 1985; Barr *et al,* 1989). Nevertheless, the risk of acquiring HIV through saliva is said to be very low because the saliva is said to contain less quantity of HIV, which can cause infection (CDC, 1997). Because of the potential contact with blood during "French" or "Open-Mouth Kissing" CDC (National Centre for HIV/STD Control and Prevention) recommends against engaging in this activity with a person known to be infected (CDC, 1997; Berry and Shea, (1997). However, CDC has investigated only one case of HIV infection that may be an attitude to contact with blood during open mouth kissing (Crombie *et al,* 1998).

4.1 Role of opportunistic infections in development of aids

Opportunistic infections are typically observed only in individuals with a dysfunctional immune system (Madigan *et al.* 2009**).** The immune system can be weakened or compromised by malnutrition, alcoholism, cancer, diabetes, leukaemia, HIV/AIDS, trauma from surgery or injury, an altered microbiota from prolonged use of antibiotics (e.g. virginal candidiasis), and immune suppression led by drugs, hormones, genetic deficiencies, cancer therapy and old age (Joanne, 2008). Infection with HIV progressively reduces the effectiveness of the immune system by infecting primarily vital cells in the human immune system such as helper-T cells (to be specific, $CD4^+$ T cells), macrophages, and dendritic cells, leading to low levels of $CD4^+$ T cells. When $CD4^+$ T cell numbers decline below a critical level, cell-mediated immunity is lost, and the body becomes progressively more susceptible to malignancies and a mirage of infections, the opportunistic infections.

The geometric increase in the prevalence rates of the dual infections, tuberculosis and sexually transmitted diseases (STIs) have been identified as major factors driving the HIV epidemic in Nigeria. Untreated/poorly managed STIs create opportunity for viral entry. Similarly, the presence HIV activates latent TB and vice versa, which rather complicates HIV spread. Other driving factors worth enumerating include absence of quality medi-care, and health education programs particularly at the local levels.

4.2 Sexually transmitted infections

Sexually transmitted infections are a major global cause of acute illness, infertility, long term disability and death, with severe medical and psychological consequences for millions of men, women and children. The World Health Organization states that: "in developing countries, STIs and their complications are amongst the top five disease categories for which adults seek health care. In women of childbearing age, STIs (excluding HIV) are second only to maternal factors as causes of disease, death and healthy life lost". The presence of an untreated STI can also "increase the risk of both acquisition and transmission of HIV by a factor of up to 10". Unlike HIV, many STIs can be treated and cured relatively easily and cheaply if diagnosed early enough. However, diagnosis of STIs particularly among the local populace has become a herculean task as a result of indiscriminate use of antibiotics and/or drug abuse, which has increased the incidence in drug resistant strains. To fight these epidemics, Nigerian health authorities must act to expand access to testing and treatment facilities; to educate people about safer sex and risk reduction; and to counter the prejudice surrounding STIs.

The WHO estimates that 340 million new cases of syphilis, gonorrhea, chlamydia and trichomoniasis occurred throughout the world in 1999 in men and women aged 15-49 years. The largest number of new infections occurred in the region of South and Southeast Asia, followed by sub-Saharan Africa and Latin America and the Caribbean. The highest rate of new cases per 1,000 population occurred in sub-Saharan Africa (UNAIDS/WHO, 2004).

Prevalence rates of syphilis among women in the developing countries, is estimated at 100 times higher than in developed, industrialized world. The dissimilitude is due to socioeconomic factors, primarily poverty and its twin evil, lack of employment opportunity for the productive age group. These necessitate the influx of young men into urban, and quickly lead to increased demand for sexual services, provided very often by commercial sex workers as documented by Dibua (2009). The women at home in turn, resort to similar occupation to subsidize their income, with the resultant spread of several diseases including STIs. Other prevailing and devastating factors in Nigeria include lack of infrastructure and adequate information about STIs, illiteracy, and limited access to medi-care. Many women have symptomless STIs, hence do not recognize symptoms or are too embarrassed, shy or afraid to seek adequate medical attention. Several others rely on native doctors and traditional healing methods and end up compounding the infection, ending up in multi resistant pathogens. Similarly, the social stigma associated with STIs, as well as the absence of cost effective treatment in government hospital/clinics necessitates the turmoil that encourages the patronage of native doctors and quacks. As a result of unrecognized and untreated STIs, women suffer severe complications such as pelvic inflammatory diseases (PID), ectopic pregnancy and infertility; men become sterile; new-born are left blind.

4.3 Dangers of the STIs/HIV interaction

Several control strategies have been mounted by both national and international health oriented organizations against sexually transmitted diseases during the past decade due primarily to the fact that infection with several STIs is strongly believed to predispose or enhance HIV infection. It is now a general opinion that the presence of an STI can lead to tenfold increase of the risk of HIV infection.

An STI may increase susceptibility to HIV infection by causing genital lesions that facilitate viral entry, or by increasing the number of target cells (viral load) for HIV (activated lymphocytes or monocytes), causing infected individuals to reach peak infectivity at an earlier time. Genital ulcer disease cause enhanced HIV-1 transmission by amplifying viral replication (shedding) or independently increasing immunosuppression, giving rise to bursts of viremia, and subsequently, development of more rapid immunodeficiency. Sero-prevalence studies conducted in some African STI clinics indicate that these ulcers are more frequently cause by *Haemophilus ducreyi* infection, which is of less occurrence in the Western world. It was also shown that in Africa, the risk of HIV infection is higher with genital ulcers caused by Syphilis, Herpes Simplex, and *Chlamydia trachomatis* infections. Epstein Barr virus (EBV) and Cytomegalovirus (CMV), though not directly associated with genital lesions, result in activation of target cells, hence are co-factors though their single and pair-wise effect has not been documented in Nigeria.

The shedding of HIV in genital fluids is increased by discharge from, and the inflammatory to sexually acquired infections, rendering the HIV sero-positive individuals more infective at the moment of the infection with STIs. The CD4 lymphocytes (the white blood cells targeted by HIV) in the mucus membrane lining the womb (endocervic) where the infection often occurs in women, is observed to increased incommensurably during a gonoccocal or chlamydial infection. Research has shown that treating an STI can reduce the secretion of HIV. In one study, HIV virus was isolated in only half as many HIV-positive men after treating them for gonorrhea. In another, there was a 100-fold decrease in the amount of virus detected in the ejaculate of a man after treatment for chlamydial urethritis (Dallabetta, 1999). Other epidemiological studies indicated that the risk of HIV infection was higher with genital ulcers (caused by syphilis, chancroid or herpes). The clearest evidence STIs have significant impact on HIV transmission is the result of a community-based randomized clinical trial from the London School of Hygiene and Tropical Medicine, the Tanzania National Institute of Medical Research and the African Medical and Research Foundation (AMREF). The investigation showed a 42 percent reduction in new HIV infections in communities where improved STD treatment was effected

The foregoing outline the synergy between HIV and STIs. While HIV enhances the span of several STIs, Some STIs in turn intensifies the infective rate of HIV. It therefore becomes evident that effective and worthwhile intervention strategies aimed at preventing HIV infection in Nigeria particularly among the high risk groups are rooted in the prevention and control of sexually transmitted infections - STIs.

4.4 HIV and TB, the dual epidemic

HIV epidemic has breathed new life into an old enemy - Tuberculosis even in Nigeria. HIV spurs the spread of TB and increases the tuberculosis risk for the whole population. One-third of the world's population, or two billion people, carry the TB bacteria, more than 9 million of whom become sick each year with "active" TB which can be spread to others. "Latent TB" disease cannot be spread (WHO, 2010). TB has highest prevalence in conditions of poverty and overcrowding. In such communities as in most African countries, people typically become infected in childhood, but a healthy immune system wards off the infection. Hence, people can remain infected for life with dormant, un-infectious TB, and are called TB carriers. The carriers remain healthy, but transmit the germs to the close contacts.

With the emergence of HIV, the depleted immune system due to the virus is predisposed to TB infection. Hence, the risk of developing active TB is 30-50 folds higher for people infected with TB alone. TB disproportionately affects people in resource-poor settings, particularly those in Asia and Africa (WHO, 2009). Clearly TB is the single most important opportunistic disease related to HIV infection in the developing world, and in Africa. Twenty-two countries are considered "high-burden countries (HBCs)," accounting for approximately 80% of new TB cases each year; most HBCs are in Africa and Asia. India, China, South Africa, Nigeria, and Indonesia have the highest number of new TB cases in the world. In 2008, the global TB incidence rate was 139 per 100,000 population, down from a peak of 143 per 100,000 in 2004 (U.S. Global Health Policy, 2010). About 78% of co-infections were in Africa, the region hardest hit by HIV. South Africa alone accounted for 32% of the total number of HIV positive TB cases in the Africa region.3. Of the 1.8 million people who died from TB in 2008, an estimated 500,000 were HIV-positive. Overall, one-third of the world's population is currently infected with the TB bacillus. 5-10% of people who are infected with TB bacilli (but who are not infected with HIV) become sick or infectious at some time during their life. People with HIV and TB infection are much more likely to develop TB (WHO, 2010).

TB and HIV are frequently referred to as co- or dual-epidemics due to their high rate of co-infection (UNAIDS 2006). TB is the dominant infection in one third or more of AID patients (De Cock *et al,* 1992). The proposal that all HIV - positive patients in the US with CD4 cell counts less than 200 (0.20 x 109/L - 200 ml) be considered cases of AIDS (CDC, 1992) irrespective of disease presentation, would resolve the discussion about when TB becomes an AIDS-defining illness but would be impossible to apply in the developing world.

4.5 HIV and TB - a deadly synergy

HIV and TB form a lethal combination, each speeding the other's progress. HIV weakens the immune system. Someone who is HIV-positive and infected with TB bacilli is many times more likely to become sick with TB than someone infected with TB bacilli that is HIV-negative. TB is a leading cause of death among people who are HIV-positive. In Africa, HIV is the single most important factor contributing to the increase in the incidence of TB since 1990 (WHO, 2010).

Interest in the study of the dual epidemic has emerged as a result of the following:

- One-third of the world population is living with HIV. 80% of the adult population in the developing and under-developed countries, especially in conditions of poverty and overcrowding carry the tubercle bacilli.
- TB adds to HIV burden by shortening life expectancy, while HIV spurs the spread of TB.
- Range of infectivity of TB (spread via aerosol) is wider than HIV. TB can infect 10-15 people if untreated within 1 year. TB carriers who are also infected with HIV are 30-15 times more likely to develop active TB than those without HIV since HIV weakens their immune system.
- Spread of HIV in a community where TB carriers live implies parallel epidemics of AIDS and TB faced by the population.
- TB cases have doubled or even tripled in some countries of Africa. These caseloads are great health hazards stretching the health care system to breaking point.
- TB is the leading killer of HIV- positive Africans. More than 5 million of the 13 million Africans now alive with HIV are expected to develop TB, and over 4 million will die untidy deaths.
- HIV infected people who also have the tubercle bacilli are unusually prone to developing active tuberculosis.

4.5.1 In HIV infected people

- TB is harder to diagnose than in HIV-negative people, only 35-50% of HIV positive people have pulmonary TB, detectable from first a sputum simple others have "extra-pulmonary disseminated TB" which can be diagnosed only with special laboratory facilities.
- TB progresses faster (than AIDS) in HIV-infected people and is more fatal.
- TB occurs earlier in the course of HIV infections than other opportunistic infections, at a CD4 cell count of 350.
- The epidemiology of TB has been profoundly influenced by the epidemic of HIV infection in most developing countries.
- TB is an earlier opportunistic disease in the course of HIV infection. Wherever the infection with *M. tuberculosis* is common, predominantly in the developing world, TB rapidly becomes the major implication of HIV infection where HIV begins to spread.
- The highest rates of TB incidence and HIV specific mortality occurs in Sub Saharan African (Murray *et al*, 1990).

4.5.2 Burden of HIV/TB

- Infection with HIV will increase the number of TB cases directly promoting reactivation of TB.
- It will increase the caseload to man uncertain degree by increasing secondary transmission from the increased number of active cases.
- Untreated, a sputum-smear positive patient infects 10-15 other people in a year (Murray *et al*, 1990)

- Primary TB infections in HIV- positive persons will run a more aggressive course and cause disease more frequently.
- About 10% HIV seroprevalence will result in a three-fold increase in adult TB cases.
- Published data of TB in HIV-positive persons range from 3.1 to 7.9 per 100 person-year. If applied to Africa, between 95,000 and 359,000 cases of TB occur annually in HIV-positive persons.

5. Conclusion

HIV epidemic has become a reality in Nigeria. Understanding the dynamics and variability of HIV infection in a community is a major step in tracking down HIV transmission in the area. This study elucidates target issues in HIV epidemic such as global and national prevalence, associated sociocultural and socioeconomic predisposing factors, transmission modes, risk groups, and AIDS-related opportunistic infections including other sexually transmitted infections and tuberculosis with the aim to encourage further research on the dynamics and mechanisms of HIV transmission which will foster HIV Prevention and Control strategies. Primary prevention of HIV/AIDS pandemic can best be achieved through education changes in sexual behaviour (abstinence or reduction of sexual partners). Treatment of other sexually transmitted diseases was shown to reduce HIV infection in a large controlled trial form Tanzania. Among persons already infected with HIV early detection of the infection provides the greatest opportunity for Counselling, partner referral, prevention, and other services. Increased rate of HIV infection has been inextricably linked to socioeconomic factors (poverty) that place women at disadvantaged position (Ainsworth *et al,* 1994). Alleviation of poverty and women emancipation programs may contribute towards effective HIV control and/or prevention. Similarly, wider prevention of perinatal transmission, screening of blood and heat treatment of blood products to destroy the virus should be fostered particularly in resource poor villages and peri-urban centres (Ullrich, 2003). HIV infected mothers should avoid breast-feeding to reduce transmission of the virus to their children using alternative feeding options available (WHO, 1992). All women who have been potentially exposed should seek HIV antibody testing before becoming pregnant and, if the test is positive, should consider avoiding pregnancy. Further action needed include: education of intravenous drug users concerning the need to avoid sharing the needles and syringes, abstinence from casual sex and strict monogamous relationship, education on protected sexual behavior and practices. Effectiveness of Condom remains issue of debate. The Food and Drug Administration (FDA) of America indicated that proper and consistent use of latex or polyurethane (a type of plastic) condoms when engaging in sexual intercourse--vaginal, anal, or oral, greatly reduce a person's risk of acquiring or transmitting sexually transmitted diseases, including HIV. Nevertheless, fidelity and abstinence remain significant preventive measures.

6. References

Ainsworth, M. & Over, M.A (1994). The economic impact of AIDS in Africa. *AIDS in Africa,* pp. 559-585.

Akinsete, I., Nasidi, A. S., Egbewunmi, A. et al. (1989). Seroprevalence of HIV- Infection in Various Groups Tested at the Lagos University Teaching Hospital, Lagos, Nigeria, between. *IV Internet Conf.: AIDS and Assoc. Cancers in Africa,* Marseille, Oct. 18-20, Poster 400

Ammann, A.J., Wara, D.W. & Dritz, S. (1983). Acquired immunodeficiency in an infant: possible transmission by means of blood products. *Lancet,* 1: 965-958.

AVERT HIV/AIDS Nigeria. (2010). http://www.avert.org/aids-nigeria.htm

Berry, M.M., & Shea, T. (1997). Oral sex and HIV transmission. *Journal of Acquired Immune Deficiency Syndrome,* 14: 475-7.

Busch, M.P., Young, M.J. & Samson, S.M. (1991). Risk of human immunodeficiency virus (HIV) transmission by blood transfusions before the implementation of HIV-1 antibody screening. *Transfusion,* 31: 4 -11.

Center for Disease Control and Prevention (CDC) (1982). Possible transfusion-associated acquired immune deficiency syndrome (AIDS) - California. *Mortality and Morbidity Weekly Report,* 1: 652-65.

Center for Disease Control and Prevention (CDC) (1987). Revision of the CDC Surveillance Case Definition for Acquired Immunodeficiency Syndrome. *Journal of American Medical Association,* 258: 1143-1145.

Center for Disease Control and Prevention (CDC) (1992). Revised classification system for HIV infection and expanded surveillance case definition for AIDS among adolescents and adults. MMWR. 41 (no.17:961-2.

Center for Disease Control and Prevention (CDC) (1993). Recommendations on prophylaxis and therapy for disseminated *Mycobacterium avium* complex for adults and adolescents infected with human immunodeficiency virus. *Mortality and Morbidity Weekly Report,* 42: 3-20.

Center for Disease Control and Prevention (CDC) (1997). Evaluation of safety devices for preventing percutaneous injuries among health-care workers during phlebotomy procedures - Minneapolis St. Paul, New York City, and San Francisco. *Mortality and Morbidity Weekly Report,* 46: 21-25.

CIA World Fact-book, (2010). https://www.cia.gov//Library/publications/the-world-fact-book/fields/2155/html

Conley, L. J. & Holmerg, S.D. (1992). Transmission of AIDS from blood screened negative for antibody to the human immunodeficiency virus. *New England Journal of Medicine,* 326: 1499-1502

Crombie, R. & Silverstein, R. L. (1998). Identification of a CD36-related thrombosporidin 1-binding domain in HIV-1 envelope glycoprotein gp120: relationship to HIV-1 specific inhibitory factors in human saliva. *Journal of Experimental Medicine,* 198: 25-35.

Dallabetta, G. (1999). Treating sexually transmitted diseases to control HIV transmission. Current Option in Infectious Diseases, 10: 22-25.

De Cock, K.M., Soro, B. Coulibaly, I.M. & Lucas, S.B. (1992). Tuberculosis and HIV infection in sub-Saharan Africa. *Journal of American Medical Association,* 268: 1581-1587

Dibua U. (2010). Socio-Economic And Socio-Cultural Predisposing Risk Factors To HIV/AIDS: Case Study of Some Locations In Eastern Nigeria. *The Internet Journal of Tropical Medicine; Volume* 6 Number 2.

Ezumah, N.E. (2003). Gender Issues in the Prevention and Control of STIs and HIV/AIDS; Lessons from Awka and Agulu, Anambra State, Nigeria. *African Journal of Reproductive Health*, 7:89: 99

Federal Ministry of Health (FMOH), 1999) HIV/Syphilis Sentinel Sero-prevalence Survey in Nigeria. Technical Report. National AIDS/STD Control Programme, Nov. Pp. 1-53

Federal Ministry of Health (FMOH). (2001). A Technical Report on 2001 National HIV/Syphilis Sero-Prevalence Sentinel Survey among Pregnant Women Attending Antenatal Clinics in Nigeria. Abuja: NASCP, Nigeria

Federal Ministry of Health (FMOH). (2007). Integrated Bio-Behavioural Surveillance Survey Among Most at Risk Populations in Nigeria. Abuja: National AIDS/STIs Control Programme (NASCP), Nigeria (IBBSS 2007)

Federal Ministry of Health. (2009). National HIV/AIDS and Reproductive Health Survey. Abuja (NARHS 2007), Nigeria

Fleming, D.T. & Wasserheit, J.N. (1999). From epidemiological synergy to public health policy and practice: the contribution of other sexually transmitted diseases to sexual transmission of HIV infection. *Sexually Transmitted Infections*,75: 3–17.

Fox, P.C. & Wolff, A. (1988). Salivary inhibition of HIV-1 infectivity: functional properties and distribution in men, women, and children. *Journal of American Dental Asso*ciation 118: 709-11.

Fultz, P.N. (1986). Components of saliva inactivate human immunodeficiency virus [letter]. *Lancet*, 2: 215.

Garner, J.S. and Simmons, B. P. (1983). Guidelines for isolation precautions in hospitals. *Infectious Control*, 4: 245-253.

Gilmore, N. (1996). Blood and blood product safety. In: Mann J, Tarantola D, eds. *AIDS in the World*. II. Oxford: Oxford University Press, 287-301.

Heald, A.E., & Ransohoff, D.F. (1990). Phlebotomy practices/needles stick injuries/Hepatitis B status/among interns in a Dublin Hospital *Irish Medical Journal*, 85: 102-104.

Henry, K. & Campbell, S. (1995). Needle stick/sharps injuries and HIV exposure among health care workers. National estimates based on a survey of U.S. Hospitals. *Minn. Med* . 78: 41-44.

Ho, D.D. & Byington, R. E.. (1985). Infrequency of isolation of HIV-III virus from saliva in AIDS [Letter]. *New England Journal of Medicine*, 313: 1606-1672.

Joanne W.M., Linda M.S., Christopher J.W. (2008). Prescott, Harley, Klen's Microbiology. Seventh Edition. McGrow Hill. Boston. Pg 1016.

John, G.C. & Kreiss, J. (1996). Mother to child transmission of human immunodeficiency virus type 1. *Epidemiological Review*, 8: 149-157.

Madigan M.T., Martinko J.M., Dunlap P.V., Clark D.P. (2009). Brock's Biology of Microorganisms 12th Edition. Pearson Benjamin Cummings. San Francisco. Pg 993.

Minkoff, H., Nanda., D., Merez, R. & Fikrig, S. (1990). Pregnancies resulting in infants with acquired immunodeficiency syndrome or AIDS related complex *Obstetric gynecology*, 69: 285.

Murray, C.J.L., Stylblo, K. & Rouillon, A. (1990). Tuberculosis in developing countries: burden, intervention and cost. *Bulletin of the International Union Against Tuberculosis and Lung Disease*, 65: 6-24.

NASCP Abuja. (2008). Federal Ministry of Health Report on the 2008 National HIV/Syphilis Seroprevalence Sentinel Survey among Pregnant Women Attending Antenatal Clinics in Nigeria. Abuja: Nigeria.

Ogbuagu, S.U. & Charles, J.O. (1993). Survey of sexual networking in Calabar. *Health Transition Review*. 3 (Suppl): 105-19.

Peckham, C. & Gibb, D. (1995). Mother to child transmission of the human Immunodeficiency virus. *New England Journal of Medicine*, 1: 133:298-302

Population Reference Bureau. (2009). HIV Data Fact Sheet Reference Bureau

Quinn, T.C., Overbaugh, J. (2005). HIV/AIDS in women: an expanding epidemic. *Science*, 308: 1582–83

Schwartz, S.K. & Kellogg, T.A. (1995). Temporal trends in human immunodeficiency virus seroprevalence and sexual behavior at San Francisco Municipal Sexually Transmitted Disease Clinic, 1989-1992. *American Journal of Epidemiology*, 142: 314-22.

Southern, S. & P.J. Southern. (1997). Oral Transmission of HIV during long-term breastfeeding. HIV-1 Infection, Mucosal Immunity and Pathogenesis. *Natcher Conference Center NIH*, October [abstract p.51]

Ullrich, D. (2003). HIV/AIDS and Urban Poverty in South Africa, An *Update* pp. 11-19.

UNAIDS, 2006. *Report on the global AIDS epidemic*. Geneva, http://www.unaids.org:80/en/KnowledgeCentre/HIVData/GlobalReport/Default.asp, accessed 5 May 2008).

UNAIDS. (2009). Report: Modes of HIV Transmission in Nigeria: Analysis of the Distribution of New HIV Infections in Nigeria and recommendations for Prevention

UNAIDS/WHO. (2004). Epidemiological Fact-Sheets on HIV/AIDS and Sexually Transmitted Infections, Update

UNAIDS/WHO. (2007). *AIDS epidemic update*. Geneva http://www.unaids.org/en/KnowledgeCentre/HIVData/EpiUpdate/EpiU pd Archive/2007, accessed 5 May)

UNAIDS/WHO (2008). UNAIDS/ Reference Group on HIV/AIDS Estimates, Modelling and Projections. Estimated number of adults and children living with HIV

World Health Organization (WHO). (1986). Acquired immunodeficiency syndrome (AIDS). *Weekly Epidemiological Records*, 61: 69-73.

World Health Organization (WHO) (1992). Global AIDS Case Surveillance. World Health Statistics, *Annual Review*, 30-2

World Health Organization WHO. (2009). Rapid advice: Antiretroviral Therapy for HIV infection in adults and adolescents

World Health Organisation (WHO). (2010). Gender inequalities in HIV. August
http://www.who.int/en/

4

Pearls and Pitfalls of HIV-1 Serologic Laboratory Testing

Jiasheng Shao[1], Yunzhi Zhang[1], Yi-Wei Tang[2] and Hongzhou Lu[1]
[1]*Department of Infectious Diseases, Shanghai Public Health Clinical Center, Fudan University, Shanghai,*
[2]*Departments of Pathology and Medicine, Vanderbilt University Medical Center, Nashville, TN,*
[1]*People's Republic of China*
[2]*USA*

1. Introduction

Detection of HIV-specific antibodies forms the corner stone for laboratory diagnosis of HIV infections. Serologic methods are routinely used to determine whether a host is infected with HIV, to evaluate the status of infections, and to assist monitoring antiretroviral therapy. Primary diagnosis of HIV infection is commonly accomplished by serology via detection of HIV antibody using a screening enzyme immunoassay (EIA) or a rapid assay, followed by a subsequent confirmatory Western blot (WB) test. Used in a point of care testing (POCT) format, rapid HIV antibody tests have filled an essential need in HIV testing especially in resource-limited settings. Detuned antibody assays allow for the distinction between recent and distant HIV-1 infections, which have been used mainly for epidemiology surveillance and investigations. In addition to clinical diagnosis of HIV infection, serology remains the mainstay for screening donated blood and blood products prior to transfusion to ensure that recipients receive the safest possible blood products. In this chapter, we will review pearls and pitfalls of serologic methods currently being used in routine HIV diagnosis and screening. Rational use of HIV serologic testing will be illustrated by clinical case presentations.

2. Cases from clinical settings

2.1 Case 1

A 45-year-old single man presents to a primary care unit with complaints of 'having a prostate problem". He wants to find out whether he has the same condition because his father and elder brother have the same problem. He tells doctors that he has always been in good health except for urinary symptoms. Approximately 1 year ago, he paid a medical visit due to a sore throat. When the patient is asked more closely about other symptoms besides the sore throat, he said that skin rash, coughs, malaise are included. He was prescribed a course of antibiotics and spent a week at home before returned to work. However, it took almost 2 weeks to recover fully. The patient accepts routine HIV testing and other tests specific for STIs are also obtained on the basis of his history. The patient is tested with the standard blood test. He is told that the HIV test results are negative when he returns for follow-up 2 weeks later. He comments that after being made aware of his personal risks, he convinced his wife to be tested (who is negative); because they both had other sex partners with an unknown sex and drug use history during their separation. Although family members and alleged partners, including spouses, should not be notified of a specific person's tests result, the CDC recommends as part of partner services that they should be independently encouraged to have HIV testing as part of routine care (CDC, 2008).

2.2 Case 2

A 21-year-old man comes to the outpatient clinic with complaints of 'burning while urinating' for the past 3 days. Symptoms such as fevers, flank pain, or penile discharge have been denied. He had several sexual partners over the past 6 months. He uses condoms with his casual partners but prefers not to do so with his primary partner. He attributes his present symptoms to condom breakage during sexual intercourse with a casual partner. He tells that he has sex only with men, but denies use of injection drugs. He has never been tested for HIV. Reasons for previously declining are that he 'is usually careful' and, besides, 'Magic Johnson has it and he looks good.' After some discussion, the patient states that he has had blood drawn at emergency department visits at other hospitals in the past several years. However, he did not return for the test results and assumed that because he was not contacted about the results, all tests, including any for HIV, must be negative. However, he states that he is unemployed and frequently stays with friends at different locations. The patient initially declines HIV screening. He has a family member who works at the local health department and is very concerned that this person would have access to his results if he tested positive. State laws require that positive confirmatory HIV test results be reported to the surveillance division of the respective health department. However, access to test results is restricted to a very few individuals who have signed confidentiality agreements. Additionally, as noted after being reassured about test confidentiality, the patient agrees to screening. His rapid HIV test is reactive. This result was confirmed by follow-up testing. Linkage of patients newly diagnosed HIV positive to further care is very important and relatively brief interventions can be effective (Craw, JA., et al., 2008).

On the basis of other laboratory indices, such as CD4 count and viral load, it appears that the patient has been infected for many years.

2.3 Case 3

A 16-month-old boy presented with prolonged fever and oral candidiasis for the past 6 month. He was a term infant delivered by cesarean section without complications. He was breast-fed for the first 6 days of life and then switched to bottle-feeding. At one month of age, he developed oral candidiasis and was treated with mycostatin, but no effect was observed. Subsequently, he was hospitalized due to prolonged fever and cough and diagnosed with Pseudomonas aeruginosa infection by sputum culture. His cytomegalovirus and adenovirus IgM antibody tests were positive. Ultrasound examination of the abdomen revealed hepatosplenomegaly. His mother was HIV antibody positive one week before delivery, which was subsequently confirmed by a Genetic System HIV-1 Western-blot. Her

CD4+ cell count was 212/mm^3 and viral load was 1.6×10^6 copies/ml. The boy had a rapid HIV-1/2 antibody test performed twice in serum at age 5- and 7-month, which were negative. The Abbott rapid test was repeated at age 7- and 8-month during his hospitalization and the results remained negative; however, HIV-1/2 antibody was detected in his serum by an enzyme-linked immunosorbent assay (TNA-Abb, Dainabot Co., Tokyo, Japan) at the time of readmission when he was 7-mo old. HIV-1 Western-blot was performed in plasma at the Shanghai Centers for Disease Control and prevention, which revealed the presence of a single HIV gp120 band. His HIV viral loads ranged from 1.5 to 2.2×105 copies/ml in plasma during his hospitalization (Zhang, YZ., et al., 2008).

2.4 Case 4

A 26-year-old woman presents to a community-based facility because she suspects that she is pregnant. She has not had a menstrual period for 2 months. She has been married for 5 years, but has no child. The pregnant test is positive. The patient has a family history of sickle cell disease, and she asks about the diseases that she and her unborn child will be screened for as part of the initial prenatal evaluation. The patient was informed of the various screening tests routinely included in the initial prenatal evaluation. Although an HIV test is included in the general consent for obstetric care, she declines. She remarks that she has been monogamous for 5 years and had a negative test 'back then.' She reports having had some marital difficulties 'like all couples,' but she is not concerned about contracting HIV because she 'has never used drugs and is not gay.' Besides, her husband 'would kill me if I ever gave him something'. After the patient spent time discussing her reasons for declining testing and these concerns were addressed by the provider, she realized that she was not being singled out for an HIV test and agreed to screening. The result of the rapid HIV test was negative. She breathes a sigh of relief and discloses that some of her marital problems were due to her husband's infidelity.

3. Discussion and comments

It is estimated currently that 21% of HIV cases in the United States are undiagnosed (Campsmith, ML., et al., 2010). Recent studies showed that missed opportunity visits, i.e., when HIV screening is not included as a routine part of the appraisal or is not offered when it should have been, are very common
(Althoff, KN., et al., 2010; Duffus, WA., et al., 2009). In addition, there will always be a new generation of individuals at risk for HIV acquisition. Screening should be offered regardless of perceived behavioral risk, and the opportunity should not be lost to educate those who test negative. To redirect local health jurisdictions in taking a broader approach to HIV testing in their communities, the CDC published revised recommendations for routine HIV testing in healthcare settings in 2006 (Branson, BM., et al., 2006). These recommendations include routine screening of 13- to 64-year-old patients. However, it may be prudent to screen beyond the recommended older age limit if history suggests continued sexual activity. All patients being screened should be asked about specific behaviors associated with increased risk such as sexual practices, including multiple partners, condom use, and use of performance-enhancing medications and about injection drug use (Adimora, AA., et al., 2003). The CDC further recommends that routine screening take place in all healthcare

facilities and institutions, unless prevalence of undiagnosed HIV infection in the patient population has been documented to be <0.1%. If such data are unavailable, routine screening should occur until it has been prospectively established that diagnostic yield is <1 per 1000 patients screened. When a yield of < 1 per 1000 is present, routine screening is no longer warranted and targeted testing should be used. Other recommendations for routine screening include any patient initiating treatment for tuberculosis (Taylor, Z., et al. 2005), because of the increased incidence of coinfection and the requisite modification to HIV therapy in case of coinfection in developing countries (Jiang, XY., et al., 2008). Any patient seeking treatment for an STD should be screened at each visit for a new complaint. Testing should be performed whether the patient is known or suspected to have specific behavioral risks for HIV infection. Repeat screening of persons not likely to be at high risk for HIV should be based on clinical judgment. Individuals at high risk for HIV should be screened at least annually. Indications of high risk include (1) injection drug users and their sex partners, (2) persons who exchange sex for drugs or money, (3) sex partners of HIV-infected individuals, (4) men who have sex with men (MSM), (5) heterosexuals who themselves or whose sex partners have had more than 1 sex partner since their most recent HIV test. Any identified risk exposure within the past 3-6 months should prompt rescreening within the next 3-6 months. If risk behavior continues, periodic testing in 3-6 months is recommended.

A meta-analysis of 11 independent findings (6 comparing HIV-aware persons with independent groups of unaware individuals; 5 comparing seroconverters before and after learning status) demonstrated that HIV-infected individuals were likely to reduce unprotected anal or vaginal intercourse after learning their positive serostatus. After adjusting data to focus on partners not already infected, the analysis showed a 68% reduction in reports of unprotected anal or vaginal intercourse (Marks, G., et al. 2005). This is important because greater than 80% of HIV cases diagnosed in the United States are among individuals who report sexual exposure (CDC, 2010).

The cost-effectiveness of routine HIV screening has also been demonstrated. Recently, published papers concerning the cost-effectiveness of HIV screening concluded that even when the prevalence of HIV infection in specific populations is substantially lower than 1%, screening for HIV is cost-effective relative to other established screening programs (Farnham, PG., et al., 2008). Sanders indicated that screening was also cost-effective in comparison with other commonly accepted screening programs, even when the known population prevalence of HIV was substantially lower than 1% (Sanders, GD., et al., 2005).

Immediately after infection occurs, there is a rapid rise in plasma viremia with the virus being disseminated widely in the body. During the period from initial infection to complete seroconversion (referred to as primary HIV infection), routine tests for HIV antibody are unable to detect the new infection (Fiebig, EW., et al., 2003). This high concentration of the virus has important public health implications because the HIV diagnosis could be missed, and it is a period of extreme infectiousness (Wawer, MJ., et al. 2005).

It has been shown that the majority of seropositive patients do not present with symptoms suggestive of HIV infection. Because of their nonspecific nature, it requires a high index of suspicion to associate the symptoms of acute retroviral syndrome (ARS) with primary HIV infection. The signs and symptoms of ARS can develop within days or occur up to weeks after initial exposure. Although these can last from a few days to more than 10 weeks, symptom duration is usually less than 2 weeks (Hecht, FM., et al., 2002). Fever, fatigue, rash, and pharyngitis are the most common symptoms of ARS. Other symptoms include lymphadenopathy, myalgia, headache, arthralgia, aseptic meningitis, weight loss, depression, night sweats, gastrointestinal distress, and oral or genital ulcers. Differential diagnosis includes infectious mononucleosis, secondary syphilis, acute hepatitis A or B, roseola or other viral exanthems, and toxoplasmosis. The occurrence and severity of symptoms during primary HIV infection correlate with the rapidity of clinical and immunologic decline. The nonspecific nature of these symptoms poses a major challenge for diagnosis, and emphasizes the need to obtain an accurate history of possible HIV exposure. For example, primary HIV infection should be considered in any patient with possible exposure presenting with fever of unknown cause (Pincus, JM., et al., 2003). This was especially pronounced in episodic care settings, such as STD clinics, emergency departments and urgent care facilities. The implementation of rapid testing for routine screening can substantially reduce the number of individuals who fail to learn test results, and minimize the expenses allocated to locate persons identified as HIV infected.

3.1 HIV testing with rapid technology

With the rapid test, as with the standard (conventional) HIV test, the provider should recommend testing, provide information about the test and an explanation of the window period, and give the patient an opportunity to decline or opt out of HIV testing; guides are available online
(http://www.cdc.gov/hiv/topics/research/respect-2/counseling/pdf/RESPECT2Standard TestingCounselingProtocol.pdf).
A number of US Food and Drug Administration (FDA)-approved rapid HIV testing products are available
(http://www.cdc.gov/hiv/topics/testing/rapid/rt-comparison.htm).
Providers who will be administering the test should be trained, either by the manufacturer or the local health department, in how to use the product available at their facilities. Rapid testing is done in a single session, so a patient should be assessed for their readiness to receive results on the same day. Positive rapid test results are preliminary and must be confirmed by Western blot or direct immunofluorescence assay before a diagnosis of HIV infection is established. However, negative results are considered conclusive and follow-up is not generally required (CDC, 2004).
As previously stated, because of the same-day availability of the results, rapid testing is very suitable for patients who are unlikely to return for their results. It is also the test of choice when an immediate treatment decision needs to be made (e.g., untested woman in labor, occupational or sexual exposure). In order to reduce the mortality, morbidity, and transmission among groups most affected
(http://www.cdc.gov/hiv/topics/surveillance/resources/slides/mortality/index.htm), it is important to understand and address the reasons for late testing for HIV. Persons diagnosed with AIDS concurrently or soon after (e.g., 3 or fewer years) receiving their initial HIV test results continue to represent a significant number of missed opportunities for diagnosis and prevention. Although there has been a steady increase in the CD4 counts of infected individuals at initial presentation, a large North American data set found that the average remained below 350 cells/μL, whereas 500 cells/μL is the lower threshold for

treatment initiation recommended by the US Department of Health & Human Services HIV treatment guidelines, as of December 2009 (http://www.aidsinfo.nih.gov/contentfiles/AdultandAdolescentGL.pdf). Data from 34 states showed that 38.3% of people who tested positive had progressed to AIDS 1 year or less after initial diagnosis of their HIV infection, and 45% had an AIDS diagnosis within 3 years (Shouse, RL., et al., 2009).

The percentage of individuals with AIDS occurring within 3 years after diagnosis increased with age, ranging from 22.7% in adolescents (13-19 years old) to 63.2% in those older than 60 years of age. Racial disparities were also noted (42.6% whites; 42.9% multiple/unknown race; 46.1% black/African American; 46.1% American Indian/Alaskan native; 48.4% Hispanic/Latino, and 50.4% Asian). A greater proportion of adolescent boys/men (46.9%) compared with adolescent girls/women (41.5%) developed AIDS within 3 years.

Possible reasons for late testing include stigma and homophobia as well as lack of access to testing facilities. Individuals may not seek HIV testing because they do not consider themselves at risk. Also, healthcare providers may not recognize the risk factors for HIV infection or the signs and symptoms of ARS, i.e., the signs and symptoms of primary HIV infection.

3.2 HIV serologic testing for men who have sex with men (MSM)

National HIV Behavioral Surveillance (NHBS) system estimates and monitors risk behaviors and collects data from metropolitan areas. According to the 2008 NHBS report, nearly 1 in 5 MSM were infected with HIV and 44% were unaware of their serostatus (CDC, 2010), 19% of MSMs were HIV infected, with the highest rates of prevalence among blacks (28%) followed by Hispanics (18%) and whites (16%). Increasing age and lower levels of income and education also were associated with higher prevalence rates. Poverty is also recognized as an important risk factor for HIV infection, and a greater proportion of MSM with no health insurance and those who had not visited a healthcare provider during the preceding year were unaware of their infection; 55% of those unaware of their infection were not tested during the preceding 12 months.

HIV prevalence was highest among black MSM < 30 years of age. However, the majority of young black and Hispanic MSM in each age group were unaware of their HIV infection. Thus, available data suggest that HIV prevalence among MSM remains high; many HIV infected MSMs are unaware of their serostatus; and minority MSM are disproportionately affected by HIV. The NHBS data underscore the specific need for increased HIV testing efforts directed toward all MSM, especially minorities. It has been demonstrated that about 25% of individuals testing HIV positive and 33% of those testing negative did not return for results of standard testing (Kendrick, SR., et al., 2005).

3.3 HIV serologic testing for children

Most children were infected with HIV-1 through vertical transmission of the virus. The route of HIV-1 can occur in utero, at the time of labor and delivery, and breastfeeding. Before treatment or interventions to prevent transmission were available, the rate of MTCT of HIV-1 in the United States was approximately 25%. And now, both clinical and laboratory-based methods for the diagnosis of HIV-1 infection in children have been developed. Laboratory-based methods include both immunologic and virological assays. Evaluations of clinical staging systems for the diagnosis of HIV-1 infection in children in sub-Saharan Africa, especially in young infants, have suggested limited sensitivity (Jones, SA., et al., 2005). Laboratory-based methods for the diagnosis of HIV-1 infection can be divided into 2 groups: immunologic and virological. The former includes (1) Detection of HIV-1 Antibodies, (2) Enzyme-Linked Immunosorbent Assays, (3) Rapid Tests which is to detection of IgG antibodies against HIV-1, (3) Semi-quantitative Antibody Assays, (4) Western Blot Assays, (5) Indirect Immunofluorescence Assays, (6) Analysis by Flow cytometry. Virological assay includes HIV-1 Culture, HIV-1 DNA Assays, HIV-1 RNA Assays and p24 Antigen Assays (Read, JS, 2007).

Rapid HIV tests provide results in min, use minimal laboratory equipment, and have been widely used especially in resource-poor settings since their introduction. However, false-negative results have happened, especially when the tests are used in infants. The case showed above demonstrates that the rapid HIV antibody test can result in false-negative results in infants. There are at least two possible explanations for the child's negative rapid HIV-1 antibody results. First, the primary antibody production has been suppressed by the presence of maternal IgG antibodies (Karlsson, MC., et al., 1999).

Secondly, mothers living with HIV were highly immunosuppressed; therefore, the low level of maternally-derived circulating HIV-1 IgG was only detected by HIV-EIA and Western blot. While the antigen components used in the rapid assay merit further investigation, our data indicate that the HIV rapid assay test is not reliable in screening for HIV infection in infants aged <18 months. Due to passive transfer of maternal antibody during pregnancy, infants born to HIV-infected mothers remain antibody-positive into the second year of life, even if they are not infected. For this reason, standard HIV antibody tests cannot reliably confirm HIV infection in infants until after maternal antibodies have disappeared. Tests that can diagnose pediatric HIV infection accurately during the first year of life include HIV-PCR assays, HIV culture, and repeat p24 antigen tests (Shah, I. et al., 2006). The sensitivity and the specificity of an HIV DNA PCR at birth have been estimated to be 50% and 99%, respectively. The sensitivity of the test improves dramatically in the first weeks of life and reaches a sensitivity of 90% or better when used in infants who are older than 1-mo of age. Two negative tests by PCR or viral culture after 3-mo of age would indicate that a child is not infected and would be more useful than screening serology. Although HIV DNA PCR and HIV RT-PCR are important tests in this clinical situation, they must be interpreted carefully. Several studies demonstrate a high sensitivity for both tests; however, specificities vary among reports. Also, HIV PCR testing should be repeated at regular, defined intervals, preferably lasting until the HIV antibody status of the infant is resolved (Sahni, AK., et al., 2005). HIV RNA amplification assays may be better at detecting HIV-infected infants than DNA PCR. In a cohort study, qualitative nucleic acid sequence-based amplification (NASBA) assay was shown to be highly specific and more sensitive than DNA PCR. NASBA results from infected children were compared with DNA PCR results from the same blood samples taken during the first 3 mo of life from HIV-infected and uninfected children. Sensitivity, specificity, and predictive values were calculated. The conclusion was that qualitative RNA assays (including RT-PCR) may be useful for diagnosing and excluding perinatal HIV infection in children after the first week of life for such purposes as initiating antiretroviral therapy and other treatment, resolving parental uncertainty, determining timing of transmission, and providing endpoints for intervention trials. Infants born to HIV-infected mothers are at great risk of becoming infected with HIV during labor and delivery. HIV is present in breast-milk, and the risk of transmission during breast-feeding depends on several factors including infant age, pattern of breast-feeding, breast-feeding duration, breast health, maternal viral load, and maternal immune status. HIV rapid assay may not be sensitive enough for testing HIV antibodies in infants who are less than 18-mo old. Other sensitive assays, including fourth-generation EIA as well as nucleic acid amplification-based assays should be used.

3.4 HIV serologic testing for pregnant women

Major successes have been achieved in prevention of (mother-to-child transmission) MTCT of HIV-1 in the United States; the MTCT rate has decreased to less than 2% with antiretroviral treatment of HIV-1–infected pregnant women and, for women who do not yet require treatment of their HIV-1 infection, with the use of the following efficacious interventions to prevent transmission: antiretroviral prophylaxis, cesarean section before labor and before rupture of membranes, 12 and complete avoidance of breastfeeding.

The CDC recommends that all pregnant women receive universal HIV testing as early as possible during prenatal care, with repeat testing in the third trimester in certain circumstances, such as those exhibiting signs or symptoms of infection, those with high-risk behaviors, and those living in or receiving care in areas with a high incidence or prevalence of HIV (identifies 1 HIV infection for every 1000 pregnant women tested). The screening preferably should occur at the first obstetric visit, after the patient has been informed that an HIV test will be performed unless declined (the opt-out screening model). Permission for HIV testing should be included as part of the general consent for healthcare. Clinicians should provide pregnant women with appropriate information in regard to HIV infection, risk factors, and reasons for testing, and transmission risk to ensure an informed decision about screening. Reasons for declining HIV testing should be addressed. If a woman has an unknown test history during prenatal care or undocumented serostatus at labor and delivery, she should be screened at the time of labor or immediately postpartum with a rapid HIV test, unless testing is declined. The majority of women with undocumented HIV testing or serostatus have few or no prenatal care visits. Rapid point-of-care testing during labor has been shown to be effective and accepted, with acceptance rates of 86% among those approached for testing during labor and delivery (Jamieson, DJ., et al., 2007).

The HIV test result of an expectant mother should be documented in her chart as well as in the medical record of her newborn. After appropriate maternal consent is given, maternal and pediatric healthcare providers should both be aware of the mother's HIV serostatus. This is necessary so that appropriate prophylaxis and testing of an HIV-exposed infant can occur, as well as proper management of any potential complications. It is important for pregnant women to know their serostatus as early as possible in the course of pregnancy to prevent transmission to infants and partners (Mofenson, L., et al., 2006; 55).

In 2005, approximately 92% of all HIV/AIDS cases in children younger than 13 years of age were due to vertical (mother-to-child) transmission. In the United States, the use of combination antiretroviral therapy during pregnancy has reduced the transmission rate from approximately 20%-30% to < 2%. Transmission to fetuses and infants can also be prevented through antiretroviral therapy, cesarean delivery, and avoiding breast-feeding. Transmission to partners and others can be prevented by changing previous risk behaviors, such as no or inconsistent condom use and by reducing viral load through antiretroviral treatment.

All patients, including all pregnant women, should be given the option to decline HIV testing. However, the clinician should discuss the reasons for declining testing and document the decision in the medical record. Risks for HIV and reasons for testing should be thoroughly reviewed. A woman may decline HIV testing for many reasons: She may not believe that she is at risk for HIV. Fear also may be influencing her decision, whether it is fear of being HIV positive, fear of discrimination if positive, or fear of partner retribution. Often, women think that they are not at risk for HIV due to a poor understanding of HIV and its risk factors. Women may also be unaware of their partners' HIV or STD risk, which also influences HIV transmission (Witte, SS., et al., 2010).

Other reasons for refusing HIV screening include scheduling conflicts; concerns over cost; health insurance; confidentiality; and other reasons, such as having a previous negative test. Identified issues should be addressed as fully as possible by the provider, with the intent of overcoming barriers and alleviating specific concerns about screening. HIV testing should continue to be recommended at subsequent prenatal visits if this has been refused in earlier visits. However, refusing HIV testing should never affect the level or quality of prenatal care provided to the patient.

4. References

Adimora, AA., Schoenbach, VJ. & Martinson, FE. (2003). Concurrent partnerships among rural African Americans with recently reported heterosexually transmitted HIV infection. Journal of Acquired Immune Deficiency Syndromes, Vol.34, No.4, pp.423-429, ISSN 1525-4135

Althoff, KN., Gange, SJ. & Klein, MB. (2005). Late presentation for human immunodeficiency virus care in the United States and Canada. Clinical Infectious Diseases, Vol. 50, No.11, pp.1512-1520, ISSN 1058-4838

Branson, BM., Handsfield, HH. & Lampe, MA. (2006). Centers for Disease Control and Prevention (CDC). Revised recommendations for HIV testing of adults, adolescents, and pregnant women in health-care settings. Recommendations and Reports: Morbidity and Mortality Weekly Report, Vol. 55, No.11, pp (RR14).1-17, ISSN 1545-8601

Campsmith, ML., Rhodes, PH.. & Hall, HI. (2010). Undiagnosed HIV prevalence among adults and adolescents in the United States at the end of 2006. Journal of Acquired Immune Deficiency Syndromes, Vol.47, No.5, pp.619-624, ISSN 1525-4135

Centers for Disease Control and Prevention. HIV surveillance reports. Diagnoses of HIV infection and AIDS in the United States and dependent areas, 2008. Page last updated: June 14, 2010. Available from:

http://www.cdc.gov/hiv/topics/surveillance/resources/reports Accessed October 28, 2010

Centers for Disease Control and Prevention (CDC). (2004). Protocols for confirmation of reactive rapid HIV tests. Morbidity and Mortality Weekly Reports, Vol. 53, pp.221-222, ISSN 1545-8601

Centers for Disease Control and Prevention (CDC). (2010). Prevalence and awareness of HIV infection among men who have sex with men -21 cities, United States, 2008. Morbidity and Mortality Weekly Reports, Vol.59, pp.1201-1207, ISSN 1545-8601

Centers for Disease Control and Prevention (CDC). (2008). Recommendations for partner services programs for HIV infection, syphilis, gonorrhea, and chlamydial infection. Recommendations and Reports: Morbidity and Mortality Weekly Report, Vol. 57(RR-9), pp.1-83, ISSN 1545-8601

Craw, JA., Gardner, LI. & Marks, G. (2008). Brief strengths-based case management promotes entry into HIV medical care: results of the Antiretroviral Treatment Access Study-II. Journal of Acquired Immune Deficiency Syndromes, Vol. 47, No.11, pp.597-606, ISSN 1525-4135

Duffus, WA., Weis, K. & Kettinger, L. (2009). Risk-based HIV testing in South Carolina health care settings failed to identify the majority of infected individuals. AIDS Patient Care and STDS, Vol.23, No.5, pp.339-345, ISSN 1087-7449

Farnham, PG., Hutchinson, AB. & Sansom, SL. (2008). Comparing the costs of HIV screening strategies and technologies in health- care settings. Public Health Reports, Vol. 123 (suppl3), pp.51-62, ISSN 0033-3549

Fiebig, EW., Wright, DJ. & Rawal, BD. (2003). Dynamics of HIV viremia and antibody seroconversion in plasma donors: implications for diagnosis and staging of primary HIV infection. AIDS, Vol.17, No.13, pp.1871-1879, ISSN 1473-5571

Hecht, FM., Busch, MP. & Rawal, B. (2002). Use of laboratory tests and clinical symptoms for identification of primary HIV infection. AIDS, Vol.16, No.8, pp.1119-1129, ISSN 1473-5571

http://www.cdc.gov/hiv/topics/research/respect-2/counseling/pdf/RESPECT2StandardTestingCounselingProtocol.pdf

http://www.cdc.gov/hiv/topics/testing/rapid/rt-comparison.htm

http://www.cdc.gov/hiv/topics/surveillance/resources/slides/mortality/index.htm

http://www.aidsinfo.nih.gov/contentfiles/AdultandAdolescentGL.pdf

Jamieson, DJ., Cohen, MH. & Maupin, R. (2007). Rapid human immunodeficiency virus-1 testing on labor and delivery in 17 US hospitals: the MIRIAD experience. American Journal of Obstetrics and Gynecology, Vol.197 (suppl3), pp.S72-S82, ISSN 0002-9378

Jiang, X., Lu, H. & Zhang Y. (2008). A cross-sectional study of HIV and tuberculosis coinfection cases in mainland China. Southern Medical Journal, Vol.101, No.9, pp.914-917, ISSN 0038-4348

Jones, SA., Sherman, GG. & Coovadia, AH. (2005). Can clinical algorithms deliver an accurate diagnosis of HIV infection in infancy? Bulletin of World Health Organization, Vol.83, No.7, pp.559–560, ISSN 0042-9686

Karlsson, MC., Wernersson, S. & Diaz de Stahl T. (1999). Efficient IgG-mediated suppression of primary antibody responses in Fcgamma receptor-deficient mice. Proceeding of the National Academy of Science of United States of America, Vol.96, No.5, pp.2244-2249, ISSN 1091-6490

Kendrick, SR., Kroc, KA. & Withum, D. (2005). Outcomes of offering rapid point-of-care HIV testing in a sexually transmitted disease clinic. Journal of Acquired Immune Deficiency Syndromes, Vol.38, No.2, pp.142-146, ISSN 1525-4135

Marks, G., Crepaz, N. & Senterfitt, JW. (2005). Meta-analysis of high-risk sexual behavior in persons aware and unaware they are infected with HIV in the United States: implications for HIV prevention programs. Journal of Acquired Immune Deficiency Syndromes, Vol.39, No.4, pp.446-453, ISSN 1525-4135

Mofenson, L., Taylor, AW. & Rogers, M. (2006). Achievements in public health: reduction in perinatal transmission of HIV infection -United States, 1985-2005. Morbidity and Mortality Weekly Report, Vol.55, pp.592-597, ISSN 0149-2195

Pincus, JM., Crosby, SS. & Losina, E. Acute human immunodeficiency virus infection in patients presenting to an urban urgent care center. Clinical Infectious Diseases, 2003; 37:1699-1704

Read, JS. (2007). Diagnosis of HIV-1 infection in children younger than 18 months in the United States. Pediatrics, Vol.120, No.6, pp.1547-1562, ISSN 0031-4005

Sahni, AK., Gupta, RM. & Jena, J. (2005). Early detection of HIV-1 in infants by PCR. Indian Journal of Pathology and Microbiology, Vol.48, No.1, pp.49-52, ISSN 0974-5130

Sanders, GD., Bayoumi, AM. & Sundaram, V. (2005). Cost-effectiveness of screening for HIV in the era of highly active antiretroviral therapy. The New England Journal of Medicine, Vol.352, No.6, pp.570-585, ISSN 1533-4406

Shah, I. (2006). Efficacy of HIV PCR techniques to diagnose HIV in infants born to HIV infected mothers–an Indian perspective. Journal of Association of Physicians of India, Vol.54, pp.197-199, ISSN 0004-5772

Shouse, RL., Kajese, T. & Hall, HI. (2009). Late HIV testing-34 states, 1996-2005. Morbidity and Mortality Weekly Report, Vol.58, pp.661-665, ISSN 1545-8601

Taylor, Z., Nolan, CM. & Blumberg, HM. (2005). American Thoracic Society, Centers for Disease Control and Prevention, Infectious Diseases Society of America. Controlling tuberculosis in the United States: recommendations from the American Thoracic Society, CDC, and the Infectious Diseases Society of America. Recommendations and Reports: Morbidity and Mortality Weekly Report, Vol.54 (RR12), pp.1-81, ISSN 1545-8601

Wawer, MJ., Gray, RH. & Sewankambo, NK. (2005). Rates of HIV-1 transmission per coital act, by stage of HIV-1 infection, in Rakai, Uganda. Journal of Infectious Diseases, Vol.191, No.9, pp.1403-1409, ISSN 1528-8366

Witte, SS, El-Bassel, N. & Gilbert, L. (2010). Lack of awareness of partner STD risk among heterosexual couples. Perspectives on Sexual and Reproductive Health, Vol.42, No.1, pp.49-55, ISSN 1931-2393

Zhang, YZ., Wang, J. & Wilson, GJ. (2008). Negative results of a rapid antibody test for HIV in a 16-month-old infant with AIDS. Annals of Clinical and Laboratory Science, Vol.38, No.3, pp.293-295, ISSN 1550-8080

5

The Sub-Saharan African HIV Epidemic - "Successes and Challenges"

Roos E. Barth and Andy I.M. Hoepelman
University Medical Centre Utrecht,
Department of Internal Medicine and Infectious Diseases,
The Netherlands

1. Introduction

The global impact of the human immunodeficiency virus (HIV) pandemic is enormous. To date, more than 25 million lives have been claimed by the acquired immunodeficiency syndrome (AIDS) and over 33 million people are currently estimated to be HIV-infected. Ninety-five percent of these people infected with HIV live in developing countries. Sub-Saharan Africa is the region that is hit hardest by the HIV pandemic.

During the quarter century since the first reports of a novel immunodeficiency syndrome in 1981, great advances have been made in HIV diagnosis, prevention and care. The first protease inhibitor (PI) was approved in 1996, marking the start of the highly active antiretroviral therapy (HAART) era. From then on, HIV-infections were no longer inevitably associated with AIDS and death, but could be viewed as a chronic condition [Merson, 2006; Sepkowitz, 2006]. Currently, the antiretroviral armamentarium includes over 20 different drugs and more are in the pipeline. The use of HAART can result in effective, long-term suppression of the virus with consequent recovery of the patient's immune system. Unfortunately, complete HIV eradication is still not feasible. Moreover, it is apparent that the virus generally resurges to pre-treatment levels within months after ART withdrawal. Patients therefore need a life-long commitment to their treatment.

The logistic and monetary costs associated with such long-term HIV-care are high. HIV monitoring and treatment was therefore initially only available in resource-rich countries. Great efforts and large funds were needed to make ART more widely available. This awareness and initiatives, such as the "United States' President's Emergency Plan for AIDS Relief" and the "Global fund for AIDS, TB and Malaria", resulted in an unprecedented roll-out of treatment since the turn of the millennium [United Nations]. The increase in HIV-infected individuals receiving ART has been especially large In Sub-Saharan Africa where over the last decade, many ART programs took off, treating millions of HIV-infected patients. Despite these impressive accomplishments however, monitoring and research facilities in low-income countries (LICs) still lag behind.

There are great differences between HIV care in resource-rich and LICs. First, due to limited resources, the number of clinics, health care providers and other necessities for quality health care are lower in LICs compared to high-income countries. Second, HIV is generally transmitted via heterosexual contact in African countries, whereas homosexual contacts and intravenous drug use are the main routes of transmission in western countries. Moreover,

due to differences in genetic make up there may be different reactions to the virus and its treatment between different populations. Third, the virus itself differs between various geographical areas. While subtype B is the main HIV subtype in Europe and the United States, it is rarely seen in Sub-Saharan Africa, where subtype C is the prevailing HIV subtype.
The on-treatment HIV-RNA-level is associated with a patients' clinical outcome. Therefore, western guidelines recommend regular HIV-RNA monitoring in all patients receiving ART. Roll-out strategies in LICs on the other hand were initially mainly focused on providing as many patients with antiretroviral drugs (ARVs) as possible, thereby limiting the resources left for laboratory monitoring. As regular HIV-RNA testing is not feasible in many, Sub-Saharan African ART programs, treatment decisions are frequently solely based on clinical or immunological parameters. However, the correlation between these parameters and virological outcomes appears to be marginal [Kantor et al., 2009; Keiser et al., 2009; Reynolds et al., 2009b]. Moreover, making predictions on long-term treatment outcomes is difficult, as the virological effects of these programs are not clear and other surrogate markers for clinical outcomes are not available.
Despite the above mentioned difficulties, great progress has been made regarding HIV care in Sub-Sahara Africa. However, challenges remain. Both successes and challenges regarding prevention and treatment of HIV as well as viral resistance development and treatment of co-morbidities will be addressed in the following chapter.

2. Prevention

In 2007, the WHO announced that the HIV-epidemic seemed to be levelling off. Still, over 33 million people are estimated to be HIV-infected globally, with 2.6 million people becoming newly infected annually. The overall adult HIV prevalence in Sub-Saharan Africa is estimated to be over five percent, with prevalence rates up to twenty-five percent in some countries [UNAIDS, 2009]. This however means that the vast majority (more than ninety percent) is still HIV-negative. Keeping these people free from HIV, as well as preventing new generations from becoming infected, is a major challenge and should remain a priority on the HIV-care agenda.

2.1 Prevention of mother to child transmission

One of the great advances in HIV preventive-care has been the "prevention of mother to child transmission" (PMTCT) strategies. Testing pregnant women for the presence of HIV and subsequently providing those that are infected, as well as their new-born babies, with ARVs has the potential of reducing vertical HIV transmission rates to below one percent [Paintsil and Andiman, 2007; Paintsil and Andiman, 2009]. Short-course ARVs or single-dose nevirapine (SDNVP) are frequently used for PMTCT instead of complete ART regimens in low-income countries (LICs). Such regimens have shown to be efficacious in averting many infant-HIV infections. Still, with transmission rates ranging from one to above ten percent, results are lagging behind those observed in resource-rich settings [Boeke and Jackson, 2008; Chigwedere et al., 2008; Leroy et al., 2008; Palombi et al., 2007; Tonwe-Gold et al., 2007]. Moreover, administration of SDNVP can lead to the selection of non-nucleoside reverse transcriptase- (NNRTI-) associated resistance mutations. There is evidence that fewer mutations are selected when other ARVs are added to the SDNVP [Arrive et al., 2007; Chi et al., 2007a]. However, the optimal combination of drugs and best time for treatment initiation in order to create a feasible and effective PMTCT strategy for

LICs, still need to be defined [Chi et al., 2007b; Lockman et al., 2007]. In addition to improving the efficacy of PMTCT programmes, the PMTCT coverage needs to be expanded. Many resource-limited countries still have a limited PMTCT-coverage; in South Africa for example only sixty percent of HIV-infected pregnant women have access to this simple, cost-effective strategy and figures are worse for several other LICs [Abdool Karim et al., 2009; Paintsil and Andiman, 2009]. These data show that, even though much progress is made in the field of PMTCT, improvements are urgently needed to prevent even more infant-HIV infections and deaths.

2.2 Vaccines

Historically, vaccine development is one of the fields in health care where major progress is achieved. Many infectious diseases were effectively prevented and some nearly eradicated. Unfortunately, results of HIV vaccine research are unrelentingly negative. Many candidate vaccines were developed, but the results proved unsatisfactory and major vaccination studies were stopped [Johnston and Fauci, 2008]. Despite these failures, some vaccines are still being tested. Most of these are directed at stimulating the immune system [Fauci et al., 2008]. Still, finding an effective vaccine in the near future does not seem likely.

2.3 Circumcision

Several other preventive strategies were analyzed and implemented, resulting in variable success rates. Male circumcision was put forward to prevent heterosexual HIV transmission since a lower female HIV prevalence was observed in Sub-Saharan African countries with high levels of male circumcision [Auvert et al., 2005; Williams et al., 2006]. However, epidemiological evidence of a direct protective effect of male circumcision on women becoming infected with HIV is limited according to some [Weiss et al., 2009]. To date, most consider male circumcision to have a significant, albeit partial, efficacy in reducing heterosexual HIV transmission [Doyle et al.; Smith et al.]. To what extend expanding circumcision coverage will contribute to combating the global HIV epidemic, still needs to be determined.

2.4 Post- and pre-exposure prophylaxis

Post-exposure prophylaxis (PEP) is a successful prevention method after incidental needle or sex accidents. In Sub-Saharan Africa however, where heterosexual contact drives the HIV epidemic, PEP provision is limited and will not substantially influence the HIV statistics. Pre-exposure prophylaxis (PrEP) on the other hand may prove to be a promising strategy. An effective agent that can be used safely by women prior to sexual intercourse and without the need for agreement from a partner would be a major contributor to preventive HIV care [Al-Jabri and Alenzi, 2009]. However, until now trials of microbicide candidates have shown disappointing results; some even suggested a boosted risk of infection as more vaginal lesions were observed in treated patients [Al-Jabri and Alenzi, 2009; Wilson et al., 2008]. Possibly gels that incorporate ARVs will be more effective as PrEP. Studies are being set up and hopefully results will come available in the coming years [Grant et al., 2008].

2.5 Antiretroviral treatment as a preventive measure

In spite of these preventive strategies it is not likely that the high HIV incidence will change in the near future. Some strategies are only partly effective and many remain grossly underused [USAID, UNAIDS, WHO, CDC and the POLICY project; Kerr et al.]. More importantly, the development of a preventive vaccine seems to be nearly impossible and HIV-eradication can not be realised with current treatment strategies. Still, provision of ART surpasses the obvious benefits it has on an individual level. Treating HIV can be used as an essential part of prevention efforts. For heterosexual contact and for mother-to-child-transmission a clear dose-response effect was found between HIV-RNA levels and risk of HIV transmission [Fang et al., 1995; Quinn et al., 2000; Tovanabutra et al., 2002]. As these are the main routes of HIV transmission in Sub-Saharan Africa, it seems likely that bringing down individual HIV-RNA levels can make a substantial contribution to reducing the number of new infections. Indeed, such positive effects were described previously, suggesting cost-saving effects of ART due to the reduction of HIV transmission, in addition to the clear benefits of such treatment on an individual basis [Granich et al., 2009; Mayer and Venkatesh; Montaner et al., 2006]. Up till now, the roll-out of ART has not clearly reduced HIV-incidence. If a preventive effect of ART becomes more apparent as treatment-coverage increases, and as patients receive care for longer periods of time, will largely depend on the number of patients experiencing virological failure.

2.6 Awareness

Creating awareness about the risks of unprotected sex and other potential transmission routes, as well as providing information on advances that have been made in HIV care, is of utmost importance in reducing the stigma's associated with HIV and in motivating people to do an HIV-test. An elevated level of awareness may lead to patients seeking care at a less advanced stage of disease. As a result, chances of a good clinical response to ART will be greater. Moreover, the period that patients will have high viral loads and therefore are highly infectious, will be shorter if patients have their HIV tested and treated at an earlier stage. Continued monitoring of HIV incidence, and possibly mathematical modelling studies, are needed to further calculate the preventive and cost-saving effects of ART expansion programmes.

3. Treatment

HIV leads to AIDS and death when left untreated. ART provides clear benefits for those infected and rendered HIV-infection a manageable chronic condition. Access to treatment increased considerably over the last decade. Still, by the end of 2008, less than half of the people in need of treatment in Sub-Saharan Africa actually received ART [UNAIDS 2009] and the United Nations endorsed target of "universal access by 2010" has not been met [WHO, 2006b]. It was recognized that access to treatment is especially limited for certain groups of people, such as those living in rural settings [Crowley et al., 2009]. Therefore, continued efforts are needed to increase the availability of ART even further.

3.1 When to start ART

When to start ART in HIV-infected individuals remains a controversial issue. Initially, treatment was deferred until CD4 counts dropped to below 200 cells/mm^3 in most LICs [Wood et al., 2005]. In western settings it is common practice to initiate ART earlier, when CD4 counts are less than 350 or even 500 cells/mm^3, as various studies suggest improved treatment outcomes at higher CD4 thresholds [Braithwaite et al., 2008; Emery et al., 2008; Kitahata; Sterne]. Benefits of an earlier treatment start may be even greater in LICs compared to high-income countries, due to higher rates of opportunistic diseases and mortality there. However, the number of people eligible for ART will increase as CD4 treatment-initiation thresholds move up, putting extra pressure on the already fragile health care facilities and limited resources. A mathematical modelling study on the other hand reported that an increase of the CD4 treatment-initiation threshold (to 350 cells/mm^3) would reduce morbidity and mortality while remaining cost-effective, in the South African context [Walensky et al., 2009]. Moreover, the WHO recently adjusted its guidelines, recommending to start treatment at CD4 counts of 350 cells/mm^3 or less for all HIV-infected individuals [Crowley et al., 2009]. However, definite results from ongoing, international trials assessing when to initiate ART in resource-limited settings will not be available for several years.

3.2 Treatment outcomes

Overall, on-treatment, short-term outcomes of Sub-Saharan African ART programs that have access to HIV-RNA monitoring, are promising and similar to those initially observed in western settings. However, high early attrition (composed of all-cause mortality and patients being lost to follow up) is frequently observed, negatively influencing intention-to-treat results. Within a few years after treatment start, virological failure is observed in only fifteen percent of patients. It should be borne in mind though, that applied failure criteria are generally more lenient than those used in western settings [Barth RE, 2010b]. Long-term outcome data are still limited, but seem promising as well.

First-line ART regimens in Sub-Saharan Africa are generally NNRTI-based. Boosted PIs may also be used in treatment-naïve patients. Compared to an NNRTI-based first-line regimen this resulted in a slightly reduced treatment efficacy, but fewer resistance mutations [Riddler et al., 2008; von Wyl et al., 2007]. A review on clinical trials also showed that fewer nucleoside reverse transcriptase inhibitor- (NRTI)-associated resistance mutations were present in case of boosted PI-based regimen failure compared to NNRTI-based regimens [Gupta et al., 2008]. The answer to the question whether or not it is advisable to move to a PI-based first-line ART regimen in LICs will largely depend on the balance between costs, adverse events and resistance development profiles.

3.3 Adverse effects

Providing all those in need with ART is a daunting task. However, caring for those already receiving treatment poses many challenges as well. As HIV-infected people live longer, the long-term effects of the virus and its treatment become more evident. Simple, affordable treatment regimens facilitated the initial, extensive ART roll-out. However, the negative effects associated with these commonly used treatment options called for a reconsideration of widely applied treatment strategies. Mitochondrial toxicity causes neuropathy, lipodystrophy and lactic acidosis in many individuals receiving stavudine-containing ART. Therefore, it was recommended to move away from stavudine-based regimens to zidovudine or tenofovir (TDF) [Crowley et al., 2009; WHO, 2006a]. As yet, not all African countries have adopted TDF as a first-line regimen in their guidelines for financial reasons, but this may change during coming years. As TDF becomes more widely available, knowledge of its side-effects grows more important. TDF has potential nephrotoxic effects. Generally no negative effects on renal function are observed when TDF is used in a first-line ART regimen [Gallant and Moore, 2009], but little is known regarding the prevalence and nature of renal impairment in African cohorts. In one South African cohort the number of people with severe renal dysfunction was limited [Franey et al., 2009], but future studies will have to show what the long-term effects of TDF use in African patients are. Another concern with TDF use relates to the possible increased risk of bone disease. HIV-infected individuals have an increased risk of osteopenia compared to HIV-uninfected people. This risk is increased further by the use of TDF [Jacobson et al., 2008]. It is not yet clear whether patients receiving TDF also have an increased bone-fracture risk. The increased risk of cardiovascular disease and diabetes, associated with some antiretroviral drugs, will be discussed in more detail later. These and other negative effects of long-term ARV use in various populations have to be addressed in future studies.

3.4 Second line treatment

PIs are becoming more widely available in LICs since the advent of heat-stable drug formulations. They are typically used in second-line regimens, in case of treatment failure. As currently the vast majority of patients receiving ART in Sub-Saharan Africa are receiving a NNRTI-based, first-line regimen, limited data are available on the efficacy of PI-based regimens in African settings. Good, early, virological responses were reported, but a frequent occurrence of adverse events was also observed [Castelnuovo et al., 2009a; Hosseinipour et al.]. In a large trial performed in western countries (TITAN trial) over three quarters of treatment-experienced patients achieved an HIV-RNA less than 400 copies/mL after switching to either lopinavir/ritonavir or darunavir/ritonavir in combination with an optimized backbone regimen. Results were even better if patients with any prior PI-exposure were excluded from analysis [Madruga et al., 2007]. These data suggest that a boosted PI-based second-line regimen would be effective in the majority of African patients who experience treatment failure while receiving NNRTI-based first-line ART. However, the generalisability of these data is limited as defining an optimized backbone is hazardous in LICs, where fewer ARVs are available and resistance testing is not widely available. Long-term data regarding second-line efficacy in resource-limited settings are not yet available and should be a subject for future research.

3.5 New antiretroviral drugs

New drugs within traditional drug classes and new drug-classes were developed over the last years. In western countries drugs such as boosted darunavir and etravirine as well as drug-classes such as fusion and integrase inhibitors, CCR5-receptor antagonists and maturation inhibitors expanded the antiretroviral arsenal. Long-term care for HIV-infected patients frequently demands switching to third- or consecutive lines of ART. Moreover, an individualised- rather than a protocol-based approach is increasingly being used. Viral characteristics, such as HIV-subtype and presence of drug-resistance mutations, as well as host characteristics such as medical history, organ functions and genetic background, all contribute to the efficacy and toxicity of the various ARVs. Most HIV-related pharmacological research was done in resource-rich settings, where Caucasian, male patients, infected with a subtype-B virus, predominate. Important differences exist between western and non-western countries regarding both these viral- as well as these host-characteristics. Even though the new ARVs will not shortly become available on a large-scale in LICs, it will be interesting to analyse what effects such drugs have in different ethnic populations and on various HIV-subtypes. Such research hopefully provides more insight in the dynamics between drugs, viruses and hosts and increases therapeutic options for all

HIV-infected individuals in the future. Moreover, expansion of the ARV armamentarium for second- and consecutive- lines of treatment is needed to ensure treatment success in the future.

3.6 Paediatric HIV care

Ninety percent of the 2.1 million HIV-infected children worldwide live in LICs. Until recently it was estimated that few vertically HIV-infected children survived beyond the age of five years. However, despite high mortality-rates in HIV-infected infants, a substantial increase of older survivors of mother-to-child transmission is visible in Africa [Ferrand et al., 2009]. Caring for small, HIV-infected children is associated with specific challenges, such as drug-administration problems and weight-based dosing. Later, during adolescence, an increased fear for stigma and loss of social acceptance may lead to a decreased adherence to treatment. Still, paediatric ART can result in virological and immunological benefits which are comparable to those observed among children in more developed settings [Ciaranello et al., 2009]. Unfortunately, despite optimistic, initial outcomes, long-term paediatric ART is associated with frequent virological failure [Barth et al. 2010c]. Similar to adult patients, most children were receiving NNRTI-based ART. Paediatric treatment outcomes may improve when PI-based regimens are used, which have a higher genetic barrier and are therefore somewhat more forgiving in case of sub-optimal treatment adherence. However, the effects of a long-term HIV infection and many years of ART on growth and development are not yet known. Simplifying treatment regimens and limiting side effects will be crucial to retain children in care and achieve good, long-term clinical outcomes.

4. Drug-resistance development

First-line ART failure is generally caused by poor adherence to the drugs. Various issues are linked to poor adherence. Drug toxicity is a major contributor, but other factors such as co-morbidities, insufficient drug supply, stigma, pill burden and traditional beliefs can play a role in drug-adherence. Contrasting initial fears, observed adherence rates in African ART programmes are good [Mills et al., 2006]. Still, around 15 percent of patients receiving first-line treatment in Sub-Saharan Africa experience virological failure within a few years after treatment initiation [Barth RE, 2010b].

In western guidelines it is recommended to perform resistance testing in case of virological failure in order to determine an optimal second-line regimen with a sufficiently high genetic barrier. Regular resistance testing is not feasible in most African clinics. In western countries, most HIV-infected individuals are infected with HIV-1, subtype B. This is in stark contrast with Sub-Saharan African countries, were less than one percent of patients subtype-B virus. Various non-B subtypes are prevalent, with subtype-C being most prevalent. Therefore, treatment outcome data and genotypic resistance data from western studies can not simply be extrapolated to African settings.

Available resistance data of people experiencing virological failure in LICs typically show (multiple) NNRTI-associated mutations and the lamivudine-associated M184V mutation [Barth RE, 2010b; Barth et al., 2008; Hoffmann et al., 2009; Marconi et al., 2008]. With such drug-resistance profiles a PI-based second-line regimen will generally be effective. Actual second-line treatment outcomes may however be less good. As in many HIV-treatment programmes in LICs regular HIV-RNA testing is not feasible, and due to the delay before immunological and clinical decline becomes apparent, there may be a large number of people where virological failure remains unnoticed [Castelnuovo et al., 2009b; Kantor et al., 2009; Keiser et al., 2009; Reynolds et al., 2009b]. These people will continue their failing, first-line regimen. This is important, as a delay in treatment modification after virological failure is associated with an increased mortality [Petersen et al., 2008]. Moreover, an accumulation of drug-resistance mutations is observed in patients who continue first-line ARVs in spite of virological failure, limiting future treatment options [Cozzi-Lepri et al., 2007; Hoffmann et al., 2009; Reynolds et al., 2009a]. Empirically starting second-line ART in programmes with limited access to virological diagnostics, may therefore result in sub-optimal treatment outcomes, stressing the need for affordable, easy-access drug-resistance tests in LICs.

Drug-resistant HIV not only decreases the efficacy of new ART regimens in patients harbouring such a virus; transmission of resistant strains in the community may also limit first-line treatment outcomes of newly infected individuals [Barth et al., 2008; Kuritzkes et al., 2008; Wensing et al., 2005]. Fortunately, transmission of drug-resistant viruses is still limited in the African continent. Published primary resistance rates are generally well-below the WHO cut-off rate of five percent [Bartolo et al., 2009; Bussmann et al., 2005; Derache et al., 2008]. The prevalence of drug-resistant viruses will probably increase in LICs though, as ARVs become more widely available in those countries. Regular monitoring of primary resistance is needed to predict whether currently used treatment regimens will remain effective in the majority of patients.

5. Co-morbidities

Many other, both communicable and non-communicable, diseases can cause morbidity and mortality in HIV-infected individuals. Diagnosing and treating such co-morbidities are of utmost importance when caring for people with HIV. Below, a few of these diseases will be briefly addressed.

5.1 Tuberculosis

Concomitant with the HIV epidemic, South Africa has one of the worst TB epidemics of the world [Abdool Karim et al., 2009; WHO, 2009]. The HIV/TB co-infection rate is estimated to be as high as 70%, causing morbidity and mortality in many. However, making a definite TB diagnosis is hazardous, especially in HIV-infected individuals. In immuno-compromised patients, sputum-smear-negative and non-pulmonary TB are frequent, limiting the utility of commonly available TB diagnostics. Culturing mycobacterium tuberculosis, the golden standard when making a TB diagnosis, is often omitted due to the time and money needed for these tests. Therefore, there is a clear need for accurate, simple and low-cost diagnostic tests for the detection of TB infection.

The use of ART causes a great reduction in the risk of developing TB in the long term [Badri et al., 2002]. However, the incidence of TB increases soon after ART initiation, following the restoration of immune responses [Bonnet et al., 2006; Lawn et al., 2005; Moore et al., 2007]. As a result, TB is an important cause of the high mortality during the first months of ART, observed in many HIV treatment programmes [Brinkhof et al., 2007; Koenig et al., 2009; Lawn et al., 2008; Manabe et al., 2009].

The WHO declared that "urgent and extraordinary means" are needed in order to combat this massive disease burden, and it set targets for cure and case detection rates [WHO, 2009]. Unfortunately, in South Africa these targets are far from being met. Case detection rates are only 62% instead of the WHO minimum target of 70% and cure rates are only 58% instead of the intended 85% [Abdool Karim et al., 2009]. These worrying figures are partly due to the expansion of multi- and even extensively- drug-resistant TB (MDR and XDR). Case-fatality rates are much higher in case of drug-resistant TB, compared with sensitive mycobacterial infections. Exogenous, nosocomial re-infections are thought to drive the spread of drug-resistant TB. Drug-susceptibility testing is needed to identify those in need of stricter isolation and broader anti-tuberculosis treatment regimens. However, susceptibility testing is currently only done in a subgroup of re-treatment cases and even if such testing is performed, it often takes long before results are available. The development of cheap, fast HIV-tests was an important contribution to the massive scaling up of HIV-care. Such easy-access tests are also needed to make a rapid TB diagnosis and to differentiate drug-resistant from normally susceptible infections [Lawn et al.]. Hopefully efforts to optimize diagnostic and treatment strategies, combined with a better integration of HIV- and TB-care will eventually result in a reversal of the TB epidemic.

5.2 Hepatitis

Apart from TB, hepatitis B (HBV) and C (HCV) co-infections are commonly observed in HIV-infected individuals. As ART roll-out continues, life expectancy of HIV-infected individuals in resource-limited countries improves. As a result, long-term effects of such hepatitis co-infections, like liver cirrhosis and hepato-cellular carcinomas, become more evident. HBV as well as HCV are highly prevalent in African, HIV-infected individuals (15% and 7% respectively', but there is a wide geographical variation in HBV and HCV prevalence [Barth et al. 2010a].

In western countries HIV infection is strongly associated with an increased incidence of both HBV and HCV [Burnett et al., 2005; Rockstroh et al., 2005; Thio, 2009]. This association is attributed to shared routes of transmission: mostly (homo)sexual contact in the case of HBV and intravenous drug use (IVDU) for hepatitis C [Cooper et al., 2009; Lavanchy, 2004; Modi and Feld, 2007]. In African countries HBV acquisition is assumed to occur during early childhood. As the route of HIV transmission in Africa is mainly via heterosexual contact, at a later point in life, it can be expected that the association between both infections is limited. However, reliable data on the mode and age of HBV acquisition amongst HIV-infected individuals in Africa are lacking. The predominant mode of HCV transmission in Africa is not yet established. However, IVDU seems to be less influential as in western countries [Cooper et al., 2009; Lavanchy, 2004; Modi and Feld, 2007]. Due to the different times and modes of transmission, the observed association between HIV and the hepatic viruses is less evident in Sub-Saharan Africa. Still, the burden of HIV/hepatitis co-infections in that region is high, as all these viruses are highly endemic. According to WHO estimates, 22.5 million HIV-infected people lived in Sub-Saharan Africa by the end of 2007 [WHO, 2007]. When geographical variations in HBV and HIV prevalence are not taken into account, an HBV prevalence of 15% would mean that 3.4 million HBV/HIV co-infected people live in this region.

HIV accelerates the progression of HBV and HCV related liver disease. Evidence that such co-infections are also associated with an increased mortality came available only recently [Chen et al., 2009; Nikolopoulos et al., 2009]. It is to be expected that HBV and HCV related cirrhosis and malignancies will become even more evident during coming years, as ART roll-out carries on and life-expectancy for HIV-individuals improves.

Knowledge on a patients' HBV/HCV status can help clinicians interpret clinical problems and lab results. More importantly, such information can guide decisions on which ARVs can best be prescribed in co-infected patients. The vast majority of first-line ART regimens in Sub-Saharan Africa contain lamivudine. Lamivudine has long been approved for the treatment of chronic HBV. However, it has a poor resistance profile. Around half of HBV-isolates show drug-resistance mutations after 2-3 years of lamivudine use [Liaw et al., 2000; Lok et al., 2000]. Tenofovir is not yet widely available in Sub-Saharan Africa, but its use may increase during coming years. This nucleotide analogue has been approved for the treatment of HBV in 2008. Rates of HBV suppression in mono-infected patients are impressive and drug-resistance development seems to be limited [Marcellin et al., 2008]. Another problem regarding lamivudine use in HIV/HBV co-infected patients can arise when lamivudine is being stopped. A paradoxical HBV 'flare up' can occur, potentially causing liver tissue destruction [Lim et al., 2002].

Treating HCV infections is not feasible in most African settings due to the high costs and intensive monitoring associated with currently available therapies. Still, knowledge on a possible HCV co-infection is useful. Screening policies for liver cirrhosis and hepato-cellular carcinomas can be installed and the use of hepato-toxic agents can be minimized.

5.3 Non-communicable diseases

The unprecedented increase in ART roll-out which took place over the last decade shows what can be achieved with the joined efforts of international organisations, governments, non-governmental organisations and many enthusiastic, hard-working people. An extensive expansion of health care infrastructures was realized in many countries in order to reach and treat the millions of HIV-infected individuals. Large funds were made available to make ART free of charge for most patients. After being enrolled in an HIV-treatment programme, patients are frequently also provided with other medical care, like the diagnostics for and treatment of opportunistic infections. For HIV-negative persons on the other hand, medical care is frequently less readily available and costly. This may lead to disparities between individuals with HIV and those who are suffering from other (chronic) illnesses. Instead of increasing the gap between medical care that is available to HIV-infected and HIV-uninfected individuals, we should try to extend the benefits of the improved health care systems to other target groups. As in the established market economies, non-communicable disorders are the leading cause of death in adults in low- and middle-income countries. Ischemic heart disease and cerebrovascular accidents are the most frequent causes of death. Risk factors such as hypertension, diabetes, smoking and obesity are major contributors to this disease burden [Chopra et al., 2009; Gill et al., 2009; Lopez et al., 2006; Murray and Lopez, 1997; Sliwa and Mocumbi, 2009]. Sub-Saharan Africa includes countries with the highest non-communicable disease burden, such as South Africa. Poor people living in urban areas are affected most, but the burden is clearly rising in rural communities [Mayosi et al., 2009]. This rise is partly due to demographic changes; people grow older despite the negative effect of the HIV epidemic.

As ART roll-out continues, cardiovascular diseases will become even more evident due to a decline in HIV-related mortality. Moreover, an increased incidence of inflammatory circulatory disorders is observed in HIV-infected individuals and the use of PIs and certain NRTIs is associated with a greater risk of insulin resistance, lipodystrophy and dyslipidaemia [Friis-Moller et al., 2007; Grunfeld et al., 2009; Hsue et al., 2009]. Despite these worrying figures, attention for the prevention and treatment of non-communicable diseases in African countries has been limited because most efforts were directed at combating the

HIV and tuberculosis epidemics. However, there is a growing recognition that an integrated chronic care model is needed to combat both epidemics of communicable and non-communicable diseases in Sub-Saharan Africa. Surveillance, treatment and prevention strategies need to be improved [Unwin et al., 2001].

6. Finance

Over the last decade more funds have been raised to combat the HIV epidemic than have ever been made available for a single disease. The above described successes would never have been achieved without these funds. However, due to the number of HIV-infected people and the chronic nature of the disease, there remains a continued need for large amounts of money. Expansion of preventive strategies, earlier and wider access to ART, increased availability of laboratory testing, and improved health care facilities for both HIV-infected and HIV-uninfected individuals are all urgently needed, but costly. HIV-care is generally sponsor-based, making it sensitive to global economic instability. Currently, the economic crisis, and possibly donor fatigue, are negatively influencing the amount of money donors are willing to spend on the worldwide HIV epidemic [Ewing, 1990]. Therefore, using the available resources as efficiently as possible is of utmost importance. Prioritizing is needed when treatment capacity is limited, but leads to many difficult ethical and humanitarian dilemmas. Rather than considering the costs associated with expanding HIV care, we should consider the costs of not treating all HIV-infected individuals. A recent modelling study argues that by spending the available money wisely, but rapidly, eradication of AIDS will be feasible. Holding money in reserve now, could lead to extra, unnecessary infections and therefore extra costs in the future [Smith et al., 2009]. Moreover, the loss of large numbers of people who are in their working age and the resulting increase in HIV-related orphans has an enormous negative impact on economies and future generations. Therefore, continued attention and funds are still needed to control the HIV epidemic and to hopefully make HIV care more affordable in the future.

7. Conclusion

Since the start of the HIV epidemic, much progress has been made regarding global HIV-care. The joint efforts of people, organisations and governments around the world made it possible to reverse a previously fatal disease to a chronic condition and to prevent many from becoming newly infected. This is a great accomplishment. Still, the time to "sit back and relax" has by no means been reached. As in LICs large-scale ART has only been available for a couple of years, the long-term effects of HIV infections and their treatment in different groups of people are still unknown. Where initial programmes were mainly focussed on treating as many HIV-infected people as possible, future studies need to focus on the long-term care. There are important differences, both in host as in viral factors, between the western and African HIV epidemics. The long-term treatment effects, adverse events and viral resistance profiles in African ART programmes therefore need to be analyzed. In addition to the currently available strategies, new preventive methods and treatments are under development. Testing their efficacy and making them available in LICs should be another focus of future research. Moreover, by extending the focus beyond HIV-care and trying to improve the care for other important chronic diseases, HIV scale-up may generate substantial benefits for the broader health system in many countries.

8. Acknowledgement

We would like to thank Hugo Tempelman and all the people working at Ndlovu Medical Centre for their hard work in order to achieve a better standard of HIV care in Sub-Saharan Africa and for supporting research in a rural, South African setting.

9. References

United Nations. 2001. Declaration of Commitment on HIV/AIDS. "Global crisis - Global action."New York: United Nations, 2001. Accessed at: http://www.un.org/ga/aids/docs/aress262.pdf.

USAID, UNAIDS, WHO, CDC and the POLICY project. 2004. Coverage of selected services for HIV/AIDS prevention, care and support in low and middle income countries in 2003. Accessed at: http://www.who.int/hiv/pub/prev_care/en/coveragereport_2003.pdf.

Abdool Karim SS, Churchyard GJ, Abdool Karim Q, Lawn SD. 2009. HIV infection and tuberculosis in South Africa: an urgent need to escalate the public health response. Lancet 374(9693):921-933.

Al-Jabri AA, Alenzi FQ. 2009. Vaccines, virucides and drugs against HIV/AIDS: hopes and optimisms for the future. Open AIDS J 3:1-3.

Arrive E, Newell ML, Ekouevi DK, Chaix ML, Thiebaut R, Masquelier B, Leroy V, Perre PV, Rouzioux C, Dabis F. 2007. Prevalence of resistance to nevirapine in mothers and children after single-dose exposure to prevent vertical transmission of HIV-1: a meta-analysis. Int J Epidemiol 36(5):1009-1021.

Auvert B, Taljaard D, Lagarde E, Sobngwi-Tambekou J, Sitta R, Puren A. 2005. Randomized, controlled intervention trial of male circumcision for reduction of HIV infection risk: the ANRS 1265 Trial. PLoS Med 2(11):e298.

Badri M, Wilson D, Wood R. 2002. Effect of highly active antiretroviral therapy on incidence of tuberculosis in South Africa: a cohort study. Lancet 359(9323):2059-2064.

Barth RE, Huijgen Q, Taljaard J, Hoepelman AI. 2010a. Hepatitis B/C and HIV in sub-Saharan Africa: an association between highly prevalent infectious diseases. A systematic review and meta-analysis. Int J Infect Dis 14(12):e1024-1031.

Barth RE SvdLM, Schuurman R, Hoepelman AIM, Wensing AJM. 2010b. Virological follow up of adult patients in antiretroviral treatment programmes in Sub-Saharan Africa: a Review. Lancet Infect Dis: 10(3):155-166.

Barth RE, Tempelman HA, Smelt E, Wensing AM, Hoepelman AI, Geelen SP. 2010c. Long-Term Outcome of Children Receiving Antiretroviral Treatment in Rural South Africa: Substantial Virologic Failure on First-Line Treatment. Pediatr Infect Dis J.

Barth RE, Wensing AM, Tempelman HA, Moraba R, Schuurman R, Hoepelman AI. 2008. Rapid accumulation of nonnucleoside reverse transcriptase inhibitor-associated resistance: evidence of transmitted resistance in rural South Africa. Aids 22(16):2210-2212.

Bartolo I, Rocha C, Bartolomeu J, Gama A, Fonseca M, Mendes A, Cristina F, Thamm S, Epalanga M, Silva PC, Taveira N. 2009. Antiretroviral drug resistance surveillance among treatment-naive human immunodeficiency virus type 1-infected individuals in Angola: evidence for low level of transmitted drug resistance. Antimicrob Agents Chemother 53(7):3156-3158.

Boeke CE, Jackson JB. 2008. Estimate of infant HIV-free survival at 6 to 8 weeks of age due to maternal antiretroviral prophylaxis in Sub-Saharan Africa, 2004-2005. J Int Assoc Physicians AIDS Care (Chic Ill) 7(3):133-140.

Bonnet MM, Pinoges LL, Varaine FF, Oberhauser BB, O'Brien DD, Kebede YY, Hewison CC, Zachariah RR, Ferradini LL. 2006. Tuberculosis after HAART initiation in HIV-positive patients from five countries with a high tuberculosis burden. Aids 20(9):1275-1279.

Braithwaite RS, Roberts MS, Chang CC, Goetz MB, Gibert CL, Rodriguez-Barradas MC, Shechter S, Schaefer A, Nucifora K, Koppenhaver R, Justice AC. 2008. Influence of alternative thresholds for initiating HIV treatment on quality-adjusted life expectancy: a decision model. Ann Intern Med 148(3):178-185.

Brinkhof MW, Egger M, Boulle A, May M, Hosseinipour M, Sprinz E, Braitstein P, Dabis F, Reiss P, Bangsberg DR, Rickenbach M, Miro JM, Myer L, Mocroft A, Nash D, Keiser O, Pascoe M, van der Borght S, Schechter M. 2007. Tuberculosis after initiation of antiretroviral therapy in low-income and high-income countries. Clin Infect Dis 45(11):1518-1521.

Burnett RJ, Francois G, Kew MC, Leroux-Roels G, Meheus A, Hoosen AA, Mphahlele MJ. 2005. Hepatitis B virus and human immunodeficiency virus co-infection in sub-Saharan Africa: a call for further investigation. Liver Int 25(2):201-213.

Bussmann H, Novitsky V, Wester W, Peter T, Masupu K, Gabaitiri L, Kim S, Gaseitsiwe S, Ndungu T, Marlink R, Thior I, Essex M. 2005. HIV-1 subtype C drug-resistance background among ARV-naive adults in Botswana. Antivir Chem Chemother 16(2):103-115.

Castelnuovo B, John L, Lutwama F, Ronald A, Spacek LA, Bates M, Kamya MR, Colebunders R. 2009a. Three-year outcome data of second-line antiretroviral therapy in Ugandan adults: good virological response but high rate of toxicity. J Int Assoc Physicians AIDS Care (Chic Ill) 8(1):52-59.

Castelnuovo B, Kiragga A, Schaefer P, Kambugu A, Manabe Y. 2009b. High rate of misclassification of treatment failure based on WHO immunological criteria. Aids 23(10):1295-1296; author reply 1296.

Chen TY, Ding EL, Seage Iii GR, Kim AY. 2009. Meta-analysis: increased mortality associated with hepatitis C in HIV-infected persons is unrelated to HIV disease progression. Clin Infect Dis 49(10):1605-1615.

Chi BH, Sinkala M, Mbewe F, Cantrell RA, Kruse G, Chintu N, Aldrovandi GM, Stringer EM, Kankasa C, Safrit JT, Stringer JS. 2007a. Single-dose tenofovir and emtricitabine for reduction of viral resistance to non-nucleoside reverse transcriptase inhibitor drugs in women given intrapartum nevirapine for perinatal HIV prevention: an open-label randomised trial. Lancet 370(9600):1698-1705.

Chi BH, Sinkala M, Stringer EM, Cantrell RA, Mtonga V, Bulterys M, Zulu I, Kankasa C, Wilfert C, Weidle PJ, Vermund SH, Stringer JS. 2007b. Early clinical and immune response to NNRTI-based antiretroviral therapy among women with prior exposure to single-dose nevirapine. Aids 21(8):957-964.

Chigwedere P, Seage GR, Lee TH, Essex M. 2008. Efficacy of antiretroviral drugs in reducing mother-to-child transmission of HIV in Africa: a meta-analysis of published clinical trials. AIDS Res Hum Retroviruses 24(6):827-837.

Chopra M, Lawn JE, Sanders D, Barron P, Abdool Karim SS, Bradshaw D, Jewkes R, Abdool Karim Q, Flisher AJ, Mayosi BM, Tollman SM, Churchyard GJ, Coovadia H. 2009. Achieving the health Millennium Development Goals for South Africa: challenges and priorities. Lancet 374(9694):1023-1031.

Ciaranello AL, Chang Y, Margulis AV, Bernstein A, Bassett IV, Losina E, Walensky RP. 2009. Effectiveness of pediatric antiretroviral therapy in resource-limited settings: a systematic review and meta-analysis. Clin Infect Dis 49(12):1915-1927.

Cooper CL, Mills E, Wabwire BO, Ford N, Olupot-Olupot P. 2009. Chronic viral hepatitis may diminish the gains of HIV antiretroviral therapy in sub-Saharan Africa. Int J Infect Dis 13(3):302-306.

Cozzi-Lepri A, Phillips AN, Ruiz L, Clotet B, Loveday C, Kjaer J, Mens H, Clumeck N, Viksna L, Antunes F, Machala L, Lundgren JD. 2007. Evolution of drug resistance in HIV-infected patients remaining on a virologically failing combination antiretroviral therapy regimen. Aids 21(6):721-732.

Crowley S, Rollins N, Shaffer N, Guerma T, Vitoria M, Lo YR. 2009. New WHO HIV treatment and prevention guidelines. Lancet.

Derache A, Maiga AI, Traore O, Akonde A, Cisse M, Jarrousse B, Koita V, Diarra B, Carcelain G, Barin F, Pizzocolo C, Pizarro L, Katlama C, Calvez V, Marcelin AG. 2008. Evolution of genetic diversity and drug resistance mutations in HIV-1 among untreated patients from Mali between 2005 and 2006. J Antimicrob Chemother 62(3):456-463.

Doyle SM, Kahn JG, Hosang N, Carroll PR. The impact of male circumcision on HIV transmission. J Urol 183(1):21-26.

Emery S, Neuhaus JA, Phillips AN, Babiker A, Cohen CJ, Gatell JM, Girard PM, Grund B, Law M, Losso MH, Palfreeman A, Wood R. 2008. Major clinical outcomes in antiretroviral therapy (ART)-naive participants and in those not receiving ART at baseline in the SMART study. J Infect Dis 197(8):1133-1144.

Ewing T. 1990. AIDS programme faces donor fatigue. Nature 346(6285):595.

Fang G, Burger H, Grimson R, Tropper P, Nachman S, Mayers D, Weislow O, Moore R, Reyelt C, Hutcheon N, Baker D, Weiser B. 1995. Maternal plasma human immunodeficiency virus type 1 RNA level: a determinant and projected threshold for mother-to-child transmission. Proc Natl Acad Sci U S A 92(26):12100-12104.

Fauci AS, Johnston MI, Dieffenbach CW, Burton DR, Hammer SM, Hoxie JA, Martin M, Overbaugh J, Watkins DI, Mahmoud A, Greene WC. 2008. HIV vaccine research: the way forward. Science 321(5888):530-532.

Ferrand RA, Corbett EL, Wood R, Hargrove J, Ndhlovu CE, Cowan FM, Gouws E, Williams BG. 2009. AIDS among older children and adolescents in Southern Africa: projecting the time course and magnitude of the epidemic. Aids 23(15):2039-2046.

Franey C, Knott D, Barnighausen T, Dedicoat M, Adam A, Lessells RJ, Newell ML, Cooke GS. 2009. Renal impairment in a rural African antiretroviral programme. BMC Infect Dis 9:143.

Friis-Moller N, Reiss P, Sabin CA, Weber R, Monforte A, El-Sadr W, Thiebaut R, De Wit S, Kirk O, Fontas E, Law MG, Phillips A, Lundgren JD. 2007. Class of antiretroviral drugs and the risk of myocardial infarction. N Engl J Med 356(17):1723-1735.

Gallant JE, Moore RD. 2009. Renal function with use of a tenofovir-containing initial antiretroviral regimen. Aids 23(15):1971-1975.

Gill GV, Mbanya JC, Ramaiya KL, Tesfaye S. 2009. A sub-Saharan African perspective of diabetes. Diabetologia 52(1):8-16.

Granich RM, Gilks CF, Dye C, De Cock KM, Williams BG. 2009. Universal voluntary HIV testing with immediate antiretroviral therapy as a strategy for elimination of HIV transmission: a mathematical model. Lancet 373(9657):48-57.

Grant RM, Hamer D, Hope T, Johnston R, Lange J, Lederman MM, Lieberman J, Miller CJ, Moore JP, Mosier DE, Richman DD, Schooley RT, Springer MS, Veazey RS, Wainberg MA. 2008. Whither or wither microbicides? Science 321(5888):532-534.

Grunfeld C, Delaney JA, Wanke C, Currier JS, Scherzer R, Biggs ML, Tien PC, Shlipak MG, Sidney S, Polak JF, O'Leary D, Bacchetti P, Kronmal RA. 2009. Preclinical atherosclerosis due to HIV infection: carotid intima-medial thickness measurements from the FRAM study. Aids 23(14):1841-1849.

Gupta R, Hill A, Sawyer AW, Pillay D. 2008. Emergence of drug resistance in HIV type 1-infected patients after receipt of first-line highly active antiretroviral therapy: a systematic review of clinical trials. Clin Infect Dis 47(5):712-722.

Hoffmann CJ, Charalambous S, Sim J, Ledwaba J, Schwikkard G, Chaisson RE, Fielding KL, Churchyard GJ, Morris L, Grant AD. 2009. Viremia, resuppression, and time to resistance in human immunodeficiency virus (HIV) subtype C during first-line antiretroviral therapy in South Africa. Clin Infect Dis 49(12):1928-1935.

Hosseinipour MC, Kumwenda JJ, Weigel R, Brown LB, Mzinganjira D, Mhango B, Eron JJ, Phiri S, van Oosterhout JJ. Second-line treatment in the Malawi antiretroviral programme: high early mortality, but good outcomes in survivors, despite extensive drug resistance at baseline. HIV Med 11(8):510-518.

Hsue PY, Hunt PW, Wu Y, Schnell A, Ho JE, Hatano H, Xie Y, Martin JN, Ganz P, Deeks SG. 2009. Association of abacavir and impaired endothelial function in treated and suppressed HIV-infected patients. Aids 23(15):2021-2027.

Jacobson DL, Spiegelman D, Knox TK, Wilson IB. 2008. Evolution and predictors of change in total bone mineral density over time in HIV-infected men and women in the nutrition for healthy living study. J Acquir Immune Defic Syndr 49(3):298-308.

Johnston MI, Fauci AS. 2008. An HIV vaccine--challenges and prospects. N Engl J Med 359(9):888-890.

Kantor R, Diero L, Delong A, Kamle L, Muyonga S, Mambo F, Walumbe E, Emonyi W, Chan P, Carter EJ, Hogan J, Buziba N. 2009. Misclassification of first-line antiretroviral treatment failure based on immunological monitoring of HIV infection in resource-limited settings. Clin Infect Dis 49(3):454-462.

Keiser O, MacPhail P, Boulle A, Wood R, Schechter M, Dabis F, Sprinz E, Egger M. 2009. Accuracy of WHO CD4 cell count criteria for virological failure of antiretroviral therapy. Trop Med Int Health 14(10):1220-1225.

Kerr T, Kaplan K, Suwannawong P, Jurgens R, Wood E. 2004. The Global Fund to Fight AIDS, Tuberculosis and Malaria: funding for unpopular public-health programmes. Lancet 364(9428):11-12.

Kitahata MG, S: Moore, R. North American AIDS Cohort Collaboration on Research and Design. Initiating rather than deferring HAART at a CD4+ count >500cells/mm3 is associated with imporved survival [Abstract 71]. Montreal, Quebec, Canada, 8-11 February 2009.

Koenig SP, Riviere C, Leger P, Joseph P, Severe P, Parker K, Collins S, Lee E, Pape JW, Fitzgerald DW. 2009. High mortality among patients with AIDS who received a diagnosis of tuberculosis in the first 3 months of antiretroviral therapy. Clin Infect Dis 48(6):829-831.

Kuritzkes DR, Lalama CM, Ribaudo HJ, Marcial M, Meyer WA, 3rd, Shikuma C, Johnson VA, Fiscus SA, D'Aquila RT, Schackman BR, Acosta EP, Gulick RM. 2008. Preexisting resistance to nonnucleoside reverse-transcriptase inhibitors predicts virologic failure of an efavirenz-based regimen in treatment-naive HIV-1-infected subjects. J Infect Dis 197(6):867-870.

Lavanchy D. 2004. Hepatitis B virus epidemiology, disease burden, treatment, and current and emerging prevention and control measures. J Viral Hepat 11(2):97-107.

Lawn SD, Badri M, Wood R. 2005. Tuberculosis among HIV-infected patients receiving HAART: long term incidence and risk factors in a South African cohort. Aids 19(18):2109-2116.

Lawn SD, Edwards DJ, Wood R. Reducing the burden of tuberculosis presenting during the initial months of antiretroviral therapy in resource-limited settings. Clin Infect Dis 50(1):124-125; author reply 125.

Lawn SD, Harries AD, Anglaret X, Myer L, Wood R. 2008. Early mortality among adults accessing antiretroviral treatment programmes in sub-Saharan Africa. Aids 22(15):1897-1908.

Leroy V, Ekouevi DK, Becquet R, Viho I, Dequae-Merchadou L, Tonwe-Gold B, Rouet F, Sakarovitch C, Horo A, Timite-Konan M, Rouzioux C, Dabis F. 2008. 18-month effectiveness of short-course antiretroviral regimens combined with alternatives to breastfeeding to prevent HIV mother-to-child transmission. PLoS One 3(2):e1645.

Liaw YF, Leung NW, Chang TT, Guan R, Tai DI, Ng KY, Chien RN, Dent J, Roman L, Edmundson S, Lai CL. 2000. Effects of extended lamivudine therapy in Asian patients with chronic hepatitis B. Asia Hepatitis Lamivudine Study Group. Gastroenterology 119(1):172-180.

Lim SG, Wai CT, Rajnakova A, Kajiji T, Guan R. 2002. Fatal hepatitis B reactivation following discontinuation of nucleoside analogues for chronic hepatitis B. Gut 51(4):597-599.

Lockman S, Shapiro RL, Smeaton LM, Wester C, Thior I, Stevens L, Chand F, Makhema J, Moffat C, Asmelash A, Ndase P, Arimi P, van Widenfelt E, Mazhani L, Novitsky V, Lagakos S, Essex M. 2007. Response to antiretroviral therapy after a single, peripartum dose of nevirapine. N Engl J Med 356(2):135-147.

Lok AS, Hussain M, Cursano C, Margotti M, Gramenzi A, Grazi GL, Jovine E, Benardi M, Andreone P. 2000. Evolution of hepatitis B virus polymerase gene mutations in hepatitis B e antigen-negative patients receiving lamivudine therapy. Hepatology 32(5):1145-1153.

Lopez AD, Mathers CD, Ezzati M, Jamison DT, Murray CJ. 2006. Global and regional burden of disease and risk factors, 2001: systematic analysis of population health data. Lancet 367(9524):1747-1757.

Madruga JV, Berger D, McMurchie M, Suter F, Banhegyi D, Ruxrungtham K, Norris D, Lefebvre E, de Bethune MP, Tomaka F, De Pauw M, Vangeneugden T, Spinosa-Guzman S. 2007. Efficacy and safety of darunavir-ritonavir compared with that of lopinavir-ritonavir at 48 weeks in treatment-experienced, HIV-infected patients in TITAN: a randomised controlled phase III trial. Lancet 370(9581):49-58.

Manabe YC, Breen R, Perti T, Girardi E, Sterling TR. 2009. Unmasked tuberculosis and tuberculosis immune reconstitution inflammatory disease: a disease spectrum after initiation of antiretroviral therapy. J Infect Dis 199(3):437-444.

Marcellin P, Heathcote EJ, Buti M, Gane E, de Man RA, Krastev Z, Germanidis G, Lee SS, Flisiak R, Kaita K, Manns M, Kotzev I, Tchernev K, Buggisch P, Weilert F, Kurdas OO, Shiffman ML, Trinh H, Washington MK, Sorbel J, Anderson J, Snow-Lampart A, Mondou E, Quinn J, Rousseau F. 2008. Tenofovir disoproxil fumarate versus adefovir dipivoxil for chronic hepatitis B. N Engl J Med 359(23):2442-2455.

Marconi VC, Sunpath H, Lu Z, Gordon M, Koranteng-Apeagyei K, Hampton J, Carpenter S, Giddy J, Ross D, Holst H, Losina E, Walker BD, Kuritzkes DR. 2008. Prevalence of HIV-1 drug resistance after failure of a first highly active antiretroviral therapy regimen in KwaZulu Natal, South Africa. Clin Infect Dis 46(10):1589-1597.

Mayer KH, Venkatesh KK. Antiretroviral therapy as HIV prevention: status and prospects. Am J Public Health 100(10):1867-1876.

Mayosi BM, Flisher AJ, Lalloo UG, Sitas F, Tollman SM, Bradshaw D. 2009. The burden of non-communicable diseases in South Africa. Lancet 374(9693):934-947.

Merson MH. 2006. The HIV-AIDS pandemic at 25--the global response. N Engl J Med 354(23):2414-2417.

Mills EJ, Nachega JB, Buchan I, Orbinski J, Attaran A, Singh S, Rachlis B, Wu P, Cooper C, Thabane L, Wilson K, Guyatt GH, Bangsberg DR. 2006. Adherence to antiretroviral therapy in sub-Saharan Africa and North America: a meta-analysis. Jama 296(6):679-690.

Modi AA, Feld JJ. 2007. Viral hepatitis and HIV in Africa. AIDS Rev 9(1):25-39.

Montaner JS, Hogg R, Wood E, Kerr T, Tyndall M, Levy AR, Harrigan PR. 2006. The case for expanding access to highly active antiretroviral therapy to curb the growth of the HIV epidemic. Lancet 368(9534):531-536.

Moore D, Liechty C, Ekwaru P, Were W, Mwima G, Solberg P, Rutherford G, Mermin J. 2007. Prevalence, incidence and mortality associated with tuberculosis in HIV-infected patients initiating antiretroviral therapy in rural Uganda. Aids 21(6):713-719.

Murray CJ, Lopez AD. 1997. Mortality by cause for eight regions of the world: Global Burden of Disease Study. Lancet 349(9061):1269-1276.

Nikolopoulos GK, Paraskevis D, Hatzitheodorou E, Moschidis Z, Sypsa V, Zavitsanos X, Kalapothaki V, Hatzakis A. 2009. Impact of hepatitis B virus infection on the progression of AIDS and mortality in HIV-infected individuals: a cohort study and meta-analysis. Clin Infect Dis 48(12):1763-1771.

Paintsil E, Andiman WA. 2007. Care and management of the infant of the HIV-1-infected mother. Semin Perinatol 31(2):112-123.

Paintsil E, Andiman WA. 2009. Update on successes and challenges regarding mother-to-child transmission of HIV. Curr Opin Pediatr 21(1):94-101.

Palombi L, Marazzi MC, Voetberg A, Magid NA. 2007. Treatment acceleration program and the experience of the DREAM program in prevention of mother-to-child transmission of HIV. Aids 21 Suppl 4:S65-71.

Petersen ML, van der Laan MJ, Napravnik S, Eron JJ, Moore RD, Deeks SG. 2008. Long-term consequences of the delay between virologic failure of highly active antiretroviral therapy and regimen modification. Aids 22(16):2097-2106.

Quinn TC, Wawer MJ, Sewankambo N, Serwadda D, Li C, Wabwire-Mangen F, Meehan MO, Lutalo T, Gray RH. 2000. Viral load and heterosexual transmission of human immunodeficiency virus type 1. Rakai Project Study Group. N Engl J Med 342(13):921-929.

Reynolds SJ, Kityo C, Mbamanya F, Dewar R, Ssali F, Quinn TC, Mugyenyi P, Dybul M. 2009a. Evolution of drug resistance after virological failure of a first-line highly active antiretroviral therapy regimen in Uganda. Antivir Ther 14(2):293-297.

Reynolds SJ, Nakigozi G, Newell K, Ndyanabo A, Galiwongo R, Boaz I, Quinn TC, Gray R, Wawer M, Serwadda D. 2009b. Failure of immunologic criteria to appropriately identify antiretroviral treatment failure in Uganda. Aids 23(6):697-700.

Riddler SA, Haubrich R, DiRienzo AG, Peeples L, Powderly WG, Klingman KL, Garren KW, George T, Rooney JF, Brizz B, Lalloo UG, Murphy RL, Swindells S, Havlir D, Mellors JW. 2008. Class-sparing regimens for initial treatment of HIV-1 infection. N Engl J Med 358(20):2095-2106.

Rockstroh JK, Mocroft A, Soriano V, Tural C, Losso MH, Horban A, Kirk O, Phillips A, Ledergerber B, Lundgren J. 2005. Influence of hepatitis C virus infection on HIV-1 disease progression and response to highly active antiretroviral therapy. J Infect Dis 192(6):992-1002.

Sepkowitz KA. 2006. One disease, two epidemics--AIDS at 25. N Engl J Med 354(23):2411-2414.

Sliwa K, Mocumbi AO. 2009. Forgotten cardiovascular diseases in Africa. Clin Res Cardiol.

Smith DK, Taylor A, Kilmarx PH, Sullivan P, Warner L, Kamb M, Bock N, Kohmescher B, Mastro TD. Male circumcision in the United States for the prevention of HIV infection and other adverse health outcomes: report from a CDC consultation. Public Health Rep 125 Suppl 1:72-82.

Smith RJ, Li J, Gordon R, Heffernan JM. 2009. Can we spend our way out of the AIDS epidemic? A world halting AIDS model. BMC Public Health 9 Suppl 1:S15.

Sterne. When to start consortium. When should HIV-1infected infected persons initiate ART? Collaborative analysis of HIV cohort studies [Abstract 72LB]. Montreal, Quebec, Canada, 8-11 February 2009.

Thio CL. 2009. Hepatitis B and human immunodeficiency virus coinfection. Hepatology 49(5 Suppl):S138-145.

Tonwe-Gold B, Ekouevi DK, Viho I, Amani-Bosse C, Toure S, Coffie PA, Rouet F, Becquet R, Leroy V, El-Sadr WM, Abrams EJ, Dabis F. 2007. Antiretroviral treatment and prevention of peripartum and postnatal HIV transmission in West Africa: evaluation of a two-tiered approach. PLoS Med 4(8):e257.

Tovanabutra S, Robison V, Wongtrakul J, Sennum S, Suriyanon V, Kingkeow D, Kawichai S, Tanan P, Duerr A, Nelson KE. 2002. Male viral load and heterosexual transmission of HIV-1 subtype E in northern Thailand. J Acquir Immune Defic Syndr 29(3):275-283.

UNAIDS. 2005a. Financing the expanded response to AIDS: HIV vaccine and microbicide research and development. Accessed at:

http://data.unaids.org/UNAdocs/financingresdevvaccinemicrobicide_report_en.pdf.

UNAIDS. 2005b. Resource needs for an expanded response to AIDS in low- and middle-income countries. Accessed at: http://data.unaids.org/pub/Report/2005/jc1239_resource_needs_en.pdf.

UNAIDS. 2009. AIDS epidemic update. http://www.unaids.org/en/media/unaids/contentassets/dataimport/pub/report/2009/jc1700_epi_update_2009_en.pdf.

Unwin N, Setel P, Rashid S, Mugusi F, Mbanya JC, Kitange H, Hayes L, Edwards R, Aspray T, Alberti KG. 2001. Noncommunicable diseases in sub-Saharan Africa: where do they feature in the health research agenda? Bull World Health Organ 79(10):947-953.

von Wyl V, Yerly S, Boni J, Burgisser P, Klimkait T, Battegay M, Furrer H, Telenti A, Hirschel B, Vernazza PL, Bernasconi E, Rickenbach M, Perrin L, Ledergerber B, Gunthard HF. 2007. Emergence of HIV-1 drug resistance in previously untreated patients initiating combination antiretroviral treatment: a comparison of different regimen types. Arch Intern Med 167(16):1782-1790.

Walensky RP, Wolf LL, Wood R, Fofana MO, Freedberg KA, Martinson NA, Paltiel AD, Anglaret X, Weinstein MC, Losina E. 2009. When to start antiretroviral therapy in resource-limited settings. Ann Intern Med 151(3):157-166.

Weiss HA, Hankins CA, Dickson K. 2009. Male circumcision and risk of HIV infection in women: a systematic review and meta-analysis. Lancet Infect Dis 9(11):669-677.

Wensing AM, van de Vijver DA, Angarano G, Asjo B, Balotta C, Boeri E, Camacho R, Chaix ML, Costagliola D, De Luca A, Derdelinckx I, Grossman Z, Hamouda O, Hatzakis A, Hemmer R, Hoepelman A, Horban A, Korn K, Kucherer C, Leitner T, Loveday C, MacRae E, Maljkovic I, de Mendoza C, Meyer L, Nielsen C, Op de Coul EL, Ormaasen V, Paraskevis D, Perrin L, Puchhammer-Stockl E, Ruiz L, Salminen M, Schmit JC, Schneider F, Schuurman R, Soriano V, Stanczak G, Stanojevic M, Vandamme AM, Van Laethem K, Violin M, Wilbe K, Yerly S, Zazzi M, Boucher CA. 2005. Prevalence of drug-resistant HIV-1 variants in untreated individuals in Europe: implications for clinical management. J Infect Dis 192(6):958-966.

WHO. 2006a. antiretroviral therapy for HIV infection in adults and adolescents: recommendations for a public health approach. p accessed at: http://www.who.int/hiv/pub/guidelines/artadultguidelines.pdf.

WHO. 2006b. Global access to HIV therapy tripled in past two years, but significant challenges remain. p Accessed at: http://www.who.int/hiv/mediacentre/news57/en/index.html.

WHO. 2007. AIDS epidemic update. http://www.unaids.org/en/KnowledgeCentre/HIVData/EpiUpdate/EpiUpdArchive/2007/.

WHO. 2009. Global Tuberculosis control report. p Accessed at: http://www.who.int/tb/publications/global_report/2009/update/tbu_2009.pdf.

Williams BG, Lloyd-Smith JO, Gouws E, Hankins C, Getz WM, Hargrove J, de Zoysa I, Dye C, Auvert B. 2006. The potential impact of male circumcision on HIV in Sub-Saharan Africa. PLoS Med 3(7):e262.

Wilson DP, Coplan PM, Wainberg MA, Blower SM. 2008. The paradoxical effects of using antiretroviral-based microbicides to control HIV epidemics. Proc Natl Acad Sci U S A 105(28):9835-9840.

Wood E, Hogg RS, Harrigan PR, Montaner JS. 2005. When to initiate antiretroviral therapy in HIV-1-infected adults: a review for clinicians and patients. Lancet Infect Dis 5(7):407-414.

6

AIDS and Opportunistic Infections

Aydin Çiledağ and Demet Karnak
Ankara University School of Medicine, Chest Disease Department, Cebeci-Ankara, Turkey

1. Introduction

Pulmonary parenchymal complications remain the main cause of morbidity and mortality in human immunodeficiency virus (HIV) infected patients (McGuinness, 1997). Early diagnosis and treatment of these complications are important to improve survival.

HIV impairs the immune system, leading the infected person susceptible to a variety of infections, called opportunistic infections, a leading cause of mortality and morbidity in patients with HIV/AIDS. The effect of HIV on the immune system is monitored by measuring the CD4 (T-helper) lymphocyte count in the blood. Depletion of CD4 cell count is a hallmark of disease progression in AIDS. CD4 cell count is essential to decide about the timing of initiation of antiretroviral therapy and for prophylaxis of opportunistic infections.

It has been known that the lungs are principal targets of HIV-associated complications and persons with HIV infection are at an increased risk for opportunistic pneumonias, neoplasms, and other pulmonary conditions. The spectrum of pulmonary manifestations in patients infected with HIV is broad, including many infectious and noninfectious complications. Pneumonia is the leading HIV-associated infection. In a recent report in which 762 patients with HIV/AIDS were analyzed, pulmonary infections was found as the most prevalent infections (Huang et al., 2010). It is estimated that 65% of the patients infected with HIV will present pulmonary involvement as their first clinical manifestation of the syndrome and that approximately 80% of these patients will present some kind of pulmonary involvement in the course of the disease (Suffredini & Masur, 1988).

This section is related with the pulmonary infectious complications of HIV/AIDS.

2. Bacterial infections

Bacterial respiratory infections are one of the most common causes of respiratory complaints in HIV-positive patients.

Although HIV infection is most closely associated with altered cell-mediated immunity, a number of additional immune deficiencies may occur in association with HIV infection (Daley, 1993; Davis et al, 1993; Noskin & Glassroth, 1996). It usually includes a poor antibody response due to B cell dysfunction and defects in chemotaxis, phagocytosis and intracellular killing by monocytes, macrophages and neutrophils. Moreover, HIV-infected individuals may experience impairment of local defenses, manifested by a depression of specific IgA at the mucosal surfaces. These immune abnormalities all contribute to an increased risk of bacterial infection among HIV-infected persons.

Combination antiretroviral therapy (ART) is associated with a decreased risk for bacterial pneumonia and during the combination ART era the incidence of community-acquired bacterial pneumonia among HIV-infected patients has declined (Crothers et al., 2010). Antiretroviral regimens contain an HIV protease inhibitor (Sullivan et al., 2000) and the use of trimethoprim-sulfamethoxazole as prophylaxis for *Pneumocystis jiroveci* pneumonia may be associated with decreased risk for bacterial pneumonia (Kohli et al., 2006). However, community-acquired pneumonia represents a frequent cause of morbidity and is associated with an increased mortality in HIV-infected patients also in the ART era.

Bacterial pneumonia may be the first manifestation of underlying HIV infection and thus the presence of HIV infection should be considered in any person presenting with bacterial pneumonia, especially if the individual has no other risk factors for pneumonia or if the pneumonia is recurrent. Recurrent bacterial pneumonia (defined as two or more episodes within 12 months) is included as an AIDS-defining illness in the 1993 CDC Expanded Surveillance Case Definition for AIDS (Centers for Disease Control and Prevention, 1993).

The incidence of bacterial pneumonia among persons with HIV infection is greater than that among persons without HIV. It has been estimated that one third of all persons with AIDS will develop at least one episode of severe bacterial pneumonia over the course of their HIV infection (Noskin & Glassroth, 1996). Afessa et al. (Afessa et al., 1998) found bacterial pneumonia to be the most frequent pulmonary complication (42%) in an autopsy series of 233 HIV-infected individuals. In a recent autopsy study, in which 250 autopsies of HIV/AIDS patients who died of acute respiratory failure was analyzed, bacterial bronchopneumonia was present in 36% (91 cases) (Soeiro et al., 2008). According to another study, the incidence of pneumococcal pneumonia is five to 18 times greater than that in the general population, and the development of pneumococcal septicemia is 100 times greater (Janoff et al., 1992). In a multicenter, prospective, observational study, Hirschtick et al. monitored 1130 HIV-positive and 167 HIV-negative adults for up to 64 months for pulmonary disease and they found that, there were 237 episodes of bacterial pneumonia among the HIV-positive participants (rate, 5.5 per 100 person-years), as compared with 6 episodes among the HIV-negative participants (rate, 0.9 per 100 person years; $p<0.001$). They also showed that, the rate of bacterial pneumonia increased with decreasing CD4 lymphocyte counts (2.3,6.8, and 10.8 episodes per 100 person-years in the strata with more than 500, 200 to 500, and fewer than 200 cells per cubic millimeter, respectively; $p \leq 0.022$ for each comparison) (Hirschtick et al., 1995). Bacterial pneumonia is more common in smokers with HIV than in nonsmokers and injection drug use more than doubles the risk of bacterial lower respiratory infections compared with those who acquired HIV through sexual exposure (Fangman & Sax, 2008). Other risk factors are a low socioeconomic, alcohol abuse status, comorbidities (including cardiovascular, renal disease malnutrition, and hepatic cirrhosis), low CD4 cell counts (<200 cells/ml), uncontrolled HIV replication and not receiving ART (Madeddu et al., 2010).

Similar to that in the general population, *Streptococcus pneumoniae* and *Haemophilus* species are the most frequently identified causes of community-acquired bacterial pneumonia (Hirschtick et al., 1995; Madeddu et al., 2008; Schneider, 1999). *Staphylococcus aureus, Escherichia coli,* and *Pseudomonas aeruginosa* account for most of the remainder of cases (Afessa & Green, 2000; Baron & Hollander, 1993; Madeddu et al., 2008). Risk factors for *S. aureus* include recent viral or influenza infection and use of injection drugs. Methicillin-resistant *S. aureus* which may be acquired in health care setting or in the community is increasingly common. *P. aeruginosa* has been increasingly recognized as an important source of bacterial pneumonia in HIV-infected individuals, particularly in those with advanced HIV/AIDS (CD4 cell count less than 50 cells/µL), underlying structural lung disease (bronchiectasis), neutropenia, indwelling catheters, receipt of corticosteroid therapy, multiple antibiotic therapy, and severe malnutrition. Atypical pathogens such as *Legionella pneumophila, Mycoplasma pneumoniae,* and *Chlamydophila* species are less frequent causes of pneumonia (Sandkovsky et al., 2008). Other less causes of pneumonia include *Rhodococcus equi, Nocardia* species *Bartonella henselae* and *quintana. Rhodococcus equi,* an aerobic gram-positive, may cause focal consolidation, endobronchial disease and cavitation, and is usually associated with low CD4 cell count (100 cells/µl) in HIV/AIDS patients. *Nocardia asteroides* may cause nodules, consolidation, cavitation, pleural effusions, empyema and intrathoracic lymphadenopathy in HIV-infected persons.

In contrast with community-acquired pneumonia, the two most common bacterial causes of hospital- acquired pneumonia in patients with HIV are *P. Aeruginosa* and *S. Aureus,* while *S pneumoniae* and *K. Pneumoniae* are other relatively frequent causes (Crothers et al., 2010).

The clinical features of bacterial pneumonia in HIV-infected persons is similar to those in immunocompetent persons and includes acute onset of fever, dyspnea, dry or productive cough, chills and chest pain. Physical findings consist of fever, tachypnea, tachycardia, rales or rhonchi, and other signs of consolidation and occasionally pleural effusion (Huang & Crothers, 2009). Bacterial pneumonia in HIV-infected patients can occur at all levels of CD4 cell count, and an inverse relationship between the incidence of pneumonia and the CD4 cell count has been observed (Hirschtick et al., 1995). However, patients with higher CD4 cell counts are more likely to present with a typical clinical picture, in contrast, patients with low CD4 cell count often present an atypical clinical picture (Madeddu et al., 2010).

The most common radiographic pattern in bacterial pneumonia is focal consolidation, which typically presents in either a segmental or lobar distribution (Boiselle et al., 1997; Gold et al., 2002; Kuhlman, 1999; Selwyn et al., 1998; Sider et al. 1993). In two studies of HIV-infected individuals with bacterial pneumonia, focal consolidation was observed in approximately 45–60% of patients (Boiselle et al., 1997; Magnenat et al., 1991). Most persons with *S. pneumoniae* or *Haemophilus* pneumonia present with unilateral, focal, segmental or lobar consolidation. Lobar pneumonia is seen most commonly in *S. pneumoniae* pneumonia. A variety of gram (+) and gram (-) bacteria, most commonly *Staphylococcus, Streptococcus, Pseudomonas, Klebsiella, Enterobacter,*and *Haemophilus,* may cause bronchopneumonia.

In almost half of the cases of bacterial pneumonia, a radiographic pattern other than focal consolidation is observed (Brecher et al., 2003). Solitary or multiple lung nodules, cavitary pulmonary lesions are other radiologic findings often associated with bacterial pneumonia in HIV-infected patients. *P. aeruginosa* or *S. aureus* are most common bacterial causes of cavitary nodules or cavitary consolidation, while less common bacterial causes include *N. asteriodes* and *R. equi* infections. HIV-infected patients had an increased risk for complicated parapneumonic effusions, especially if due to *S. pneumoniae* or *S. aureus.*

Although conventional radiographs are the mainstay of imaging of bacterial respiratory infections in HIV-infected persons, CT provides more information about nodules, cavities, and pleural fluid collections. Hence, CT may be useful for further characterizing atypical radiographic findings, for diagnosing complications of infection such as abscess or empyema.

The diagnostic approach to bacterial pneumonia in HIV-infected patients is similar to that of HIV-negative patients. Current US guidelines recommend that persons hospitalized with suspected bacterial pneumonia should undergo diagnostic evaluation for specific pathogens (Centers for Disease Control and Prevention, 2009). The diagnostic tests include gram stain and culture of sputum, blood cultures and thoracentesis should be performed in patients with pleural effusions. Bronchoscopy should be done to support or establish correct diagnosis via taking wash, brush or biopsy. In patients in whom the diagnosis is unclear, other supplemental testing such as a modified acid-fast stain (for *Nocardia* and *Rhodacoccus*) or a urinary legionella antigen can be appropriate (Fangman & Sax, 2008). In pneumococcal pneumonia, pneumococcal urinary antigen testing offers the potential for early, specific diagnosis.

Although numerous guidelines (BTS guidelines, 2001; Mandell et al., 2007; Woodhead et al., 2005) for the management of community-acquired pneumonia (CAP) in HIV-negative patients have been developed by scientific societies, to date, no specific guidelines have been developed for HIV-infected patients. However, the principle of the treatment of bacterial pneumonia is similar in both HIV positive and negative patients (Fangman & Sax, 2008). The choice of antimicrobial agent should be based on the results of a sputum gram stain, the clinical and radiologic presentation, severity of the illness, presence of co-morbid disease and knowledge of local microbiology and resistance patterns. Duration of the therapy is generally similar or a bit longer than to that of HIV negative patients.

Although the emergence of antimicrobial resistant organisms is a global problem, in HIV-infected patients, there is limited data on the prevalence and the impact of drug resistant bacteria on the clinical course of the disease. The rate of penicillin-resistant *S. pneumoniae* in HIV-infected patients is reported to be higher than in HIV-noninfected patients (Madeddu et al., 2009). However, in a recent report, no obvious difference in pneumococci resistance patterns has been found between HIV-positive and negative patients (Stephan et al., 2009). Also, in a study in which the trend of *S. pneumoniae* antibiotic resistance has been evaluated, a near significant decrease in penicillin-resistant strains in the late-HAART compared with of pre and early-HAART era has been found (Grau et al., 2009). Patients on TMP-SMX prophylaxis for Pneumocystis pneumonia may be more likely to have penicillin and TMP-SMX resistant *S. pneumoniae.* With the widely use of TMP-SMX prophylaxis, *an increase in* resistance to *TMP-SMX* in other bacteria has also been reported (Marin et al., 1999).

Prevention strategies of bacterial pneumonia should address on several problems such as the role of cigarette smoking, alcohol abuse and ongoing injection drug use, hepatic and renal comorbidities, late presentation of HIV diagnosis, highly active antiretroviral therapy (HAART) lack of compliance, and virus effects and immunological failure. Combination antiviral therapy should be considered for all patients with recurrent bacterial lower respiratory tract infections. HIV patients not receiving HAART are clearly at an increased risk of bacterial pneumonia. Vaccination strategies are still controversial in HIV infected individuals. On the one hand, some studies showed a good response and a reduction in new cases among vaccinated patients, on the other, some reports found no evidence of efficacy. However, pneumococcal vaccine is recommended for all HIV patients who have a CD4 cell count greater than 200 cells/µl. The influenza vaccine should be given to all persons with HIV infection annually prior to influenza season. Trimethoprim-sulfamethoxazole, when administered daily for PCP prophylaxis, can reduce the frequency of bacterial respiratory infections (French et al., 2000; Loeliger et al., 1995; Rodriguez-Barradas et al., 1992).

3. Mycobacterial infections

Tuberculosis (TB) remains an important cause of morbidity and mortality among persons with HIV infection. Pulmonary TB is still the commonest form. In HIV infected persons, the estimated annual risk of developing active TB ranges from 35 to 162 per 1,000 person-years, compared to 12.9 per 1,000 person-years for those without HIV infection (Centers for Disease Control and Prevention, 2009). The World Health Organization (WHO) estimated that, in 2007, of the 9.27 million new cases of TB worldwide, 1.37 million occured in persons with HIV (World Health Organization, 2009). In 2008, nearly 1 of 3 TB-related deaths (29%) worldwide was considered to be related to HIV infection, and TB contributed to 26% of the estimated deaths due to HIV infection. HIV has increased the incidence of TB by up to sevenfold in African countries (Williams et al., 2010). Countries in southern Africa are particularly affected, with over 50% of TB patients diagnosed each year being co-infected with HIV (Corbett et al., 2003; World Health Organization, 2007). In 2007, countries in sub-Saharan Africa accounted for nearly 80% of the estimated global burden of HIV infection-associated TB. It has been reported that, TB is the commonest cause of death in hospitalized HIV-infected adults in sub-Saharan Africa (Sani et al., 2006; Lucas et al., 1993; Nelson et al., 1993) and in another report, among HIV-infected patients not on ART, it was the commonest cause of adult hospitalization, in Nigeria (Habib et al., 1998).

TB disease in persons with HIV infection can develop immediately after exposure (i.e. primary disease) or as a result of progression after establishment of latent TB infection. The risk of progression to active TB is highest in those with HIV coinfections (Lawn et al., 2011). While the lifetime risk of reactivation latent TB infection is 5% in HIV negative persons, the risk among HIV-infected persons has been estimated to be 10% per year. The interaction between HIV infection and tuberculosis is complex: HIV infection, by decreasing interferon-gamma production, increases the risk for the development of active TB disease. Following the initial exposure, the rate of progression of TB infection to active disease is higher than 40% in HIV positive patients compared to approximately 5% in HIV negative patients (Havlir & Barnes, 1999). On the other hand, *M. tuberculosis* enhances HIV replication and accelerates the natural progression of HIV infection by increasing cytokine production (in particular tumor necrosis factor-alpha).

TB disease occurs among HIV-infected persons at all CD4 T lymphocyte counts, but the incidence increases as the count decreases. Also, the clinical, radiographic, and histopathologic presentation of HIV-related TB disease is influenced by the degree of immunodeficiency. With CD4 T lymphocyte counts >350 cells/μL, HIV positive TB appears like TB among HIV negative persons. The majority of patients have disease limited to the lungs. However, extrapulmonary disease is more common in HIV positive cases than in HIV negative ones and those with advanced immunosuppression (CD4 T lymphocyte count <200 cells/μL) are more likely to have extrapulmonary or disseminated disease.

Although HIV positive persons with TB may have the classic symptoms of TB (eg, productive cough, chest pain, shortness of breath, hemoptysis, fever, night sweats, and/or weight loss), many such patients have few symptoms or have symptoms that are even less specific.

The radiographic findings of TB also depend on the degree of immunosuppression (Marchiori et al., 2005). In patients who have CD4 cell counts above 350-400 cells/μL, the findings tend to be similar to those without HIV infection. Most of these persons present with a classic reactivation TB radiographic pattern consisting of unilateral or bilateral upper lung zone reticulonodular infiltrates with or without cavitation. In more severely immunocompromised patients, the radiologic manifestations tend to resemble those of primary disease including areas of consolidation, miliary disease, pleural effusion, and lymph node enlargement (Laissy et al., 1998). Cavitation is less common but intrathoracic adenopathy is more common in these individuals with advanced HIV/AIDS. Up to 20% of severely immunocompromised AIDS patients with pulmonary TB have radiographs that show normal findings (Boiselle et al., 2002). The small nodules and lymph node enlargement are the usual findings at high resolution CT.

The diagnostic approach to TB in HIV positive person is same with those HIV negative ones. The gold standard diagnostic test for TB remains the isolation and identification of *M. Tuberculosis* by culture (Crothers et al., 2010). It is more sensitive than sputum smear, allowing detection of TB in sputum smear negative cases such as HIV positive patients. In a setting in South Africa, 49% of sputum smear negative HIV patients were sputum culture positive. All cultures positive for *M. Tuberculosis* should be sent for susceptibility testing to identify drug resistance.

Typically, diagnostic evaluation of suspected TB includes 2 to 3 sputum specimens sent for acid fast bacillus (AFB) smear and, mycobacterial culture. The quality and number of collected specimens affect diagnostic results. A systemic review in 2007 concluded that, the average sensitivity of the first sputum slide (53,5%) increased following the addition of second slide (64.9%), but not further with a third slide (Mase et al., 2007). Sputum smear microscopy is the primary tool for TB diagnosis. However, a lower sensitivity in HIV-patients is often seen due to their lower sputum bacillary load. Sputum microscopy may also be false-negative if the sputum concentration of mycobacteria is below 10,000 organisms/mL. Alternative sample processing methods may increase sensitivity. A systemic review showed that centrifugation or overnight sedimentation with chemical processing increases sputum smear sensitivity (Steingart et al., 2006). Fluorescent microscopy (FM) is an alternative way to Ziehl-Neelsen (ZN) staining for the detection of AFB. The procedure is thought to be faster, more-cost effective, and more sensitive than ZN. In a study from Kenya, FM was twice as sensitive as ZN in HIV positive cases using the culture as a gold standard (Kivihya-Ndugga et al., 2003). An Indian study reported 26% more TB cases detected when FM was used compared to ZN in a population including 15% HIV positive patients (Prasanthi & Kumari, 2005). In many cases, especially those with advanced immunosuppression and low CD4 cell-counts, are unable to produce sputum spontaneously. In such patients, sputum induction by inhalation hypertonic solution should be performed. Mycobacterial blood cultures can be obtainable, especially in persons whose CD4 cell count is below 200 cells/µL and/or persons with evidence of disseminated disease.

Nucleic-acid amplification (NAA) tests are useful in providing rapid identification of *M. tuberculosis* from sputum smear-positive specimens, but false-negative results can occur among patients with TB disease. The positive predictive value of NAA tests are decreased in persons who have sputum smear-negative results. Several reports indicate that in HIV patients, NAA tests may also be helpful for diagnosing TB when used on blood and urine (Kibiki et al., 2007; Rebollo et al., 2006; Torrea et al., 2005). Despite its possible advantages, NAA diagnostics remain expensive, technically demanding and prone to contamination, especially in high-volume settings (Rewata et al., 2009).

Current estimates are that one third of the world's population is infected with *M. Tuberculosis*. Yet, to date, there is no gold standard for diagnosis of latent TB infection (LTBI). Traditionally, the tuberculin skin test (TST) has been used to measure delayed hypersensitivity reaction following intradermal injection of purified protein derivative (PPD). However, its use in the diagnosis of LTBI lacks both specificity and sensitivity. More recently, IFN-γ release assays (IGRA) such as QuantiFERON-TB Gold In-Tube and T-SPOT. TB has been developed (Lalvani et al., 2001). IGRA improve the specificity of LTBI diagnosis by measuring cytokine production by immune cells to *M. tuberculosis*-specific proteins, transcribed from genes not found in Bacile Calmette-Guerin (BCG) and most other environmental mycobacteria. Early secreted antigenic target-6 and culture filtrate-10 are the two best studied to date and can improve the sensitivity of LTBI diagnosis to 96% compared with 69% achieved by TST.

In principle, the treatment of TB in individuals with HIV infection should be the same as that for patients with TB who do not have HIV disease. Currently, treatment guidelines recommend that the duration of TB therapy should be the same for both HIV positive and HIV negative cases (Blumberg et al., 2003; Hopewell et al., 2006; World Health Organization, 2003). Standard first-line therapy for TB with a 4-drug intensive treatment phase of 2 months, followed by 4 months of treatment with a 2-drug regimen, is highly effective in patients with HIV infection–related TB. Initial treatment of presumed drug-sensitive TB consists of isoniazid (INH), rifampin (RIF) or rifampicin (RFB), pyrazinamide (PZA), and ethambutol (EMB). Pyridoxine (B6 vitamin) should also be given to avoid peripheral neuropathy side effect of INH. Persons with cavitary lung disease whose 2-month repeat sputum culture remains positive should receive additional initial phase treatment for a month or an additional 3-4 months of treatment (total of 9-12 months). Consultation with a TB expert should be obtained in persons with known drug-resistant (multi drug-resistant, MDR, or extensively drug-resistant, XDR) TB and in persons who are failing standard 4-drug therapy, where drug-resistance is suspected. When results of species identification and susceptibility become available, drug selection can be tailored as needed. Because of the severity of TB disease among immunocompromised patients, directly observed therapy (DOT) is strongly recommended for patients with HIV–related TB.

It has been reported that trimethoprim-sulfamethoxazole, given a month after initiation of anti-TB therapy, reduced mortality by 46% among HIV1- and HIV2 coinfected patients with TB (Wiktor et al., 1999). Use of trimethoprim-sulfamethoxazole appeared to reduce the risk of death by preventing gastrointestinal and respiratory infections. As a result, the WHO and the United Nations Joint Programme on HIV/AIDS (UNAIDS), recommend that patients with HIV infection–related TB be treated with trimethoprim-sulfamethoxazole during and after treatment for TB (Sterling et al., 2010).

HIV infection is associated with high rates of recurrent TB, particularly in developing countries. However, in such settings, recurrent disease is more likely to be attributable to exogenous reinfection than to relapse. A course of isoniazid after completion of standard anti-TB treatment has been associated with lower rates of TB recurrence, particularly among HIV-infected persons. Although this strategy has been proven to be effective in settings with a high incidence of TB and HIV infection, it is often not provided because of logistical constraints (Sterling et al., 2010).

Among HIV-infected persons who receive a diagnosis of TB and do not receive HAART, the mortality rate is high (as high as 91% among persons with AIDS). Initiation of HAART is associated with improved survival among all HIV infected persons, including those with TB. It is therefore recommended that HIV-infected patients with TB receive treatment for both diseases, regardless of their CD4 lymphocyte count. However, the optimal timing of HAART initiation in relation to the time of anti-TB therapy initiation is unclear, but it is generally recommended to wait at least 2 weeks or longer depending on the degree of immunocompromised status (Centers for Disease Control and Prevention, 2009).

In persons on ART, drug interactions can occur particularly between the rifamycins and both protease inhibitors and non-nucleoside reverse transcriptase inhibitors. As a result of this interaction, decreased drug levels are associated with the development of resistance by both HIV and *M. tuberculosis*, whereas increased drug levels are associated with toxicity. In addition, persons receiving dual therapy for HIV infection and TB may develop the immune reconstitution syndrome. This shows a paradoxical reaction presenting as a temporary exacerbation of clinical and radiographic features which appears to be more common among those starting ART within 6 weeks of initiating anti-TB therapy and among those with disseminated TB.

TB prevention strategies with known efficacy include rapid identification and treatment of active TB cases (in source patients), infection-control measures to reduce nosocomial transmission of TB, isoniazid preventive therapy during latent TB infection, and ART to reduce the incidence of TB among HIV-infected patients (Chamie et al., 2010). Prevention of HIV infection is necessary to control TB. ART is one of the most potent tools in TB prevention, and increasing ART access in countries with a high TB burden is a necessary step in reducing TB incidence. Observational cohort studies have shown reductions in the risk of TB among persons receiving ART (Lawn et al., 2009). Treatment of latent TB, primarily studied using isoniazid preventive therapy in HIV-infected patients who have positive tuberculin skin test results, clearly reduces the incidence of active TB. In persons with HIV, ≥5 mm of induration at 48-72 hours is considered to represent a positive purified protein derivative (PPD) or TST. IFN-γ release assays (IGRAs) can also be used to diagnose LTBI. Since HIV infection is associated with a high risk for progression to TB, current guidelines recommend that persons with either a positive TST or IGRA should be considered infected with *M. tuberculosis* (Centers for Disease Control and Prevention, 2009). Persons with HIV infection should receive INH either daily or twice weekly plus pyridoxine for 9 months.

3.1 Non-tuberculous mycobacteria

Since the beginning of the AIDS epidemic, nontuberculous mycobacterial (NTM) infections have been reported with increasing frequency in HIV-infected patients. The majority of these infections have been caused by members of the *Mycobacterium avium complex* (MAC). Occasionally, *M. kansaii M. xenopi, M. fortuitum, M.chelonae or M. sherrisii* also causes pulmonary disease. MAC includes at least two species, *Mycobacterium avium* and *Mycobacterium intracellulare* and also *M. avium* is composed of several subspecies. In a report including a total of 2,269 cases with AIDS and disseminated nontuberculous mycobacterial infection; in 96% of cases, infection was caused by MAC (Horsburgh & Selik, 1989). However, Raszka et al. reported that, among the 92 patients infected with HIV and NTM organisms identified; MAC was recovered from 50 (77%) of the 65 NTM-positive cultures of blood or bone marrow, while MAC and other non-avium NTM accounted for 18% and 5% of the isolates, respectively and the authors concluded that those data demonstrate that HIV-positive patients develop disseminated disease with NTM other than *M. avium* more frequently than has been previously reported (Raszka et al., 1995).

The disease may manifest as disseminated infection, soft tissue infection, chronic pneumonia, or hypersensitivity pneumonitis, and isolated MAC pulmonary disease is very rare. Most patients have disseminated multiorgan infection. The risk of developing disseminated MAC increases as the CD4 lymphocyte count declines and more than 95% of cases occur when the lymphocyte count is 50 cells/μ/L or less. Unlike TB, disseminated MAC is usually a primary infection and is often preceded by a period of respiratory or gastrointestinal colonization after ingestion or inhalation of contamined food or water. The clinical findings of disseminated MAC include fever, anorexia, night sweats, weight loss, abdominal pain, hepatosplenomegaly, lymphadenopathy, chronic diarrhea and anemia. The radiologic findings of pulmonary MAC include consolidation, cavities, nodules, bronchiectasis and adenopathy (Erasmus et al., 1999). While focal infiltration is extremely rare, a frequent finding is endobronchial lesion without pneumonia (Mehle et al., 1989; Salama et al., 2003). Pleural involvement in nontuberculous mycobacterium infection has also been reported rarely (Haider et al., 2009).

The diagnosis of pulmonary MAC is based on clinical, microbiological, and radiographic findings (Griffith et al., 2007). It is based on compatible clinical signs and symptoms coupled with the isolation of MAC from cultures of blood, bone marrow, or other normally sterile tissue or body fluids. The positive culture of sputum or BAL for MAC, may not be indicative for either pulmonary or disseminated disease. Culture of blood is the most useful diagnostic procedure to evaluate MAC infection. The sensitivity of blood cultures for disseminated MAC has ranged from 86% to 98%. Recently, Singh et al studied a rapid PCR method for the species-specific diagnosis of *M. tuberculosis* and its differentiation from other mycobacteria, and the authors concluded that, the combination of genus-specific PCR primers with the novel early-secreted antigen-6 primer set could provide accurate and rapid diagnosis of mycobacteriosis (Singh et al., 2007).

The therapy for pulmonary disease due to MAC includes three oral antimicrobials: a macrolide (clarithromycin or azithromycin), ethambutol, and a rifamycin (rifampin or rifabutin). Clarithromycin is the preferred first agent, but azithromycin can be substituted if needed, although its in vitro activity is less than clarithromycin. Ethambutol is the recommended second agent and should be combined with one of these macrolides. Rifabutin is also recommended as a third agent of combination therapy (Benson et al., 2003; Gordin et al., 1999). In a study in which clarithromycin (500 mg bid.) plus ethambutol (1,200 mg/d), with or without rifabutin (300 mg/d) was evaluated, rifabutin was found to no impact on bacteriologic response or survival but may protect against development of clarithromycin resistance in those who respond to therapy (Gordin et al., 1999). In another multicenter, randomized trial, Benson et al. reported that the addition of rifabutin to clarithromycin plus ethambutol, had improved the survival (Benson et al., 2003). A third or fourth drug among the fluoroquinolones (ciprofloxacin or levofloxacin) or parenteral amikacin may be given if rifabutin cannot be used or in patients with advanced immunosuppression and high mycobacterial burden (Centers for Disease Control and Prevention, 2009). Duration of treatment is for 12 months beyond the time that the patient's cultures convert to negative, which usually equates to 18 to 24 months of therapy (Kasperbauer & Daley, 2008).

4. Fungal infections

4.1 *Pneumocystis jiroveci*

PCP (shortened for Pneumocystis pneumonia) caused by *Pneumocystis jiroveci* (formerly classified as *P. carinii*), still remains the most common opportunistic infection in patients infected with HIV. Once thought to be a parasite, genomic analysis revealed that *P. jiroveci* is in fact a fungus that infects only humans. Before the widespread use of primary PCP prophylaxis and effective ART, PCP occurred in 70%–80% of patients with AIDS. The use of combination antiretroviral therapy and PCP prophylaxis has contributed to the dramatic declines. Nevertheless, despite a decrease of its overall incidence as a result of use of combination ART and PCP prophylaxis, PCP remains the most frequent AIDS-defining diagnosis in the United States (Thomas, 2004). Pneumocystosis would cause life-threatening pneumonia in patients without chemoprophylaxis, without HAART or unaware of their HIV infection.

The risk factors for the development of PCP among HIV-infected persons include a CD4 lymphocyte count less than 200cells/μL (approximately 90-95% of cases), a history of PCP and oropharyngeal candidiadis (Phair et al., 1990; Stansell et al., 1997). Clinical presentation of patients affected with *Pneumocystis* pneumonia differs among HIV and non-HIV immunosuppressed patients. HIV patients tend to present with subacute onset of progressive dyspnea, nonproductive or minimally productive cough, low-grade fever and malaise. However, up to 7% of these patients can be asymptomatic. In contrast, patients that are immunocompromised but HIV-negative usually present more acutely, with substantial dyspnea, fever, chills and some may initially present in urgent need of mechanical ventilation. The fulminant pneumonia observed among non-HIV-infected patients is less common. Approximately 90% of patients with PCP have an elevated serum LDH level, but this may occur with other pulmonary diseases, especially mycobacterial and fungal infections (Rosen, 2008). Other tests, including S-adenosylmethionine levels, KL-6 and beta-D-glucan, have been reported as the diagnostic tests for PCP (Skelly et al., 2008; Tasaka et al., 2007). Hypoxemia, the most characteristic laboratory abnormality, might range from mild-to-moderate (room air arterial oxygen [pO_2] of >70 mm/Hg or alveolar-arterial O_2 difference, [A-a] DO_2 <35 mm/Hg) to moderate-to-severe levels (pO_2 <70 mm/Hg or [A-a] DO_2 >35 mm/Hg). Recently, Sage et al. studied the prognostic value of C-reactive protein (CRP) in HIV-infected patients with PCP and reported that, higher CRP values were more suggestive of bacterial infection, but the finding lacked specificity and was not useful in distinguishing between PCP and other causes of respiratory infection. Moreover, in patients with PCP higher CRP values were associated with more severe disease and a poor outcome, suggesting CRP measurement might be used prognostically (Sage et al., 2010).

The chest X-ray (CXR) usually shows bilateral, symmetrical reticular or granular opacities. Less frequently, PCP may present with unilateral or asymmetrical opacities. Some patients with PCP have nodular densities, lobar consolidation or normal CXR findings. Cystic abnormalities and spontaneous pneumothorax in patients with known or suspected HIV infection are usually caused by PCP, but may also be caused by TB. Cavitation or pleural effusion is uncommon in the absence of other pulmonary pathogens or malignancy, and the presence of a pleural effusion might indicate an alternative diagnosis. At times clinical symptomatology, specifically in the absence of significant CXR findings, initiates more sensitive radiological approaches such as high-resolution chest CT. The most typical findings on chest CT are bilateral ground glass opacities. Less-common features can include reticular, granular, and cystic lesions.

Since *Pneumocystis* cannot be cultured, the gold standard for diagnosis is microscopic visualization of the organism of the characteristics cysts or trophic forms on stained respiratory specimens including expectorated or induced sputum, pulmonary secretions obtained by nasotracheal suction, percutaneous aspiration of the lung parenchyma; via flexible bronchoscopy including BAL, washing, brushing and transbronchial biopsy; or via thoracoscopic or open-lung biopsy (Carmona & Limper, 2011). Induced sputum can be the first diagnostic procedure. The reported diagnostic sensitivities of various methods are; induced sputum <50 to >90%, bronchoscopy with bronchoalveolar lavage 90%-99%, transbronchial biopsy 95%-100%, and open lung biopsy 95%-100%. PCR-based techniques have also been employed and have been reported to be more sensitive and less specific leading to higher false-positive rates. Therefore, clinical correlation is always necessary. Since messenger RNA (mRNA) is less stable than DNA, if the patient is not actively infected with viable organisms, the mRNA should be largely degraded and no longer detected. Hence, new techniques that detect (mRNA) have been proposed as surrogate markers for organism viability. Recent data from HIV patients with suspected *Pneumocystis* pneumonia using reverse-transcriptase PCR targeting a heat shock protein of *Pneumocystis* mRNA (Phsb1) have yielded a diagnostic sensitivity and specificity of 100% and 86%, respectively, in BAL specimens (de Oliveira et al., 2007).

In patients without known contraindications, trimethoprim-sulfamethoxazole (TMP-SMX) is the drug of choice regardless of the severity of disease. The standard dose is 15-20mg/kg/day of TMP and 75-100 mg/kg/day of SMX. However in a recent study, it has been reported that, treatment of PCP in adult HIV-infected patients with trimethoprim 10 mg/kg/day-sulfamethoxazole 50mg/kg/day appears to have comparable efficacy to treatment (Thomas et al., 2009).

For severe cases, the intravenous (IV) form is preferred over the oral formulation. However, IV regimen can be switched to oral route, once clinical improvement is achieved. Standard treatment for PCP is 21 days; some persons will have responded well before this time and therapy can often be stopped and others will remain symptomatic and require continued therapy. Dose reductions are necessary for patients with renal and liver failure. Alternatives to TMP-SMX include intravenous or aerosolized pentamidine, clindamycin plus primaquine, trimethoprim plus dapsone and atovaquone solution. Aerosolized pentamidine has been associated with the development of disseminated disease, likely due to poor systemic levels. The IV formulation of pentamidine has better coverage and greater efficacy than the aerosolized route. However, it is at times poorly tolerated due to side effects that include hypotension, hypoglycemia and pancreatitis (Carmona & Limper, 2011). Another important aspect of *Pneumocystis* treatment is the use of corticosteroids. The administration of corticosteroids at the beginning of the therapy reduces the likelihood of respiratory failure, the deterioration of oxygenation, and death in patients with moderate-to-severe pneumonia. Patients usually benefit from therapy especially with respiratory insufficiency (Rosen, 2008).

4.2 Histoplasmosis

Histoplasmosis is caused by the dimorphic fungus *Histoplasma capsulatum* and the infection causes significant morbidity and mortality in HIV-infected individuals. *Histoplasma capsulatum* is reported to exist throughout the world, although the Mississippi and Ohio River catchments of the United States represent areas of greatest endemicity (Kauffman, 2007). It is the most frequent opportunistic infection due to HIV in French Guiana, along with tuberculosis, and the first cause of AIDS-related death (Couppie et al., 2004; Lewden et al., 2004). Disseminated histoplasmosis usually occurs among persons with CD4 lymphocyte counts <150 cells/μL; while localized pulmonary histoplasmosis might occur when CD4 lymphocyte counts >300 cells/μL (Centers for Disease Control and Prevention, 2009).

In HIV-infected patients the most common clinical presentation is disseminated multiorgan disease. Common symptoms include fever, chills, anorexia, fatigue, weight loss, cough, chest pain, and dyspnea and specific symptoms and signs related to organ involvement. In a study of 200 cases of AIDS-related histoplasmosis, most patients had fever, lymphadenopathies, and pulmonary and digestive symptoms whereas neurological signs and skin/mucosal locations were less common (Huber et al., 2008). The radiologic findings of patients with pulmonary involvement are diffuse interstitial or reticulonodular infiltrates. The patients with disseminated histoplasmosis may have normal CXR. Several laboratory abnormalities include increased lactate dehydrogenase, elevated liver enzymes, especially alkaline phosphatase, markedly increased ferritin, and pancytopenia.

Although the isolation and identification of fungus provides a definitive diagnosis, isolation can take 2–4 weeks and hence, the *Histoplasma* polysaccharide antigen (HPA) test is an initial test for the diagnosis of disseminated histoplasmosis (Centers for Disease Control and Prevention, 2009). Detection of circulating HPA in urine, serum, and other body fluids has an increasingly important role in the rapid diagnosis of disseminated histoplasmosis. Sensitivity is greater in urine than serum and the sensitivity of the urine assay for the diagnosis of disseminated histoplasmosis is approximately 90% (Wheat et al., 2002). In patients who have other fungal infections, including coccidioidomycosis, blastomycosis, paracoccidioidomycosis, and penicilliosis false positive reactions for HPA in urine may occur. The HPA test is often negative in isolated pulmonary disease. In such patients, direct examination and culture of sputum, BAL, or transbronchial biopsy can be performed. Bone marrow, lymph node, liver, or a skin or mucous membrane lesion provides other diagnostic sources.

Amphotericin B, either the deoxycholate formulation or liposomal amphotericin B is currently considered the drug of choice in HIV-positive patients with severe or disseminated histoplasmosis. Once clinical improvement was achieved, Amphotericin can be switched to itraconazole to complete at least a 12-month therapy course.

4.3 Aspergillosis

Aspergillosis, an infrequent but commonly fatal infection among HIV-infected patients, is a mycotic disease caused by *Aspergillus* species, usually *Aspergillus fumigatus*. In a review including 342 cases of pulmonary aspergillosis among HIV-infected patients, *Aspergillus fumigatus* was the most common pathogen (95% of the cases), while strains of *Aspergillus flavus, Aspergillus niger,* and *Aspergillus terreus* were less common (Mylonakis et al., 1998).

The major risk factors for aspergillosis include, neutropenia and steroid treatment, whereas the other risk factors are low CD4 lymphocyte count, previous pneumonia, opportunistic infections, especially those involving the lungs, such as PCP and CMV infection and use of broad spectrum antibacterial therapy, alcohol and marijuana. Clinical manifestations of aspergillus infections include: allergic bronchopulmonary aspergillosis, intracavitary aspergilloma, chronic forms of pulmonary aspergillosis, tracheobronchitis and rhinosinusitis, and invasive pulmonary aspergillosis as the most severe clinical presentation. The two major syndromes that have been described are: respiratory tract disease, associated with fever, cough, dyspnea, stridor or wheezing caused by airway constriction and invasive parenchymal infection which is usually fatal.

Although the prevalence of invasive aspergillosis among patients infected with HIV is lower than in other immunocompromised patients (Mylonakis et al., 1998), invasive pulmonary aspergillosis is still a life-threatening opportunistic infection in the advanced stage of HIV infection. Most patients have a CD4 lymphocyte count lower than 50 cells/μL. Holding et al. reported that, among 35,252 HIV-infected patients, the incidence of aspergillosis was 350/100.000 (Holding, 2000).

The radiologic findings include cavities, nodules and localized or diffuse infiltrates. Since its presence in nasopharyngeal secretions, sputum and BAL fluid may represent contamination or colonization, the definitive diagnosis of aspergillosis requires identification of the fungus on a biopsy specimen with the documentation of tissue invasion and the presence of appropriate clinical signs and symptoms. In a report, among 45 patients with AIDS and respiratory cultures positive for aspergillus, invasive pulmonary aspergillosis was documented in only four of these patients (Pursell et al., 1992). However, a presumptive diagnosis of respiratory tract disease can be made in the absence of a tissue biopsy if *Aspergillus spp.* are cultured from a respiratory sample, a compatible lesion or syndrome is present, and no alternative causative process is identified. Although serum galactomannan antigen testing and PCR-based techniques may be useful, they have not been studied in patients with HIV.

Voriconazole is the first-line recommended therapy for invasive aspergillosis. Conventional or lipid formulations of Amphotericin B, caspofungin and posaconazole are the other alternatives for antifungal therapy.

4.4 Coccidioidomycosis

Coccidioidomycosis is a fungal disease caused by, *Coccidioides immitis* and *Coccidioides posadasii.* The disease is endemic in southwestern US and northern Mexico (Pappagianis, 1988). Although coccidioidomycosis is uncommon in HIV-infected patients, in endemic regions, it is a common opportunistic infection in HIV-infected individuals. In a study performed by Masannat et al, among 257 HIV-infected patients seen over a 64-month period, 29 cases (11.3%) of coccidioidomycosis were identified (Masannat & Ampel, 2010). The incidence of coccidioidomycosis has declined as a result of ART (Woods et al., 2000).

The risk factors for coccidioidomycosis include low CD4 cell counts (<250 cells/μL), black race, a history of oropharyngeal or esophageal candidiasis, whereas a reduced risk is associated with protease inhibitor therapy.

The most common clinical presentations of coccidioidomycosis in HIV-infected patients are disseminated disease, diffuse pneumonia and meningitis. Disseminated coccidioidomycosis, defined as disease that has spread beyond the thoracic cavity, is frequent among patients with HIV infection and associated with generalized lymphadenopathy, skin nodules or ulcers, peritonitis, liver abnormalities, and bone and joint involvement. The most common radiographic finding of coccidioidomycosis is reticulonodular infiltrates. Focal infiltrates are less common. The other findings include nodules, adenopathy, cavities and pleural effusion.

The mainstays of diagnosis of coccidioidomycosis are serologic testing, histopathological identification, and culture (Ampel, 2005). In cases of pulmonary coccidioidomycosis, results of culture of respiratory specimens (sputum, BAL fluid, or transbronchial biopsy) are frequently positive. The diagnosis can be established by also, demonstration of the typical spherule on histopathological examination of involved tissue. Although, serologic tests are useful, it is less reliable for patients with HIV infection than for immunocompetent patients and the results may not always be positive.

Amphotericin B is the preferred initial therapy for patients with isolated pulmonary disease and disseminated disease without meningeal involvement (Centers for Disease Control and Prevention, 2009). Amphotericin B should be continued until clinical improvement, and then the therapy can be switched to fluconazole or itraconazole. In patients with mild disease such as focal pneumonia, fluconazole or itraconazole may be alternative agents. Flucanozole is the recommended drug for coccidioidal meningitis, since the reported success of this agent is approximately 80% (Galgiani et al., 1993).

4.5 Candidiasis

Mucocutaneous candidiasis is frequently one of the first signs of HIV infection and 90% of patients with AIDS will develop oropharyngeal candidiasis at some time during their illness (Vazquez, 2000). However, pulmonary candidiasis is an uncommon manifestation among HIV-infected patients. In 1987, data from the Centers for Disease Control AIDS data base indicated a 50% prevalence of oropharyngeal *candida* infection, a 10% rate of esophageal infection, and 5% rate of bronchopulmonary infection among AIDS patients (Selik et al., 1987). Due to the rare occurence of pulmonary candidiasis, clinical features among HIV-infected patients are not well documented.

4.6 Blastomycosis

Blastomycosis is a fungal infection acquired via inhalation of *Blastomyces dermatitidis*. The majority of cases occur in central, southeastern, and mid-Atlantic areas of the United States. Of the endemic fungi, blastomycosis is an uncommon disease among HIV-infected patients.

The most common clinical manifestation of blastomycosis in immunocompetent hosts include skin and lung involvement which mimic those of bacterial infection. However, it is potentially much more severe and is characterized by disseminated multiple organ involvement including frequent involvement of the central nervous system, adult respiratory distress syndrome and/or miliary pulmonary involvement. In the largest case series reported to date, among 15 HIV-infected patients, the patterns of the disease was localized pulmonary involvement in seven patients, disseminated or extrapulmonary blastomycosis in eight patients and in 40% of patients central nervous system involvement was observed (Pappas et al., 1992).

In HIV-infected patients, blastomycosis tends to occur in persons CD4 counts less than 200 cells/mm^3. In the largest case series mentioned above, among 15 patients, only one patient had a CD4 lymphocyte count greater than 200 cells/μL (Pappas et al., 1992).

The definitive diagnosis requires culture of respiratory specimens or tissue samples. The visualization of characteristic budding yeast form is also highly suggestive for diagnosis. Sputum analysis in most cases aids in the diagnosis, but bronchoscopy and/or tissue biopsy should be considered if the suspicion of blastomycosis is high and sputum analysis is inconclusive, negative or not possible (Patel et al., 1999). There is no serologic test for blastomycosis that has been validated in HIV-infected patients.

Intravenous amphotericin B is the drug of choice in patients with severe or disseminated blastomycosis. Amphotericin should be continued until a total of 1.5 to 2.5 g dose. Then, with the improvement of patient, the therapy can be switched to oral itraconazole.

4.7 Cryptococcosis

Cryptococcosis is a disease caused by *Cryptococcus neoformans* a unique environmental fungus and an encapsulated budding yeast. In AIDS patients *Cryptococcus neoformans,* serotype D and in particular serotype A, is the major cause of cryptococcosis throughout the world (Sugar, 1991).

Although the lungs are the portal of entry of the infection, the most common clinical presentation of cryptococcosis among HIV-infected patients is meningitis. In a study performed by Chuck et al., 84% of patients with HIV infection and cryptococcosis had meningitis, whereas 4% of patients had isolated pneumonia (Chuck & Sande, 1989). The majority of cases of cryptococcal disease occur in persons with a CD4 cell count below 200 cells/µL, usually below 50 cells/µL. In a series of 15 HIV-infected patients with pulmonary cryptococcosis, the CD4 lymphocyte count was low in all cases (median, 24/µL) (Ballou et al., 1997). With the use of combination ART, the incidence of cryptococcosis has dramatically declined.

The clinical manifestations of pulmonary cryptococcosis include fever, cough, dyspnea, expectoration, chest pain and hemoptysis. The most common radiographic finding is diffuse interstitial opacities, while others are focal interstitial abnormalities, alveolar opacities, adenopathies, cavitary lesions, and pleural effusions. Solitary pulmonary nodules, pulmonary masses, a milliary pattern and pneumothorax have also been reported.

The inital diagnostic test for cryptococcosis is cryptococcal antigen test, which is sensitive and specific. However, patients with isolated pulmonary disease may have a negative result. The test can be performed on serum, cerebrospinal fluid and respiratory samples. Blood fungal cultures are also specific and should be performed. The diagnosis of pulmonary cryptococcosis can be made by culture of sputum, BAL fluid, pleural fluid and transbronchial biopsy specimen. The measurement of cryptococcal antigen in the BAL can be a rapid, simple way to make the diagnosis (Baughman et al., 1992).

The treatment of meningitis and pneumonia is same and the recommended initial treatment for acute disease is amphotericin B, usually combined with flucytosine, for a 2-week duration followed by fluconazole (400 mg daily) alone for an additional 8 weeks (Centers for Disease Control and Prevention, 2009). Following this period, as a maintenance therapy, fluconazole (200 mg daily) for life or until the CD4 cell count rises above 200 cells/µL for at least 6 months should be continued.

4.8 Penicilliosis

Penicilliosis is caused by *Penicillium marneffei,* a dimorphic fungus which is endemic in Southeast Asia. Although it was a rare and sporadic disease before the HIV pandemic, penicilliosis is now the third most common AIDS-defining illness (after TB and cryptococcosis) in South East Asia (Fisher et al., 2004).

Although direct inoculation through skin can occur, inhalation is the main route of exposure. Most of the patients show absolute CD4 count less than 100 cells/µL (Maniar et a., 2005).

Penicillium marneffei can cause focal or disseminated infection. The common presenting symptoms and signs of infection are: fever of unknown origin, anemia, weight loss, hepatosplenomegaly, lymphadenopathy and skin eruptions. The skin lesions commonly appear as papules (characteristically with central umbilication, resembling molluscum contagiosum), nodules, or necrotic lesions, and they are predominantly located over the face and upper trunk (Ustianowski et a., 2008). The most common radiographic finding is interstitial opacities, the other findings may include nodules, cavities and pleural effusion. In a study from Taiwan, in which etiology of cavitary lung lesions in patients with HIV infection was evaluated, fungi were the most common etiology (42.0%), followed by bacteria (29.6%) and mycobacteria (25.9%) and of the fungal pneumonias, 19 (55.9%) were caused by *Penicillium marneffei* as the most common agent (Lin et al., 2009). Definitive diagnosis requires culture of the pathogenic fungus from clinical specimens. Among all the clinical specimens studied, the bone marrow gives the highest yield for culture, approaching 100%, followed by skin biopsy (90%) and blood culture (76%) (Supparatpinyo et al., 1994). Serologic testing including various types of antigen and antibody testing specific to *P. marneffei* have been described but is of limited utility in penicilliosis (Wong & Wong, 2011).

PCR assay specific for *P. marneffei* has been developed in research setting but is not available for routine clinical use (Pornprasert et al., 2009).
The mainstay of therapy is amphotericin B (2 weeks) followed by itraconazole (10 weeks). Since relapse is common, secondary prophylaxis should be maintained until a CD4 count of greater than 200 cells/µL for at least 6 months.

5. Viral infections

Although a variety of viruses can cause pulmonary disease in HIV-infected patients, cytomegalovirus (CMV) is the most frequent agent of viral pneumonia. Pneumonia due to herpes simplex virus, varicella zoster virus, adenovirus, respiratory syncytial virus and parainfluenza virus is uncommon.

5.1 Cytomegalovirus

Cytomegalovirus (CMV) disease is a frequent opportunistic infection that usually occurs in the late stages of HIV infection as a result of reactivation of latent infection rather than new infection. It has been reported that, before ART, 21–44% of patients developed CMV-associated disease at some point during the course of HIV infection and with the use of ART, the incidence of CMV disease has declined by 75–80%, and it is now estimated to be 0.75–3.2 cases per 100 person-years (Jabs et al., 2007; Salmon-Ce´ron et al., 2000; Salzberger et al., 2005). The most common clinical manifestations of CMV are retinitis and gastrointestinal disease (colitis or esophagitis). CMV pneumonia is uncommon and has been observed in only 0.24–8% of HIV-infected patients (Erice et al., 2003; Rodriguez-Barradas et al., 1996). Most of the patients have CD4 count less than 50 cells/µL. The chest radiograph findings include diffuse interstitial infiltrates, alveolar infiltrates or rarely pleural effusion.
In HIV-infected patients, the presence of CMV in BAL fluid is not usually predictive of CMV pneumonia and a definitive diagnosis depends on the documentation of CMV infection in lung tissue specimens. Diagnosis of CMV pneumonitis should be made in the setting of pulmonary interstitial infiltrates and identification of multiple CMV inclusion bodies in lung tissue, and the absence of other pathogens. Neither BAL fluid nor transbronchial biopsy culture are sufficient to make the diagnosis of CMV pneumonitis (Huang & Crothers, 2009).
Although there is limited data, the treatment options for CMV pneumonia include ganciclovir, foscarnet, cidofovir or valganciclovir. The duration of therapy is unknown, but a 2-3 weeks course is recommended.

6. Parasitic infections

Although, *Toxoplasma gondii, Strongyloides stercoralis,* microsporidia, cryptosporidium can cause pneumonia, among HIV-infected patients, parasitic pneumonia is an uncommon disease.

6.1 *Toxoplasma gondii*

Toxoplasma gondii, is the most common cause of parasitic pneumonia. Cerebral toxoplasmosis is the most common form of clinical manifestation, followed by ocular toxoplasmosis and pulmonary toxoplasmosis. As a result of widespread utilization of trimethoprim-sulphamethoxazole as primary PCP prophylaxis in AIDS patients, which is also effective against *Toxoplasma gondii,* there has been a fall in the prevalence of pulmonary toxoplasmosis. Pulmonary toxoplasmosis (PT) is most commonly seen in patients with advanced disease (Renold et al., 1992). In an autopsy study of 78 cases of toxoplasmosis, the risk factors were founded as; intravenous drug addiction, homosexuality or bisexuality and multiple blood transfusions (Hofman et al., 1993). Bilateral interstitial infiltrates is the most frequent finding on chest radiography; however, other abnormalities including nodular densities and pleural effusion and/or pneumothorax may also occur. An elevated LDH is a common laboratory finding. In a large study of 64 HIV-infected patients with PT, the clinical features usually included fever, cough, and dyspnea and the radiological findings were mainly diffuse interstitial infiltrates (Rabaud et al., 1996). Since clinical and radiological abnormalities are not specific, the diagnosis of pulmonary toxoplasmosis is difficult. The diagnosis can be established by direct examination (by Giemsa staining or indirect immunofluorescence with a monoclonal antibody to membrane antigen P-30) and/or tissue or BAL fluid culture. Although, PCR for detecting *T. gondii* in BAL samples have been studied, the diagnostic utility of this test is unclear (Lavrard et al., 1995; Petersen et al., 2006). The treatment of PT is similar to that for central nervous system disease and the first-line treatment is pyrimethamine plus sulfadiazine. Leucovorin is recommended for the hematologic toxicities associated with pyrimethamine. Clindamycin plus pyrimethamine is the alternative regimen.

6.2 Other parasites

Strongyloides stercoralis is an intestinal nematode which usually induces a silent or limited intestinal infection in immunocompetent hosts. It can also cause hyperinfection syndrome or disseminated disease in immunocompromised patients (Kramer et al., 1990). However, disseminated infection of *Strongyloides stercoralis* to the lung is extremely rare (Armignacco et al., 1989; Glezerov & Masci, 1990; Gomples et al., 1991; Makris et al., 1993). The common symptoms and signs are dyspnea, cough, sputum, wheezing and hemoptysis. In patients with the hyperinfection syndrome and massive *Strongyloides* infection, adult respiratory distress syndrome with respiratory failure that requires mechanical ventilation may develop. Chest radiography findings include reticulonodular pattern, diffuse bilateral interstitial opacities and alveolar opacities. The diagnosis is established by the identification of *Strongyloides* larvae on BAL fluid. The recommended treatment is ivermectin plus albendazole.

Microsporidia and cryptosporidium are other parasities which can rarely cause respiratory tract disease. Cryptosporidiosis is a disease caused by a coccidial parasite of the genus *Cryptosporidium*. Pulmonary cryptosporidiosis is a rare complication of intestinal cryptosporidiosis in HIV-infected patients (Corti et al., 2008). The most frequent symptoms are cough, fever and dyspnea. Several respiratory infectious agents, mainly *P. carinii* and *Cytomegalovirus* may coexist (Brea Hernando et al., 1993). The major clinical manifestation of microsporidiosis is the involvement of gastrointestinal tract like cryptosporidiosis and it can rarely cause pulmonary symptoms (Remadi et al., 1995). The diagnosis of both diseases is made by the visualization of the organism on the respiratory specimen.

7. Conclusion

Human immunodeficiency virus (HIV), the cause of AIDS, has in the 30 years since its discovery spread rapidly to every region in the world. Since the beginning of epidemic, more than 65 million people have been infected with HIV and about 25 million people died from

AIDS. The lungs are principal target of HIV-associated complications and, accordingly, a major source of morbitidy and mortality. The spectrum of pulmonary manifestations includes bacterial infections, viral infections, mycobacterial infections, protozoal infections, fungal infections, malignancies (eg, Kaposi sarcoma, lymphoma), and other disorders (eg, pulmonary hypertension, lymphocytic interstitial pneumonitis). Among HIV-associated pulmonary complications, opportunistic pneumonias are major cause of morbitidy and mortality.

8. References

Afessa B, Green W, Chiao J & Frederick W. (1998). Pulmonary complications of HIV infection: autopsy findings. *Chest* 113(5):1225–9.

Afessa B & Green W. (2000). Bacterial pneumonia in hospitalized patients with HIV infection. the Pulmonary Complications, ICU Support, and Prognostic Factors of Hospitalized Patients with HIV (PIP) Study. *Chest* 117(4):1017–22.

Ampel NM. (2005). Coccidioidomycosis in Persons Infected with HIV Type 1 *Clin Infec Dis* 41(8):1174–8.

Armignacco O, Capecchi A, De Mori P & Grillo LR. (1989). *Strongyloides* hyperinfection and the acquired immunodeficiency syndrome. *Am J Med* 86(2):258.

Ballou E, Couderc LJ, Molina JM, Cahite I, Wolff M, Saimot AG & Caubarrere I. (1997). Pulmonary cryptococcosis during HIV infection. 15 cases. *Rev Mal Respir* 14(5):365-70.

Baron AD & Hollander H. (1993). *Pseudomonas aeruginosa* bronchopulmonary infection in late human immunodeficiency virus disease. *Am Rev Respir Dis* 148(4):992–6.

Baughman RP, Rhodes JC, Dohn MN, Henderson H & Frame PT. (1992). Detection of cryptococcal antigen in bronchoalveolar lavage fluid: a prospective study of diagnostic utility. *Am Rev Respir Dis* 145(5):1226-9.

Benson CA, Williams PL, Currier JS, Holland F, Mahon LF, MacGregor RR, Inderlied CB, Flexner C, Neidig J, Chaisson R, Notario GF & Hafner R; AIDS Clinical Trials Group 223 Protocol Team. (2003) A prospective, randomized trial examining the efficacy and safety of clarithromycin in combination with ethambutol, rifabutin, or both for the treatment of disseminated *Mycobacterium avium* complex disease in persons with acquired immune deficiency syndrome. *Clin Infect Dis* 37(9):1234–43.

Blumberg HM, Burman WJ, Chaisson RE, et al. (2003). American Thoracic Society/Centers for Disease Control and Prevention/Infectious Diseases Society of America: treatment of tuberculosis. *Am J Respir Crit Care Med* 167(4):603–62.

Boiselle PM, Tocino I, Hooley RJ, Pumerantz AS, Selwyn PA, Neklesa VP & Lange RC. (1997). Chest radiograph diagnosis of *Pneumocystis carinii* pneumonia, bacterial pneumonia and pulmonary tuberculosis in HIV-positive patients: accuracy, distinguishing features, and mimics. *J Thorac Imaging* 12(1):47–53.

Boiselle PM, Aviram G & Fishman JE. (2002). Update on lung disease in AIDS. *Semin Roentgenol* 37(1):54–71.

Brea Hernando AJ, Bandres Franco E, Mosqueral Lozano JD, Lantero Benedito M & Ezquerra Lezcano M. (1993). Pulmonary cryptosporidiosis and AIDS. Presentation of a case and review of the literature. *An Med Interna* 10(5):232-6.

Brecher CW, Aviram G & Boiselle P. (2003). CT and Radiography of Bacterial Respiratory Infections in AIDS Patients *AJR* 180(5):1203-9.

British Thoracic Society Standards of Care Committee. (2001). BTS guidelines for the management of community acquired pneumonia in adults. *Thorax* 56 (Suppl 4):IV1–64.

Carmona EM & Limper AH. (2011). Update on the diagnosis and treatment of *Pneumocystis* pneumonia. *Ther Adv Respir Dis* 5(1):41-59.

Centers for Disease Control and Prevention: (1993). 1993 revised classification system for HIV infection and expanded surveillance case definition for AIDS among adolescant and adults. *JAMA* 269(6):729-30.

Chamie G, Luetkemeyer A, Charlebois E & Havlir DV. (2010). Tuberculosis as Part of the Natural History of HIV Infection in Developing Countries. *Clin Infect Dis* 50(3):245–54.

Chuck SL & Sande MA. (1989). Infection with Cryptococcus neoformans in the acquired immunodeficiency syndrome. *N Engl J Med* 322(10):794-9.

Corbett EL, Watt CJ, Walker N, Maher D, Williams BG, Raviglione MC & Dye C. (2003). The growing burden of tuberculosis. Global trends and interactions with the HIV epidemic. *Arch Intern Med* 163 (9):1009–21.

Corti M, Villafane MF, Muzzio E, Bava J, Abuin JC & Palmieri OJ. (2008). Pulmonary cryptosporidiosis in AIDS patients. *Rev Argent Microbiol* 40(2):106-8.

Couppie´ P, Sobesky M, Aznar C, Bichat S, Clity E, Bissuel F, El Guedj M, Alvarez F, Demar M, Louvel D, Pradinaud R & Carme B. (2004). Histoplasmosis and acquired immunodeficiency syndrome: a study of pronostic factors. *Clin Infect Dis* 38(1):134–8.

Crothers K, Morris A, Huang L. (2010). Pulmonary complications of human immunodeficiency virus infection. In: Mason R, Broaddus CW, Martin RT, King ET, Schraufnagel DE, Murray JF, Nadel JA (eds). *Textbook of Respiratory Medicine*. Phiadelphia: Saunders Elsevier, 5th Edition, pp:1914-49

Daley CL. (1993). Bacterial pneumonia in HIV-infected patients. *Semin Respir Infect* 8(2):104–15.

Davis L, Beck JM & Shellito J. (1993). Update: HIV infection and pulmonary host defenses. *Semin Respir Infect* 8(2):75–85.

de Oliveira A, Unnasch T.R, Crothers K, Eiser S, Zucchi P, Moir J, Berad CB, Lawrence GG & Hunag L. (2007). Performance of a molecular viability assay for the diagnosis of Pneumocystis pneumonia in HIV-infected patients. *Diagn Microbiol Infect Dis* 57(2):169-76.

Erasmus J, McAdams HP, Farrell MA & Patz EF. (1999). Pulmonary Nontuberculous Mycobacterial Infection: Radiologic Manifestations. *Radiographics* 19(6):1487-505.

Erice A, Tierney C, Hirsch M, Caliendo AM, Weinberg A, Kendall MA & Polsky B; AIDS Clinical Trials Group Protocol 360 Study Team. (2003). Cytomegalovirus (CMV) and human immunodeficiency virus (HIV) burden, CMV end-organ disease, and survival in subjects with advanced HIV infection (AIDS Clinical Trials Group Protocol 360). *Clin Infect Dis* 37(4):567–78.

Fangman JW & Sax PE. (2008). Human immunodeficiency virus and pulmonary infections. In: Fishman AP, Elias JA, Fishman AJ, Grippi AM, Senior RM, Pack AI (eds). *Fishman's pulmonary diseases and disorders, fourth edition*. China: The McGraw Hill Companies 2241-64.

Fisher MC, Aanensen D, de Hoog S & Vanittanakom N. (2004). Multilocus microsatellite typing system for Penicillium marneffei reveals spatially structured populations. *J Clin Microbiol* 42(11):5065–9.

French N, Nakiyingi J, Carpenter LM, Lugada E, Watera C, Moi K, Moore M, Antvelink D, Mulder D, Janoff N, Whitworth J & Gilks CF. (2000). 23-valent pneumococcal polysaccharide vaccine in HIV-1-infected Ugandan adults: double-blind, randomized and placebo controlled trial. *Lancet* 355(9221):2106–11.

Galgiani JN, Catanzaro A, Cloud GA, Higgs J, Friedman BA, Larsen RA & Graybill JR. (1993). Fluconazole therapy for coccidioidal meningitis. *Ann Intern Med* 119(1):28–35.

Glezerov V & Masci JR. (1990). Disseminated strongyloidiasis and other selected unusal infections in patients with the acquired immunodeficiency syndrome. *Prog AIDS Pathol* 2:137-42.

Gold JA, Rom WN & Harkin TJ. (2002). Significance of abnormal chest radiograph findings in patients with HIV-1 infection without respiratory symptoms. *Chest* 121(5):1472–7.

Gomples MM, Todd J, Peters BS, Main J & Pinching AJ. (1991). Disseminated strongyloidiasis in AIDS: uncommon but important. *AIDS* 5(3):329-32.

Gordin FM, Sullam PM, Shafran SD, Cohn DL, Wynne B, Paxton L, Perry K & Horsburgh CR. (1999). A randomized, placebo-controlled study of rifabutin added to a regimen of clarithromycin and ethambutol for treatment of disseminated infection with *Mycobacterium avium* complex. *Clin Infect Dis* 28(5):1080–5.

Grau I, Ardanuy C, Linares J, Podzamcer D, Schulze MH & Pallers R. (2009) Trends in mortality and antibiotic resistance among HIV-infected patients with invasive pneumococcal disease. *HIV Med* 10(8):488–95.

Griffith DE, Aksamit T, Brown-Elliott BA, et al. (2007). An official ATS/IDSA statement: diagnosis, treatment, and prevention of nontuberculous mycobacterial diseases. *Am J Respir Crit Care Med* 175(4):367–416.

Habib AG, Keshinro IB, Gebi UI, Olatunde BOM, Onyemelukwe GC & Kangave D. (1998). Clinical presentation of HIV-infection in northern Nigeria and its relationship to CD4 + T-cell counts. *Nigerian Medical Practitioner* 35:3–8.

Haider A, Schliep T & Zeana C. (2009). Nontuberculous Mycobacterium Disease With Pleural Empyema in a Patient With Advanced AIDS. *Am J Med Sci* 338(5):418–20.

Havlir DV & Barnes P. (1999). Tuberculosis in patients with human immunodeficiency virus infection. *N Engl J Med* 340(5):367-73.

Hirschtick RE, Glassroth J, Jordan MC, Wilcosky TC, Wallace JM, Kvale PA, Markowitz N, Rosen MJ, Mangura BT & Hopewell PC. (1995). Bacterial pneumonia in persons infected with the human immunodeficiency virus. *N Eng J Med* 333(13):845–51.

Holding KJ, Dworkin MS, Wan PC, Hanson DL, Klevens RM, Jones JL & Sullivan PS. (2000). Aspergillosis among people infected with human immunodeficiency virus: incidence and survival. Adult and Adolescent Spectrum of HIV Disease Project. *Clin Infect Dis* 31(5):1253-7.

Hofman P, Michiels JF, Saint-Paul MC, Marty P, Durant J, Fuzibet JG, Mouroux J, Le Fichoux Y & Loubiere R. (1993). Toxoplasmosis in AIDS patients. Pathoclinical study of 78 cases. *Ann Pathol* 13(4):233-40.

Hopewell PC, Pai M, Maher D, Uplekar M & Raviglione MC. (2006). International standards for tuberculosis care. *Lancet Infect Dis* 6(11):710–25.

Horsburgh CR & Selik RM. (1989). The epidemiology of disseminated nontuberculous mycobacterial infection in the acquired immunodeficiency syndrome (AIDS). *Am Rev Respir Dis* 139(1):4-7.

Huang LF, Tang XP, Cai WP, Chen XJ, Lei CL, Li LH & Zhang FC. (2010). An analysis of opportunistic infection in 762 patients with human immunodeficiency virus infection in Guangdong areas. *Zhonghua Nei Ke Za Zhi* 49(8):653-6.

Huang L & Crothers AK. (2009). HIV-associated Opportunistic Pneumonias. *Respirology* 14(4):474–485.

Huber F, Nacher M, Aznar C, Pierre-Demar M, El Guedj M, Vaz T, Vantilcke V, Mhamat A, Magnien C, Chauvet E, Carme B & Couppie P. (2008). AIDS-related Histoplasma capsulatum var. capsulatum infection: 25 years experience of French Guiana *AIDS* 22(9):1047–53.

Jabs DA, Van Natta ML, Holbrook JT, Kempen JH, Meinert CL & Davis MD. (2007). Longitudinal study of the ocular complications of AIDS: 1. Ocular diagnoses at enrollment. *Ophthalmology* 114(4):780–6.

Janoff EN, Breiman RF, Daley CL & Hopewell PC. (1992). Pneumococcal disease during HIV infection: epidemiologic, clinical and immunologic perspectives. *Ann Intern Med* 117(4):314–24.

Kauffman CA. (2007). Histoplasmosis: a clinical and laboratory update. *Clin Microbiol Rev* 20(1):115-32.

Kasperbauer SH & Daley Cl. (2008). Diagnosis and Treatment of Infections due to Mycobacterium avium Complex. *Semin Respir Crit Care Med* 29(5):569-76.

Kibiki GS, Mulder B, van der Ven AJ, Sam N, Boeree MJ, van der Zanden A & Dolmans WM. (2007). Laboratory diagnosis of pulmonary tuberculosis in TB and HIV endemic settings and the contribution of real time PCR for M. tuberculosis in bronchoalveolar lavage fluid. *Trop Med Int Health* 12(10):1210-7.

Kivihya-Ndugga, LE., van Cleeff MR, Githui WA, Nganga LW, Kibuga DK, Odhiambo JA & Klatser PR. (2003). A comprehensive comparison of Ziehl-Neelsen and fluorescence microscopy for the diagnosis of tuberculosis in a resource-poor urban setting. *Int J Tuberc Lung Dis* 7(12):1163-71.

Kramer MR, Gregg PA, Goldstein M, Liamas R & Kreiger PS. (1990). Disseminated strongyloidiasis in AIDS and non-AIDS immunocompromised hosts:diagnosis by sputum and bronchoalveloar lavage. *South Med J* 83(10);1226-9.

Kohli R, Lo Y, Homel P, Flanigan TP, Gardner LI, Howard AA, Rompalo Am, Moskoleva G, Schuman P & Schoenbaum EE; HER Study Group. (2006). Bacterial pneumonia, HIV therapy and disease progression among HIV-infected women in the HIV. Epidemiologic Research (HER) study. *Clin Infect Dis* 43(1):90-8.

Kuhlman JE. (1999). Imaging pulmonary disease in AIDS: state of the art. *Eur Radiol* 9(3):395–408.

Laissy JP, Cadi M, Boudiaf ZE, Casalino E, Crestani B, Boyvert E, Aubier M & Schouman-Claeys E. (1998). Pulmonary tuberculosis: computed tomography and high-resolution computed tomography patterns in patients who are either HIV-negative or HIV-seropositive. *J Thorac Imaging* 13(1):58–64.

Lalvani A, Nagvenkar P, Udwadia Z, Pathan AA, Wilkinson KA, Shastri JS, Ewer K, Hill AV, Mehta A & Rodrigues C. (2001). Enumeration of T cells specific for RD1-encoded antigens suggests a high prevalence of latent Mycobacterium tuberculosis infection in healthy urban Indians. *J Infect Dis* 183(3):469–77.

Lavrard I, Chouaid C, Roux P, Poirot JL, Marteau M, Lemarchand B, Meyohas MC & Olivier JL. (1995). Pulmonary toxoplasmosis in HIV-infected patients: usefulness of polymerase chain reaction and cell culture. *Eur Respir J* 8(5):697-700.

Lawn SD, Little F, Bekker LG, Kaplan R, Campbel E, Orrel C & Wood R. (2009). Changing mortality risk associated with CD4 cell response to antiretroviral therapy in South Africa. *AIDS* 23(3):335–42.

Lawn SD, Wood R & Wilkinson RJ. (2011). Changing Concepts of "Latent Tuberculosis Infection" in Patients Living with HIV Infection. *Clin Dev Immunol* 2011/980594

Lewden C, Sobesky M, Cabie A, Couppie´ P, Boulard F, Bissuel F, May T, Morlat P, Chene G, Lamaury I & Salmon D. (2004). Causes of death among HIV-infected adults in French Guiana and the West Indies in the area of highly active antiretroviral therapy (HAART). *Med Mal Infect* 34(7):286–92.

Lin CY, Sun HY, Chen MY, Hseih SM, Sheng WH, LoYC, Hung CC & Chang SC. (2009). Aetiology of cavitary lung lesions in patients with HIV infection. *HIV Med* 10(3):191-8.

Loeliger AE, Rijkers GT, Aerts P, Been-Tiktak A, Hoepelman AI, van Dijk H & Borleffs JC. (1995). Deficient antipneumococcal polysaccharide responses in HIV-seropositive patients. *Immunol Med Microbiol* 12(1):33–41.

Lucas SB, Hounnou A, Peacock C, Beaumel A, Djomond G, N'Gbichi JM, Yeboue K, Honde M, Diomande M & Giordano C. (1993). The mortality and pathology of HIV infection in a West African city. *AIDS* 7(12):1569-79.

Madeddu G, Laura Fiori M & Stella Mura S. (2010). Bacterial community-acquired pneumonia in HIV-infected patients. *Curr Opin Pulm Med* 16(3):201–7.

Madeddu G, Porqueddu EM, Cambosu F, Saba F, Fois AG, Pirina P & Mura MS. (2008). Bacterial community acquired pneumonia in HIV-infected inpatients in the highly active antiretroviral therapy era. *Infection* 36(3):231–6.

Madeddu G, Fois GA, Pirina P & Mura MS. (2009). Pneumococcal pneumonia: clinical features, diagnosis and management in HIV-infected and HIV noninfected patients. *Currt Opin Pulm Med* 15(3):236–42.

Magnenat J-L, Nicod LP, Auckenthaler R & Junod AF. (1991). Mode of presentation and diagnosis of bacterial pneumonia in human immunodeficiency virus-infected patients. *Am Rev Respir Dis* 144(4):917–22.

Makris NA, Sher S, Bertoli C & Latour MG. (1993). Pulmonary strongyloidiasis: An unusal opportunistic pneumonia in a patient with AIDS. *AJR* 161(3):545-7.

Mandell LA, Wunderink RG, Anzueto A, Bartlett JG, Campbell GD, Dean NC, Dowel SF, File TM, Musher DM, Niederman MS, Torres A & Whitney CG. (2007). Infectious Diseases Society of American/American Thoracic Society consensus guidelines on the management of community-acquired pneumonia in adults. *Clin Infect Dis*; 44 (Suppl 2):27–72.

Maniar JK, Chitale AR, Miskeen A, Shah K & Maniar A. (2005). Penicillium marneffei infection: an AIDS-defining illness. *Indian J Dermatol Venerol Leprol* 71(3):202-4.

Martin JN, Rose DA, Hadley WH, Perdreau-Remington F, Lam PK & Gerberding JL. (1999). Emergence of Trimethoprim-Sulfamethoxazole Resistance in the AIDS Era. *J Infect Dis* 180(6):1809-18.

Masannat FY & Ampel NM. (2010). Coccidioidomycosis in patients with HIV-1 infection in the era of potent antiretroviral therapy. *Clin Infect Dis* 50(1):1–7.

Mase SR, Ramsay A, Ng V, Henry M, Hopewell PC, Cunningham J, Urbanczik R, Perkins MD, Aziz MA & Pai M. (2007). Yield of serial sputum specimen examinations in the diagnosis of pulmonary tuberculosis: a systematic review. *Int J Tuberc Lung Dis* 11(5):485-95.

Marchiori E, Müller NL, Souza AS, Escuissato DL, Gasparetto EL & Fanquet T. (2005). Pulmonary Disease in Patients with AIDS: High-Resolution CT and Pathologic Findings. *AJR Am J Roentgenol* 184(3):757–64.

McGuinness G. (1997). Changing trends in the pulmonary manifestations of AIDS. *Radiol Clin North Am* 35(5):1029–82.

Mehle ME, Adamo JP, Mehta AC, Wiederman HP, Keys T & Longworth DL. (1989). Endobronchial *Mycobacterium avium-intracellulare* infection in a patient with AIDS. *Chest* 96(1):199-201.

Mylonakis E, Barlara TF, Flanigan T & Rich JD. (1998). Pulmonary aspergillosis and invasive disease in AIDS: review of 342 cases. *Chest* 114(1):251-62.

Mylonakis E, Mileno MD, Flanigan T, De Orchis DF & Rich J. (1998). Pulmonary invasive aspergillosis in patients infected with the human immundeficiency virus: report of two cases. *Heart Lung* 27(1):63-6.

Nelson AM, Perriens JH, Kapita B, Okonda L, Lusamuno N, Kalengayi MR, Angrit P, Quinn TC& Mullick FG. (1993). A clinical and pathological comparison of the WHO and CDC case definitions for AIDS in Kinshasa, Zaire: is passive surveillance valid? AIDS 7(9):1241-5.

Noskin GA & Glassroth J. (1996). Bacterial pneumonia associated with HIV-1 infection. *Clin Chest Med* 17(4):713–23.

Pappas PG, Pottage JC, Powderly WG, Fraser WJ, Stratton CW, McKenzie S, Tapper ML, Chmel H, Bonebrake FC, Blum R, et al. (1992). Blastomycosis in patients with the acquired immunodeficiency syndrome. *Ann Inter Med* 116(10):847-53.

Pappagianis D. (1988). Epidemiology of coccidioidomycosis. Curr Top Med Mycol 2:199–238.

Patel RG, Patel B, Petrini MF, Carter RR & Griffith J. (1999). Clinical presentation, radiographic findings, and diagnostic methods of pulmonary blastomycosis: a review of 100 consecutive cases. *South Med J* 92(3):289-95.

Petersen E, Edvinsson B, Lundgren B, Benfield T & Evengård B. (2006). Diagnosis of pulmonary infection with Toxoplasma gondii in immunocompromised HIV-positive patients by real-time PCR. *Eur J Clin Microbiol Infect Dis* 25(6):401-4.

Phair J, Munoz A, Detels R, Kaslow R, Rinaldo C & Saah A. (1990). The risk of *Pneumocystis carinii* pneumonia among men infected with human immunodeficiency virus type-1. Multicenter AIDS Cohort Study Group. *N Engl J Med* 322(3):161-5.

Pornprasert S, Praparattanapan J, Khamwan C, Pawichai S, Pimsarn P, Samleerat T, Leechanachai P & Supparatpinyo K. (2009). Development of TaqMan real-time polymerase chain reaction for the detection and identification of Penicillium marneffei. *Mycoses* 52(6):487–92.

Prasanthi, K. & A.R. Kumari. (2005). Efficacy of fluorochrome stain in the diagnosis of pulmonary tuberculosis co-infected with HIV. *Indian J Med Microbiol* 23(3):179-81.

Pursell KJ, Telzak EE & Armstrong D. (1992). Aspergillus species colonization and invasive disease in patients with AIDS. *Clin Infect Dis* 14(1):141-8.

Rabaud C, May T, Lucet JC, Leport C, Ambroise-Thomas A & Canton P. (1996). Pulmonary toxoplasmosis in patients infected with human immunodeficiency virus: A French National Survey. *Clin Infect Dis* 23(6):1249-54.

Remadi S, Durnais J, Wafa K & MacGee W. (1995). Pulmonary microsporidiosis in a patient with the acquired immunodeficiency syndrome. A case report. *Acta Cytol* 39(6):1112-6.

Rodriguez-Barradas MC, Musher DM, Lahart C, Lacke C, Groover J, Watson D, Baughn R, Cate T &Crofoot G. (1992). Antibody to capsular polysaccharides of Streptococcus pneumoniae after vaccination of human immunodeficiency virus-infected subjects with 23-valent pneumococcal vaccine. *J Infect Dis* 165(3):553–6.

Raszka WW, Skilman LP, McEvoy PL & Robb ML. (1995). Isolation of nontuberculous, non-avium mycobacteria from patients infected with human immunodeficiency virus. *Clin Infect Dis* 20(1):73-6.

Rebollo MJ, San Juan Garrido R, Folgueira D, Palenque E, Diaz-Pedroche C, Lumbreras C, & Aquado JM. (2006). Blood and urine samples as useful sources for the direct detection of tuberculosis by polymerase chain reaction. *Diagn Microbiol Infect Dis* 56(2): 141-6.

Renold C, Sugar A, Chave JP, Perrin L, Delavelle J, Pizzolato G, Burkhard P, Gabriel V & Hirschel B. (1992). Toxoplasma encaphalitis in patients with the acquired immunodeficiency syndrome. *Medicine (Baltimore)* 71(4):224-39.

Rewata L, Rutherford M, Apriani L, Janssen W, Rahmadi A, Parwati I, Yuwono A & van Crevel RV. (2009). Improving diagnosis of pulmonary tuberculosis among HIV/AIDS patients: literature review and experience in a teaching hospital in Indonesia. *Acta Med Indones* 41(1):57-64.

Rodriguez-Barradas MC, Stool E, Musher DM, Gathe J Jr, Goldstein J, Genta RM & Yoffe B. (1996). Diagnosing and treating cytomegalovirus pneumonia in patients with AIDS. *Clin Infect Dis* 23(1):76–81.

Rosen MJ. (2008). Pulmonary complications of HIV infection. *Respirology* 13(2):181–90.

Sage EK, Noursadeghi M, Evans HE, Parker SJ, Copas AJ, Edwards SG & Miller RF. (2010). Prognostic value of C-reactive protein in HIV-infected patients with Pneumocystis jirovecii pneumonia. *Int J STD AIDS* 21(4):288-92.

Salama C, Policar M & Venkataraman M. (2003). Isolated pulmonary *Mycobacterium avium complex* infection in patients with human immunodeficiency virus infection: Case reports and literature review. *Clin Infect Dis* 37(3):35-40.

Salmon-Ceron D, Mazeron MC, Chaput S, Boukli N, Senechal B, Houhou N, Katlama C, Matheron S, Fillet AM, Gozlan J, Leport C, Jeantils V, Freymuth F & Costagliola D. (2000). Plasma cytomegalovirus DNA, pp65 antigenaemia and a low CD4 cell count remain risk factors for cytomegalovirus disease in patients receiving highly active antiretroviral therapy. *AIDS* 14(8):1041–9.

Salzberger B, Hartmann P, Hanses F, Uyanik B, Cornely OA, Wohrmann A & Fatkenheuer G. (2005). Incidence and prognosis of CMV disease in HIV-infected patients before and after introduction of combination antiretroviral therapy. *Infection* 33(5-6):345–9.

Sandkovsky U, Sandkovsky G, Suh J,Smith B, Sharp V & Polsky B. (2008). *Legionella* Pneumonia and HIV: Case Reports and Review of the Literature. *AIDS Patient Care STDS* 22(6):473-81.

Sani MU, Mohammed AZ, Adamu B, Yusuf SM, Samalia AA & Borodo MM. (2006). AIDS mortality in a tertiary health institution: A four-year review. *J Natl Med Assoc* 98(6):862-6.

Schneider RF. (1999). Bacterial pneumonia. *Semin Respir Infect* 14(4):327–32.

Selik RM, Starcher ET & Curran JW. (1987). Opportunistic diseases reported in AIDS patients: frequencies, associations, and trends. *AIDS* 1(3):175-82.

Selwyn PA, Pumerantz AS, Durante A, Alcabes PG, Gourevitch MN, Boiselle PM & Elmore JG. (1998). Clinical predictors of *Pneumocystis carinii* pneumonia, bacterial pneumonia, and tuberculosis in hospitalized patients with HIV-infected patients. *AIDS* 12(8):885–93.

Sider L, Gabriel H, Curry DR & Pham MS. (1993). Pattern recognition of the pulmonary manifestations of AIDS on CT scans. *Radiographics* 13(4):771–84.

Singh S, Gopinath K, Shahdad S, Kaur M, Singh B & Sharma P. (2007). Nontuberculous mycobacterial infections in Indian AIDS patients detected by a novel set of ESAT-6 polymerase chain reaction primers. *Jpn J Infect Dis* 60(1):14-18.

Skelly MJ, Holzman RS & Merali S. (2008). S-adenosylmethionine levels in the diagnosis of *Pneumocystis carinii* pneumonia in patients with HIV infection. *Clin Infect Dis* 46(3):467-71.

Soeiro AM, Hovnanian AD, Parra ER, Canzian M & Capelozzi VL. (2008). Post-mortem histological pulmonary analysis in patients with HIV/AIDS. *Clinics* 63(4):497-502.

Stansell JD, Osmond DH, Charlebois E, LaVange L, Wallace JM, Alexander BW, Glassroth J, Kvale PA, Roosen MJ, Reichman LB, Turner JR & Hopewell PC. (1997). Predictors of *Pneumocystis carinii* pneumonia in HIV-infected persons. Pulmonary Complications of HIV Infection Study Group. *Am J Respir Crit Care Med* 155(1):60-6.

Steingart KR, Ng V, Henry M, Hopewell PC, Ramsay A, Cunningham J, Cuningham J, Urbanczik R, Perkins MD, Aziz MA & Pai M. (2006). Sputum processing methods to improve the sensitivity of smear microscopy for tuberculosis: a systematic review. *Lancet Infect Dis* 6(10):664-74.

Stephan C, Just-Nübing G, Franck S, Bickel M, Shah PM, Babacan E & Staszewski S. (2009). No obvious difference in Streptococcus pneumoniae antibiotic resistance profiles--isolates from HIV-positive and HIV-negative patients. *Med Klin (Munich)* 103(2):69-74.

Sterling TR, Pham PA & Chaisson RE. (2010). HIV infection–related tuberculosis: clinical manifestations and treatment. *Clin Infect Dis* 50(3):223–30.

Suffredini AF & Masur H. (1988). Pulmonary dysfunction in patients infected with human immunodeficiency virus. In: Pennington JE, editors. *Respiratory infections: diagnosis and management*. 2nd ed. New York: Ra ven Press; pp:241-63.

Sugar AM. (1991). Overview: Cryptococcosis in the patient with AIDS. *Mycopathologia* 114(3):153-7.

Sullivan JH, Moore RD, Keruly JC & Chaisson RE. (2000). Effect of antiretroviral therapy on the incidence of bacterial pneumonia in patienys with advanced HIV infection. *Am J Respir Crit Care Med* 162(1): 64-7.

Supparatpinyo K, Khamwan C, Baosoung V, Nelson KE & Sirisanthana T. (1994). Disseminated Penicillium marneffei infection in Southeast Asia. *Lancet* 344(8915):110–3.

Tasaka S, Hasegawa N, Kobayashi S, Yamada W, Nishimura T, Takeuchi T & Ishizaka A. (2007). Serum indicators for the diagnosis of pneumocystis pneumonia. *Chest* 131(4):1173-80.

The National Institutes of Health (NIH) the Centers for Disease Control and Prevention (CDC). (2009). The HIV Medicine Association of the Infectious Diseases Society of America (HIVMA/IDSA). Guidelines for Prevention and Treatment of Opportunistic Infections in HIV-Infected Adults and Adolescents. *MMWR* 58:-207.

Thomas CF Jr & Limper AH. (2004). Pneumocystis pneumonia. *N Engl J Med* 350(24):2487–98.

Thomas M, Rupali P, Woodhouse A & Ellis-Pegler R. (2009). Good outcome with trimethoprim 10 mg/kg/day-sulfamethoxazole 50 mg/kg/day for Pneumocystis jirovecii pneumonia in HIV infected patients. *Scand J Infect Dis* 41(11-12):862-8.

Torrea G, Van de Perre P, Ouedraogo M, Zougba A, Sawadogo A, Dingtoumda B, Diallo B, Defer MC, Somvie I, Zanetti S & Sechi LA. (2005). PCR-based detection of the Mycobacterium tuberculosis complex in urine of HIV-infected and uninfected pulmonary and extrapulmonary tuberculosis patients in Burkina Faso. *J Med Microbiol* 54(1):39-44.

Vazquez JA. (2000). Therapeutic Options for the Management of Oropharyngeal and Esophageal Candidiasis in HIV/AIDS Patients. *HIV Clinical Trials* 1(1):47–59.

Ustianowski AP, Sieu TP & Day JN. (2008). Penicillium marneffei infection in HIV. *Curr Opin Infect Dis* 21(1):31–36.

Wheat LJ, Garringer T, Brizendine E & Connolly P. (2002). Diagnosis of histoplasmosis by antigen detection based upon experience at the histoplasmosis reference laboratory. *Diagn Microbiol Infect Dis* 43(1):29–37.

Wiktor SZ, Sassan-Morokro M, Grant AD, Abouya L, Karon JM, Maurice C, Diamond G, Ackah A, Domoua K, Kdio A, Yapi A, Combe P, Tossou O, Roels TH, Lackritz EM, Coulibaly D, De Cock KM, Coulibaly IM & Greenberg AE. (1999). Efficacy of trimethoprim-sulphamethoxazole prophylaxis to decrease morbidity and mortality in HIV-1-infected patients with tuberculosis in Abidjan, Cote d'Ivoire: a randomised controlled trial. *Lancet* 353(9163):1469–75.

Williams BG, Granich R, De Cock KM, Glaziou P, Sharma A & Dye C. (2010). Antiretroviral therapy for tuberculosis control in nine African countries. *Proc Natl Acad Sci USA* 107(45):19485-9. Epub 2010 Oct 25.

Woodhead M, Blasi F, Ewig S, Huchon G, Leven M, Ortqvist A, Schaberg T, Torres A, van der Heijden G & Verheij TJ. (2005). Guidelines for the management of adult lower respiratory tract infections. *Eur Respir J* 26(6):1138–80.

Woods CW, McRill C, Plikaytis BD, Rosenstein NE, Mosley D, Boyd D, England B, Perkins BA, Ampel NM & Hajeh RA. (2000). Coccidioidomycosis in human immunodeficiency virus-infected persons in Arizona, 1994-1997: incidence, risk factors, and prevention. *J Infect Dis* 181(4):1428-34.

Wong SY & Wong KF. (2011). Penicillium marneffei Infection in AIDS. *Patholog Res Int* 10;2011:764293.

World Health Organization. (2003). Global Tuberculosis Programme. Treatment of tuberculosis: guidelines for national programmes, 3rd ed. Geneva.

World Health Organization. (2008). Global tuberculosis control. Surveillance, planning, financing. Report 2007. WHO/HTM/TB/2005.376. Geneva.

World Health Organization (2009). Global Tuberculosis Control: Epidemiology, Strategy, Financing (WHO/HTM/TB/2009.411). Geneva.

7

Pneumocystis jirovecii Pneumonia in AIDS Patients

Jose M. Varela[1], Francisco J. Medrano[1],
Eduardo Dei-Cas[2,3] and Enrique J. Calderón[1]
[1]*Instituto de Biomedicina de Sevilla and CIBER de Epidemiología y Salud Pública, Internal Medicine Service, Virgen del Rocío University Hospital. Seville,*
[2]*Parasitology-Mycology Service (EA4547), Centre of Biology Pathology, Lille-2 University Hospital Centre, Faculty of Medicine, Univ. Lille Nord de France,*
[3]*Biology & Diversity of Emerging Eukaryotic Pathogens, Institut Pasteur de Lille, Lille,*
[1]*Spain,*
[2,3]*France*

1. Introduction

Pneumocystis pneumonia (PcP) in humans is caused by the opportunistic eukaryotic pathogen *Pneumocystis jirovecii* (previously known as *Pneumocystis carinii* f. sp. *hominis*), which has recently been reclassified as a fungus because its cell wall composition and gene sequences (Edman, 1988, Stringer, 1989). This atypical uncultured fungus remains a major cause of illness and death in patients who have HIV infection. PcP has been the most common AIDS-defining opportunistic infection in the United States and Europe during more than two decades. Before 1989, 60-80% of AIDS patients presented with PcP, and the infection was estimated to be the cause of the death of 20-25% of these patients (Dei-Cas, 2000). Nowadays, despite the introduction of *Pneumocystis* chemoprophylaxis and advances in the treatment of HIV infection, mainly the development of highly active anti-retroviral therapy (HAART), PcP remains as a major opportunistic infection in patients with AIDS. While, the incidence of PcP among individuals with HIV infection has decreased in developed countries, the prevalence of AIDS-related PcP in developing countries remains high and poorly controlled. AIDS-related PcP continues to be an overwhelming illness among individuals who are unaware of their HIV infection, those without access to antiretroviral therapy, among patients who are intolerant or nonadherent to therapy, those who do not comply with prophylactic medications and in cases of failure of prophylaxis, probably relate to the emergence of drug-resistant strains (Calderon, 2010b).

2. Epidemiology

Pneumocystis jirovecii is probably one of the more frequent infectious agents faced by humans in everyday life. Today, it is recognized as an extracellular, obligate, host-specific, yeast-like parasitic fungus virtually restricted to lung tissue that can be directly transmitted among susceptible hosts by the airborne route. It is established that human PcP in not a zoonotic disease, and this notion has important implications for the epidemiology of *P. jirovecii* (Calderon, 2009). Although early studies reported the isolation of *Pneumocystis* DNA from the air surrounding apple orchards and the surface of pond water, no *Pneumocystis* forms were identified in environmental samples by microscopic analysis, and it is uncertain whether there is an ecological niche for *Pneumocystis* outside mammalian hosts (Wakefield, 1996). Animal sources of *P. jirovecii* can be excluded, because the *Pneumocystis* organisms that infect mammalian species are characterized by strong, close host-species specificity (Aliouat-Denis, 2008). Thus far, the human being is the only known reservoir host for *P. jirovecii,* and humans probably acquire the infection only from other humans (Calderon, 2009).

Serologic studies have shown that specific serum anti-*Pneumocystis* antibody can be detected in most children early in life, indicating frequent exposure to this organism (Respaldiza, 2004). On the basis of this finding, disease in immunocompromised persons has long been thought to result from reactivation of latent infection acquired in childhood. However, animal and human studies have shown that elimination of *Pneumocystis* often occurs after infection, implying that the persistence of latent organisms is limited (Morris, 2002). Recent demonstration of *P. jirovecii* transplacental transmission may explain the accumulating evidence that the primary infection is widely acquired very early in the life and support the commonly held view that human infants are a major natural reservoir for *P. jirovecii,* since they can remain colonized as their immune response matures (Montes-Cano, 2009).

Colonization with *P. jirovecii* in adults has recently gained attention as an important issue for understanding the complete cycle of human *Pneumocystis* infection (Calderón, 2010a). In general, colonization is defined as isolation of an infectious agent that does not result in sufficient damage to cause clinical disease, but that may alter host homeostasis. In the specific case of *Pneumocystis,* colonization is currently defined as the detection of the organism or its DNA in respiratory samples from subjects without signs or symptoms of pneumonia (Morris, 2008).

Among adults, *Pneumocystis* colonization has been well documented in both HIV-infected and non–HIV-infected individuals, and certain populations appear to have a higher risk of colonization. Studies have shown that individuals who have an underlying HIV-infection or another cause of immunosuppression and those who are not immunosuppressed but have chronic lung disease may often be colonized by *P. jirovecii* (Calderón, 2009). These groups at risk for carriage probably represent a major species-specific reservoir of infection, although transient *Pneumocystis* colonization has been also identified in healthy individuals that could behave as a sort of dynamic reservoir for future *Pneumocystis* infection in other susceptible subjects (Medrano, 2005).

Several outbreaks of PcP have been reported in hospitals. Molecular analyses of *Pneumocystis* in some of these studies suggested nosocomial acquisition of the infection (de Boer, 2007, Olsson, 2001, Rabodonirina, 2004). In addition, *Pneumocystis* colonization has been found more frequently in health care workers in close occupational contact with patients with PcP than in those who had no occupational exposure (Vargas, 2000, Miller 2001). On the other hand, a recent study has provided molecular evidence that airborne transmission of *P. jirovecii* from colonized immunocompetent carrier hosts to susceptible persons may occur (Rivero, 2008). Therefore, interindividual airborne transmission seems to occur in humans in both hospitals, as a nosocomial infection, and in the community.

3. Pathogenesis

Basic knowledge on *Pneumocystis* has been hampered by the lack of a reliable in vitro culture system. However, through the use of molecular techniques and experimental models of PcP in immunosuppressed animals, many progresses have been made over the last decades in our understanding of the complex pathophysiology and pathogenesis of this fungal infection.

At the histopathological level has been shown that the proliferation of *Pneumocystis* is accompanied by anatomical and physiological changes. In animal models, alterations in alveolar-capillary permeability are followed by degenerative changes in type I pneumocytes, restorative hypertrophy of type II pneumocytes and diffuse alveolar damage leading to pulmonary fibrosis (Walzer, 1993). Studies in humans have also shown changes in the permeability of the alveolar-capillary membrane, pulmonary diffusing capacity and vital capacity in total lung (Coleman et al., 1984). These changes depend on the ability of *Pneumocystis,* demonstrated in animal models to induce in the very early stages of the infection alveolar macrophage activation, increased pro-inflammatory cytokines and changes in pulmonary surfactant even when small amounts of microorganisms are present (Prevost et al., 1998).

In the infected host, *Pneumocystis* organisms dwell almost exclusively within lung alveoli. Within some hours after experimental intra-tracheal infection, Pneumocystis trophic forms attach to the alveolar epithelial cells. The host immune response against the infection involves complex interactions between CD4+ and CD8+ T-cells, alveolar macrophages, neutrophils and soluble mediators that facilitate clearance of the infection. Disease only occurs when cellular and/or humoral immunity is defective.

3.1 Interactions of *Pneumocystis* with alveolar host cells

Trophic forms adhere tightly to alveolar type I cells through interdigitation of their membranes with those of the host. The binding of *Pneumocystis* to the epithelium is facilitated by interactions with proteins of the alveolar fluid, such as fibronectin and vitronectin that bind to the surface of *Pneumocystis* and mediate the attachment to integrin receptors present on the alveolar epithelium. In infected tissues, type I alveolar cells with adherent *Pneumocystis* appear vacuolated and eroded (Benfield et al., 1997). However, studies of cultured lung epithelial cells have shown that the adherence of *Pneumocystis* alone does not disrupt the structure or barrier function of alveolar epithelial cells, although proliferative repair of the epithelium is reduced. It is therefore unlikely that the adherence of *Pneumocystis* to alveolar epithelium is by itself responsible for the diffuse alveolar damage in severe pneumonia (Benfield et al., 1997; Thomas & Limper, 2007). Rather, the inflammatory responses in the host are primarily responsible for the compromise of the alveolar-capillary surface (Thomas & Limper, 2007).

Electron microscopic studies have shown that *Pneumocystis* organisms are embedded in protein-rich alveolar exudates, which contain abundant fibronectin, vitronectin, and hydrophilic surfactant proteins A and D. In contrast, hydrophobic surfactant protein B and C are reduced during PcP. Both surfactant protein A and surfactant protein D interact with the Major Surface Glycoprotein (MSG) components of the surface at *Pneumocystis*. Surfactant protein A modulates the interactions of *Pneumocystis* with the alveolar macrophages. In contrast, surfactant protein D mediates the aggregation of the *Pneumocystis* organisms, but because the aggregated organisms are extremely poorly taken up by macrophages, they may escape elimination. Pulmonary surfactant phospholipids, which contribute to the low surface tension in the alveoli, are reduced during PcP, and abnormalities in the composition and function of the surfactant are the result of the host's inflammatory response to *Pneumocystis*, rather than direct effects of the organisms on the surfactant components (Wright et al., 2001; Thomas & Limper, 2007).

3.2 Innate immunity (alveolar macrophages and neutrophils)

Although parasite attachment to lung epithelial cells is essential for *Pneumocystis* infection and propagation, invasion of host cells does not occur (Krajicek et al., 2009). Alveolar macrophages are the first line of host defence to control the infection, since they are the principal phagocytes mediating the uptake and direct degradation of both trophic forms and cysts forms in the lung (Kelly & Shellito, 2010). Macrophages display several potential receptors for glucans, including CD11b/CD18 integrin (CR3), dectin-1, and toll-like receptor 2. The activation of macrophages by *Pneumocystis* is augmented by host proteins such as vitronectin and fibronectin that bind the glucan components on the organism (Vassallo et al., 2001). When there are not opsonins in the epithelial-lining fluid, the uptake of *Pneumocystis* is mediated mainly through the macrophage mannose receptors, pattern-recognition molecules that interact with the surface mannoprotein, MSG (also called glycoprotein A). After they have been taken up by macrophages, *Pneumocystis* organisms are incorporated into phagolysosomes and degraded. Macrophages produce a large variety of proinflammatory cytokines, chemokines, and eicosanoid metabolites in response to phagocytosis of *Pneumocystis*. Although these mediators participate in eradicating *Pneumocystis*, they also promote pulmonary injury (Limper et al., 1997).

Neutrophils alone are unable to control the infection. Unlike other opportunistic fungal infections, *Pneumocystis* disease is rare in patients with neutropenia. Neutrophils are associated with inflammation and, therefore, have been implicated in severity of disease. In fact, decreased pulmonary function and local lung inflammation and damage have been correlated with elevated neutrophil counts in HIV-infected patients with PcP (Kelly & Shellito, 2010). The neutrophils recruited into the lungs release reactive oxidant species, proteases, and cationic proteins, which directly injure capillary endothelial cells and alveolar epithelial cells (Thomas & Limper, 2004).

3.3 Adaptive immunity (T cells and B cells)

Both cellular and humoral immune systems are important in defence against *Pneumocystis* infection.

The activity of CD4+ T cells is pivotal in the host's defences against *Pneumocystis*, since most HIV-infected patients with PcP have CD4+ T-cell counts below 200 cells/mm^3. CD4+ lymphocytes as memory cells coordinate and orchestrate the host inflammatory responses by means of the recruitment and activation of other immune effector cells, including monocytes and macrophages, which are responsible for elimination of the organism. Macrophage-derived TNF-α and interleukin-1 are believed to be necessary for initiating pulmonary responses to *Pneumocystis* infection that are mediated by CD4+ cells. The cells proliferate in response to *Pneumocystis* antigens and generate cytokine mediators, including lymphotactin and interferon gamma (IFN-γ). Lymphotactin, a chemokine, acts as a potent chemoattractant for further lymphocyte recruitment in PcP.

Although T lymphocytes are essential for the clearance of *Pneumocystis*, experimental data suggest that T-cell responses may also result in substantial pulmonary impairment during pneumonia. For instance, in severe combined immunodeficiency (SCID) mice infected with *Pneumocystis*, normal oxygenation and lung function occur despite active infection until the late stages of the disease. When the immune systems in these animals are reconstituted with the use of intact spleen cells, an intense T-cell–mediated inflammatory response ensues, resulting in substantially impaired gas exchange (Wright et al., 1999b). In the absence of brisk lung inflammation, *Pneumocystis* has little direct effect on pulmonary function. In a similar manner, in patients who have undergone bone marrow transplantation the clinical onset of PcP and of most marked alterations in lung function occur during engraftment (Thomas & Limper, 2004).

The CD8+ T cells seem to play also an important role in control of *Pneumocystis* infection since in experimental animal models depletion of both CD4+ and CD8+ cells results in a more severe PcP than only depletion of CD4+ cells. However, their role may be less important than CD4+ T cells since CD8+ T-cell-depleted animals can still clear the infection (Lu & Lee, 2008). *Pneumocystis* infection results in the marked accumulation of CD8+ T lymphocytes in the lung. Although not as extensively investigated as CD4+ T cells, insights into the role of CD8+ T cells in host defence against *Pneumocystis* have been achieved, but that is not nearly enough. Recent data provide the concept that CD8+ T cells, most likely those of the Tc1 phenotype, are critical for clearance of some fungal organisms including *Pneumocystis*, particularly in the context of CD4+ T-cell deficiency or dysfunction. CD8+ T cells have also been shown to play a detrimental role in *Pneumocystis* infection. CD8+ T cells are considered to be part of the damaging inflammatory response in CD4+ T-cell-depleted mice. The presence of CD8+ T cells affected surfactant function and it also has been shown to exacerbate TNF-α production (Steele et al., 2005).

Lastly, a significant role of humoral immune response in the host defence against *Pneumocystis* is supported by the observations that SCID animals require B cells to clear the infection (Burns et al., 1990), and that patients with agammaglobulinemia develop PcP despite of an intact cellular immune system (Alibrahim et al., 1998; Lu & Lee, 2008). B lymphocytes appears to play an important role in the generation of CD4+ memory cells in response to *Pneumocystis* (Lu & Lee, 2008).

3.4 Cytokine and chemokine networks

Various pro-inflammatory cytokines including IFN-γ, tumour necrosis factor alpha (TNF-α), interleukin (IL)-8, IL-1 and IL-6 and chemokines such as RANTES (Regulated upon Activation normal T-cell Expressed, and Secreted), macrophage inflammatory protein (MIP)-1α, MIP-1β and MIP-2 release by macrophages, neutrophils, epithelial cells and lymphocytes are involved in the host immune response and lung damage during *Pneumocystis* disease (Calderon et al., 2007).

INF-γ has a critical role for control lung inflammation during PcP, although is not directly toxic to *Pneumocystis* organisms. This cytokine is produced primarily by CD4+ T cells. There is an indirect correlation between IFN-levels and severity of PcP (Kelly & Shellito, 2010). IFN-γ strongly activates the macrophage production of TNF-α, superoxides, and reactive nitrogen species, each of which is implicated in the host defence against *Pneumocystis* (Wright et al., 1999a).

TNF-α is a potent pro-inflammatory cytokine secreted primarily by macrophage that promotes the recruitment of neutrophils, lymphocytes, and monocytes. Although their recruitment is important for clearance of the organisms, these cells injure the lung by releasing oxidants, cationic proteins, and proteases. TNF-α also induces the production of other cytokines and chemokines, including IL-8 and IFN-γ, which stimulate the recruitment and activation of inflammatory cells during *Pneumocystis* infection (Wright et al., 2004). The cell wall of *Pneumocystis* contains abundant beta-glucans, and studies have confirmed that the production of TNF-α by alveolar macrophages is mediated by recognition of the beta-glucan components of *Pneumocystis*. IL-8 is correlated with both neutrophil infiltration of the lung and impaired gas exchange during severe PcP (Thomas & Limper, 2004).

The most important function of chemokines is to recruit effector cells to the site of injury. Many studies have found an increase in chemokine expression during PcP. In a SCID experimental model of PcP it has been found that expression levels of RANTES, MIP-1α, MIP-1β and MIP-2 were all upregulated after lymphocyte reconstitution of the SCID animal. In addition, the time course of chemokine expression correlates *Pneumocystis* clearance, but also with the lung inflammation (Wright et al., 1999a). Thus, the role of chemokines is essential for the resolution of infection, but overexpression may also result in a hyperinflammatory state and lung damage (Kelly & Shellito, 2010).

4. Clinical presentation and chest radiology

In patients infected with HIV, PcP is a common AIDS-defining illness and occurs most frequently in subjects with a CD4+ count less than 200 cells per mm^3. The symptoms of PcP are nonspecific and PcP in patients with HIV infection tends to run a more subacute indolent course and tends to present much later, often after several weeks of symptoms, compared with PcP associated with other immunocompromising conditions. A more acute illness with symptoms including a cough productive with purulent sputum should suggest an alternate infectious diagnosis, such as bacterial pneumonia or tuberculosis

Patients with PcP often develop dyspnea (95%), which increases over time; cough productive of clear sputum or non-productive cough; low grade or no fever; malaise, and sometimes chest tightness or pain. However, the clinical picture in individual patients is variable and many infectious and non-infectious processes can present identically. Also, the general hallmarks of this disease such as fever, shortness of breath, and diffuse infiltrates do not invariably occur, especially early in the course while the disease is mild (Thomas & Limper, 2004). Acute dyspnea with pleuritic chest pain may indicate the development of a pneumothorax, which has been presented in 2% to 4% of patients (Sepkowitz et al., 1991). In all cases, a high index of suspicion and a thorough history are key factors in early detection of PcP. Physical examination may reveal tachypnea, tachycardia, and cyanosis. Lung auscultation usually reveals few abnormalities with dry cackles or rhonchi present in less than 50% of patients. Individuals with PcP can be hypoxemic with respiratory alkalosis but can also have normal alveolar-arterial gradients if identified early in the natural history of their disease. Elevated serum levels of lactate dehydrogenase (LDH) have been related with PcP and probably reflects lung parenchymal damage but is not specific and elevations can be seen in many pulmonary and non-pulmonary conditions. In general, laboratory abnormalities are less severe in HIV-infected patients than in non-HIV immunosuppressed patients (Hughes, 2004).

Classically, chest radiographic features of PcP are bilateral, symmetric, fine reticular interstitial infiltrates involving the perihilar areas (figure 1a), becoming more homogenous and diffuse as the severity of the infection increases (Thomas & Limper, 2004). Less frequently, PcP may present with unilateral or asymmetrical opacities. Thin-walled cysts or pneumatocele are seen in 10-20% of cases. Pleural effusions and intrathoracic adenopathy are rare. Patients who receive aerosolized pentamidine have an increased frequency of upper-lobe infiltrates, pneumothorax, or cystic lesions. Early in the course of PcP, the chest radiograph may be normal in up to 25% of cases (Schliep & Yarrish, 1999).

A high-resolution computed tomography scan is more sensitive than chest radiograph and is helpful when the chest radiography findings are equivocal. The typical appearance is patchy areas of ground-glass attenuation with a background of interlobular septal thickening or cystic lesions predominating in perihilar areas (figure 1b), even then chest radiographic findings are normal (Nyamande et al., 2007). While such findings are suggestive, they are not diagnostic. However, a negative high-resolution computed tomography scan may allow exclusion of PcP in patients with HIV.

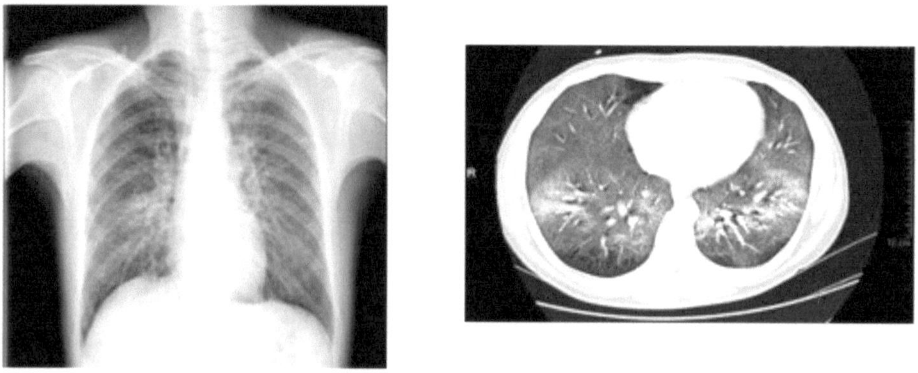

Fig. 1. Radiographic findings of *Pneumocystis* pneumonia in a patient with AIDS. (1a, left) Chest x-ray of a *Pneumocystis* pneumonia showing diffuse infiltrations in both lung fields. (1b, right) Chest high-resolution CT scan of a patient with AIDS revealing diffuse ground glass opacities and thickened alveolar septum in both lungs.

Extrapulmonary manifestations of *P. jirovecii* infection (extrapulmonary pneumocystosis) are distinctly unusual but they has been reported primarily among HIV-infected patients, particularly those who receive aerosolized pentamidine for prophylaxis of PcP and in those with advanced HIV infection who are not taking any prophylaxis. Mainly, during the terminal stage of HIV-related disease *Pneumocystis* organisms may disseminate from the lungs to other organs where they induce secondary visceral lesions. However, sometimes pulmonary infection may not be apparent when extrapulmonary lesions are detected. Lymph nodes, spleen, kidneys, liver, thyroid and bone marrow are the most commonly infected organs, but microorganisms have been also found in the brain, pancreas, skin, heart, muscle and other organs (Ng et al, 1997). For HIV-infected patients, extrapulmonary pneumocystosis limited to the choroid layer or ear (external auditory canal or middle ear) has a better prognosis, with good response to specific treatment, than disseminated pneumocystosis in multiple noncontiguous sites. Lesions are frequently nodular and may contain necrotic material or calcification. Extrapulmonary pneumocystosis in solid organs appears on computed tomography scan as focal, hypodense lesions with well-defined borders and central or peripheral calcification (Schliep & Yarrish, 1999).

Immunorestitution disease (IRD) is defined as an acute symptomatic or paradoxical deterioration of a (most probably) preexisting infection that is temporally related to the recovery of the immune system and it is due to immunopathological damage associated with the reversal of immunosuppressive processes. PcP manifesting as a form of IRD has been described in both HIV and non-HIV immunosuppressed patients (Cheng et al., 2004; Jagannathan et al., 2009; Mori et al., 2009). Among HIV-infected patients, PcP manifesting acutely during the initiation of HAART is a well-recognized phenomenon (Wislez et al., 2001). AIDS-related PcP patients seem to be at risk of clinical deterioration due to IRD if antiretroviral therapy is started within one to two weeks after the initiation of treatment for PcP (Wislez et al., 2001). The onset of clinical deterioration is associated with an increase in the CD4+ lymphocyte count and a reduction in the HIV viral load (Wislez et al., 2001).

5. Prognosis

Despite treatment, mortality of PcP still remains high. Several studies highlight that mortality rates are declining in patients with PcP. However, in other studies, PcP has remained the leading cause of death among those nor receiving o failing to comply with HAART or PcP prophylaxis. Predictors of mortality include older age, recent injection drug use, increased total bilirrubin, low serum albumin, and alveolar-arterial oxygen gradient >50 mm Hg (Fei et al, 2009).

6. Management PcP

There is no universally agreed approach on to the initial management of patients with suspected PcP. Many institutions treat patients with suspected PcP empirically, while others pursue a definitive microbiological diagnosis (Huang, 2004). Since PcP can be rapidly progressive and the mortality rate remains high, early therapy is essential (Calderon et al, 2004; Roblot, 2005). Identification of patients having PcP into mild, moderate or severe disease allows to guide the choice of the drug for the treatment of PcP, as well as, to decide if adjuvant corticosteroids are indicated (table 1) (Miller et al., 1996). In AIDS-related PcP, the typical duration of therapy is at least 21 days because of the risk for relapse with shorter treatment duration. Patients generally improved after 4 to 8 days of therapy. Although the overall prognosis of patients whose degree of hypoxemia requires intensive care unit (ICU) admission or mechanical ventilation remains poor, survival in up to 50% of patients requiring ventilatory support has been reported. Patients with reasonable functional status and severe PcP should be offered ICU admission or mechanical ventilation (CDC, 2009).

	Mild	**Moderate**	**Severe**
Symptoms and signs	Dyspnoea on exertion, with or without cough and sweats	Dyspnoea on minimal exertion and occasionally at rest. Cough and fever	Dyspnoea and tachypnoea at rest. Persistent fever and cough
Arterial oxygen tension (PaO2) at rest	> 11.0 kPa (82.7 mmHg)	8.0 to 11.0 kPa (60-82.7 mmHg)	< 8.0 kPa (60 mmHg)
Arterial oxygen saturation (SaO2) at rest	> 96%	91 to 96%	< 91%
Chest radiograph	Normal, or minor perihiliar shadowing	Diffuse interstitial shadowing	Extension interstitial shadowing with or without diffuse alveolar shadowing

Modified of Miller RF, et al., 1996.

Table 1. Grading of severity of *Pneumocystis* pneumonia.

7. Diagnosis of PCP

7.1 Microscopic detection of *Pneumocystis*

The single most important diagnostic tool for *Pneumocystis* infection is a high clinical suspicion. However, specific diagnosis of PcP requires documentation of the microorganism in respiratory specimens. Since *Pneumocystis* cannot be cultured, the diagnosis of PcP relies on microscopic detection of *Pneumocystis* organisms on stained respiratory specimens. Conventional stains such as toluidine blue O (TBO), Grocott's methenamine silver nitrate

(GMS), or methanol Giemsa methods (figure 2) can be used to identify the organism (cysts or trophic forms) but immunofluorescent staining is the most common technique currently used. TBO or GMS stains facilitate rapid parasite detection, even at low magnification, in all kinds of clinical specimens. However, these dyes also stain the cell wall of yeasts or other fungi. For this reason, a good strategy to identify *Pneumocystis* organisms accurately in clinical specimens is to systematically associate the examination of both TBO- or GMS-stained smears and methanol-Giemsa-stained smears from the same specimen (table 2). Actually, methanol-Giemsa (or other equivalent panoptical Giemsa-like stains) makes it possible, on the one hand, to distinguish *Pneumocystis* organisms from other microorganism and, on the other hand, to identify the different *Pneumocystis* life-cycle stages. In fact, Giemsa and other stains with similar cytological affinities, such as Diff Quick or RAL-555, cause the parasite nuclei to stain pinkish purple and the cytoplasm to stain blue (Dei-Cas et al, 1998). They do not stain cystic or sporocytic walls, which appear like a clear peripheral halo around cystic forms. These polychrome stains make it possible accurately to distinguish *Pneumocystis* trophic or cystic forms from other fungi and also from host cells or cell debris. On the whole, the biggest advantage of methanol-Giemsa or Giemsa-like stain methods consists in staining trophic forms and sporocytes, which remain unidentified in TBO- or GMS-stained smears (Dei-Cas et al, 1998).

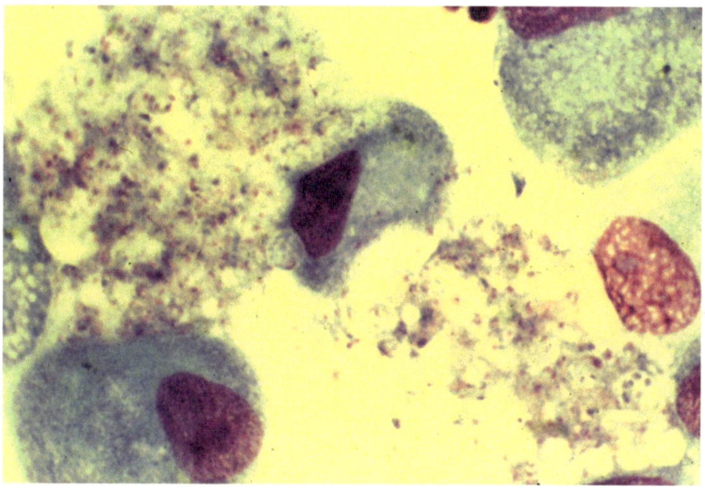

Fig. 2. Stain with methanol–Giemsa stain

Efficiency and cost-effectiveness of the different microscopic stains evoked here vary according to experience of groups, technical protocols, type and quality of the samples, local incidence of PcP, and the number of organisms present (Chouaid et al., 1995) (table 2). It is generally accepted, however, that association of methods that stain cystic cell wall (e.g. TBO or GMS) with panoptical techniques (methanol-Giemsa or analogous staining methods) is usually required (Dei-Cas et al., 2006). Moreover, it is usually recognized that specific antibody staining is mainly helpful to detect *Pneumocystis* organisms in non-BAL smears (e.g. induced sputum, expectorated sputum, gastric wash) and to clarify conflicting light microscopic observations (Aderaye et al., 2008; Cruciani et al., 2002; Kovacs et al., 1998; Limawongpranee et al., 2007).

Typically, the respiratory specimens are obtained by sputum induction or fiberoptic bronchoscopy with bronchoalveolar lavage (BAL). Sputum induction by inhalation of a hypertonic saline solution is the quickest and least-invasive method for definitively diagnosing PcP with a sensitivity between 50-90% and specificity of 99-100%. Sputum induced may also be less sensitive in patients receiving aerosolized pentamidine for prophylaxis. All of the direct organism visualization methods can lead to false-negative results, consequently, a negative sputum induction cannot rule out a diagnosis of PcP. If sputum induction is nondiagnostic or cannot be performed, then bronchoscopy with BAL is the next step. A BAL that is negative for *Pneumocystis* rules out the diagnosis of PcP.

In order to detect *Pneumocystis* organisms in histological sections from lung or other organs, pathologists target usually the cystic forms, since trophic ones are uneasily identifiable in paraffin-embedded tissues. They use therefore GMS and, less frequently, TBO staining procedures adapted to tissue sections. Trophic forms can however be identified in epon-embedded semi-thin sections stained with toluidine blue or other stains (Dei-Cas et al., 1998; Durand-Joly et al., 2000). Furthermore, *Pneumocystis*-specific fluorescein-, phosphatase or peroxidase-labeled monoclonal antibodies available from many suppliers may help to identify *Pneumocystis* organisms in BAL, induced sputum or tissue samples (table 2).

Technique	**Suitable kind of sample**	**Needed experience**	**Sensitivity**	**Specificity**	**Advantages**	**Drawbacks**	**Recommended combination with:**
Microscopy:							
PC/IC	BALF wet smear	very good	variable	good	rapidity	needs confirmation by other methods	panoptical stain
GMS/TBO	BALF air-dried cytospin smear or biopsy (histological section)	average	high	average	cost; rapidity	false positive (poor experienced staffs); identifies only the cystic stages	panoptical stain
Panoptical stains*	BALF air-dried cytospin smear	very good	average	very high	cost; rapidity; identify all *Pneumocystis* stages	limited sensitivity (poor experienced staffs)	GMS/TBO
FL Mab	BALF, IS or sputum air-dried cytospin smear	good	high	good	good sensitivity/ specificity	cost; time-consuming	-
IP/AP Mab	biopsy (histological section), air-dried cytospin smear	good	good	good	good specificity	cost; time-consuming	-
PCR	BALF, IS, OW, NPA, biopsy	average	very high	very high	Helpful in HIV-negative patients; rapidity (real-time PCR assays); non-invasive	cost; positive in colonized patients	-

Technique	Suitable kind of sample	Needed experience	Sensitivity	Specificity	Advantages	Drawbacks	Recommended combination with:
					sampling; genotyping		
BG	serum	average	good	low	rapidity; post-therapeutic control	positive in other deep fungal infections	other tests
KL-6	serum	average	good	low	-	positive in other pulmonary infections	
Serum *Pneumocystis* antibody assay	serum	average	depending on antigen and assay	depending on antigen and assay	helpful in epidemiology studies	positive in people without PcP	other tests

*Giemsa or Giemsa-like stains. BALF: Bronchoalveolar lavage fluid; BG: serum beta-1,3-glucan; FL Mab: fluorescein-labeled Pneumocystis monoclonal antibody; GMS: Grocott-methenamine silver stain; IP/AP Mab: immuneperoxidase/alkaline-phosphatase labeled monoclonal antibody; IS: induced sputum; PC/IC: phase contrast/interference contrast; TBO: toluidine blue stain. KL-6: Mucin like glycoprotein.

Table 2. Laboratory diagnostic methods for *Pneumocystis* pneumonia.

7.2 Molecular detection of *Pneumocystis*

Many *Pneumocystis* PCR assays have been developed during the last two decades. PCR tool revealed highly efficacious to amplify *Pneumocystis* DNA from diverse kinds of clinical specimens (BALF, IS, expectorated sputum, oropharyngeal or nasopharyngeal wash samples, biopsy specimens) (figure 3) (de la Horra et al., 2006; Durand-Joly et al., 2005; Olsson et al., 1993; Wakefield et al., 1990). In the clinical laboratory, the use of molecular methods is mainly warranted to increase the sensitivity of *P. jirovecii* detection in clinical specimens in order to establish earlier PcP diagnosis, detecting low parasite rates, mainly in non-HIV infected patients with PcP, and detecting *Pneumocystis* DNA in noninvasive samples (Durand-Joly et al., 2005; Respaldiza et al., 2006) (table 2). Moreover, PCR assays followed by direct sequencing or other strategies were used for typing *Pneumocystis* isolates in order to identify parasite strains and to explore correlation between specific genotypes and virulence, transmissibility or drug susceptibility. PCR, especially nested PCR assays applied to noninvasive samples, have also been used to detect *Pneumocystis* colonization either in susceptible individuals or in apparently healthy people, including health care workers in hospitals (Durand-Joly et al., 2003; Medrano et al., 2005; Nevez et al., 2008).

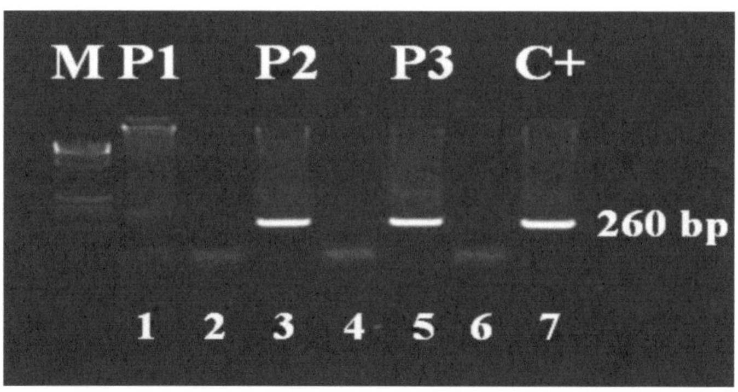

Fig. 3. Nested PCR (mtLSU rRNA region) results.

M: molecular mass marker. Lane 1 (P1) negative specimen. Lanes 3 and 5 (P2, P3) positive specimens of oral wash in cystic fibrosis patients. Lane 7 (C+) positive control. Lanes 2, 4 and 6 negative controls (water).

For PcP diagnosis in humans, conventional or real-time PCR assays based on the amplification of the large subunit of mitochondrial ribosomal DNA (mtLSUrDNA) (Wakefield et al., 1990) are the most commonly used, but many other sequences have been targeted (Major Surface Glycoprotein, Internal Transcribed Spacers, Thymidylate Synthase, Dihydrofolate Reductase, heat-shock protein 70, etc.) (Durand-Joly et al., 2005; Hugett et al., 2008). Comparative evaluating studies are uneasy to perform because of different clinical contexts, sampling methods, laboratory reagents or technical strategies used to DNA extraction, amplification or analysis of results (Durand-Joly et al., 2005).

In general, conventional or real-time *Pneumocystis* PCR assays have represented a significant advance in PcP laboratory diagnosis. Actually, highly sensitive and specific PCR tools, especially real-time PCR assays, improved the clinical diagnosis of PcP allowing an accurate, early diagnosis of *Pneumocystis* infection (Durand-Joly et al., 2005), which should lead to a decreased duration from onset of symptoms to treatment. This period has a recognized impact on prognosis since PcP-associated respiratory failure requiring mechanic ventilation entails significant mortality (Huang, 2004). In addition, PCR assay may reveal PcP in patients with negative microscopic test. For instance, among 62 HIV-negative patients with clinical PcP diagnosed in the Lille University Hospital between 1998 and 2001, 30 patients (48%) had positive PCR results with negative microscopic tests (Durand-Joly, 2002).

Notably, molecular techniques play a significant role when they are applied to noninvasive specimens as IS, oropharyngeal wash (OW, obtained by gargling 10 ml of 0.9% NaCl for >60 seconds) (Respaldiza et al., 2006) or nasopharyngeal aspirates (NPA) (Richards et al. 1994). When DNA sequences used as primers or probe have been adequately defined, the analytical specificity of *Pneumocystis*-PCR assays applied to noninvasive or to BALF samples should usually be of 100% (Durand-Joly et al., 2005). With regard to sensitivity, *Pneumocystis*-mtLSUrDNA PCR showed high analytical sensitivity for the detection of *Pneumocystis* organisms on BALF samples from AIDS patients, with a detection threshold of 0.5–1 organism/μl^{-1} (Tamburrini et al., 1998). The sensitivity of PCR assays applied to OW (or other noninvasive samples) is certainly lower (<80%) than that of PCR on BALF samples (>95%) (Tsolaki et al., 2008). However, OW can be easily repeated in order to monitor the evolution of infection and, potentially, the therapeutic response (Tsolaki et al., 2008).

A significant problem of *Pneumocystis* PCR assays is raised by *Pneumocystis* colonization (Calderon, 2009). Actually, a positive PCR result associated with a negative microscopic test may result from either *Pneumocystis* colonization or PcP. In common practice, this difficulty is often solved on the basis of a careful clinical, radiological and laboratory assessment of the patient pathological condition, as it is usually done to other infectious diseases, especially when their agents are opportunistic pathogens. However, the alternative of quantifying parasite rates was also explored (Larsen et al., 2002). Thus, a quantitative real-time PCR assay that targeted *Pneumocystis* Major Surface Glycoprotein (MSG) multigene family was applied to OW samples, and revealed significant differences between PcP patients and *Pneumocystis* colonized subjects in the number of MSG copies. The authors suggested a cutoff value of 50 MSG gene fragment copies/tube for distinguishing between the two conditions (Larsen et al., 2002). However, quantitative PCR results seemed difficult to use on the field. The main problem was inability to control the volume of the sample. Another difficulty is related with the kind of patients. Actually, it seems difficult to apply a same cutoff to AIDS patients, patients with other underlying diseases or individuals receiving chemoprophylaxis against *Pneumocystis*.

There is no formal agreement about an unequivocal definition of *Pneumocystis* colonization. The notion may however be characterized on the basis of clinical and experimental observations. In clinical practice, the diagnosis of *Pneumocystis* colonization or subclinical carriage is usually retained when *Pneumocystis* DNA is detected by PCR methods in respiratory samples from immunodepressed or immunocompetent subjects without symptoms or signs of *Pneumocystis* infection, and who do not progress to PcP (Morris et al., 2008) In these subjects, *Pneumocystis* organisms are only exceptionally detected by microscopy (Vidal et al., 2006). Interestingly, recent experimental data strengthened the biological significance of *Pneumocystis* colonization (Chabe et al., 2004). They demonstrated that *Pneumocystis* organisms can replicate in the lungs of immunocompetent carriers, stimulate an antibody response and be efficiently transmitted by airborne route to either naive immunocompetent hosts, who will develop a primary infection, or to immunosuppressed hosts, who may then develop PcP (Chabe et al., 2004). In addition, many evidences suggest that beyond PcP, *Pneumocystis* colonization may induce local or systemic inflammation, a condition that could aggravate chronic pulmonary diseases. For instance, *P. jirovecii* pulmonary carriage in patients with chronic obstructive pulmonary disease (COPD) could favor the progression of this disease (Calderon et al., 2007; Morris et al., 2008).

Efforts have been made to associate specific *P. jirovecii* genotypes with virulence, drug susceptibility or other medically important biological properties of parasite strains. Some studies reported some correlation between polymorphism and clinical features (Miller & Wakefield, 1999; Totet et al., 2003). Polymorphism of internal transcribed spacer (ITS1/ITS2) sequences was quite frequently used and more than 30 ITS1 genotypes and 40 ITS2 genotypes with more than 90 haplotypes (combinations of ITS1 and ITS2 types) have been reported (Beard, 2004).

Most polymorphism studies targeted mutations of the *P. jirovecii* dihydropteroate synthase (DHPS) gene, which could potentially be linked with sulfa resistance. Regarding this issue, and since effective *P. jirovecii* culture systems are unavailable, several groups have assessed putative trimethoprim-sulfamethoxazole (TMP-SMX) drug resistance by detecting *Pneumocystis* DHPS mutations. Indeed nonsynonymous DHPS point mutations at nucleotide positions 165 and 171 entail an amino acid change at positions 55 (Thr to Ala) and/or 57 (Pro to Ser) (Friaza et al., 2009). Such mutations confer resistance to sulfa drugs in other organisms, including *Escherichia coli*, *Streptococcus pneumoniae* and *Plasmodium falciparum*. The *P. jirovecii* DHPS mutant form has also been shown to be more resistant to sulfamethoxazole in a *Saccharomyces cerevisiae* model (Iliades et al., 2004), but it is still uncertain if *Pneumocystis* DHPS mutations lead to drug resistance in patients (Huang et al., 2000, 2004; Nahimana et al., 2004). Such mutations were shown to be associated with the use of TMP-SMX or dapsone (two DHPS inhibitors), the duration of sulfa or dapsone prophylaxis and with geographic areas in which sulfamethoxazole or dapsone were commonly used for PcP prophylaxis (Huang et al., 2004; Kazanjian et al., 2000). However, results of studies searching specifically to establish an association between the presence of *P. jirovecii* DHPS mutations and clinical outcomes, such as treatment failure or death, are contradictory (Alvarez-Martinez et al., 2008, Helweg-Larsen et al., 1999; Huang et al., 2004,

Stein et al., 2004; van Hal et al., 2009). Outstandingly, most PcP patients carrying *P. jirovecii* isolates with DHPS mutations responded well to TMP-SMX treatment and survived probably because these mutations may confer a low-level of resistance to sulfa-drugs that is overcome by high drug concentration achieved in lung tissues by sulfamethoxazole (Calderon et al., 2004; Huang et al., 2004).

7.3 Other laboratory diagnostic methods

7.3.1 Beta-D-glucan assay

β-1,3-glucan (BG) is the main structural component of the cell wall of all fungi, including *Pneumocystis* cysts (Thomas & Limper, 2007). Interestingly, high serum BG levels have been reported in patients with PcP (Desmet et al., 2009; Nakamura et al., 2009; Teramoto et al., 2000). Consistently, such levels decreased with effective anti-*Pneumocystis* treatment (Teramoto et al., 2000). Serum BG appeared therefore as a good marker of *Pneumocystis* infection. The potential utility of this assay was analyzed in a retrospective case-control study of patients with suspected PcP comparing BG with microscopic examination on BAL. The BG assay had a sensitivity of 92% and a specificity of 86% for detecting PcP for a ut-off level of 31.1 pg/ml (Tasaka et al., 2007). In a recent study, it has been observed that BG levels in HIV patients with PcP are higher than in non-HIV patients. This could be attributed to the fact that HIV patients have greater numbers of microorganisms that non-HIV patients (Nakamura et al., 2009).

However, BG levels could not be correlated with PcP prognosis, and false positive results could exceed more than 30% (Nakamura et al., 2009). False positive results were reported in patients undergoing bacterial septicemia, hemodialysis with cellulose dialysis membranes, treatment with immunoglobulin, glucan-containing antitumor drugs, amoxicillin-clavulanate, piperacillin-tazobactam or contact with gauze or surgical sponges containing BG (Ponton, 2009). Furthermore, since invasive fungal infections induce also an increase of serum BG, the test should often be associated with laboratory assays aiming at detecting such infections (Desmet et al., 2009). These preliminary studies suggest that in the right clinical setting serum BG may provide a useful noninvasive diagnostic adjunct for patients with *Pneumocystis* infection. However, additional information is necessary to address the general specificity of BG in diagnosing PcP versus other fungal infections in diverse immune-suppressed patient populations and to differentiate among patients with PcP and patients with *Pneumocystis* colonization.

7.3.2 KL-6

KL-6 is a mucin-like glycoprotein expressed on type II pneumocytes and bronchiolar epithelial cells. This marker has reached elevated levels in several studies in patients with PcP. However, the reported false-positive rate and level of detection were not as good as for the BG assay (Nakamura et al, 2009; Tasaka et al, 2007). Recent investigations indicate that KL-6 is more a generalized marker for alveolar epithelial injury (Sato et al, 2004) and high levels have also be found in non-fungal infections such as *legionellosis*, severe tuberculosis and respiratory syncythial virus bronchiolitis, and even in noninfectious interstitial lung disease (Inou et al., 1995; Kawasaki et al., 2009; Sukoh et al., 2001). Therefore, KL-6 elevation in PcP is thought to be related to lung damage and regeneration of epithelium lining and cannot be used as a specified marker of *Pneumocystis* infection.

7.3.3 *S*-adenosylmethionine (SAM)

Some observations suggested that S-adenosylmethionine (SAM), which is a universal methyl donor synthesized from methionine and ATP by SAM synthetase, could stimulate *Pneumocystis* in vitro growth (Clarkson et al., 2004). Since SAM was depleted from both the culture medium and the plasma of rats with PcP, it was hypothesized that *Pneumocystis* cells could scavenge SAM from host fluids due to the lack of SAM synthetase (Clarkson et al., 2004) Consistently, plasma SAM levels were found to be low in patients with PcP and to increase gradually with treatment (Skelly et al., 2003, 2008). These findings strengthened the idea of using plasma SAM levels as a non-invasive PcP diagnostic method. However, recent data showed that SAM-related issue could be more complex than previously thought. Firstly, differences in SAM levels between laboratories could be influenced by the method of measurement. Thus, Wang and colleagues using Chromatography Tandem Mass Spectrometry found generally higher plasma SAM levels than those reported before (Wang et al., 2008). The same group was unable to distinguish patients with acute PcP from the ones without PcP on the basis of plasma SAM levels, though these levels increased significantly with effective anti-*Pneumocystis* treatment. Indeed, the concern needs to be further explored because fasting status, dietary intake of methionine and other medications can affect plasma SAM concentration (Wang et al, 2008). Secondly, and contrarily to the results of previous works (Clarkson et al., 2004), *P. carinii*, *P. murina* and *P. jirovecii* have genes that encoded SAM synthetase (Sam1) (Kutty et al., 2008) . Moreover, the corresponding *Sam1* mRNA is transcribed, and the protein, which is enzymatically active, was immuno-localized in *P. murina* cells. Such data suggest strongly that *Pneumocystis* species do not depend on an exogenous source of SAM to survive (Kutty et al., 2008).

7.3.4 Serological tests

Serum antibody detection constitutes an adjunctive strategy currently used to diagnose systemic fungal infections, even in immunosupressed patients. This strategy was however only rarely used to PcP diagnosis because healthy subjects have frequently significant levels of serum anti-*Pneumocystis* antibody. Moreover, the antibody response against *Pneumocystis* infection is currently highly variable and the results reported by diverse groups are contradictory (Walzer, 2004). In contrast, *Pneumocystis* antibody assays, especially those using recombinant *Pneumocystis* antigens, constitutes an interesting tool in epidemiology (Daly et al., 2009).

8. Treatment

The recommended treatment of PcP has remained unchanged for many years, being Co-trimoxazole, an association of trimethoprim and sulfamethoxazole, the drug of choice as first line of treatment. Regarding which agent of second line must be choice preferably, data are limited (table 3). Drug related toxicities are increasing in HIV-infected patients and organ transplant recipients. Because of the potential for additive or synergistic toxicities associated with anti-*Pneumocystis* and antiretroviral therapies, certain health-care providers delay initiation of HAART until after the completion of anti-*Pneumocystis* therapy, or until at least 2 weeks after initiating anti-*Pneumocystis* therapy, despite some suggestion of potential benefit of early HAART in the treatment of patients with AIDS-related opportunistic infections (CDC, 2009; Zolopa et al., 2009). In order to a correct management of PcP is important to distinguish between progressive PcP, drug toxicity and concomitant infection if clinical deterioration is detected.

Trimethoprim-sulfamethoxazole (TMP-SMX)

TMP and SMX target sequential steps in the folate synthesis pathway. TMP inhibits dihydrofolate reductase and SMX inhibits dihydropteroate synthetase. TMP-SMX is the treatment of choice for PcP in all patients who tolerate this drug, and it achieves the most rapid clinical response of the anti-*Pneumocystis* agents (CDC, 2009; Helweg-Larsen et al., 2009). The recommended dose of TMP-SMX for adults (or children aged > 2 months) is 15 to 20 mg/kg/day of TMP and 75 to 100 mg/kg/day of SMX intravenously every 6 or 8 hours. With renal dysfunction, dosing must be reduced. The bioavailability of TMP-SMX from oral therapy is comparable to parenteral administration (CDC, 2009; Mofenson et al., 2009).

Patients who have PcP despite the use of TMP-SMX prophylaxis, are usually successfully treated with TMP-SMX. In this way, the presence of mutations in the DHPS gene of *P. jirovecii* has been associated with resistance to sulfa drugs, although the clinical outcome is uncertain (Crothers et al. 2005; Huang et al., 2004; Stein et al., 2004). Drug related toxicities from TMP-SMX are greater than that from therapy with other anti-*Pneumocystis* agents. The side effects of TMP-SMX are: rash (30-55%), (including Stevens-Johnson syndrome), fever (30-40%), leukopenia (30-40%), hepatitis (20%), thrombocytopenia (15%), azotemia (1-5%), and hyperkaliemia (Eeftinck et al., 1990; Gordin et al., 1984; Hughes et al., 1995). Nephrotoxicity occurs frequently in the renal transplantation recipient receiving full-dose of TMP-SMX. Liver transplant recipients are particularly susceptible to TMP-SMX toxicity. Leucovorin to prevent myelosuppression is not recommended because its uncertain efficacy and a higher rate of failure (CDC, 2009).

Pentamidine

Pentamidine is an aromatic diamidine that has broad spectrum anti-protozoal activity. This drug inhibits metabolism of *P* amino benzoic acid, interferes with anaerobic glycolysis, inhibits oxidative phosphorylation and impairs nucleic acid and protein synthesis. It was the first drug reported to treat PcP successfully and subsequent reports have confirmed the efficacy of intravenous pentamidine. Although intravenous pentamidine has been recommended as the main alternative to TMP-SMX for moderate to severe PcP (Gordin et al., 1984), a recent study has found a greater risk of death when pentamidine was used as first and second-line therapy for HIV-associated PcP with compared with TMP-SMX and clindamycin-primaquine (Helweg-Larsen et al., 2009). These findings could be due to toxicities related to pentamidine and the absence of an antibacterial effect, in contrast to TMP-SMX or clindamycin-primaquine, which might act against concomitant bacterial co-infection (Helweg-Larsen et al., 2009).

Pentamidine for children and adults is administered once a day at 4 mg/kg (maximum 300 mg daily) intravenously, infused slowly 1 to 2 hr in 5% glucose; due to its toxicity the dose can be reduced to 3 mg/kg. Aerosolized pentamidine should not be used because of limited efficacy and more frequent relapse, and intramuscular administration is not used due to the related complications (Conte et al., 1990). Side effects of pentamidine include azotemia, pancreatitis, hypo- or hyperglycemia, pancytopenia, electrolyte abnormalities, cardiac dysrhythmia and renal dysfunction (Conte et al., 1990). Pentamidine should be avoided in pancreas transplant recipients due to the potential for islet cell necrosis.

Clindamycin-primaquine

Clindamycin is a lincosamide antibiotic used to treat infections with anaerobic bacteria but can also be used to treat some protozoan diseases. Primaquine is an 8-aminoquinoline anti-protozoan agent. This combination is effective in adult patients with mild to moderate PcP, but data for children are not available (Toma et al., 1998). Clindamycin is given at 600 to 900 mg intravenously or 300-450 mg orally every 6 to 8 hours and primaquine is given orally at 15 to 30 mg/day. Clindamycin component can be administered intravenously in severe cases; primaquine is only available orally. Recently, clindamycin-primaquine appeared superior to pentamidine as second-line therapy for PcP in patients failing or developing toxicity with TMP-SMX (Helweg-Larsen et al., 2009). Side effects of clindamycin include rash, anemia, neutropenia and the development of *Clostridium difficile* colitis. The main toxicity of primaquine is methemoglobinemia, thus, patients should be tested for glucose-6-phosphate dehydrogenase deficiency before administration of primaquine (Larsen, 2004).

Dapsone

Dapsone is a sulfone drug that inhibits DHPS and it is used as alternative therapeutic regimen for mild-to-moderate PcP. Dapsone must be taken with TMP (Medina et al., 1990). Although this association might have similar efficacy and fewer side effects than TMP-SMX, is less recommended due to the number of pills. The dosage of dapsone for adolescents and adults is 100 mg orally once daily (among children aged < 13 years, 2 mg/kg/day). The dosage of TMP for children and adults taken orally is 15 mg/kg/day divided into three doses (CDC, 2009; Mofenson et al., 2009). The most common adverse effects associated to dapsone are methemoglobinemia and hemolysis, especially in those with glucose-6-phosphate dehydrogenase deficiency. Thus, patients should be tested for glucose-6-phosphate dehydrogenase deficiency (Larsen et al. 2004).

Atovaquone

Atovaquone is a unique naphthoquinone that target the cytochome B complex and, thus, inhibits mitochondrial electron transport. This drug was developed clinically in the 1990s and it is available only as oral agent. It is used as second-line agent for treatment of mild to moderate PcP if TMP-SMX cannot be used. The standard dosing regimen for adults is atovaquone 750 mg orally twice a day with food for increasing gastrointestinal absorption (30-40 mg/kg/day for children < 3 months and > 24 months of age; between 3-24 months of age, 45 mg/kg/day are required) (Medina et al., 1990; Mofenson et al., 2009). Mutations of the cytochrome *b* gene have occurred in atovaquone-resistant isolates of *Pneumocystis*, but the clinical significance of gene mutations has not been determined (Kazanjian et al., 2001). The advantages of atovaquone include oral administration and fewer side effects. Disadvantages are its high cost and its bioavailability, although it has been improved with the micronized suspension formulation (Baggish & Hill, 2002). The most frequently reported adverse effects are rash, nausea, diarrhea, elevation of liver enzyme levels and headache. Atovaquone does not cause bone marrow suppression (Larsen et al., 2004).

Trimetrexate

Trimetrexate is an analogue of methotrexate that is an inhibitor of dihydrofolate reductase, and *in vitro* it is 1500 times more potent than trimethoprim (Kovacs et al., 1988). This drug is effective for treating PcP but is available only in an intravenous formulation. Because this drug also inhibits human folate metabolism, leucovorin must be administered concomitantly to prevent cytopenias (Larsen et al., 2004). A clinical trial showed that trimetrexate is less effective but better tolerate than TMP-SMX against AIDS-related PcP (Sattler et al., 1994). Trimetrexate with folinic acid have been approved for use in patients with moderately severe PcP, however, it is not longer available commercially. The dosage recommended for treatment of PcP is trimetrexate, 45 mg/m^2 intravenously once daily, plus leucovorin 20 mg/m² orally or intravenously four times daily (Sattler et al., 1994).. Leucovorin therapy must extend for 72 hours past the last dose of trimetrexate. For adults, trimetrexate may alternatively be dosed on a mg/kg basis, depending on the patient's body weight: <50 kg, 1.5 mg/kg; 50-80 kg, 1.2 mg/kg, and >80 kg, 1.0 mg/kg. Also, leucovorin may be dosed on a mg/kg basis (<50 kg, 0.6 mg/kg, and >50 kg 0.5 mg/kg) administered every 6 hours. Despite the suggestion that leucovorin impairs the efficacy of TMP-SMX, there is no indication that the coadministration of leucovorin impairs the efficacy of trimetrexate for PcP (Larsen et al., 2004). In some cases trimetrexate plus leucovorin could be used as salvage treatment for PcP (Short et al., 2009).

Adjunctive therapies

The use of corticosteroids may reduce pulmonary inflammation response caused by the lysis of *Pneumocystis* in the lung after initiating treatment of PcP. Corticosteroids have been related with a significant benefit in terms of preventing deterioration in oxygenation in the first seven days of therapy, mortality, and reduction of intubations in AIDS patients (Briel et al., 2005). Corticosteroids are indicated in HIV-infected patients with a moderate-to-severe PcP who have hypoxemia (the partial pressure of arterial oxygen under 70 mm Hg with the patient breathing room air or an alveolar-arteriolar gradient greater than 35). In these cases, corticosteroids should be administered as early as possible within 72 hours after starting anti-*Pneumocystis* therapy (Thomas & Limper, 2004; CDC, 2009). Recommended dose are showed in table 3.

	Moderate to severe *Pneumocystis* pneumonia		
Therapeutic use	**Drug**	**Dose**	**Route**
First line	Trimethoprim- Sulfamethoxazole	15-20 mg/Kg daily divided into 3 or 4 doses 75-100 mg/Kg daily divided into 3 or 4 doses	Intravenous
Second line	Primaquine plus Clindamycin	30 mg daily 600-900 mg three times daily	Oral Intravenous
Second line	Pentamidine	4 mg/Kg daily (3 mg/Kg if toxicities)	Intravenous
Salvage therapy	Trimetrexate plus Leucovorin	45 mg/m² daily 20 mg/m² four times daily	Intravenous Intravenous or oral
Adjunctive therapy	Prednisone Methylprednisolone	Days 1–5: 80 mg daily divided into 2 doses Days 6–10: 40 mg daily Days 11–21: 20 mg daily 75% of prednisone dose	Oral Intravenous
	Mild to moderate *Pneumocystis* pneumonia		
First line	Trimethoprim- Sulfamethoxazole	15-20 mg/Kg daily divided into 3 doses 75-100 mg/Kg daily divided into 3 doses	Oral
Second line	Dapsone plus Trimethoprim	100 mg daily 15-20 mg/Kg daily divided into 3 doses	Oral Oral or intravenous
Second line	Primaquine plus Clindamycin	15-30 mg daily 300-450 mg 3 or 4 times daily	Oral Oral
Second line	Atovaquone	750 mg two times daily	Oral with food

Table 3. Drugs therapy for treatment of *Pneumocystis* pneumonia in adults according to severity

Novel agents

Novel agents undergoing clinical investigation include echinocandins and pneumocandins, which target synthesis of beta 1,3 glucan, a cell wall compound of *Pneumocystis* and other fungi.

Caspofungin is an echinocandin that acts on the cell wall by inhibiting β-1,3-glucan synthesis and it has been approved for several fungal infections as *Candida* and *Aspergillus* species. Caspofungin has shown activity against *Pneumocystis* in experimental animal models and it has strong activity on cyst forms and weak activity on trophic forms (Powles et al., 1998). Due to TMP-SMX affects only the trophic forms, it has been suggested that the association of TMP-SMX and caspofungin by fully inhibiting the organism life cycle, may provide a synergistic activity against *Pneumocystis.* According to this, it has been reported cases of PcP where the association of caspofungin and TMP-SMX achieved a complete cure of PcP (Utili et al., 2007). However, this promising therapeutic approach needs to be assessed by controlled clinical trials.

9. Prevention

Many studies have demonstrated that PcP can largely be prevented by administration of chemoprophylaxis to susceptible individuals (Di Cocco et al., 2009; Green et al., 2007; Podzamcser et al., 1995; Rodriguez & Fishman, 2004) and according with the American Thoracic Society recommendations patients infected with HIV (Huang et al., 2006) need to receive prophylaxis to prevent disease depending on specific risks to the patient's system. Recommendations for chemoprophylaxis should be based on weighing the efficacy against the risk of adverse events, the risk of developments of antimicrobial resistance, and the cost of the intervention (Roblot et al., 2005). Medications recommended for chemoprophylaxis against PcP are listed in table 4.

9.1 Primary prophylaxis

The majority of recommendations are based in studies performed in HIV-infected patients. Guidelines recommend starting primary prophylaxis against PcP in HIV-infected adolescents and adults, including pregnant and patients under HAART, when the CD4 cell count is less than 200 cells/mm^3 or the patient has a history of oropharyngeal candidiasis. Patients with a CD4 cell percentage of <14% or a history of an AIDS-defining illness should be considered for chemoprophylaxis (CDC, 2009). Prophylaxis recommendations for HIV-infected children are age-based. Chemoprophylaxis should be provided for children 6 years or older based on adults guidelines, for children aged 1 to 5 years if CD4 counts are less than 500 cells/mm^3 or CD4 percentage is less than 15%, and for all HIV-infected infants younger than 12 months (Zolopa et al., 2009).

TMP-SMX is the recommended prophylactic agent in both primary and secondary prophylaxis for PCP, because of its high efficacy, relative safety, low cost, and broad antimicrobial spectrum (CDC, 2009; Di Cocco et al., 2009; Roblot et al., 2005; Rodriguez & Fishman, 2004). TMP-SMX also is effective in preventing *Toxoplasma gondi, Isospora belli, Cyclospora cayetanensis* and some bacterial infections such us, *Streptococcus pneumoniae, Salmonella, Haemophilus, Staphylococcus,* common gram-negative gastrointestinal and urinary pathogens (Rodriguez & Fishman, 2004). Either one single-strength tablet daily or one double-strength tablet daily are the preferred regimens, but the first regimen might be better tolerated than the second (CDC, 2009). An alternative choice can be one double-strength tablet three times per week (CDC, 2009; Roblot et al., 2005). TMP-SMX at a dose of one double-strength tablet daily confers cross-protection against toxoplasmosis and selected common respiratory bacterial infections. Lower doses of TMP-SMX also likely confer such protection (CDC, 2009; Di Cocco et al., 2009).

For patients who have an adverse reaction that is not life threatening, prophylaxis with TMP-SMX should be reinstituted. These patients might better tolerate reintroduction of the drug with a gradual increase in dose or reintroduction of TMP-SMX at a reduced dose or frequency (CDC, 2009). If TMP-SMX is not tolerated, a second choice would be dapsone given 100 mg daily, dapsone 50 mg daily plus pyrimethamine 50 mg weekly plus leucovorin 25 mg weekly or dapsone 200 plus pyrimethamine 75 mg plus leucovorin 25 mg weekly, aerosolized pentamidine 300 mg monthly administered by an ultrasonic or jet-nebulizer, and atovaquone 1500 mg daily (CDC,2009). Dapsone is effective and inexpensive but

Drug	Dose for adults	Dose for children	Route	Comments
Trimethoprim-Sulfamethoxazole	160/800 mg (DS tablet) per day or 3 times per week 80/400 mg (SS tablet) per day	150/750 mg/m^2 body surface area (max: 320/1600 mg) as single or 2 divided doses 3 times per week	Oral	First choice Weekly regimen is recommended if daily therapy in not tolerated
Dapsone	100 mg per day	2 mg/Kg body weight (max: 100 g) per day 4 mg/Kg body weight (max: 200 g) per week	Oral	Alternative choice Ensure patient does not have Glucose-6 phosphate dehydrogenase deficiency
Pentamidine	300 mg per month	300 mg per month (aged ≥ 5 years)	Aerosol	Alternative choice
Atovaquone	1500 mg per day	30-45 mg/Kg body weight according to age per day	Oral	Alternative choice Take with high-fat meals for maximal absorption
Dapsona + Pyrimethamine + Leucovorin	50 mg per day 50 mg per week 25 mg per week		Oral Oral Oral	Alternative choice Ensure patient does not have Glucose-6 phosphate dehydrogenase deficiency Effective in preventing toxoplasmosis
Dapsona + Pyrimethamine + Leucovorin	200 mg per week 75 mg per week 25 mg per week		Oral Oral Oral	Alternative choice Ensure patient does not have Glucose-6 phosphate dehydrogenase deficiency Effective in preventing toxoplasmosis

Table 4. Prophylaxis regimens for *Pneumocystis* pneumonia.

associated with more serious adverse effects than atovaquone (El-Sadr et al., 1998). Atovaquone is effective, safe and it is effective against *Toxoplasma gondii* but it is more expensive (Rodriguez & Fishman, 2004). The widespread concept that TMP-SMX is contraindicated for prophylaxis in patients treated with methotrexate might be obsolete because the safety of one single-strength tablet daily or one double-strength tablet thrice-weekly has been proved in clinical studies (Langford et al., 2003). However, these patients need to receive folate supplementation besides blood counts and liver-function tests should be closely monitored (Roblot, 2005).
Primary prophylaxis should be discontinued for HIV-infected adult and adolescent patients who have responded to HAART with an increase in CD4 counts major than 200 cells/mm^3 during more than 3 months (Lopez Bernaldo et al., 2001). Prophylaxis should be reintroduced if the CD4 cell count decreases to less than 200 cells/mm^3.

9.2 Secondary prophylaxis

HIV-infected adults and adolescents patients who have developed previous episodes of PcP should receive secondary prophylaxis (Thomas & Limper, 2004). Chemoprophylaxis should be discontinued for adult and adolescent patients when CD4 cell count increases to more than 200 cells/mm^3 for a period of 3 months as a result of HAART (Lopez Bernaldo et al., 2001). Prophylaxis should be reintroduced if the CD4 count decreases again to less than 200 cells/mm^3. If PcP recurs at a CD4 count higher than 200 cells/mm^3, continuing PcP prophylaxis for life would be prudent (CDC, 2009).

10. Conclusions

Pneumocystis jirovecii is an atypical fungus that causes PcP mainly in HIV-infected individuals. Today, PcP is still a major cause of morbidity and mortality among AIDS patients, and constitutes a worldwide problem to public health. While the incidence of PcP among HIV infected individuals has decreased in developed countries, the prevalence of AIDS-related PcP in developing countries remains high and poorly controlled. The epidemiology of this infection is only beginning to be understood. The accumulating evidence suggests that *P. jirovecii* is a highly infectious organism with low virulence that takes advantage of hosts as temporary reservoirs of infection. In this sense, colonization with *P. jirovecii* (that is infection without disease) has recently gained attention as a important issue for understanding the complete cycle of human *Pneumocystis* infection. The clinical presentation in HIV-infected patients may differ from that in other immunosuppressed patients and its diagnosis continues to be challenging. Clinicians must be familiar with its presentation and management because mild cases are sometimes difficult to diagnose. The emergence of highly sensitive and specific molecular methods for PcP diagnosis have represented a significant advance in order to establish earlier PcP diagnosis, detect low parasite rates, and detect *Pneumocystis* DNA in non-invasive samples. Co-trimoxazole is the most effective medication for its prevention and treatment but other alternative medications are also available. Future clinical research should include studying the transmission and epidemiology of PcP in populations worldwide, improving the diagnosis of PcP, improving regimens for prophylaxis and treatment in various patient populations, and determining the significance of the DHPS mutations in various populations and in different geographic locations. Furthermore, the threat of emerging resistance to available anti-*Pneumocystis* drugs highlights the need to continue investigating the biology of this organism in the hope of developing novel treatment strategies.

11. References

Aderaye G, Woldeamanuel Y, Asrat D, *et al.* (2008). Evaluation of Toluidine Blue O staining for the diagnosis of *Pneumocystis jiroveci* in expectorated sputum sample and bronchoalveolar lavage from HIV-infected patients in a tertiary care referral center in Ethiopia. *Infection*, Vol. 36, pp. 237-243, ISSN 0300-8126

Alvarez-Martínez MJ, Moreno A, Miró JM *et al.* (2008). *Pneumocystis jirovecii* pneumonia in Spanish HIV-infected patients in the combined antiretroviral therapy era: prevalence of dihydropteroate synthase mutations and prognostic factors of mortality. *Diagn Microbiol Infect Dis*, Vol. 62, pp. 34-43, ISSN 0732-8893

Alibrahim, A., Lepore, M., Lierl, M. et al. (1998). *Pneumocystis carinii* pneumonia in an infant with X-linked agammaglobulinemia. *J Allergy Clin Immunol*, Vol.101, pp. 552–553, ISSN 0091-6749

Aliouat-Denis CM, Chabé M, Demanche C, Aliouat el M, Viscogliosi E, Guillot J, et al. (2008). *Pneumocystis* species, co-evolution and pathogenic power. *Infect Genet Evol*, Vol. 8, pp. 708-26, ISSN 1567-1348

Baggish AL, Hill DR. (2002). Antiparasitic agent atovaquone. *Antimicrob Agents Chemother*, Vol. 46, pp. 1163-1173. ISSN 0066-4804

Beard CB. (2004). Molecular typing and epidemiological insights. In: *Pneumocystis carinii Pneumonia (3rd edition)*. Walzer PD, Cushion MT (eds.), Marcel Dekker, Inc., New York, 479-504. ISBN 0-8247-5451-4

Benfield, TL., Prento, P., Junge, J. et al. (1997). Alveolar damage in AIDS-related *Pneumocystis carinii* pneumonia. *Chest*, Vol.111, No.5, (May 1997), pp. 1193-1199, ISSN 0012-3692

Briel M, Boscacci R, Furrer H, Bucher HC. (2005). Adjunctive corticosteroids for *Pneumocystis jiroveci* pneumonia in patients with HIV infection: a meta-analysis of randomised controlled trials. *BMC Infect Dis*, Vol. 5, pp. 101. ISSN 1471-2334

Burns, SM., Read, JA., Yap, PL. et al. (1990). Reduced concentrations of IgG antibodies to *Pneumocystis carinii* in HIV infected patients during active Pneumocystis carinii infection and the possibility of passive immunisation. *J Infect*, Vol.20, pp. 33–39. ISSN 0163-4453

Calderon E, de la Horra C, Montes-Cano MA, Respaldiza N, Martín-Juan J, Varela JM. (2004). Resistencia genotípica a sulfamidas en pacientes con neumonía por *Pneumocystis jiroveci*. *Med. Clin. (Barc)*, Vol. 122, pp. 617-619, ISSN 0025-7753

Calderon EJ, Rivero L, Respaldiza N *et al.* (2007). Systemic inflammation in patients with chronic obstructive pulmonary disease who are colonized with *Pneumocystis jirovecii*. *Clin Infect Dis*, Vol. 45, pp. 17-19, ISSN 1058-4838

Calderon EJ. (2009). Epidemiology of *Pneumocystis* infection in human. *J Mycol Med*, Vol. 19, pp. 270-275, ISSN 1156-5233

Calderon EJ. (2010a). *Pneumocystis* infection: seeing beyond the tip of the iceberg. *Clin Infect Dis*, Vol. 50, pp. 354-356, ISSN 1058-4838

Calderon EJ, Gutiérrez-Rivero S, Durand-Joly I, Dei-Cas E. (2010b). *Pneumocystis* infection in humans: diagnosis and treatment. *Expert Rev Anti Infect Ther*, Vol. 8, pp. 683-701, ISSN 1478-7210

Centers for Disease Control and Prevention. (2009). Guidelines for Prevention and Treatment of Opportunistic Infections in HIV-Infected Adults and Adolescents. *MMWR*, Vol. 58, pp. 1-216, ISSN 0149-2195

Chabé M, Dei-Cas E, Creusy C *et al.* (2004). Immunocompetent hosts as a reservoir of *Pneumocystis* organisms: histological and RT-PCR data demonstrate active replication. *Eur J Clin Microbiol Infect Dis*, Vol. 23, pp. 89-97, ISSN 0934-9723

Cheng VC, Hung IF, Wu AK, Tang BS, Chu CM, & Yuen KY. (2004). Lymphocyte surge as a marker for immunorestitution disease due to *Pneumocystis jiroveci* pneumonia in HIV-negative immunosuppressed hosts. *Eur J Clin Microbiol Infect Dis,* Vol. 23, pp. 512-514, ISSN 1058-4838

Chouaid C, Housset B, Lebeau B. (1995). Cost-analysis of four diagnostic strategies for *Pneumocystis carinii* pneumonia in HIV-infected subjects. *Eur Respir J*, Vol. 8, pp. 1554-1558, ISSN 0903-1936

Clarkson AB, Merali S. (2004). Polyamines, Iron, and *Pneumocystis carinii*. In: *Pneumocystis carinii Pneumonia (3rd edition)*, Walzer PD, Cushion MT (eds.), Marcel Dekker, Inc., New York, 577-605. ISBN: 0-8247-5451-4

Coleman, DL., Doder, PM., Goleen, JA. et al. (1984). Correlation between serial pulmonary function test and fiberoptic bronchoscopy in patients with *Pneumocystis carinii* pneumonia and the acquired immune deficiency syndrome. *Am Rev Respir Dis*, Vol.129, pp. 491-493, ISSN 0003-0805

Conte JE, Jr., Chernoff D, Feigal DW, Jr., et al. (1990). Intravenous or inhaled pentamidine for treating *Pneumocystis carinii* pneumonia in AIDS: a randomized trial. *Ann Intern Med*, Vol. 113, pp. 203-209, ISSN 0003-4819

Crothers K, Beard CB, Turner J, et al. (2005). Severity and outcome of HIV-associated *Pneumocystis* pneumonia containing *Pneumocystis jirovecii* dihydropteroate synthase gene mutations. *AIDS*, Vol. 19, pp. 801-805, ISSN 0269-9370

Daly K, Koch J, Respaldiza N *et al.* (2009). Geographical variation in serological responses to recombinant *Pneumocystis jirovecii* major surface glycoprotein antigens. *Clin Microbiol Infect*, Vol. 15, pp. 937-942, ISSN 1469-0691

de Boer MG, Bruijnesteijn van Coppenraet LE, Gaasbeek A, et al. (2007). An outbreak of *Pneumocystis jiroveci* pneumonia with 1 predominant genotype among renal transplant recipients: interhuman transmission or a common environmental source? *Clin Infect Dis*, Vol. 44, pp. 1143-9, ISSN 1058-4838

Dei-Cas E, Fleurisse L, Aliouat EM *et al.* (1998). Morphological and ultrastructural methods for *Pneumocystis*. *FEMS Immunol. Med Microbiol*, Vol. 22, pp. 185-189, ISSN 0928-8244

Dei-Cas E. (2000). *Pneumocystis* infections: the iceberg?. *Med Mycol*, Vol. 38, pp. 23-32, ISSN 1369-3786

Dei-Cas E, Chabé M, Moukhlis R *et al.* (2006). *Pneumocystis oryctolagi* sp. nov., an uncultured fungus causing pneumonia in rabbits at weaning: review of current knowledge, and description of a new taxon on genotypic, phylogenetic and phenotypic bases. *FEMS Microbiol. Rev*, Vol. 30, pp. 853-871, ISSN 0168-6445

de la Horra C, Varela JM, Friaza V, et al. (2006). Comparison of single and touchdown PCR protocols for detecting *Pneumocystis jirovecii* DNA in paraffin-embedded lung tissue samples. *J. Eukaryot. Microbiol*, Vol. 53, (Suppl 1), pp. 98-99, ISSN 1066-5234

Desmet S, Van Wijngaerden E, Maertens J *et al.* (2009). Serum (1-3)-beta-D-glucan as a tool for diagnosis of *Pneumocystis jirovecii* pneumonia in patients with human immunodeficiency virus infection or hematological malignancy. *J Clin Microbiol,* Vol. 47, pp. 3871-3874, ISSN 0095-1137

Di Cocco P, Orlando G, Bonanni L, et al. (2009). A systematic review of two different trimetoprim-sulfamethoxazole regimens used to prevent *Pneumocystis jirovecii* and no prophylaxis at all in transplant recipients: appraising the evidence. *Transplant Proc,* Vol. 41, pp. 1201-1203, ISSN 0041-1345

Durand-Joly I, Wakefield AE, Palmer RJ *et al.* (2000). Ultrastructural and molecular characterization of *Pneumocystis carinii* isolated from a rhesus monkey (*Macaca mulatta*). *Med Mycol,* Vol. 38, pp. 61-72, ISSN 1369-3786

Durand-Joly I. (2002). Épidémiologie moléculaire de la pneumocystose humaine. Caractérisation génétique et phénotypique de *Pneumocystis jirovecii* et espèces proches. *Thesis Dissertation.* Lille, France.

Durand-Joly, I., Soula, F., Chabe, M *et al.* (2003). Longterm colonization with *Pneumocystis jirovecii* in hospital staffs: a challenge to prevent nosocomial pneumocystosis. *J Eukaryot Microbiol,* Vol. 50 (Suppl.), pp. 614–615,ISSN 1066-5234

Durand-Joly I, Chabé M, Soula F, Delhaes L, Camus D, Dei-Cas E. (2005). Molecular diagnosis of *Pneumocystis* pneumonia (PcP). *FEMS Immunol. Med Microbiol,* Vol. 45, pp. 405-410, ISSN 0928-8244

Edman JC, Kovacs JA, Masur H, Santi DV, Elwood HJ, Sogin ML. (1988). Ribosomal RNA sequence shows *Pneumocystis carinii* to be a member of the fungi. *Nature,* Vol. 334, pp. 519-22, ISSN 0028-0836

Eeftinck Schattenkerk JK, Lange JM, van Steenwijk RP, Danner SA. (1990). Can the course of high dose cotrimoxazole for *Pneumocystis carinii* pneumonia in AIDS be shorter? A possible solution to the problem of cotrimoxazole toxicity. *J Intern Med,* Vol. 227, pp. 359-362, ISSN 1365-2796

Fei MW, Kim EJ, Sant CA, et al. (2009). Predicting mortality from HIV-associated *Pneumocystis* pneumonia at illness presentation: an observational cohort study. *Thorax,* Vol. 64, pp. 1070-1076, ISSN 0028-4793

Friaza V, Montes-Cano MA, Respaldiza N, Morilla R, Calderón EJ, de la Horra C. (2009). Prevalence of dihydropteroate synthase mutations in Spanish patients with HIV-associated *Pneumocystis* pneumonia. *Diagn Microbiol Infect Dis,* Vol. 64, pp. 104-105, ISSN 0732-8893

Gordin FM, Simon GL, Wofsy CB, Mills J. (1984). Adverse reactions to trimethoprim-sulfamethoxazole in patients with the acquired immunodeficiency syndrome. *Ann Intern Med,* Vol. 100, pp.495-499, ISSN 0003-4819

Green H, Paul M, Vidal L, Leibovici L. (2007). Prophylaxis of *Pneumocystis* pneumonia in immunocompromised non-HIV-infected patients: systematic review and meta-analysis of randomized controlled trials. *Mayo Clin Proc,* Vol. 82, pp. 1052-1059, ISSN 0025-6196

Helweg-Larsen J, Benfield TL, Eugen-Olsen J, Lundgren JD, Lundgren B. (1999). Effects of mutations in *Pneumocystis carinii* dihydropteroate synthase gene on outcome of AIDS-associated *P. carinii* pneumonia. *Lancet,* Vol. 354, pp. 1347–1351, ISSN 0140-6736

Helweg-Larsen J, Benfield T, Atzori C, Miller RF. (2009). Clinical efficacy of first- and second-line treatments for HIV-associated *Pneumocystis jirovecii* pneumonia: a tri-centre cohort study. *J Antimicrob Chemother*, Vol. 64, pp. 1282-1290, ISSN 0305-7453

Huang L, Beard CB, Creasman J *et al.* (2000). Sulfa or sulfone prophylaxis and geographic region predict mutations in the *Pneumocystis carinii* dihydropteroate synthase gene. *J Infect Dis*, Vol. 182, pp. 1192–1198, ISSN 0022-1899

Huang L. (2004). Clinical presentation and diagnosis of *Pneumocystis* pneumonia in HIV-infected patients. In: *Pneumocystis carinii Pneumonia, 3rd edition*, Walzer PD, Cushion MT (eds.), Marcel Dekker, Inc., New York, 349-406. ISBN 0-8247-5451-4

Huang L, Crothers K, Atzori C *et al.* (2004). Dihydropteroate synthase gene mutations in *Pneumocystis* and sulfa resistance. *Emerg Infect Dis*, Vol. 10, pp. 1721–1728, ISSN 1080-6059

Huang L, Morris A, Limper AH, Beck JM; ATS *Pneumocystis* Workshop Participants. (2006). An Official ATS Workshop Summary: Recent advances and future directions in *Pneumocystis* pneumonia (PCP). *Proc Am Thorac Soc*, Vol. 3, pp. 655-664, ISSN 1546-3222

Huggett JF, Taylor MS, Kocjan G *et al.* (2008). Development and evaluation of a real-time PCR assay for detection of *Pneumocystis jirovecii* DNA in bronchoalveolar lavage fluid of HIV-infected patients. *Thorax*, Vol. 63, pp. 154-159, ISSN 0028-4793

Hughes WT, LaFon SW, Scott JD, Masur H. (1995). Adverse events associ¬ated with trimethoprim-sulfamethoxazole and atovaquone during the treatment of AIDS-related *Pneumocystis carinii* pneumonia. *J Infect Dis*, Vol. 171, pp. 1295-1301, ISSN 0022-1899

Hughes WT. (2004). *Pneumocystis* Pneumonitis in Non-HIV-Infected Patients: Update. In: *Pneumocystis carinii Pneumonia (3rd edition)*. Walzer PD, Cushion MT (eds.), Marcel Dekker, Inc., New York, 407-434, ISBN 0-8247-5451-4

Iliades P, Meshnick SR, Macreadie IG. (2004). Dihydropteroate synthase mutations in *Pneumocystis jiroveci* can affect sulfamethoxazole resistance in a *Saccharomyces cerevisiae* model. *Antimicrob Agents Chemother*, Vol. 48, pp. 2617-2623, ISSN 0066-4804

Inoue Y, Nishimura K, Shiode M, et al. (1995). Evaluation of serum KL-6 levels in patients with pulmonary tuberculosis. *Tuber Lung Dis*, Vol. 76, pp. 230-233, ISSN 0962-8479

Jagannathan P, Davis E, Jacobson M, & Huang L. (2009). Life-threatening immune reconstitution inflammatory syndrome after *Pneumocystis* pneumonia: a cautionary case series. *AIDS*, Vol. 23, pp. 1794-1796, ISSN 0269-9370

Kawasaki Y, Aoyagi Y, Abe Y, et al. (2009). Serum KL-6 levels as a biomarker of lung injury in respiratory syncytial virus bronchiolitis. *J Med Virol*, Vol. 81, pp. 2104-2108, ISSN 0146-6615

Kazanjian P, Armstrong W, Hossler PA *et al.* (2000). *Pneumocystis carinii* mutations are associated with duration of sulfa or sulfone prophylaxis exposure in AIDS patients. *J Infect Dis*, Vol. 182, pp. 551–557, ISSN 0022-1899

Kazanjian P, Armstrong W, Hossler P.A, et al. (2001). *Pneumocystis carinii* cytochrome b mutations are associated with atovaquone exposure in patients with AIDS. *J Infect Dis*, Vol. 183, pp. 819-822, ISSN 0022-1899

Kelly, MN. & Shellito, JE. (2010). Current understanding of *Pneumocystis* immunology. *Future Microbiol*, Vol.5, pp. 43-65, ISSN 1746-0913

Kovacs JA, Ng VL, Masur H *et al.* (1988). Diagnosis of *Pneumocystis carinii* pneumonia: improved detection in sputum with use of monoclonal antibodies. *N Engl J Med,* Vol. 318, pp. 589-593, ISSN 0028-4793

Krajicek. BJ., Limper, AH., & Thomas, CF. (2008). Advances in the biology, pathogenesis and identification of *Pneumocystis* pneumonia. *Curr Opin Pulm Med.* 2008; Vol. 14, pp. 228-234, ISSN 1070-5287

Krajicek, BJ., Thomas, CFJr. & Limper, AH. (2009). *Pneumocystis* pneumonia: current concepts in pathogenesis, diagnosis, and treatment. *Clin Chest Med,* Vol.30; pp. 265-278, ISSN 0272-5231

Kutty G, Hernandez-Novoa B, Czapiga M, Kovacs JA. (2008). *Pneumocystis* encodes a functional S-adenosylmethionine synthetase gene. *Eukaryot Cell,* Vol. 7, pp. 258–267, ISSN 1535-9786

Langford CA, Talar-Williams C, Barron KS, Sneller MC. (2003). Use of cyclophosphamide-induction methotrexate-maintenance regimen for the treatment of Wegener's granulomatosis: extended follow-up and rate of relapse. *Am J Med,* Vol. 114, pp. 463–469,ISSN 0002-9343

Larsen HH, Masur H, Kovacs JA *et al.* (2002). Development and evaluation of a quantitative, touchdown, real-time PCR assay for diagnosing *Pneumocystis carinii* pneumonia. *J Clin Microbiol,* Vol. 40, pp. 490–494, ISSN 0095-1137

Larsen HH, Masur H, Kovacs JA. (2004). Current regimens for treatment and prophylaxis of *Pneumocystis jiroveci* pneumonia. In: *Pneumocystis carinii Pneumonia, 3rd edition,* Walzer PD, Cushion MT (eds.), Marcel Dekker, Inc., New York, 505-538, ISBN 0-8247-5451-4

Limper, AH., Hoyte, JS. & Standing, JE.. (1997). The role of alveolar macrophages in *Pneumocystis carinii* degradation and clearance from the lung. *J Clin Invest,* Vol.99, pp. 2110-2107, ISSN 0021-9738

Lopez Bernaldo de Quiros JC, Miro JM, Peña JM, et al. (2001). A randomized trial of the discontinuation of primary and secondary prophylaxis against *Pneumocystis carinii* pneumonia after highly active antiretroviral therapy in patients with HIV infection. *N Engl J Med,* Vol. 344, pp. 159-167, ISSN 0028-4793

Lu, JJ. & Lee CH. (2008). *Pneumocystis* pneumonia. *J Formos Med Assoc,* Vol.107, pp. 830-842, ISSN 0929-6646

Medina I, Mills J, Leoung G, et al. (1990). Oral therapy for *Pneumocystis carinii* pneumonia in the acquired immunodeficiency syndrome: a controlled trial of trimethoprim-sulfamethoxazole versus trimethoprim-dapsone. *N. Engl. J. Med,* Vol. 323, pp. 776-782, ISSN 0028-4793

Medrano FJ, Montes-Cano M, Conde M, et al. (2005). *Pneumocystis jirovecii* in general population. *Emerg Infect Dis,* Vol. 11, pp. 245-250, ISSN 1080-6059

Miller RF, Le Noury J, Corbett EL, Felton JM, De Cock KM. (1996). Pneumocystis carinii infection: current treatment and prevention. J Antimicrob Chemother. Vol. 37, Suppl B, pp. 33-53, ISSN 0305-7453

Miller RF, Wakefield AE. (1999). *Pneumocystis carinii* genotypes and severity of pneumonia. *Lancet,* Vol. 353, pp. 2039-2040, ISSN 0140-6736

Miller RF, Ambrose HE, Wakefield AE. (2001). *Pneumocystis carinii* f. sp. hominis DNA in immunocompetent health care workers in contact with patients with *P. carinii* pneumonia. *J Clin Microbiol,* Vol. 39, pp. 3877-3882, ISSN 0095-1137

Mofenson LM, Brady MT, Danner SP, et al. (2009). Guidelines for the Prevention and Treatment of Opportunistic Infections among HIV-exposed and HIV-infected children: recommendations from CDC, the National Institutes of Health, the HIV Medicine Association of the Infectious Diseases Society of America, the Pediatric Infectious Diseases Society, and the American Academy of Pediatrics. *MMWR Recomm Rep*, Vol. 58 (RR-11), pp. 1-166, ISSN 1057-5987

Montes-Cano MA, Chabe M, Fontillon-Alberdi M, de La Horra C, Respaldiza N, Medrano FJ, et al. (2009). Vertical transmission of *Pneumocystis jirovecii* in humans. *Emerg Infect Dis*, Vol. 15, pp. 125-127, ISSN 1080-6059

Mori S, Polatino S, & Estrada-Y-Martin RM. (2009). *Pneumocystis*-associated organizing pneumonia as a manifestation of immune reconstitution inflammatory syndrome in an HIV-infected individual with a normal CD4+ T-cell count following antiretroviral therapy. *Int J STD AIDS*; Vol. 20. pp. 662-665, ISSN 0956-4624

Morris A, Beard CB, Huang L. (2002). Update on the epidemiology and transmission of *Pneumocystis* carinii. *Microbes Infect*, Vol. 4, pp. 95-103, ISSN 1286-4579

Morris A, Wei K, Afshar K, Huang L. (2008). Epidemiology and clinical significance of *Pneumocystis* colonization. *J Infect Dis*, Vol. 97, pp. 10-17, ISSN 0022-1899

Nahimana A, Rabodonirina M, Bille J, Francioli P, Hauser PM. (2004). Mutations of *Pneumocystis jirovecii* dihydrofolate reductase associated with failure of prophylaxis. *Antimicrob Agents Chemother*, Vol. 48, pp. 4301-4305, ISSN 0066-4804

Nakamura H, Tateyama M, Tasato D *et al.* (2009). Clinical utility of serum beta-D-glucan and KL-6 levels in *Pneumocystis jirovecii* pneumonia. *Intern Med*, Vol. 48, pp. 195-202, ISSN 1349-7235

Nevez G, Chabé M, Rabodonirina M *et al.* (2008). Nosocomial *Pneumocystis jirovecii* infections. *Parasite*, Vol. 15, pp. 359-365, ISSN 1776-1042

Ng VL, Yajko DM, Hadley WK. (1997). Extrapulmonary pneumocystosis. *Clin Microbiol Rev*, Vol. 10, pp. 401-418, ISSN 0893-8512

Nyamande, K., Lalloo, UG., & Vawda, F. (2007). Comparison of plain chest radiography and high-resolution CT in human immunodeficiency virus infected patients with community-acquired pneumonia: a sub-Saharan Africa study. *Br J Radiol*, 2007; Vol. 80, pp. 302-306, ISSN 0007-1285

Olsson M, Elvin K, Löfdahl S, Linder E. (1993). Detection of *Pneumocystis carinii* DNA in sputum and bronchoalveolar lavage samples by polymerase chain reaction. *J Clin Microbiol*, Vol. 31, pp. 221-226, ISSN 0095-1137

Olsson M, Eriksson BM, Elvin K, Strandberg M, Wahlgren M. (2001). Genotypes of clustered cases of *Pneumocystis carinii* pneumonia. *Scand J Infect Dis*, Vol. 33, pp. 285-289, ISSN 0036-5548

Podzamczer D, Salazar A, Jimenez J, et al. (1995). Intermittent trimethoprim-sulfamethoxazole compared with dapsone-pyrimethamine for the simultaneous primary prophylaxis of *Pneumocystis* pneumonia and toxoplasmosis in patients infected with HIV. *Ann Intern Med*, Vol. 122, pp. 755–761, ISSN 0003-4819

Pontón J. (2009). Utilidad de los marcadores biológicos en el diagnóstico de la candidiasis invasora. *Rev Iberoam Micol*, Vol. 26, pp. 8-14, ISSN 1130-1406

Powles MA, Liberator P, Anderson J, et al. (1998). Efficacy of MK-991 (L- 743,872), a semisynthetic Pneumocandin, in murine models of *Pneumocystis carinii*. *Antimicrob Agents Chemother*, Vol. 42, pp. 1985-1989, ISSN 0066-4804

Prevost, MC., Escamilla, R., Aliouat, EM., et al. (1998) Pneumocystosis pathophysiology. *FEMS Immunol Med Microbiol*, Vol. 28, pp. 123-128, ISSN 0928-8244

Richards CG, Wakefield AE, Mitchell CD. (1994). Detection of *Pneumocystis* DNA in nasopharyngeal aspirates of leukaemic infants with pneumonia. *Arch Dis Child*, Vol. 71, pp. 254–255, ISSN 1743-0585

Sato H, Callister ME, Mumby S, et al. (2004). KL-6 levels are elevated in plasma from patients with acute respiratory distress syndrome. *Eur Respir J*, Vol. 23, pp. 142-145, ISSN 0903-1936

Schliep, TC., Yarrish, RL. (1999). *Pneumocystis carinii* pneumonia. *Semin Respir Infect*, 1999; Vol. 14, pp. 333-343, ISSN 0882-0546

Sepkowitz., KA., Telzak, EE., & Gold, JW, et al. (1991). Pneumothorax in AIDS. *Ann Intern Med*, 1991; Vol. 114, pp. 455-459, ISSN 0003-4819

Short CE, Gilleece YC, Fisher MJ, Churchill DR. (2009). Trimetrexate and folinic acid: a valuable salvage option for *Pneumocystis jirovecii* pneumonia. *AIDS*, Vol. 23, pp. 1287-1290, ISSN 0269-9370

Sukoh N, Yamamoto H, Kikuchi E, et al. (2001). A case of severe Legionella pneumonia monitored with serum SP-A, SP-D, and KL-6. *Nihon Kokyuki Gakkai Zasshi*, Vol. 39, pp. 126-130, ISSN 0301-1542

Rabodonirina M, Vanhems P, Couray-Targe S, et al. (2004). Molecular evidence of interhuman transmission of *Pneumocystis* pneumonia among renal transplant recipients hospitalized with HIV-infected patients. *Emerg Infect Dis*, Vol. 10, pp. 1766-1773, ISSN 1080-6059

Respaldiza N, Medrano FJ, Medrano AC, Varela JM, de la Horra C, Montes-Cano M, et al. (2004). High seroprevalence of *Pneumocystis* infection in Spanish children. *Clin Microbiol Infect*, Vol. 10, pp. 1029-1031, ISSN 1198-743X

Respaldiza N, Montes-Cano MA, Friaza V, et al. (2006). Usefulness of oropharyngeal washings for identifying *Pneumocystis jirovecii* carriers. *J Eukaryot Microbiol*, Vol. 53, (Suppl 1), pp. 100-101, ISSN 1066-5234

Rivero L, de la Horra C, Montes-Cano MA, Rodríguez-Herrera A, Respaldiza N, Friaza V, et al. (2008). *Pneumocystis jirovecii* transmission from immunocompetent carriers to infant. *Emerg Infect Dis*, Vol. 14, pp. 1116-1118, ISSN 1080-6059

Roblot, F. (2005). Management of *Pneumocystis* pneumonia in patients with inflammatory disorders. *Expert Rev Anti Infect. Ther*, Vol. 3, pp. 435-444, ISSN 1478-7210

Rodriguez, M., Fishman, JA. (2004). Prevention of infection due to *Pneumocystis* spp. in human immunodeficiency virus-negative immunocompromised patients. *Clin Microbiol Rev*, 2004; Vol. 17, pp. 770-82, ISSN1098-6618

Sattler FR, Frame P, Davis R, et al. (1994). Trimetrexate with leucovorin versus trimethoprim-sulfamethoxazole for moderate to severe episodes of *Pneumocystis carinii* pneumonia in patients with AIDS: a prospective, controlled multicenter investigation of the AIDS Clinical Trials Group Protocol 029/031. *J Infect Dis*, Vol. 170, pp. 165-172, ISSN 0022-1899

Skelly M, Hoffman J, Fabbri M, Holzman RS, Clarkson AB Jr, Merali S. (2003). S-adenosylmethionine concentrations in diagnosis of *Pneumocystis carinii* pneumonia. *Lancet*, Vol. 361, pp. 1267–1268, ISSN 0140-6736.

Skelly MJ, Holzman RS, Merali S. (2008). S-adenosylmethionine levels in the diagnosis of *Pneumocystis carinii* pneumonia in patients with HIV infection. *Clin Infect* Dis, Vol. 46, pp. 467–471, ISSN 1058-4838

Stein CR, Poole C, Kazanjian P, Meshnick SR. (2004). Sulfa use, Dihydropteroate sythase mutations, and *Pneumocystis jirovecii* pneumonia. *Emerg Infect Dis,* Vol. 10, pp. 1760-1765, ISSN 1080-6059

Steele, C., Shellito, JE. & Kolls, JK. (2005). Immunity against the opportunistic fungal pathogen *Pneumocystis. Medical Mycology,* Vol. 43; pp. 1-19, ISSN 1369-3786

Stringer SL, Stringer JR, Blase MA, Walzer PD, Cushion MT. (1989). *Pneumocystis carinii*: sequence from ribosomal RNA implies a close relationship with fungi. *Exp Parasitol,* Vol. 68, pp. 450-456, ISSN 0014-4894

Tamburrini E, Mencarini P, Visconti E, et al. (1998). Potential impact of *Pneumocystis* genetic diversity on the molecular detection of the parasite in human hosts. *FEMS Immunol Med Microbiol,* Vol. 22, pp. 37-49, ISSN 0928-8244

Tasaka S, Hasegawa N, Kobayashi S, et al. (2007). Serum indicators for the diagnosis of pneumocystis pneumonia. *Chest,* Vol. 131, pp. 1173-1180, ISSN 0012-3692

Teramoto S, Sawaki D, Okada S, Ouchi Y. (2000). Markedly increased plasma (1-->3)-beta-D-glucan is a diagnostic and therapeutic indicator of *Pneumocystis carinii* pneumonia in a non-AIDS patient. *J Med Microbiol,* Vol. 49, pp. 393-394, ISSN 0022-2615

Thomas, CF., Limper, AH. (2004). *Pneumocystis* pneumonia. *N Engl J Med,*. 2004; Vol. 350, pp :2487-2498. ISSN 0028-4793

Thomas CF Jr, Limper AH. (2007). Current insights into the biology and pathogenesis of *Pneumocystis* pneumonia. *Nat Rev Microbiol,* Vol. 5, pp. 298-308, ISSN 1740-1526

Toma E, Thorne A, Singer J, et al. (1998). Clindamycin with primaquine vs. Trimethoprim-sulfamethoxazole therapy for mild and moderately severe *Pneumocystis carinii* pneumonia in patients with AIDS: a multicenter, double-blind, randomized trial. *Clin Infect Dis,* Vol. 27, pp. 524-30, ISSN 1058-4838

Totet A, Pautard JC, Raccurt C, Roux P, Nevez G. (2003). Genotypes at the internal transcribed spacers of the nuclear rRNA operon of *Pneumocystis jirovecii* in nonimmunosuppressed infants without severe pneumonia. *J Clin Microbiol,* Vol. 41, pp. 1173-1180, ISSN 0095-1137

Tsolaki AG, Miller RF, Wakefield AE. (1999). Oropharyngeal samples for genotyping and monitoring response to treatment in AIDS patients with *Pneumocystis carinii* pneumonia. *J. Med. Microbiol,* Vol. 48, pp. 897-905, ISSN 0022-2615

van Hal SJ, Gilgado F, Doyle T *et al.* (2009). Clinical significance and phylogenetic relationship of novel Australian *Pneumocystis jirovecii* genotypes. *J Clin Microbiol,* Vol. 47; pp. 1818-1823, ISSN 0095-1137

Vassallo, R., Kottom, TJ., Standing, JE. et al. (2001). Vitronectin and fibronectin function as glucan binding proteins augmenting macrophage responses to *Pneumocystis carinii. Am J Respir Cell Mol Biol,* Vol.25, pp. 203-211, ISSN1044-1549

Vidal S, de la Horra C, Martín J, *et al.* (2006). *Pneumocystis jirovecii* colonisation in patients with interstitial lung disease. *Clin Microbiol Infect,* Vol. 12, pp. 231-235, ISSN 1058-4838

Utili R, Durante-Mangoni E, Basilico C, Mattei A, Ragone E, Grossi P. (2007). Efficacy of caspofungin addition to trimethoprim-sulfamethoxazole treatment for severe

Pneumocystis pneumonia in solid organ transplant recipients. *Transplantation*, Vol. 84, pp. 685-688, ISSN 0041-1345

Vargas SL, Ponce CA, Gigliotti F, et al. (2000). Transmission of Pneumocystis carinii DNA from a patient with *P. carinii* pneumonia to immunocompetent contact health care workers. *J Clin Microbiol*, Vol. 38, pp. 1536-1538, ISSN 0095-1137

Wakefield AE, Pixley FJ, Banerji S *et al.* (1990). Detection of *Pneumocystis carinii* with DNA amplification. *Lancet*, Vol. 336, pp. 451–453, ISSN 0140-6736

Wakefield AE. (1996). DNA sequences identical to *Pneumocystis carinii* f. sp. carinii and *Pneumocystis carinii* f. sp. hominis in samples of air spora. *J Clin Microbiol*, Vol. 34, pp. 1754-1759, ISSN 0095-1137

Walzer, PD. (1993). *Pneumocystis carinii*: recent advances in basic biology and their clinical application. *AIDS*, Vol.7, pp. 1293-1305, ISSN 0269-9370

Walzer PD. (2004). Immunological Features of *Pneumocystis* Infection in Humans. In: *Pneumocystis carinii Pneumonia, 3rd edition*, Walzer PD, Cushion MT (eds.), Marcel Dekker, Inc., New York, 451-477, ISBN 0-8247-5451-4

Wang P, Huang L, Davis JL *et al.* (2008). A hydrophilic-interaction chromatography tandem mass spectrometry method for quantitation of serum s-adenosylmethionine in patients infected with human immunodeficiency virus. *Clin Chim Acta*, Vol. 396, pp. 86-88, ISSN 0009-8981

Wazir, JF., Ansari, NA. (2004). *Pneumocystis carinii* infection. Update and review. *Arch Pathol Lab Med*, 2004; Vol. 128, pp. 1023-1027, ISSN 0003-9985

Wislez M, Bergot E, Antoine M, et al. (2001). Acute respiratory failure following HAART introduction in patients treated for *Pneumocystis carinii* pneumonia. *Am J Respir Crit Care Med*, Vol. 164, pp. 847-851, ISSN 1073-449X

Wright, TW., Gigliotti, F., Finkelstein, JN., et al. (1999). Immune-mediated inflammation directly impairs pulmonary function, contributing to the pathogenesis of *Pneumocystis carinii* pneumonia. *J Clin Invest*, Vol.104, pp. 1307-1317, ISSN 0021-9738

Wright, TW., Johnston, CJ., Harmsen, AG. et al. (1999). Chemokine gene expression during *Pneumocystis carinii*-driven pulmonary inflammation. *Infect Immun*, Vol.67, pp. 3452-3460, ISSN 0019-9567

Wright, TW., Notter, RH., Wang, Z., et al. (2001). Pulmonary inflammation disrupts surfactant function during *Pneumocystis carinii* pneumonia. *Infect Immun*, Vol.69, pp. 758-764, ISSN 0019-9567

Wright, TW., Pryhuber, GS., Chess, PR., et al. (2004). TNF receptor signalling contributes to chemokine secretion, inflammation, and respiratory deficits during *Pneumocystis* pneumonia. *J Immunol*, Vol.172, pp. 2511-2521, ISSN 0022-1767

Wu AK, Cheng VC, Tang BS, et al. (2004). The unmasking of *Pneumocystis jiroveci* pneumonia during reversal of immunosuppression: case reports and literature review. *BMC Infect Dis*, Vol.4, pp.57, ISSN 1471-2334

Zolopa A, Andersen J, Powderly W, et al. (2009). Early antiretroviral therapy reduces AIDS progression/death in individuals with acute opportunistic infections: a multicenter randomized strategy trial. *PLoS One*, Vol. 4, pp. e5575, ISSN 1932-6203

8

Bacterial and Parasitic Agents of Infectious Diarrhoea in the Era of HIV and AIDS - The Case of a Semi Rural Community in South Africa

Samie A.[1], Bessong P.O.[1], Obi C.L.[2], Dillingham R.[3] and Guerrant R.L.[3]
[1]*AIDS Virus Research Laboratory, Department of Microbiology, University of Venda, Thohoyandou,*
[2]*Academic and Research Directorate, Walter Sisulu University, Nelson Mandela Drive Eastern Cape,*
[3]*Centre for Global Health, University of Virginia, Charlottesville,*
[1,2]*South Africa*
[3]*USA*

1. Introduction

Infection by the human immunodeficiency virus (HIV) is a worldwide public health concern. In the Southern African region, the HIV and AIDS pandemic has grown faster than in any other parts of the world, from infection rate, in pregnant women, of 0.8% in 1990 to 30.2% in 2005 in South Africa and 29.4% in 2009 (DOH, 2000; DOH, 2006; DOH 2010). Due to its destructive effect on the immune system, HIV infection further exposes the individual to multiple opportunistic infections. From the beginning of the HIV pandemics in the 1980s, gastrointestinal diseases have been demonstrated to be a major problem in patients with HIV and AIDS, and diarrhea is reported in up to 60% of patients with AIDS in developed countries and up to 90% in developing countries (Siddiqui et al., 2007; Silva et al., 2010). Recent studies by Bradshaw *et al.*, (2005) have indicated that HIV/AIDS is the leading cause of premature mortality for all provinces in South Africa and mortality due to pre-transitional causes, such as diarrhea, is more pronounced in the poorer and more rural provinces. In Limpopo Province as well as other poorer provinces in South Africa, diarrheal diseases are the first cause of mortality after HIV/AIDS (Bradshaw *et al.*, 2005). However, data on specific etiologies is sparse (Obi and Bessong, 2002) and such information will be crucial in the specific management of HIV and AIDS.

Although diarrheagenic organisms have been studied in different parts of the African continent, most research activities targeted specific organisms and their role in the production of diarrhea with little consideration to the presence of other organisms, their role in the production of inflammation which might be a considerable part of the pathogenesis of the organisms (Nel et al., 2010). Elsewhere, the combination of environmental factors, new ways of living and structural changes in the genetic material of most microorganisms have led to the appearance of emerging and re-emerging diseases (Lashley, 2006). Combined to the increasing recognition of a widening array of enteric pathogens associated with illnesses of the gastrointestinal tract, these factors highlight the growing need for the understanding of the epidemiology and transmission of the different organisms involved in infectious diarrhea in specific settings, using the more specific and sensitive molecular tools, for a better management of these diseases and the improvement of the quality of life of the concerned populations.

Gastrointestinal infections are major causes of morbidity and mortality throughout the world and particularly in developing countries where mortality rates due to infectious diarrhea could be as high as 56% (WHO, 2004). Children and young adults are the most affected, particularly in regions with limited resources and where hygienic measures are not strictly followed (Guerrant *et al.*, 2005; Opintan et al., 2010). In Africa, diarrhea has been estimated to be responsible for 25 to 75% of all childhood illnesses (Kirkwood, 1991), and episodes of diarrhea lead to about 14% of outpatient visits, 16% of hospital admissions, and account for an average of 35 days of illness per year in children less than five years old (Greenwood *et al.*, 1987). Causes of diarrhea in endemic areas include a wide variety of bacteria, viruses and parasites. Intestinal parasites are associated with serious clinical disease and mortality, and are known to cause malnutrition, growth, learning and physical development impairment in children. It is thus necessary to have a fairly accurate picture of the situation in order to target intervention strategies in affected areas.

It has been suggested that intestinal parasites occur at unacceptably high levels throughout South Africa. However, accurate prevalence data for the whole country are not currently available. With the exception of mapping being undertaken in KwaZulu-Natal, the medical geography of intestinal parasitic infections is stale, very fragmented and almost useless for planning, implementing and monitoring effective interventions (Fincham et al., 1997). In Cape Town, surveys at primary schools in urban and rural communities have revealed soil transmitted helminthiasis prevalence range between 7% and 83% (Kirkwood, 1991). However, there is scanty information, if any, on the prevalence of intestinal parasitic infections in the Limpopo Province.

Bacterial organisms such as *Campylobacter spp*, *Salmonella spp*, *Shigella spp* and different groups of enteropathogenic *E. coli* are well known as causes of gastrointestinal diseases all over the world. These organisms have been demonstrated in water and stools from the Vhembe district (Obi *et al.*, 2004; Larsen et al., 2011). Infections by most of these organisms can be asymptomatic, or can be treated with rehydration solutions particularly in case of viruses and some bacteria. The use of antibiotics might shorten the duration of diarrhea and limit the shedding of the organisms which otherwise might continue to pollute the environment and pose further risk of infections. Antibiotics such as erythromycin and gentamicin have been proven to be effective in some communities. However, antibiotic resistance is an overgrowing problem and there is a need to monitor the susceptibility of common bacterial isolates to drugs used in the community in order to provide guidelines for the empirical treatment of bacterial infections.

Diarrhea is a common final expression of infection with a myriad of pathogens. Appropriate management requires knowledge of the setting in which the patient became ill, the underlying disease state, presence and extent of dehydration and other clinical symptoms, travel history, known outbreaks, and pathogenic mechanism (invasive or toxigenic) and the physical findings and laboratory results at the time the patient presented with the condition (de Truchis and de Truchis, 2007; Beatty, 2010). Optimal evaluation and treatment of each of these infections (as well as of cases caused by noninfectious organisms) can limit the duration of illness, the morbidity rate, the cost of work-up, and the spread of secondary infection (Goodman and Segreti, 1999). Although the differential diagnosis of infectious diarrhea is broad, the clinical history can help guide the clinician toward the appropriate evaluation for each patient. For those patients with diarrhea of 2-3 days' duration, work-up is rarely necessary unless fever, bloody diarrhea, or severe abdominal pain is present. A detailed history of recent travel (within 6 months), recent antibiotic use (within 6-8 weeks), and contact with individuals who are ill and specific dietary ingestions during foodborne outbreaks can suggest an infectious etiology (DuPont, 1997). Infection with HIV is also a common cause of diarrhea. Therefore, medical history should include looking for risk factors for HIV and other comorbid illness that may result in immunosuppression (eg, diabetes, liver disease, organ transplantation) (Quinn *et al.*, 1983).

Clinical signs of dehydration, including dry mucous membranes, low urine output, or tachycardia, suggest severe infection. Other symptoms of severe infection include fever, severe abdominal pain, distension of the abdomen, and decreased bowel sounds. Although these findings are less helpful in determining the etiology of the diarrhea, they are helpful in deciding if the patient requires any immediate treatment or hospitalization.

Most cases of acute infectious diarrhea do not need medical evaluation or intervention because they will resolve spontaneously and rapidly (Herickstad *et al.*, 2002). However, if patients have any of the following clinical signs or presentations, they should undergo medical evaluation: (1) dehydration secondary to profuse watery diarrhea or inability to tolerate oral fluids; (2) fever (temperature >= 38.5 °C or 101.3 °F); (3) stools containing blood and mucus; (4) passage of 6 or more stools in a 24-hour period or duration of illness 48 hours or longer; (5) diarrhea with severe abdominal pain in patients 50 years of age or older; or (6) diarrhea in individuals 70 years of age or older or in those with known immunosuppression (eg, AIDS, transplant patients, patients who have recently received chemotherapy) (Guerrant *et al.*, 2001).

The distinction between inflammatory and non-inflammatory diarrhea has long been useful in the diagnosis of diarrhea and in the creation of treatment algorithms for managing diarrhea (Guerrant *et al.*, 2001; Thielman and Guerrant, 2004). The highly inflammatory diarrheas (or overt dysenteries) are caused by cultivable and potentially treatable pathogens, such as *Shigella* species, *Campylobacter jejuni*, *E. histolytica*, *C. difficile* and more recently Enteroaggregative *E. coli* and sometimes, *Salmonella* species (Huang *et al.*, 2003; Jiang et al., 2010; Hou et al., 2010). The currently available tests, microscopy for fecal leukocytes and an immunoassay for fecal lactoferrin (a simpler, quicker and more sensitive marker for the presence of fecal leukocytes), provide supporting evidence of inflammatory diarrhea and may be useful when such clinical features are equivocal (Victora *et al.*, 2000; Mercado et al, 2011). Recent studies have indicated that infections with *Cryptosporidium parvum* or *Giardia* species may result in mild intestinal inflammation that leads to detectable levels of fecal lactoferrin (Alcantara *et al.*, 2003). In equivocal cases, the negative predictive value of fecal lactoferrin testing may help to determine the need for routine bacteriologic culture for organisms such as *Campylobacter* spp, *Salmonella* spp, and *Shigella* spp (Thielman and Guerrant, 2004).

Stool cultures are considered to be the gold standard for the diagnosis of bacterial causes of gastroenteritis. However, their clinical use is limited to organisms that are routinely cultured (Choi *et al.*, 1996). The choice of the organisms to be cultured for depends on epidemiological data available for the region as well as outbreak and travel history. For example, most laboratories only attempt to culture for *Salmonella* spp, *Shigella* spp, and *Campylobacter* spp. Culture has also been used for diagnosis purposes in cases of *Entamoeba histolytica* suspicion. However this method is cumbersome and lack both sensitivity and specificity for the detection and identification of *E. histolytica* (Abd-Alla *et al.*, 1998). Considerable savings may be achieved if cultures for bacterial enteric pathogens are restricted to samples from patients hospitalized for ≤ 3 days (Valenstein *et al.*, 1996). Common organisms that can cause diarrhea, such as enteroinvasive *E. coli* and enterotoxigenic *E. coli* are not routinely looked for since these organisms can only be identified by molecular methods which are mostly restricted to research laboratories or few laboratories in developed countries. Unusual organisms such as *Yersinia* species and *Vibrio* species, which may be important in certain locations, are not routinely tested for.

Microscopy is the traditional method commonly used in developing countries for the detection of ova and trophozoites of parasites and some times can be helpful in the detection of bacterial organisms such as *Campylobacter* spp. In developed countries such as the USA, stool examination for ova and parasites is generally performed particularly if a patient is potentially immunosuppressed or returning from a developing country. However, in Africa microscopy is the mostly used method for diagnosis of parasitic infections and can be used in direct stools examination, or after staining by different methods such as the simplified Ritchie technique and Ziehl Neelsen modified coloration (Kassi *et al.*, 2004). The method used also depends on the suspected microorganism. In some cases such as in cryptosporidiosis where shedding of oocysts can be intermittent, up to 3 stool specimens may be needed for diagnosis (Goodgame *et al.*, 1993; Chappell *et al.*, 1996). By use of a modified acid-fast stain (Kinyoun), oocysts appear as red spheres of 4 - 6µm in diameter; no other organisms should be easily confused with *Cryptosporidium* species on the basis of size and appearance. Unfortunately, acid-fast staining is relatively insensitive, requiring 10,000 oocysts/g of watery stool and 500,000 oocysts/g of formed stool to make the diagnosis. Microscopy remains the best available test for acid-fast *Cyclospora cayetanensis* infections.

Traditionally, infections by *Giardia* as well as other organisms such as *E. histolytica, Dientamoeba fragilis, Balantidium coli* and other helminthes have been diagnosed by means of ova and parasite examination of fecal or small bowel specimens (including small bowel specimens obtained using the "string" test) (Stark *et al.*, 2006; Kurniawanet al., 2009). The physical characteristics of the cysts or ova may prove helpful in the differentiation of the organisms involved. For example, *Giardia* cysts are ovoid or ellipsoid and measure 11–15 µm in diameter while trophozoites are approximately the same size, with 2 anteriorly placed nuclei and 8 flagella best visualized by staining with trichrome or with the iron hematoxylin method (Shetty *et al.*, 1988; El-Naggar *et al.*, 2006). Although microscopy might be useful in a rural setting, its use is limited by its insensitivity and lack of specificity which might lead to over diagnosis of some infections such as those of *E. histolytica* (Kebede *et al.*, 2003; Nesbitt *et al.*, 2004). More sensitive methods have thus been introduced which are easier and have higher sensitivities and specificities.

The development of molecular methods has tremendously improved the detection and identification of infecting agents. A variety of PCRs have been described for the detection of different bacteria such as *Shigella, Salmonella, Campylobacter* spp, diarrheagenic *E. coli, Aeromonas* spp and *Plesiomonas* spp as well as parasitic organisms such as *Cryptosporidium, E. histolytica,* Micrsoporidia, *Cyclospora, Isospora* and *Giardia* species (Marshall *et al.*, 1999; Sturbaum *et al.*, 2001, Larsen et al., 2011) . The sensitivity of detection by PCR is greater than that by microscopy, making it of great use for detection of low numbers of parasites in stool samples (Bialek et al., 2002). PCR for the detection of Cryptosporidium species, for example, has a sensitivity of 93% and a specificity of 95%, compared with 67% and 99%, respectively, for the Direct immunofluorescence assay (DFA) assay and 68% and 58%, respectively, for

Enzyme Immuno Assay (EIA) (Bushen et al., 2004; Kar et al., 2011). In addition to identifying protozoa, the use of real-time PCR–restriction fragment–length polymorphism (RFLP) analysis can detect as few as 5 *Cryptosporidium* oocysts and can differentiate between 5 genotypes and, more recently, subtypes (Limor *et al.*, 2002). PCR-RFLP analysis is more sensitive, as it may detect 50–500 oocysts/mL of liquid stool or <1 pg of DNA and <10 oocysts from environmental samples (Sturbaum *et al.*, 2001). Detection of diarrheagenic *E. coli* such as EAEC has required a specific test for one of the characteristic virulence traits of this group of organisms. Because an entire cassette of potential virulence traits is regulated by the transcriptional activator AggR, some have proposed that genetic probes for this trait may be the single best test for EAEC at the present time, and such genetic probes have been incorporated into a multiplex PCR test (Cerna *et al.*, 2003). With the introduction of easier, more-sensitive methods that reduce labor, time, and reagent costs, the possibility of combining assays for the detection of different targets into one assay has become a possibility. A multiplex real-time PCR and an oligonucleotide microarray may be new methods for the detection of *Campylobacter* spp, *Salmonella* spp, *Shigella* spp, *E. histolytica, Giardia lamblia,* and *C. parvum,* with excellent, perhaps unprecedented, sensitivity and specificity in either fecal or water samples (Wang *et al.*, 2004; Verweij *et al.*, 2004). Work on these and potential new methods to detect fecal contamination in water may help to identify and ameliorate inadequate sanitation and contaminated water that perpetuates the devastating illness burdens associated with enteric infections around the world (Dillingham and Guerrant, 2004).

The causes of infectious diarrhea include a wide array of viruses, bacteria, and parasites, many of which have been recognized only in the last decade or two (Steiner *et al.*, 2006). The occurrence of the different pathogens depends on region. While enterotoxigenic *Escherichia coli* and rotaviruses predominate in developing areas, Norwalk-like viruses, *Campylobacter jejuni*, and cytotoxigenic *Clostridium difficile* are seen with increasing frequency in developed areas; and *Shigella, Salmonella, Cryptosporidium* species, and *Giardia lamblia* are found throughout the world (Taylor, 1993). Bacterial gastroenteritis generally produces more severe symptoms than viral infection, including more frequent and bloody stools and severe cramping. The importance of each pathogen depends on the region. In a study in Mozambique for example, diarrheagenic *Escherichia coli* (22%) were the most frequently isolated pathogens, followed by *Ascaris lumbricoides* (9.3%). Others detected pathogens included *Salmonella* spp. and *Giardia lamblia* (2.5% each) and *Campylobacter* spp. (1.7%). *A. lumbricoides* and *Strongyloides stercolaris* (100% versus 0%; P=0.008) were most frequently isolated in children older than 12 months of age (Mandomando *et al.*, 2007).

The prevalence of *Cryptosporidium* varies widely from country to country and from one region to another. In Korea, for example, Lee *et al.* (2005) reported a prevalence of 1% (among HIV patients) while in Tanzania, Houpt *et al.* (2005) described a prevalence of 17.3% amongst HIV patients. In Guinea Bissau, *Cryptosporidium parvum* had a prevalence of 7.7% and was the second most common parasite with a marked seasonal variation, with peak prevalence found consistently at the beginning of or just before the rainy seasons, May through July. In South Africa, studies by Kfir *et al.* (1995) indicated that *Giardia* cysts and *Cryptosporidium* oocysts were found in all types of water tested including surface water, sewage or treated effluents. Studies by Moodley *et al.* (1991) in Durban, South Africa showed that *Cryptosporidium* was the second most common enteric pathogen isolated from children admitted to hospital with gastroenteritis with infection rates varying between 1.2 and 20.9% according to season with the highest prevalence in the summer months, and 10%

of the children infected with *Cryptosporidium* died. However the prevalence of *Cryptosporidium* infections is not known in Limpopo Province, and particularly in the Vhembe district.

With the advent of HIV and AIDS, it has become more important to determine the distribution of parasitic infections such as *E. histolytica* and *E. dispar* amongst HIV infected individuals. In Mexico, *E. histolytica* prevalence of 25.3% in the HIV/AIDS group and 18.5% in the HIV negative group was described using PCR (Moran *et al.*, 2005). Likewise in Taiwan, persons infected with HIV were at increased risk for invasive amoebiasis and exhibited a relatively high frequency of elevated antibody titers and intestinal colonization with *E. histolytica* (Hung *et al.*, 2005). Previous studies in South Africa have been based in the Durban area in the eastern coast of the country where a prevalence of 10% using the PCR has been described (Zaki *et al.*, 2003). However no study to our knowledge has been conducted in the Limpopo Province and particularly in the Vhembe district. The first case of human microsporidial infection was described in 1959 and as early as 2 years after the identification of HIV as the causative agent of AIDS, the microsporidial species *Enterocytozoon bieneusi* was discovered in HIV-infected patients with chronic diarrhea (Desportes *et al.*, 1985). Although infections in immunocompetent patients are usually self-limiting, infections in immune compromised host can be life threatening, especially in patients with AIDS (Desportes *et al.*, 1985). Studies in Cape Town have indicated prevalence up to 22% of all *Campylobacter* spp when the filter method is used for isolation (Lastovica and Roux, 2000). In Venda, the infection level by *Campylobacter spp* was found to be around the same level (20%) amongst HIV infected individuals (Obi and Bessong, 2002). However, the isolates were not ascertained by the use of molecular methods and very few studies have determined the genetic variability of *Campylobacter* spp in Africa. Enteroaggregative *Escherichia coli* (EAEC) is an emerging diarrheagenic pathogen associated with diarrheal illnesses among patients in developed and developing countries. Recent studies have implicated EAEC in persistent diarrhea in patients infected with human immunodeficiency virus (HIV) (Wanke *et al.*, 1998; Nataro *et al.*, 2006).

Clostridium difficile is a spore-forming, anaerobic Gram positive bacillus that produces exotoxins that are pathogenic to humans. Infection can lead to asymptomatic carriage or clinical disease, ranging from mild diarrhea to life threatening pseudomembranous colitis (Cleary, 1998). *Clostridium difficile* associated disease (CDAD) is an important clinical problem that is believed to occur predominantly following hospitalisation and administration of antibiotics and especially affects the elderly (Wilcox, 1996). Community-acquired disease has been reported but the incidence is felt to be low and the rate of disease resulting in hospitalization is reported as negligible. For example a Swedish study of 5 133 cases of *C. difficile d*iarrhea defined 28% as being community acquired (Karlström *et al.*, 1998). Recent events in the USA, Canada and Europe have indicated the changing epidemiology of *Clostridium difficile* associated diarrhea (CDAD) with the occurrence of serious CDAD in otherwise healthy patients with minimal or no exposure to a health-care setting (Kuijper *et al.*, 2006; Reichardt *et al.*, 2007). However, the occurrence of *C. difficile* in developing regions such as the Vhembe district has not been reported. In the present study, molecular biology methods were used for the detection of different emerging bacterial and parasitic organisms including *Campylobacter* spp, *Arcobacter* spp, Enteroaggregative *E. coli, Clostridium difficile, Cryptosporidium* spp, *Entamoeba histolytica* and microsporidia, in relation to their pathogenicity among HIV positive and HIV negative individuals visiting different hospitals in the Vhembe district of South Africa.

2. Material and methods

2.1 Ethical Issues

Ethical approval of this research was granted by the Health, safety and Research Ethics Committee of the University of Venda. Authorization was also sought and obtained from the Department of Health and Welfare Limpopo Province, South Africa. The different hospitals and schools were then approached and the research objectives thoroughly explained to the study participants in the local language (TshiVenda) for their consent. Informed consent was obtained from all participants either directly or through their legal and competent guardians. Only consenting individuals were accepted in the study.

2.2 Study sites and sample collection

The study was conducted in the Vhembe district, of the Vhembe district, Limpopo Province, South Africa. Thohoyandou, meaning "head of the elephant" in tshiVenda, is the former capital of the independent homeland and the proud heart of the VhaVenda people. Thohoyandou is home to the University of Venda and is also the headquarters of the Vhembe district and is the tenth most populated town in the country with 584,469 people while the population of the region is approximately 1.2 million. The Vhembe district is semi urban and agriculture is the main activity practiced by the population. Main hospitals in the region include Elim, Tshilidzini, Vhufhuli (Donald Frazer) and Siloam hospitals. These hospitals deliver care directly to the population and are referral centers for smaller clinics in the region. The Vhembe district is bounded on the north by the Limpopo River, on the west by Sand River, on the south and east by the Levubu River and the remainder of the southern boundary by the farms adjoining the south of the Sinthumule location. The bulk of the people are today concentrated in locations and crown lands approximately from longitude 29*40'E-30*50'E and latitude 22*20'S-23*10'S. In normal seasons the rain starts in October/November and from that time onwards the weather becomes moist and hot, the shade temperature ranging from 80-90 degrees and north of the mountains being 110 degrees or more.

For sample collection two groups of population were considered for the study including patients attending four main public hospitals in the region namely Elim, Vhufuli, Siloam and Tshilidzini hospitals, and pupils from two public primary schools both situated in Wuwani, locality situated at about 6km from the Tshilidzini hospital. At the primary schools, the objectives of the study were explained to the parents in a meeting with the authority of the schools who then distributed the collection bottles to the pupils whose parents had agreed to the study and signed a consent form. The pupils then brought the collection bottles home and with the help of their parents collected the stool in the bottles. The samples were collected the following morning from the schools and transported without any further delay to the Laboratory of Microbiology, University of Venda. Samples that were not analysed the same day were stored at -20°C. A total of 322 stool samples were collected. 255 samples were from patients attending the three public hospitals with abdominal complaints or diarrhea while 67 were from apparently healthy pupils attending two public primary schools.

2.3 Lactoferrin latex agglutination assay

Stool supernatants were tested according to the manufacturer's specifications including appropriate kit controls (LEUKO-TEST; Tech Lab, Blacksburg, VA). Stool sample dilution was conducted as described by the manufacturer in the following way: one drop (50 µl) of stool was added to 375 µl of diluent yielding a 1:25 dilution. Using the pipette provided with the Kit, one drop of the diluted sample was mixed with one drop of sensitized latex (lactoferrin antibody-coated latex beads) or negative latex beads for 3min and the agglutination was observed for positive samples. Each test was run in parallel with a negative control as indicated by the manufacturer. Positive controls provided with the test kits were also performed. Agglutination reaction was graded with the unaided eye from 0 (no agglutination) to 4+ (large agglutination with a clear background).

2.4 Lactoferrin quantitative assay

The lactoferrin content in the lactoferrin positive stools samples was quantified using the ELISA method with the IBD scan kit from Techlab (Blacksburg, Virginia) following the instructions of the manufacturer.

2.5 Test for occult blood

The presence of occult blood in the stool samples was tested by the Hemoccult test kit (Beckman Coulter, Inc Harbor Blvd, Fullerton, CA, USA) following the instructions of the manufacturer.

2.6 Detection of pathogenic organisms

2.6.1 DNA purification

Four different methods were used and compared for the purification of total genomic DNA from stool samples. This would then allow for the detection of most parasites from the same sample and avoid conducting several DNA extractions from the same samples for the molecular detection of different pathogens. The first method involved the treatment of 200µg of stool sample by a freeze-thaw procedure using liquid nitrogen and boiling water followed by the use of the QIAamp DNA Stool Mini Kit from Qiagen (Valencia, CA, USA) according to the manufacturer's recommendations. The second method involved the use of the QIAamp DNA Stool Mini Kit, with higher temperature (95ºC) for the first incubation. The third method involved the used of alkaline treatment following a modified version of the method described by Haque *et al.*, (1998). Briefly, fifty microliters of 1M KOH and 18 µl of 1M dithiothreitol were added to 250mg or 250 µl of stool. The samples were mixed thoroughly by stirring with a pipette tip, followed by brief shaking. After incubation at 65°C for 15 min, the samples were neutralized with 8 µl of 25% HCl and buffered with 80 µl of 2M Tris-HCl (pH 8.3) and the suspension was mixed by briefly vortexing. The genomic DNA was then purified from the suspension using the QIAamp DNA Stool Mini Kit from Qiagen (Valencia, CA, USA) following the manufacturer's instructions. The last method was the use of glass beads in order to physically dreak open the cells, cysts, oocysts and spore that could be in the stool samples. Following the bead beating the QIA amp DNA Stool Mini Kit from Qiagen for final DNA purification.

The comparison of all the pretreatment methods showed that a combination of two pretreatment methods including one which is either the bead beating or the alkaline treatment or freeze and thaw with a surplus stool portion added untreated and the whole used in the Qiagen with an increased temperature at 95oC for 15 min gave bettwe detectionof all pathogens including bacterial and parasites. The purified DNA was stored at -20oC until further used in the different PCR and Real time PCR procedures.

2.6.2 Detection and genotyping of *Cryptosporidium*

Cryptosporidium species detection and genotyping was conducted as previously described using a real time PCR for the screening and PCR -RFLP for genotyping (Samie et al., 2006a).

2.6.3 Detection and genetic characterisation of *Entamoeba histolytica*

Entamoeba histolytica was detected from the samples using the Techlab (TechLab, Inc. Blacksburg, VA, USA) *E. histolytica* II antigen detection kit . The identification of the different species of *Entamoeba* mainly *E. histolytica* and *E. dispar* was conducted as previously described (Samie et al., 2006b). Genotyping of *E. histolytica* was conducted as previously described through the polymorphism of the serine-rich *E. histolytica* protein (SREHP) followed by enzymatic digestion (Samie et al., 2008).

2.6.4 PCR amplification for the detection of microsporidia

The PCR method described by Fedorko *et al* (1995) and further developed by Samie et al., (2007) was used with minor modification as indicated followed by restriction analysis.

2.6.5 Detection of *Campylobacters*

2.6.5.1 Culture and maintenance of reference strains

Reference strains used in this study included *Campylobacter jejuni* subsp. jejuni (ATCC 33291), *Campylobacter coli* (ATCC 33559) , *Campylobacter concisus* (ATCC 33237), *Campylobacter fetus* subsp. *fetus* (ATCC 27374), *Campylobacter hyointestinalis* (ATCC 35217), *Campylobacter upsaliensis* (ATCC 43954), *Helicobacter pylori* (ATCC 43504), *Arcobacter butzleri* (ATCC 49616), *Campylobacter jejuni* (ATCC 33560), *Campylobacter jejuni* (ATCC 81116), *Campylobacter jejuni* (ATCC 11168), *Campylobacter coli* (ATCC 33559) and *Campylobacter lari* (ATCC 35221). The cultures were sub-cultured in blood agar supplemented with 10% tryptose and 0.1% yeast extract and were preserved in Bolton broth and 25% sterile glycerol. Prior to DNA isolation, 500 µl of the preserved culture was added to 10ml of brain Heart infusion or Bolton broth and incubated in a Microaerophilic environment for 24hours and inoculated to blood agar or mCCDA. The culture method using a charcoal based media (mCCDA) was used to detect *Campylobacter* spp from 37 diarrheal stool samples collected from Donald Frazer hospital as indicated in the Cape Town protocol (Lastovica and Le Roux, 2000) and suspected colonies were confirmed using a *Campylobacter* haemagglutination kit "Campy Dry Spot" (Oxoid, England) as recommended by the manufacturer.

2.6.5.2 PCR detection of Campylobacteria

The genomic DNA purified as described above was used for the detection of *Campylobacter* spp, *Arcobacter* spp and *Helicobacter* spp by the PCR- RFLP as described by Marshall et al (1999) and Samie et al., (2007a).

Restriction profiles were generated with *Dde*I, *Taq*I, or *Bsr*I (New England Biolabs, Inc., Beverly, Mass.) in a 20-µl reaction mixture including 10 µl of the PCR amplicon with 10 U of the restriction endonuclease following conditions recommended by the manufacturer. Ten microliters of each digest was analyzed electrophoretically at 5 V/cm for 2 h with a 3% agarose gel in 1× TAE buffer. The gels were stained in ethidium bromide and photographs were taken for the analysis of the profiles. **Further specific detection and confirmation of** *Campylobacter jejuni* **and** *coli* was conducted as previously described (Linton et al., 1997; Samie al., 2007a)

Campylobacter concisus was detected from the samples using the method described by conventional and real time PCR protocols based on the methods previously described by Matsheka et al (2001).
A real time PCR for the rapid detection of *Campylobacter concisus* was developed based on the method described by Matsheka *et al.* (2001) and Samie et al (2008) using the primers pcisus1 and pcisus6 and the iQTM SYBR® Green Supermix (Bio-Rad, CA),

2.6.5.3 Specific detection of *Helicobacter Pylori*

The specific detection of H. pylori was conducted as previously described (Samie et al., 2007b) using the primers consisting of two specific 16S rRNA oligonucleotides, designated HPF and HPR, which generates a 138-bp product.

2.6.5.4 Use of a multiplex PCR assay for the simultaneous detection and identification of *Arcobacter butzleri, Arcobacter cryaerophilus* and *Arcobacter skirrowii*

A multiplex PCR reaction described by Houf et al (2000) and modified by Samie et al was used to identify the three main *Arcobacter* species.

2.6.6 Detection of Enteroaggregative *E. coli* from stool samples

A quantitative real time PCR using SYBR-Green -490 (Bio-Rad, CA) based on the protocol described by Samie et al., (2007c) used to confirm the presence of the *AggR* gene of EAEC in the stool samples. Standard cultures with known numbers of EAEC cells were used as reference and positive controls, while water and *E. coli* K-12 were used as negative controls in each reaction. The level of positivity of the samples was indicated by the Ct values.

2.6.6.1 Multiplex PCR detection of EAEC virulence genes from stool samples

A multiplex PCR protocol previously described was used with modifications in order to determine the presence of three EAEC genes in the stool samples (Cerna *et al.*, 2003; Samie et al., 2007c). Only the presence of the correctly sized gene PCR product(s) was interpreted as a positive test.

2.6.7 Detection of *Clostridium difficile* from stool samples

A PCR protocol targeting a species-specific internal fragment of the triose phosphate isomerase (*tpi*) housekeeping gene was used as described by Lemee *et al.*, (2004) for the detection of *C. difficile* in the stool samples (Samie et al., 2008c). The presence of the binary toxin was ascertained by two different reactions using two different primer pairs for the enzymatic and the binding components of the *cdt* gene using the conditions previously described by Stubbs *et al.*, (2000). The negative regulator gene was detected by using two different primer pairs as previously described by Spigaglia and Mastrantonio (2002). The first primer pair (C1 and C2) detects a fragment of the *tcdC* gene while the second primer pair (Tim 1 and Struppi 2) amplifies and internal fragment of the first PCR product. The PCR products were observed in 2% agarose gel except for the products of the second PCR for the *tcd* gene that was run in 3% agarose gel. This helped to observe any size difference that could exist in the amplification products.

2.7 Statistical analysis

All data was analysed using the statistical package for social sciences (SPSS) program (Version 13.1). The potential relationship between the presence of the different pathogens and the pathogenesis variables such as diarrhea, intestinal inflammation (through the measurement of the intestinal lactoferrin in the stool samples) and the presence of occult blood was determined by cross tabulation and the chi squarre test, risk evaluation and the Mantel-Haenszel Common Odds Ratio Estimate was used for statistical analysis. The difference was considered significant if the p value was less than 0.05. The Pathogenicity index (PI) as well as the Inflammatory index (II) were calculated. These were the ratios of the number of samples that were diarrheal (for PI) or were positive for Lactoferrin (for II) and positive for the pathogen in consideration over the number of samples that were positive for the pathogen but not positive for lactoferrin or diarrhea. This indicates the strength of the involvement of the organisms in the specific pathogenicity (diarrhea or intestinal inflammation).

3. Results

3.1 Population demographics and characteristics of stool specimens

From a total of 322 samples from 322 individuals of whom 44 were HIV positive patients while 211 were HIV negative patients and 67 were apparently healthy school children. The age of the hospital patients varied between 2 weeks and 88 years with most patients aged between 10 and 39 years old while the school children were aged between 3 and 15 years. At the hospital 148 (58%) were females while at the schools 34 (51%) were females. Diarrhea was common among hospital patients (65%) as well as intestinal inflammation indicated by elevated lactoferrin level in the stool samples (56%), and the presence of occult blood in the stools (43%). Diarrhea was common in the age groups 0 - 2 and 2 - 5 yeas old, and also in the age groups 40 - 49 and > 60. Diarrhea was more common amongst the HIV positive group compared to the HIV negative (χ^2= 12.452, $p = 0.002 < 0.05$). Of the 44 samples collected from HIV positive individuals, 11 (25%) were non diarrheal, 32 (72.7%) were diarrheal and 1 (2.3%) had bloody diarrhea. Of the 44 HIV positive patients 27 (61.4%) were females. HIV positive individuals were found at all age groups but the highest percentage was among those older than 20 years.

3.2 Gender distribution of diarrheagenic organisms in the study population

There was no significant difference in the distribution of the different pathogens tested in the present study according to gender, except for *Campylobacter coli* and *H. pylori* both of which were more common in males compared to females (Table 1a). *C. parvum* was more common among females while *C. hominis* was more common among males, however, the difference was not significant (Table 1b). For *E. histolytica*, 16% of the females had *E. histolytica* DNA with about 4% E. *histolytica* single infection and 13% mixed infections with *E. dispar*, while 12.2% had *E. dispar* DNA alone. Of the 109 stool samples from males, 16 (14.7%) had *E. histolytica* with 2 (1.8%) *E. histolytica* alone and 14 (12.8%) mixed infections. Seven (6.4%) had *E. dispar* DNA alone. *Campylobacter concisus* was more common among females (although the difference was not statistically significant) unlike *C. coli* that was more common in males. Similarly, *Cryptosporidium parvum* was more common among males while *C. hominis* was more common among females. *Enterocytozoon bieneusi* and *Entamoeba histolytica* were all more common in females compared to males, but with no significant difference.

	C. jejuni	*C. coli*	*C. concisus*	*H. pylori*	*A. butzleri*	*A. skirrowii*	*A cryaerophilus*
Females	19 (10.4%)	7 (3.8%)	7 (3.8%)	76 (41.8%)	10 (5.5%)	4 (2.2%)	7 (3.8%)
Males	14 (10.0%)	14 (10%)	3 (2.1%)	75 (53.6%)	10 (7.1%)	2 (1.4%)	2 (1.4%)
Sub-total	33 (10.2%)	21 (6.5%)	10 (3.1%)	151 (46.9%)	20 (6.3%)	6 (1.9%)	9 (2.8%)
χ^2,	0.017	4.915	0.763	4.434	0.369	0.256	1.702
p value	0.897	0.027	0.382	0.035	0.544	0.613	0.192

Table 1a. Distribution of diarrheagenic pathogens by gender.

	C. parvum	*C. hominis*	*E. bieneusi*	*E. histolytica*	*C. difficile*	EAEC
Females	6 (4.4%)	18 (13.3%)	23 (12.6%)	22 (16.3%)	27 (14.8%)	29 (15.9%)
Males	2 (1.8%)	18 (16.5%)	13 (9.3%)	16 (14.7%)	18 (12.8%)	23 (16.4%)
Sub-total	8 (3.3%)	36 (14.8%)	36 (%11.2)	38 (15.6%)	45 (14%)	52 (16.1%)
χ^2,	1.295	0.485	0.895	0.120	0.258	0014
p value	0.255	0.486	0.344	0.729	0.612	0.905

Table 1b.

3.3 Age distribution of different pathogens in Vhembe according to sample origin

In the population studied, all age groups were affected by infections. However, patients in the age group between 3 and 5 years were the most infected particularly with organisms like *C. jejuni, H. pylori, A. butzleri* and Enteroaggregative *E. coli* for the bacterial organisms as well as *C. hominis* and *E. histolytica* among the parasites (Table 2a and 2b). Other species of *Arcobacter* did not occur among patients less than 5 years of age. *Cryptosporidium parvum* did not occur among patients aged less than 10 years (Table 2b). For *Cryptosporidium*, the age group the most affected were 2-5 years old (28.6%) 30–39 years old (23.5%), and 40–49, and 4 (27.7%). None of the samples from individuals aged >60 was positive for *Cryptosporidium*. For *E. histolytica*, the age groups most infected were 0 - 2 (33%) followed by the age group 20 - 29 (27%). *E. bieneusi* was also common among the patients aged between 3 and 5 years old. The prevalence of *A. butzleri* was lower in the older population compared to the younger populations.

3.4 Diarrhea related pathogens in the studied population

Of all the samples analyzed, 31% of diarrheal samples did not have any pathogen while 66% of the non diarrheal samples had no pathogens detected. *Helicobacter pylori* was the most commonly detected organisms using polymerase chain reaction from both diarrheal and non- diarrheal samples, However, the difference was not significant. Of the 10 bacterial organisms tested, *C. jejuni, toxigenic C. difficile,* Enteroaggregative *E. coli* and *C. coli* were the most commonly detected and associated with diarrhea among the patients in the total population. These organisms also had the highest pathogenic indexes indicating their potential involvement in diarrheal cases. Of the 4 parasitic organisms tested, *E. histolytica* and *Cryptosporidium hominis* were more common and statistically associated with diarrhea with pathogenic indexes of 8 for *E. histolytica* and 2.1 for *C. hominis*. The prevalence of the different organisms in both diarrheal and non diarrheal samples is shown in Table 3 below as well as the pathogenic indexes of the organisms. Briefly, *C. jejuni* was the most pathogenic bacterial organisms (in relation to diarrhea) while *E. histolytica* was the most diarrheagenic parasitic organism in this population.

Origin	Age group	Total	*C. jejuni*	*C. coli*	*C. concisus*	*H. pylori*	*A butzleri*	*A. skirrowii*	*A cryaerophilus*
Hospitals	0 – 2	18	2 (11.1%)	0	1 (5.5%)	9 (50%)	2(11.1%)	0	0
	3 – 5	16	3 (18.7%)	1 (6.2%)	0	9 (56.2%)	1 (6.2%)	0	0
	6 – 9	16	2 (12.5%)	0	0	8 (50%)	1 (6.2%)	0	0
	10 – 19	65	4 (6.2%)	3 (4.6%)	4 (6.1%)	29 (44.6%)	6 (9.2%)	1 (1.5%)	1 (1.5%)
	20 – 29	62	9 (14.5%)	7 (11.3%)	1 (1.6%)	26 (41.9%)	4 (6.5%)	2 (3.2%)	2 (3.2%)
	30 – 39	42	6 (14.3%)	1 (2.3%)	0	29 (69%)	4 (9.5%)	2 (4.8%)	4 (9.5%)
	40 – 49	18	4 (22.2%)	2 (11.1%)	1 (5.5%)	8 (44.4)	0	0	1 (5.5%)
	50 – 59	10	1 (10%)	2 (20%)	0	4 (40%)	0	0	0
	≥ 60	8	1 (12.5%)	2 (25%)	0	4 (50%)	1(12.5%)	0	1 (12.5%)
	Subtotal	255	32 (12.5%)	18 (7%)	7 (2.7%)	126(49.4%)	19(7.5%)	5 (2%)	9 (3.5%)
Schools	3 – 5	5	0	0	1 (20%)	4 (80%)	0	0	0
	6 – 9	4	0	0	0	1 (25%)	0	0	0
	10 – 15	58	1 (1.7%)	3 (5.2%)	2 (3.4%)	32 (55.2%)	1 (1.7%)	1 (1.7%)	0
	Subtotal	67	1 (1.5%)	3 (4.4%)	3 (4.5%)	37 (55.2%)	1 (1.5%)	1 (1.5%)	0
Total		322	33 (10.2%)	21 (6.5%)	10 (3.1%)	163 (50.6%)	20 (6.2%)	6 (1.9%)	9 (2.8%)
χ^2			7.052	0.580	0.871	0.717	4.853	0.064	2.433
P value			0.008	0.446	0.351	0.397	0.028	0.801	0.119

Table 2a

Origin	Age group	Total	*C. parvum*	*C. hominis*	*E. bieneusi*	*E. histolytica*	*C. diff*	*EAEC*
Hospitals	0 – 2	18		1 (9.1%)		3 (27.3%)	3 (16.7%)	1 (5.6%)
	3 – 5	16		4 (28.6%)	4 (25.0%)	4 (28.6%)	2 (12.5%)	5 (31.3%)
	6 – 9	16		2 (15.4%)		2 (15.4%)	1 (6.3%)	2 (12.5%)
	10 – 19	65	2 (4.3%)	5 (10.6%)	6 (9.2%)	6 (12.8%)	10 (15.4%)	11 (16.9%)
	20 – 29	62	1 (2.1%)	7 (14.6%)	11 (17.7%)	13 (27.1%)	11 (17.7%)	12 (19.4%)
	30 – 39	42	5 (14.7%)	3 (8.8%)	9 (21.4%)	5 (14.7%)	12 (28.6%)	11 (26.2%)
	40 – 49	18		2 (13.3%)	2 (11.1%)	3 (20.0%)	1 (5.6%)	5 (27.8%)
	50 – 59	10		4 (50.0%)			2 (20.0%)	3 (30.0%)
	≥ 60	8			1 (12.5%)	1 (14.3%)	1 (12.5%)	
	Subtotal	255	8 (4.1%)	28 (14.2%)	33 (12.9%)	37 (18.8%)	43 (17%)	50 (19.6%)
Schools	3 – 5	5		2 (50.0%)				2 (40.0%)
	6 – 9	4						
	10 – 15	58		6 (14.6%)	3 (5.2%)	1 (2.4%)	2 (3.4%)	
	Subtotal	67		8 (17.0%)	3 (4.5%)	1 (2.1%)	2 (3.0%)	2 (3.0%)
Total		322			36 (11.2%)	38 (15.6%)	45 (13.9%)	52 (16.1%)
χ^2								
P value								

Table 2b.

Table 2. Distribution of bacterial and parasitic agents of diarrhea in the study population according to age group.

3.5 Diarrheagenic organisms and intestinal inflammation

Intestinal inflammation was measured by the amount of lactoferrin produced in the stool samples. Previous studies have correlated the occurrence of lactoferrin in the stool samples with leukocytes which is a marker of intestinal inflammation and even better because fecal leukocytes are generally difficult to count since they die faster once out of the body. Therefore, fecal lactoferrin is the best marker of intestinal inflammation. The inflammatory index was calculated in the same manner as the pathogenic index by dividing the prevalence of the organisms in lactoferrin positive samples by that of the organisms in lactoferrin negative samples. Of all the bacterial organisms tested *Campylobacter jejuni* was the most significantly associated with intestinal inflammation. Enteroaggregative *E. coli* was the next most inflammatory bacterial organism followed by *C. coli* and *C. concisus* (Table 4). Of all the parasitic organisms tested in the present study, *E. histolytica* was significantly associated with intestinal inflammation.

Characteristics	Diarrheal stools	Non-diarrheal stools	Total	χ^2, p value	PI
No Infection	53 (31.2%)	101 (66.4%)	154 (47.8%)		
All infections					
C. jejuni	29 (17.1%)	4 (2.6%)	33 (10.2%)	**18.159 (0.000)**	**6.6**
C. coli	16 (9.4%)	5 (3.3%)	21 (6.5%)	**4.934 (0.026)**	**2.8**
C. concisus	8 (4.5%)	2 (1.4%)	10 (3.1%)	1.226(0.268)	3.2
A. butzleri	14 (8.2%)	6 (3.9%)	20 (6.2%)	2.533 (0.112)	2.1
A. skirrowii	3 (1.8%)	3 (2.0%)	6 (1.9%)	0.019 (0.890)	0.9
A. cryaerophilus	4 (2.4%)	5 (3.3%)	9 (2.8%)	0.259 (0.611)	0.7
H. pylori	91 (51.7%)	60 (41.1%)	151 (46.9%)	2.652(0.103)	1.2
C. diff	34 (19.3%)	11 (7.5%)	45 (13.9%)	**9.21 (0.002)**	2.6
Toxigenic *C. diff*	20 (11.4%)	3 (2.1%)	23 (7.1%)	**10.48 (0.001)**	5.4
Non Toxigenic C. diff	14 (8%)	8 (5.5%)	22 (6.8%)	0.768 (0.381)	1.4
EAEC	36 (21.2%)	16 (10.5%)	52 (16.1%)	**6.722 (0.010)**	2.01
Parasitic organisms					
E. histolytica	34 (27%)	4 (3.4%)	38 (15.6%)	**25.544 (0.000)**	**8**
C. parvum	4 (3.2%)	4 (3.4%)	8 (3.3%)	0.009 (0.925)	1
C. hominis	25 (19.8%)	11 (9.3%)	36 (14.8%)	**5.361 (0.021)**	**2.1**
E. bieneusi	23 (13.1%)	13 (8.9%)	36 (11.2%)	1.393 (0.238)	1.5

Table 3. Prevalence of different diarrheagenic pathogens in diarrheal and non diarrheal stool samples in the general population in the Vhembe district of South Africa as detected by different Polymerase Chain Reaction methods. The pathogenic indexes show the potential association of the organisms with diarrhea.

3.6 Occurrence of organisms and occult blood in the stool samples

Occult blood was tested in the samples and correlated with the presence of the different organisms. Of all the organisms tested, 4 bacterial species were significantly associated with occult blood and these included in order of statistical importance Enteroaggregative *E. coli*, *Campylobacter jejuni*, *C. difficile* and *Campylobacter coli*. Of all the parasitic organisms tested, only *Entamoeba histolytica* showed a statistically significant correlation with occult blood. The pathogenicity index in terms of occult blood occurrence in the stool samples in association

Characteristics	Lactoferrin positive stools	Lactoferrin negative stools	Total	χ^2, p value	OR (95%CI)	II
All infections						
C. jejuni	26 (17.4%)	7 (4.0%)	33 (10.2%)	**16.586 (0.000)**	5.231 (2.2 - 12.4)	4.4
C. coli	14 (9.6%)	7 (4.0%)	21 (6.5%)	**4.122 (0.042)**	2.561 (1 - 6.5)	2.4
C. concisus	8 (5.5%)	2 (1.1%)	10 (3.1%)	**5.002 (0.025)**	5.043 (1 - 24.1)	5
A. butzleri	11 (7.5%)	9 (5.1%)	20 (6.2%)	0.803 (0.370)	1.5 (0.6 - 3.7)	1.5
A. skirrowii	2 (1.4%)	4 (2.3%)	6 (1.9%)	0.356 (0.551)	0.597 (0.1 - 3.3)	0.6
A. cryaerophilus	3 (2.1%)	6 (3.4%)	9 (2.8%)	0.539 (0.463)	0.594 (0.1 - 2.4)	0.6
H. pylori	69 (47.3%)	82 (46.6%)	151 (46.9%)	0.014 (0.905)	1.027 (0.6 - 15)	1.01
C. diff	25 (17.1%)	23 (13.1%)	48 (14.9%)			
EAEC	32 (21.9%)	20 (11.4%)	52 (16.1%)	**6.565 (0.010)**	2.189 (1.2 - 4)	1.9
E. histolytica	27 (26%)	11 (7.9%)	38 (15.6%)	**14.875 (0.000)**	4.112 (1.9 - 8.7)	3.3
C. parvum	3 (2.9%)	5 (3.6%)	8 (3.3%)	0.089 (0.766)	0.802 (0.2 - 3.4)	0.8
C. hominis	18 (17.3%)	18 (12.9%)	36 (14.8%)	0.940 (0.332)	1.419 (0.6 - 2.8)	1.3
E. bieneusi	16 (11%)	20 (11.4%)	36 (11.2%)	0.013 (0.909)	0.960 (0.4 - 1.9)	1

Table 4. Diarrheagenic organisms and intestinal inflammation as indicated by the detection of lactoferrin in the stool samples.

with the organisms was calculated using the same formula described above for lactoferrin and diarrhea. EAEC had the highest index followed by *Campylobacter jejuni, Campylobacter coli* and *Clostridium difficile* for the bacteria and *E. histolytica* among the parasites. The summary of these results is shown in table 4. EAEC infections were significantly associated with intestinal inflammation (χ^2=6.565, P=0.010) and 61.5% of stools that were positive for EAEC genes had elevated lactoferrin compared to 42.2% for samples negative for EAEC genes. Stool samples positive for EAEC genes were more likely to have occult blood (Odd ratio=5.069; 95%CI: 2.665 - 9.644) even when the number of cells carrying the *AggR* gene was lower in the stool. Of the samples positive for at least one EAEC gene, 69.2% had occult blood compared to only 30.7% for samples negative for EAEC genes (χ^2=27.725, P<0.00001). The occult blood pathogenicity index was higher for samples containing *AggR* compared to the other two genes. In general, most bacterial and parasitic organisms tested were more common in samples with occult blood. However, the difference was not significant (P>0.05) (Table 5).

3.7 Occurrence of infections in HIV positive and HIV negative patients with or without diarrhea

In the present study, the presence of bacterial and parasitic organisms was determined according to HIV status of the patients. In order to have a better indication on how important could a pathogen be to the HIV positive group, we calculated the HIV relatedness index (HI) by dividing the prevalence of these infections in HIV positive by the prevalence of the same organism among HIV negative patients. A higher HI indicates that the organism was more common among HIV positive patients. Generally a HI higher than 2 was a good

Characteristics	Occult blood positive stools (n=119)	Occult blood negative stools (n=203)	Total	χ^2, p value	OR (95%CI)	PI
All infections						
C. jejuni	21 (17.6%)	12 (5.9%)	33 (10.2%)	**11.233 (0.001)**	3.411 (1.6 – 7.2)	2.9
C. coli	2 (10.1%)	9 (4.4%)	21 (6.5%)	**3.929 (0.047)**	2.417 (0.9 – 5.9)	2.3
C. concisus	6 (5.0%)	4 (2.0%)	10 (3.1%)	2.35 (0.125)	2.642 (0.7 – 9.5)	2.5
A. butzleri	10 (8.4%)	10 (4.9%)	20 (6.2%)	1.557 (0.212)	1.771 (0.7 – 4.3)	1.7
A. skirrowii	2 (1.7%)	4 (2.0%)	6 (1.9%)	0.034 (0.853)	0.850 (0.1 – 4.7)	0.85
A. cryaerophilus	5 (4.2%)	4 (2.0%)	9 (2.8%)	1.275 (0.241)	2.182 (0.5 – 8.2)	2.1
H. pylori	58 (48.7%)	93 (45.8%)	151 46.9(%)	0.258 (0.611)	1.125 (0.7 – 1.7)	1.06
C. diff	26 (21.8%)	22 (10.8%)	48 (14.9%)	**7.171 (0.007)**	2.300 (1.2 – 4.2)	2.01
EAEC	36 (30.3%)	16 (7.9%)	52 (16.1%)	**27.725 (0.000)**	5.069 (2.7 – 9.6)	3.8
E. histolytica	21 (23.3%)	17 (11%)	38 (15.6%)	**6.530 (0.011)**	2.453 (1.2 – 4.9)	2.1
C. parvum	4 (4.4%)	4 (2.6%)	8 (3.3%)	0.611 (0.434)	1.7 (0.7 – 4.1)	1.7
C. hominis	17 (18.9%)	19 (12.3%)	36 (14.8%)	1.938 (0.164)	1.655 (0.8 – 3.4)	1.5
E. bieneusi	18 (15.1%)	18 (8.9%)	36 (11.2%)	2.960 (0.085)	1.832 (0.9 – 3.6)	1.7

Table 5. Diarrheagenic organisms and occult blood in the stool samples.

indication that the specific pathogen was correlated with HIV infections. Of all the organisms tested in the present study, EAEC, *C. jejuni* and *C. coli* appeared to be important bacterial pathogens in HIV positive patients while *E. bieneusi* was the most common parasitic organism among HIV positive patients.

The prevalence of EAEC infection among HIV positive individuals was significantly higher (χ^2=5.360, P=0.021) with 13 (29.5%) infections than the rest of the study population with 39 (14%) infections. Of the HIV positive patients tested, 8 were positive for *E. histolytica*. Of these individuals 5 were females and three were males. Among the HIV negative individuals, 29 (13.8%) males and 28 (13.3%) females were infected (χ^2=0.754, P= 0.385). Five samples from HIV positive patients were genotyped for *E. histolytica*. Of these, 3 (60%) belonged to the same profile mostly (3 out of 4 [75%]) found in HIV positive patients with diarrhea (2 out of 3) or without diarrhea (1 out of 3). One other profile was found mostly (7 out of 8) in HIV negative patients while one other profile was unique to a HIV positive individual. In the present study, we found a higher *Campylobacter* infection rate: 18.2% and 11.4% among HIV positive patients compared to 11.4% and 6.2% in HIV negative individuals for *C. jejuni* and *C. coli* respectively. The prevalence of these *Campylobacter's* infection among HIV positive individuals was significantly higher (χ^2=5.360, P=0.021) with 13 (29.5%) infections than the rest of the study population with 39 (14%) infections. When compared to HIV negative individuals, HIV positive individuals were more likely to have microsporidiosis (χ^2=4.414, p=0.036). In the HIV negative population, males were more infected than females. However, in the HIV positive population, females were significantly more infected than males (p<0.001). In the HIV negative subgroup, *E. bieneusi* was more common in individuals without diarrhea (15.9%) than individuals with diarrhea (9.0%), but this was not statistically significant. In the HIV positive group, *E. bieneusi* was found only in diarrheal samples indicating the possible involvement of these organisms in the production of diarrhea in immunocompromised hosts. The prevalence of infection by *C. difficile* was generally higher in HIV negative individuals (14.4%) than HIV positive individuals (11.4%), but the difference was not significant (χ^2=0.289, p=0.591). However, all the toxigenic *C. difficile* in HIV positive patients were found in diarrheal samples, with elevated lactoferrin and occult blood while the non-toxigenic strains were found in stool samples negative for the lactoferrin test and for occult blood indicating that even though *C. difficile* infections are not more prevalent among HIV positive patients, they might be more susceptible to these infections.

		C. jejuni	*C. coli*	*C. concisus*	*H. pylori*	*A butzleri*	*A. skirrowii*	*A cryaerophilus*
HIV positive	Diarrheal	8 (21.1%)	5 (13.2%)	2 (5.3%)	19 (50%)	1 (2.6%)	1 (2.6%)	2 (5.3%)
	Non diarrheal	0	0	0	3 (50%)	0	0	0
	Sub-total	8 (18.2%)	5 (11.4%)	2 (4.5%)	22 (50%)	1 (2.3%)	1 (2.3%)	2 (4.5%)
HIV negative	Diarrheal	21 (15.9%)	12 (9.1%)	6 (4.5%)	68 (51.5%)	13 (9.8%)	2 (1.5%)	3 (2.3%)
	Non diarrheal	4 (2.7%)	4 (2.7%)	2 (1.4%)	61 (41.8%)	6 (4.1%)	3 (2.1%)	4 (2.7%)
	Sub-total	25 (9%)	16 (5.8%)	8 (2.9%)	129 (46.4%)	19 (6.8%)	5 (1.8%)	7 (2.5%)
	χ^2, p value	3.487 (0.062)	1.960 (0.162)	0.351 (0.553)	0.197 (0.657)	1.357 (0.244)	0.047 (0.829)	0.575 (0.448)
	PI	2	2	1.5	1.1	0.3	1.3	1.8

Table 6a

		C. parvum	*C. hominis*	*E. bieneusi*	*E. histolytica*	*C. difficile*	EAEC
HIV positive	Diarrheal	1 (3.8%)	3 (11.5%)	9 (23.7%)	4 (15.4%)	5 (13.2%)	12 (31.6%)
	Non diarrheal	0	0	0	1 (16.7%)	0	1 (16.7%)
	Sub-total	1 (3.1%)	3 (9.4%)	9 (20.5%)	5 (15.6%)	5 (11.4%)	13 (29.5%)
HIV negative	Diarrheal	2 (2.1%)	19 (20.2%)	13 (9.8%)	30 (31.9%)	28 (20.3%)	25 (18.9%)
	Non diarrheal	5 (4.2%)	14 (11.9%)	14 (9.6%)	3 (2.5%)	12 (8.6%)	14 (9.6%)
	Sub-total	7 (3.3%)	33 (15.6%)	27 (9.7%)	33 (15.6%)	40 (14.4%)	39 (14.0%)
	χ^2, p value	0.003 (0.958)	0.847 (0.357)	4.414 (0.036)	0.000 (0.993)	0.504 (0.478)	6.754 (0.009)
	PI	1	0.6	2.1	1	0.8	2.1

Table 6b.

Table 6. Distribution of bacterial and parasitic organisms among HIV positive and HIV negative patients. The statistics compare the values for the HIV positive and the HIV negative patients. The HIV relatedness index (HI) was the ratio of the occurrence of infection among HIV positive patients to the prevalence of that same infection among HIV negative patients.

4. Discussion

Intestinal bacterial and parasitic infections are common in developing countries and responsible for most acute and chronic diarrhea cases amongst HIV/AIDS patients (Silva et al., 2010). The objective of this study was to determine the prevalence and genotype distribution of bacterial and parasitic organisms in the general population including school children and among HIV positive and HIV negative individuals in the Vhembe district of South Africa; a semi urban area situated in Limpopo Province in the northern part of the country. The organisms detected include *Cryptosporidium species, Entamoeba histolytica,* Microsporidia, *Campylobacter* spp, *Arcobacter* spp, *Helicobacter pylori,* Emteroaggregative *E. coli* and *Clostridium difficile.*

According to the South African Department of Health, the HIV prevalence in the general population was 10.8% for all South Africans over the age of 2 years in 2005 (DOH, 2010). Among those between 15 and 49 years old, the estimated HIV prevalence was 16.2% in 2005. Females were more affected (13.3%) than males (8.2%). In the Limpopo Province, the prevalence in the whole population was 8%. In our study, 15.7% of the patients visiting the hospitals were positive for HIV. This is closer to the national prevalence for individuals between 15 and 49 years of age. These rates are still high compared to countries from other parts of the African continent such as Mali (1.9%), but is comparable with the rates in other countries in the Southern African sub-region such as Malawi (14.2%) and Zambia (16.5%) (Banerjee *et al.*, 2004). It is well known that chronic diarrhea is one of the major AIDS-defining illnesses in WHO Classification and occurs in 60-90% of HIV infected patients in Africa and in a Swiss Cohort Study, diarrhea was found to be an independent predictor of poor survival amongst HIV and AIDS patients (Tadesse and Kassu, 2005; Humphreys et al., 2010). In our study, diarrhea was very common and was present in 74.2% of fecal specimens submitted from cases in the HIV population and is thus in agreement with data from previous studies.

Studies in other parts of the world have indicated that *Cryptosporium* spp represented by *C. Parvum* are the most common diarrheagenic parasitic organisms, however, few studies have compared rates among HIV negative and HIV positive patients. The prevalence and species distribution of *Cryptosporidium spp* vary greatly with the regions or country studied and even within specific groups of the population. This creates a complex picture of the epidemiology of infection by these organisms whose understanding will be helpful in shaping the appropriate measures for their control. In Limpopo Province, the HIV prevalence is 16.2% as determined by the report of the Department of Health and Welfare of South Africa (DOH, 2003). Previous studies in Limpopo Province have targeted different bacterial infections in HIV/AIDS patients; however no attempt has been made to isolate parasites (Obi and Bessong, 2002). This study is thus the first to use a molecular approach for the detection, genetic diversity and pathogenicity of the bacterial and parasitic infections in the region.

The real time quantitative PCR (qPCR) is a very sensitive, specific and easy to use method for the identification and quantification of organisms from a variety of sources. The qPCR used in the present study for the detection of *Cryptosporidium* has been tested for specificity and sensitivity using stools spiked with different numbers of oocysts and proved to be highly effective (Houpt *et al.*, 2005; Taniuchi et al 2011). Studies in various tropical countries have demonstrated highest prevalence of cryptosporidiosis in children younger than 2 years. In rural areas children of between 2 - 5 years old are more exposed to infections since this is the period when they begin to be active on their own. In Zimbabwe, Simango and Mutikani (2004) demonstrated that *Cryptosporidium* was common amongst children aged less than 5 years old with infection rate of 11.2%. In India, studies conducted in twin cities of Hyderabad and Secunderabad indicated that children in the age group of six months to one year were the most vulnerable with 14.3% infections compared to 8.2% among children less than five years of age while in Malaysia the prevalence was 7.5% and 33.3% in Egypt (Nagamani et al., 2007; Al-Mekhlafi et al., 2011).

It has been demonstrated in some countries such as Mexico (Javier-Enriquez *et al.*, 1997), Brazil (Newman *et al.*, 1999; de Oliveira-Silva et al 2007), and Indonesia (Katsumata *et al.*, 2000; Moyo et al., 2011) that *Cryptosporidium* transmission in children is usually associated with the rainy season, and waterborne transmission is considered a major route in the epidemiology of cryptosporidiosis in these areas. Although water contamination with *Cryptosporidium* has been demonstrated in other parts of South Africa, such research needs to be completed in the Limpopo Province in order to confirm the source of transmission in the region. Considering the presence of *Cryptosporidium* in the hospitals as well as in the schools, it can be hypothesized that water is a widespread transmission vector in the region. A study in Peruvian children has demonstrated that cryptosporidiosis was more frequent in children from houses without a latrine or toilet (Bern *et al.*, 2002). Previous studies in Venda have also indicated poor level of hygiene in Venda (Potgieter *et al.*, 2005). However, more detailed studies need to be conducted in order to clarify the role of hygienic habits in the transmission of *Cryptosporidium* as well as other parasitic organisms in the Vhembe district.

Cryptosporidium parasitizes the small intestinal epithelium. Infection results in accelerated loss of villous enterocytes, leading to severe villous atrophy and a malabsorptive and secretory diarrhea. The most common symptom of cryptosporidiosis is watery diarrhea. Other symptoms include: dehydration, weight loss, stomach cramps or pain, fever, nausea, and vomiting. Abdel-Messih *et al.* (2005) in Egypt demonstrated that clinical findings associated with *Cryptosporidium* diarrhea included vomiting, persistent diarrhea and the need for hospitalization. Studies by Alcantara *et al.* (2003) indicated that *Cryptosporidium* was associated with inflammation as indicated by the lactoferrin test and the presence of IL8 and TNF-α. In this study, *Cryptosporidium* was also associated with inflammation and more than 59.1% of *Cryptosporidium* infections might lead to inflammation. However more detailed study is required to clarify the real impact of *Cryptosporidium* infections as well as other protozoan parasitic infections in the production of intestinal inflammation in Venda. Another study in Haiti by Kirkpatrick *et al.* (2002) indicated that malnourished children with acute cryptosporidiosis mount inflammatory (with high lactoferrin content), Th-2, and counter regulatory intestinal immune responses. Studies of Peruvian as well as Brazilian children have demonstrated malnutrition, particularly stunting with lack of growth catch-up after even asymptomatic *C. parvum* infection (Checkley *et al.*, 1998; Antonios et al., 2010).

The existence of two *Entamoeba* species morphologically identical but genetically different was suggested as early as 1925 by Brumpt. However, it was not until 1993 that enough biochemical, immunological and genetic data were gathered to re-classify *E. histolytica* into 2 separate species: *E. histolytica* which can invade the gut mucosa, causes diarrhea and extra-intestinal disease, and *E. dispar*, which causes only asymptomatic colonization (Diamond and Clark, 1993). Following the reclassification of *Entamoeba histolytica*, the epidemiology of amoebiasis needed to be redefined by the use of methods that are able to differentiate between *E. histolytica* and *E. dispar*. Thus different PCR methods have been developed with variable efficiencies. A nested PCR previously described has been successfully used to differentiate between *E. histolytica* and *E. dispar* (Haque *et al*, 1998; Ali *et al.*, 2003). Using the same method; we were able to differentiate between *E. histolytica* from *E. dispar* in samples collected from patients visiting public hospitals with gastrointestinal complaints or diarrhea; and pupils attending public primary schools in the Vhembe district. *E. histolytica* was found both in the hospital and in the Schools. However, *E. histolytica* was less common amongst primary School children aged between five and fifteen. These findings underscore the potential role of *E. histolytica* in morbidity in the study area since the association between *E. histolytica* infections and diarrhea was statistically significant ($P < 0.05$). Similar results have been found in other countries around the world such as Thailand (Haghighi *et al.*, 2003).

Infection rates as well as species diversity (ratio between the occurrence of *E. histolytica* and *E. dispar*) varied tremendously from one region to the other. In Italy, more patients were found to be infected with *E. dispar* (8.3%) than *E. histolytica* (5.6%) using PCR assays (Calderaro *et al.*, 2005). In Sweden, amoebiasis is a notifiable disease and 400–500 cases are reported annually to the Swedish Institute for Infectious Disease Control (SMI). The PCR analysis showed that 165 (79.7%) patients were positive for *E. dispar*, whereas only 10 (4.8%) patients were positive for *E. histolytica* (Lebbad and Svard, 2005). In contrast, higher rates of *E. histolytica* infections was found in Mexico as compared to *E. dispar* infections (13.8% versus 9.6%), using PCR (Ramos *et al.*, 2005). Similarly in the Philippines, 74 cases (65.48%) were positive for *E. histolytica* and 6 cases (5.30%) positive for *E. dispar* from a mental institution (Rivera *et al.*, 2006). In the Gaza strip, Palestine, *E. histolytica* was identified by PCR in 64 (69.6%) of the samples and that of *E. dispar* in 21 (22.8%) (Al-Hindi *et al.*, 2005).

In the present study, we found a rate of 15.5% for *E. histolytica* which is higher than the rate found in Durban by Gathiram and Jackson (1985). This can be explained by the fact that our population was potentially ill and thus had a higher risk of been infected which was not the case in the group without diarrhea in whom there were no mixed infections and only one asymptomatic case of *E. histolytica* was found. The antigen detection test from Techlab (Blacksburg, Virginia, USA) has previously been shown to be suitable for the diagnosis of amoebiasis in endemic areas (Abd-Alla and Ravdin, 2002). In the present study, ELISA had a high specificity. It should be noted that samples positive for PCR and negative with the ELISA test were generally mixed infections with *E. histolytica* and *E. dispar*. This might have a hindering effect on the ability of the ELISA test to detect these samples and might also be related to the pathogenicity or virulence of the strains involved. It has been indicated elsewhere that when both organisms are present in an individual, *E. dispar* generally outgrows *E. histolytica*. However, since *E. dispar* is non pathogenic, the result of the infection will probably be asymptomatic. Mixed infections have also been described in Mexico where 13% of individuals were found harboring *E. histolytica* and *E. dispar* at the same time, particularly amongst HIV positive individuals (Moran *et al.*, 2005).

The mechanisms of disease production following an infection by *E. histolytica* are not fully understood. Most *E. histolytica* infections remain asymptomatic. However, other studies have suggested that amebic colitis may be encountered during colonoscopic examination even in subjects who are asymptomatic (Okamoto *et al.*, 2005). *E. histolytica* has also been associated with traveler's diarrhea. In a study in Sweden, when the patients were divided into immigrants and travelers, the percentages with *E. histolytica* were 3.8% and 9.5%, respectively (Barwick *et al.*, 2002). In invasive amoebiasis, white blood cells can be present in the stool, and in severe cases pus can be visible, but faecal leukocyte numbers are generally not as high as in shigellosis (Speelman *et al.*, 1984). Indeed, virulent *E. histolytica* can destroy neutrophils upon contact; hence may induce inflammation but show only pyknotic leukocytes in the stools (Guerrant *et al.*, 1981; Callendar, 1933). Such a process would be expected to cause evidence of inflammation (i.e. lactoferrin) even without morphologically clear PMNs in the stool. Inflammation occurs most often and previous studies have demonstrated that fecal lactoferrin was the best way to indicate the presence of PMN in stool samples. In our study, 85.7% of samples with *E. histolytica* DNA were positive for lactoferrin with 43% of cases presenting with high level of lactoferrin while *E. dispar* positive samples had only 1 (4.3%) case with a high lactoferrin level. This further confirms the pathogenic differences between the two species. When we excluded other detected organisms, the association of *E. histolytica* with diarrhea and with lactoferrin was even stronger. Other studies had indicated low levels of lactoferrin with *E. histolytica* and *S. hematobium* infections compared to shigellosis and other UTI infections (Aly *et al.*, 2005). However, *E. histolytica* infections had not been ascertained by specific test such as PCR.

Whether risk of invasive amebiasis due to *E. histolytica* is higher among human immunodeficiency virus (HIV)-infected persons than uninfected persons remains unclear, although intestinal colonization by *E. histolytica/dispar* has been reported to be higher among HIV positive individuals (Moran *et al.*, 2005). While studies in Thailand have indicated that *E. histolytica* was more common among HIV positive patients ($P<0.001$), studies in Mexico were not conclusive on this issue (Hung *et al.*, 2005). We had recently described a much higher seroprevalence of *Entamoeba histolytica* among HIV and AIDS patients compared to HIV negative patients (Samie et al., 2010). In a study on the genetic diversity of *E. histolytica*, we found that one profile was more common among HIV positive individuals indicating that the increased susceptibility of HIV positive individual to *E. histolytica* might depend on the genetic profile of the infecting *E. histolytica* strain. In a recent study in Uzbekistan, HIV-infected patients were found to have virtually all parasites, such as *Giardia lamblia, Cryptosporidium parvum, Chilomastix mesnili, Entamoeba coli, Iodamoeba butschlii, Entamoeba histolytica/dispar, Endolimax nana, Blastocystis hominis, Enlerobius vermicularis, Ascaris lumbricoides, Hymenolepis nana,* detectable in the population of Tashkent (Nurtaev *et al.*, 2006). Of special interest was the fact that in all the forms (stages) of HIV infection, the infestation with *E. histolytical/dispar* was 10 times greater than that in non HIV infected individuals.

Since their successful isolation from stools in the 1970s *Campylobacter spp* have risen from obscurity to notoriety as important food borne agents of gastroenteritis with present isolation rates superceding those of other enteric pathogens such as *Salmonella* spp. and *Shigella* spp. in most developed countries and higher prevalence among children in the developing world (Crushell *et al.*, 2004; Fernández-Cruz et al., 2010). Although their implication in human infections has been described worldwide, their epidemiology varies in different regions of the world and the knowledge of their prevalence using molecular methods is essential for the designing of efficient control measures adapted to each area. Acute self-limited gastrointestinal illness, characterized by diarrhea, fever and abdominal cramps, is the most common presentation of *C. jejuni/C. coli* infection (Butzler, 2004). In this study we found a significant association of *C. jejuni* and *C. coli* infections with diarrhea and inflammation. *Campylobacter spp* other than *C jejuni/coli* have also been implicated in human and animal diseases (Lastovica and Skirrow, 2000; Moran, 2010). In this study, we detected *C. concisus* in 10 (3.1%) samples with 6 (60%) cases present in diarrheal stools indicating the possibility of the involvement of this *Campylobacter species* in disease production in the Vhembe district. In Cape Town, studies by Lastovica and LeRoux indicated that C. *concisus* was the second most isolated *Campylobacter* after *C. jejuni* and constituted 23.55% of all *Campylobacter* isolates (Lastovica and Le Roux, 2000).

Unlike its close phenotypically related neighbour *Campylobacter*, *Arcobacter* is not currently a major public health concern, but is considered as an emerging human pathogen, and is of significance in animal health (Snelling *et al.*, 2006; Kalischuk and Buret, 2010). In the present study 70% of *A. butzleri* containing samples was diarrheal and 55% with elevated level of lactoferrin indicating possible involvement in inflammatory processes. However more research needs to be conducted in order to confirm its involvement in human disease. *H. pylori* was found in 163 (50.6%) of all the samples among which 55.9% of *H. pylori* positive samples were diarrheal and that *Helicobacter pylori* was common among school children and hospital patients. These results are similar to previous studies that have indicated that *H. pylori* is *a* common human pathogen estimated to colonize 50% of the world's population (Van Der Hulst *et al.*, 1996). Epidemiological evidence has suggested that *H. pylori* is spread by fecal-oral and oral-oral routes. Although there are no known environmental reservoirs for *H.* pylori, *H. pylori* has been cultured from the feces (Thomas *et al.*, 1992) of infected individuals and has been detected by polymerase chain reaction (PCR) in dental plaque (Nguyen *et al.*, 1993). The prevalence found in the present study was lower compared to other recent studies in Pretoria, South Africa, where *H. pylori* was found in 84% of stomach biopsies from Healthy individuals but not in dental samples (Olivier *et al.*, 2006). It has been estimated that the relationship between chronic diarrhea, retarded growth, iron-deficient anaemia, and *H. pylori* infection in children especially from developing countries remains controversial (Raymond *et al.*, 2005). However, more research is needed in order to determine their involvement in gastric ulcers as well as any other pathogenic features in the Vhembe district.

Over the past few years, enteroaggregative *E. coli* have been increasingly characterized in developing countries and recent data have suggested that EAEC are emerging as diarrheal agents in developed nations as well (Nataro *et al.*, 2006; Opintan et al., 2010). However; the true distribution of these organisms as well as their pathogenicity is not well studied in South Africa particularly in the Vhembe district. In the present study, we detected the presence of three EAEC pathogenic genes employing a recently developed multiplex PCR. We evaluated these genes in relation to HIV status, diarrheal symptoms, intestinal inflammation, determined by elevated lactoferrin, and occult blood in a sample population composed of hospital patients with known HIV status and school children in the Vhembe district of South Africa. Different methods have been described for the detection of EAEC and have suggested the existence of two different categories of EAEC including Typical and Atypical EAEC (Jenkins *et al.*, 2006). Typical EAEC carry the pAA plasmid originally detected by the AA probe. Enteroaggregative *E. coli* have also been associated with weakened immune system such as in patients with HIV and AIDS. EAEC have been described as the most common pathogen among HIV positive patients in many countries even though the rates of infection vary from country to country. In this study we found a higher rate of EAEC infection among HIV positive patients (29.5%) compared to Senegal (West Africa) where EAEC was found in 19.6 % of HIV patients and was the most common pathogen amongst these individuals (Gassama *et al.*, 2001). In Switzerland, EAEC genes were detected in 22% of HIV positive patients with diarrhea while in Zambia, EAEC was found in both HIV patients and control even though cytotoxic phenotypes were only isolated from the AIDS patients with no evidence of seasonality in the frequency of isolation, and no evidence of long-term carriage (Kelly *et al.*, 2003; Crump et al., 2011).

Different markers of pathogenesis have been described in EAEC infections including fecal cytokines such as IL-8 and IL-1R, lactoferrin, and occult blood (Steiner *et al.*, 1998, Greenberg *et al.*, 2002). Volunteer challenge studies have demonstrated heterogeneity in the ability of EAEC isolates to cause disease and several studies have been unable to make clear associations with EAEC and diarrhea. In this study, more EAEC positive samples had elevated lactoferrin and diarrhea, and the presence of EAEC in the stools was significantly associated with occult blood ($P<0.001$). Although EAEC have been associated with bloody stool samples the relationship with occult blood has not been clearly described (Durrer *et al.*, 2000). A study in Central African Republic indicated that EAEC were the most frequently identified agents in HIV positive patients with persistent diarrhea and 42.8% of the patients with EAEC as sole pathogens had bloody diarrhea (Germani *et al.*, 1998). The presence of occult blood in the stools of individuals infected with EAEC was tested in a previous study that did not find a significant association between EAEC infection and the presence of occult blood in the stools since only 4 (31.1%) of EAEC positive stool samples had occult blood, while 27 (60.0%) of EAEC positive stool samples had lactoferrin (Bouckenooghe *et al.*, 2000). Our study is thus the first that found significant association between EAEC infections and occult blood in the stool and might indicate a different pathogenic manifestation of these organisms in this part of the world.

Studies elsewhere have indicated that the best characterized *E. coli* pathotypes require multiple genes to be fully/highly virulent. For example enterotoxigenic *E. coli* (ETEC) with heat-labile toxin (LT), heat-stable toxin (ST) and colonization factor antigens (CFAs) are the most virulent; Enteropathogenic *E. coli* (EPEC) with Bundle Forming Pilus (BFP) and the *eae* gene encoding the adhesin intimin, responsible for the intimate attachment of the bacteria to the epithelial cell are most virulent; Shiga-toxin-producing *E. coli* (STEC) with Shiga-like toxin (Stx) and eaeA, encoding intimin involved in attachment of bacteria to enterocytes and plasmid are most virulent (Qadri *et al.*, 2000 ; Rappelli *et al.*, 2001 ; Scaletsky *et al.*, 2002 ; Karch *et al.*, 2006; Turner *et al.*, 2006; Medina et al., 2010). However, the presence of multiple genes has not been associated with pathogenesis in EAEC. This study has shown that strains with all the three genes were more pathogenic in terms of diarrhea production, intestinal inflammation indicated by the lactoferrin level in the stools and occult blood.

Two species of microsporidia, *Enterocytozoon bieneusi* and *Encephalitozoon* (*Septata*) *instestinalis*, are known to cause intestinal microsporidiosis. Even though *E. bieneusi* is responsible for about 90% of reported infections (Orenstein, 1994), other microsporidial species such as the Vittaforma-like species were recently described in stool samples from both HIV positive and HIV negative individuals in Portugal (Sulaiman *et al.*, 2003). In our study, only *E. bieneusi* was detected in stool samples, even though the PCR method used could detect all of the *Encephalitozoon spp.* in addition to *E. bieneusi*. Other studies have also indicated that *E. bieneusi* was the most common microsporidia infecting HIV negative as well as HIV positive individuals (Sarfati *et al.*, 2006) and that PCR based assays can be used successfully for microsporidian species differentiation from stool specimens, thus obviating the need for invasive biopsy procedures (Liguory *et al.*, 1997).

To date, the pathogenicity of Microsporidia is not clearly defined and the mechanisms by which Microsporidia induce diarrhea in HIV patients have not been determined. A wide range of pathology has been associated with Microsporidia; these include inflammation and cell death, and symptoms such as shortness of breath, sinusitis, and diarrhea with wasting (Orenstein, 2003; Stark et al., 2009). In our study we found that even though HIV positive patients infected by *E. bieneusi* had more diarrhea than those non-infected, they actually had less inflammation as compared to the non-infected HIV positive individuals as demonstrated by the lactoferrin test. This could be explained by the occurrence of multiple infections in these individuals. The high level of lactoferrin could thus be due to infections by other organisms such as *Cryptosporidium* spp, *Entamoeba histolytica*, Enteroaggregative *E. coli*, *Clostridium difficile* and *Campylobacter jejuni / coli* also found in these stool samples. Compared to previous studies we have conducted in the same region, *E. bieneusi* was more common than *Cryptosporidium spp* among HIV patients (Samie *et al.*, 2006a). However, HIV positive patients infected with *Cryptosporidium* had more diarrhea and more lactoferrin than those who were not infected, indicating that the expected outcome would be worse with *Cryptosporidium* than with *E. bieneusi* in this population. This observation is similar to those described by Bern *et al.* (2005) in Peru, where microsporidiosis did not appear to have a major impact on survival among AIDS patients compared to cryptosporidiosis, even though some genotypes of *E. bieneusi* caused chronic diarrhea in these patients.

E. bieneusi was not associated with intestinal inflammation in our study, as demonstrated by the lactoferrin test in HIV negative and HIV positive individuals even though most HIV positive individuals without microsporidia had elevated lactoferrin, indicating high level of intestinal inflammation. This could be due to the effect of HIV itself as previously demonstrated (Kotler *et al.*, 1993; Maingat et al., 2011). This is in line with some studies where multiple small intestinal biopsies showed atrophy with acute and chronic inflammation in HIV seropositive individuals even without apparent pathogens (Orenstein *et al.*, 1992; Snijders *et al.*, 1995; Idris et al 2010). It thus suggests that microsporidia might be cause of secretory diarrhea in HIV patients while most HIV negative individuals remain asymptomatic in the Vhembe district.

This study also determined the prevalence of community acquired *C. difficile* toxigenic characteristics among hospital outpatients and school children and evaluated the association between different pathologic features and the presence and toxigenic profiles of the isolates. *C. difficile* was less frequent among apparently healthy school children. The two positive samples obtained from the schools were non toxigenic as opposed to the toxigenic strains obtained from the hospital outpatients. We also identified the existence of a mutation on the *tcdC* gene associated with increased virulence of associated *C. difficile* infections and this is in harmony with a previous repport (Cloud *et al.*, 2007). The prevalence of *C. difficile* associated diarrhea among HIV patients have been demonstrated to vary according to different studies (Cappell 1993; Lu 1994). In a study of *C difficile* associated diarrhea among HIV positive patients in Illinois, USA, CDAD was observed in 32% of all study patients with diarrhea especially those with advanced HIV disease (Pulvirenti *et al.*, 2002). Other reports have suggested that clinical manifestations and response to therapy in HIV infected patients with *C. difficile* associated diarrhea (CDAD) were similar to that of patients without HIV (DeLalla 1992; Hutin 1993; Cozart 1993) while others have noted a more severe, refractory presentation in HIV infected patients (Colarian 1988; Beaugerie 1994). In our study *C. difficile* did not appear to be associated with HIV. However like other studies, our HIV population was very little (44 patients) and was not clearly characterized in terms of CD4+ counts or HIV disease state. Thus more studies are needed to confirm the role of *C. difficile* as diarrheal agent among HIV positive patients in the Vhembe district and in South Africa in general.

Toxin-A-negative, toxin-B-positive (A- B+) *Clostridium difficile* isolates were identified in several studies (Wultanska *et al.*, 2005). We found that only 3 (6.7%) of all *C. difficile* positive samples were A-B+ variants which is lower compared to those found in horses by Arroyo *et al.*, (2007) and around the same level as those described by Pituch *et al*, (2003) in Poland were about 7% of the strains isolated from CDAD patients had the variant A-B+ isolates. Recent studies have also reported on the existence of cluster of A- B+ *C. difficile*, universally resistant to the fluoroquinolones tested including ofloxacin, ciprofloxacin, levofloxacin, moxifloxacin and gatifloxacin, with MICs > 32 mg/mL, associated with a novel transversion mutation in gyrB (Drudy *et al.*, 2006). The high prevalence of A-B+ *C. difficile* strains might have a negative impact on the detection of toxigenic *C. difficile* in stool samples when the ELISA test is used. This further underscores the importance of the implementation of molecular methods in the detection and characterization of *C. difficile* in specific settings.

5. Conclusions

The quantitative real time PCR using SYBR green is a simple and fast method for the detection of different infectious organisms including bacteria and parasites. Different pre-treatment methods can be used to improve DNA purification for the detection of bacterial and parasitic organisms in stool samples for molecular epidemiological studies. These include the alkaline treatment of the stool sample, the use of the freeze and thaw and the use of glass beads prior to DNA purification by the traditional phenol chloroform method or the use of different kits such as the Qiagen. This study has demonstrated a high prevalence of microsporidia, *Cryptosporidium* infections in the Vhembe district and its implications in the production of diarrhea and inflammation. *C. hominis* was more common and related to pathogenesis than *C. parvum*. HIV positive patients did not appear to be more likely to be infected by *Cryptosporidium*. However, more studies are needed using larger number of HIV positive samples. The study of antigenic profiles of these organisms will provide insight for the development of effective vaccines.

E histolytica appears to be common in the Vhembe district of South Africa. Mixed infections were especially frequent as opposed to other areas in the world such as Japan (Ali *et al.*, 2003). *E. dispar* was less associated with diarrhea or fecal lactoferrin and occurred more often than *E. histolytica* in the general population. Fecal lactoferrin may provide a useful indicator of acute invasive *E. histolytica* infections and could be used as screening test for inflammatory diarrhea including *E. histolytica* in the Vhembe district considering its simplicity. This study also shows the susceptibility of females infected with HIV to *E. histolytica,* which is also commonly seen in males with or without HIV. The study of genetic and antigenic profiles will shed more light on the pathogenicity of this important protozoal infection and provide insight into improved control measures such as improved water and sanitation, vaccine and drug development.

We successfully used different PCR methods for the detection and identification of Enteroaggregative E. Coli, *Campylobacter*, *Helicobacter* and *Arcobacter* spp from stool samples. Of interest was the development of a fast and efficient real time PCR using SYBR GREEN for the detection of *C. concisus*. EAEC was an important etiological agent of diarrhea in the Vhembe district, South Africa as indicated by its high prevalence among hospital patients and particularly among HIV positive patients. Furthermore, EAEC may be a treatable cause of diarrhea in patients with AIDS (Wanke *et al.*, 1998b). Toxigenic *C. difficile* was associated with pathologic conditions among the patients. Typical preventive measures against infections by these organisms include careful personal hygiene, especially promotion of hand washing through health education programs. Major therapeutic intervention for all individuals with diarrhea consists of fluid and electrolyte therapy. However, when antimicrobial therapy is appropriate, selection of a specific agent should be made based upon susceptibility patterns of the pathogen or information on local susceptibility patterns.

Quantitative real time PCR showed that a certain threshold, related to the number of cells, was needed for the EAEC to cause pathologic symptoms such as diarrhea and inflammation. HIV positive individuals are at a higher risk of infection by EAEC and had higher level of lactoferrin when compared to HIV negative individuals. This is the first study to significantly associate EAEC with the presence of occult blood in the stools which might be due to pathogenic factors such as the plasmid encoded toxin (Pet) which is highly homologous to the EspP protease of EHEC and to EspC of EPEC as well as the protein involved in colonization (Pic) .

The current study has demonstrated that *E. bieneusi* is the most common microsporidian species occurring in the Vhembe district particularly among HIV positive patients and *E. bieneusi* is a cause of secretory diarrhea among HIV positive individuals as opposed to inflammatory diarrhea. This study has demonstrated that the pathogenicity of Enteroaggregative *E. coli* could be directly related to the genetic profile of the infecting strains. This is important in the understanding of the pathogenicity of these organisms with possible effect on the development of control methods including diagnostics, drug target molecules (genes) and vaccination procedures. This study also associated EAEC infections with occult blood which might indicate a possible relation/link between the pathogenicity of this organism and that of Enterohemorrhagic *E. coli* (EHEC) often involved in hemolytic uremic syndrome (HUS) and bloody diarrhea.

The pathogenicity index determines the importance of the infecting agent as a pathogen in a specific community. The pathogenicity index indicated that *E. histolytica, Cryptosporidium hominis, C. jejuni/coli, C. concisus, Clostridium difficile* and Enteroaggregative *E. coli* were the most diarrheagenic organisms in the Vhembe population while *E. histolytica, C. jejuni/coli, C. concisus, Clostridium difficile* were the most inflammatory. Enteroaggregative *E. coli* was the most associated with occult blood followed by *E. histolytica, C. jejuni/coli,* and *Clostridium difficile*. This further indicates the importance of the lactoferrin and occult tests as screening methods for diarrheal organisms in hospitals and will probably reduce the cost of infectious diarrheal diagnosis and improve the quality of service. HIV positive patients are more susceptible to infections, therefore, the implementation of molecular methodologies is recommended for an improved diagnosis of gastrointestinal infections among these patients and the quality of their lives. Diarrheal diseases can be prevented through access to clean, safe drinking water and through proper sanitation measures, including hand washing and safe disposal of human waste. Thus increased health education in schools as well as in the communities is highly recommended and could help prevent the transmission of diarrheal diseases in the population. Proper management and treatment of waste and waste water is recommended through increased investments in water and sanitation systems at least in fast growing areas. Such strategies could alleviate a great deal of unnecessary suffering and loss of productivity; reduce the number of lives lost to these diseases, and result in significant savings in health care costs.

6. Acknowledgements

The present study was supported in part by the Pfizer and Ellison foundations through the Centre for Global Health of the University of Virginia, The National research foundation of South Africa, The International Society for Infectious diseases and the United Nations educational, scientific and cultural organization (UNESCO) and the University of Venda. Samples were collected thanks to the collaboration of primary schools' staff and the Hospitals' staff. Authorization was obtained from the Department of Health in Limpopo, South Africa.

7. References

Abd-Alla MD, and Ravdin JI (2002). Diagnosis of amebic colitis by antigen capture ELISA in patients presenting with acute amebic diarrhea in Cairo Egypt. *Tropical Medicine and International Health,* 7, 365--370.

Abd-Alla MD, Jackson TG and Ravdin JI (1998). Serum IgM antibody response to the galactose-inhibitable adherence lectin of *E. histolytica. American Journal of Tropical Medicine and Hygiene,* 59, 431-434.

Abdel-Messih IA, Wierzba TF, Abu-Elyazeed R, Ibrahim AF, Ahmed SF, Kamal K, Sanders J, French R (2005). Diarrhea associated with *Cryptosporidium parvum* among young children of the Nile River Delta in Egypt. *Journal of Tropical Pediatrics* 51, 154–159.

Alcantara CS, Yang CH, Steiner TS, Barret LJ, Lima AA, Chappell CL, Okhuysen PC, White JrAC, Guerrant RL (2003). Interleukin- 8, tumor necrosis factor alpha, and lactoferrin in immunocompetent hosts with experimental and Brazilian children with acquired cryptosporidiosis. *American Journal of Tropical Medicine and Hygiene,* 68, 325–328.

Al-Hindi A, Shubair ME, Marshall I, Ashford RW, Sharif FA, Abed AA, Kamel EG (2005). *Entamoeba histolytica* or *Entamoeba dispar* among children in Gaza, Gaza Strip? *Journal of the Egyptian Society of Parasitology,* 35(1), 59--68.

Ali IK, Hossain MB, Roy S, Ayeh-Kumi PF, Petri WA Jr, Haque R, Clark CG (2003). *Entamoeba moshkovskii* infections in children in Bangladesh. *Emerg Infect Dis* 9:580--584.

Al-Mekhlafi HM, Mahdy MA, 'azlin MY, Fatmah MS, Norhayati M (2011). Childhood *Cryptosporidium* infection among aboriginal communities in Peninsular Malaysia. Annals of Tropical Medicine and Parasitology, 105(2):135-43.

Aly SM, El-Zawawy LA, Said DE, Fathy FM, Mohamed On (2005). The utility of lactoferrin in differentiating parasitic from bacterial infections. *Journal of the Egyptian Society of Parasitology,* 35(3 Suppl):1149--1162.

Antonios SN, Tolba OA, Othman AA, Saad MA (2010). A preliminary study on the prevalence of parasitic infections in immunocompromised children. *Journal of the Egyptian Society of Parasitology,* 40(3), 617-30.

Arroyo LG, Staempfli H, Weese JS (2007). Molecular analysis of *Clostridium difficile* isolates recovered from horses with diarrhea. *Veterinary Microbiology,* 120, 179-83.

Banerjee B, Hazra S and Bandyopadhyay D (2004). Diarrhea Management Among Under Fives. *Indian Pediatrics* 41: 255 --260.

Barwick RS, Uzicanin A, Lareau S, Malakmadze N, Imnadze P, Iosava M, Ninashvili N, Wilson M, Hightower AW, Johnston S, Bishop H, Petri WA Jr, Juranek DD (2002). Outbreak of amebiasis in Tbilisi, Republic of Georgia, 1998. *American Journal of Tropical Medicine and Hygiene* , 67(6), 623--631.

Beatty GW (2010). Diarrhea in patients infected with HIV presenting to the emergency department. Emergency Medicine Clinics of North America, 28(2), 299-310.

Beaugerie L, Ngo Y, Goujard F, Gharakhanian S, Carbonnel F, Luboinski J, Malafosse M, Rozenbaum W, Le Quintrec Y (1994). Etiology and management of toxic megacolon in patients with human immuno deficiency virus infection. *Gastroenterology,* 107, 858-63.

Bern C, Kawai V, Vargas D, Rabke-Verani J, Williamson J, Chavez-Valdez R, Xiao L, Sulaiman I, Vivar A, Ticona E, Navincopa M, Cama V, Moura H, Secor WE, Visvesvara G, Gilman RH (2005). The epidemiology of intestinal microsporidiosis in patients with HIV/AIDS in Lima, Peru. *Journal of Infectious Diseases,* 191, 1658-64.

Bern C, Ortega Y, Checkley W, Roberts JM, Lescano AG, Cabrera L, Verastegui M, Black RE, Sterling C, Gilman RH (2002). Epidemiologic differences between cyclosporiasis and cryptosporidiosis in Peruvian children. *Emerging Infectious Diseases,* 8, 581–585.

Bialek R, Binder N, Dietz K, Joachim A, Knobloch J, Zelck UE (2002). Comparison of fluorescence, antigen and PCR assays to detect *Cryptosporidium parvum* in fecal specimens. Diagnostic Microbiology and Infectious Diseases, 43(4), 283-8.

Bouckenooghe AR, DuPont HL, Jiang ZD, Adachi J, Mathewson JJ, Verenkar MP, Rodrigues S, Steffen R (2000). Markers of enteric inflammation in enteroaggregative *Escherichia coli* diarrhea in travellers. *American Journal of Tropical Medicine and Hygiene,* 62, 711–713.

Bradshaw D, Nannan N, Groenewald P, Joubert J, Laubscher R, Nojilana B, Norman R, Pieterse D and Schneider M (2005). Provincial mortality in South Africa, 2000: priority-setting for now and a benchmark for the future. *South African Medical Journal,* 95 (7), 496-503.

Bushen OY, Davenport JA, Lima AB, Piscitelli SC, Uzgiris AJ, Silva TM, Leite R, Kosek M, Dillingham RA, Girao A, Lima AA, Guerrant RL (2004). Diarrhea and reduced levels of antiretroviral drugs: improvement with glutamine or alanyl-glutamine in a randomized controlled trial in northeast Brazil. *Clinical Infectious Diseases,* 38(12), 1764-70.

Butzler JP (2004). *Campylobacter,* from obscurity to celebrity. *Clin Microbiol Infect* 2004; 10:868-76.

Calderaro A, Gorrini C, Bommezzadri S, Piccolo G, Dettori G, and Chezzi C (2005). *Entamoeba histolytica* and *Entamoeba dispar*: comparison of two PCR assays for diagnosis in a non-endemic setting. *Transactions of the Royal Society of Tropical Medicine and Hygiene,* 100(5), 450--457.

Callendar GR (1933). The differential pathology of dysentery. *American Journal of Tropical Medicine and Hygiene* , 14, 207 - 233.

Cappell MS, Philogene C (1993). *Clostridium difficile* infection is a treatable cause of diarrhea in patients with advanced human immunodeficiency virus infection: a study of seven consecutive patients admitted from 1986 to 1992 to a university teaching hospital. *American Journal of Gastroenterology,* 88, 891-7.

Cerna JF, Nataro JP, Estrada-Garcia T (2003). Multiplex PCR for detection of three plasmid-borne genes of enteroaggregative *Escherichia coli* strains. *Journal of Clinical Microbiology,* 41, 2138-2140.

Chappell CL, Okhuysen PC, Sterling CR, DuPont HL (1996). *Cryptosporidium parvum*: intensity of infection and oocyst excretion patterns in healthy volunteers. *Journal of Infectious Diseases,* 173(1), 232-6.

Checkley W, Epstein LD, Gilman RH, Black RE, Cabrera L, Sterling CR (1998). Effects of *Cryptosporidium parvum* infection in Peruvian children: growth faltering and subsequent catch-up growth. *American Journal of Epidemiology,* 148, 497–506.

Choi SW, Park CH, Silva TM, Zaenker EI, Guerrant RL (1996). To culture or not to culture: fecal lactoferrin screening for inflammatory bacterial diarrhea. *Journal of Clinical Microbiology,* 34(4), 928-32.

Cleary RK (1998). *Clostridium difficile*-associated diarrhea and colitis: Clinical manifestations, diagnosis, and treatment. Diseases of the Colon & Rectum, 41, 1435–49.

Cloud J, Kelly CP (2007). Update on *Clostridium difficile* associated disease. *Curr Opin Gastroenterol* 23:4-9.

Colarian J (1988). *Clostridium difficile* colitis following antiviral therapy in the acquired immunodeficiency syndrome. *Am J Med* 84: 1081.

Cozart JC, Kalangi SS, Clench MH, Taylor DR, Borucki MJ, Pollard RB, Soloway RD (1994). *Clostridium difficile* diarrhea in patients with AIDS versus non-AIDS controls. Methods of treatment and clinical response to treatment. *J Clin Gastroenterol* 16:192-4.

Crump JA, Ramadhani HO, Morrissey AB, Msuya LJ, Yang LY, Chow SC, Morpeth SC, Reyburn H, Njau BN, Shaw AV, Diefenthal HC, Bartlett JA, Shao JF, Schimana W, Cunningham CK, Kinabo GD. Invasive bacterial and fungal infections among hospitalized HIV-infected and HIV-uninfected children and infants in northern Tanzania. Trop Med Int Health. 2011 Apr 7. doi: 10.1111/j.1365-3156.2011.02774.x.

Crushell E, Harty S, Sharif F, Bourke B (2004). Enteric *Campylobacter*: Purging Its Secrets? *Pediatr Res* 55: 3-12.

de Lalla F, Nicolin R, Rinaldi E, Scarpellini P, Rigoli R, Manfrin V, Tramarin A (1992). Prospective study of oral teicoplanin versus oral vancomycin for therapy of pseudomembranous colitis and *Clostridium difficile*-associated diarrhea. Antimicrobial Agents and Chemotherapy, 36, 2192-6.

de Oliveira-Silva MB, de Oliveira LR, Resende JC, Peghini BC, Ramirez LE, Lages-Silva E, Correia D (2007). Seasonal profile and level of CD4+ lymphocytes in the occurrence of cryptosporidiosis and cysto-isosporidiosis in HIV/AIDS patients in the Triângulo Mineiro region, Brazil. *Revista da Sociedade Brasileira de Medicina Tropical.* 40(5):512-5.

de Truchis P, de Truchis A (2007). Acute infectious diarrhea]. *Presse Medicale,* 36(4 Pt 2), 695-705.

Department of Health (DOH) (2006). National HIV and syphilis antenatal seroprevalence survey in South Africa: 2005.

Department of Health, "National HIV and Syphilis Antenatal Sero-prevalence Survey in South Africa 2000.

Department of Health, 2010. National Antenatal Sentinel HIV and Syphilis. Prevalence Survey in South Africa, 2009.

Desportes I, Le Charpentier Y, Galian A, Bernard F, Cochand-Priollet B, Lavergne A, Ravisse P, Modigliani R (1985). Occurrence of a new microsporidan: Enterocytozoon bieneusi n.g., n. sp., in the enterocytes of a human patient with AIDS. *Journal of Protozoology*, 32(2), 250-4.

Diamond LS and Clark CG (1993). A redescription of *Entamoeba histolytica* Schaudinn, 1903 (emended Walker, 1911) separating it from *Entamoeba dispar* Brumpt, 1925, Journal of Eukaryotic Microbiology, 40, 340-344.

Dillingham R, Guerrant RL (2004). Childhood stunting: measuring and stemming the staggering costs of inadequate water and sanitation. *Lancet*, 363(9403), 94-5.

Drudy D, Quinn T, O'Mahony R, Kyne L, O'Gaora P, Fanning S (2006). High-level resistance to moxifloxacin and gatifloxacin associated with a novel mutation in gyrB in toxin-A-negative, toxin-B-positive *Clostridium difficile*. *Journal of Antimicrobial Chemotherapy*, 58, 1264-7.

DuPont HL (1997). Guidelines on acute infectious diarrhea in adults. The Practice Parameters Committee of the American College of Gastroenterology. *American Journal of Gastroenterology*, 92(11), 1962-75.

Durrer P, Zbinden R, Fleisch F, Altwegg M, Ledergerber B, Karch H, Weber R (2000). Intestinal infection due to enteroaggregative *Escherichia coli* among human immunodeficiency virus-infected persons. *J Infect Dis* 182:1540-1544.

el-Naggar SM, el-Bahy MM, Abd Elaziz J, el-Dardiry MA (2006). Detection of protozoal parasites in the stools of diarrhoeic patients using different techniques. *Journal of the Egyptian Society of Parasitology*, 36(2), 487-516.

Fedorko DP, Nelson NA, Cartwright CP (1995). Identification of microsporidia in stool specimens by using PCR and restriction endonucleases. *Journal of Clinical Microbiology*, 33, 1739–1741.

Fernández-Cruz A, Muñoz P, Mohedano R, Valerio M, Marín M, Alcalá L, Rodriguez-Créixems M, Cercenado E, Bouza E. *Campylobacter* bacteremia: clinical characteristics, incidence, and outcome over 23 years. *Medicine (Baltimore)*. 2010, 89(5):319-30.

Fincham JE, Jackson TFHG, Schoeman S, Evans AC, Markus MB, Mwamba JC. Intestinal parasites in children: the need for community-based interventions. Tygerberg: Medical Research Council, 1997:1-2. (MRC policy brief no. 3).

Gassama A, Thiaw B, Dia NM, Fall F, Camara P, Hovette P, Perret JL, Gueye - Ndiaye A, Mboup S, Sow PS, Aidara-Kane A, (2001). [Infective etiology of diarrhea in adults with HIV infection in Dakar: a case-control study on 594 patients]. *Dakar Medical* 46:46-50.

Gathiram V, Jackson TF (1985). Frequency distribution of *Entamoeba histolytica* zymodemes in a rural South African population. *Lancet* 30 (8431):719--721. 35.

Germani Y, Minssart P, Vohito M, Yassibanda S, Glaziou P, Hocquet D, Berthelemy P, Morvan J, (1998). Etiologies of acute, persistent, and dysenteric diarrheas in adults in Bangui, Central African Republic, in relation to human immunodeficiency virus serostatus. *Am J Trop Med Hyg* 59:1008-1014.

Goodgame RW, Genta RM, White AC, Chappell CL (1993). Intensity of infection in AIDS-associated cryptosporidiosis. Journal of Infectious Diseases, 167(3), 704-9.

Goodman L, Segreti J (1999). Infectious diarrhea. Dis Mon. 1999 Jul; 45(7):268-99.

Greenberg DE, Jiang ZD, Steffen R, Verenker MP, DuPont HL, (2002). Markers of inflammation in bacterial diarrhea among travelers, with a focus on enteroaggregative *Escherichia coli* pathogenicity. *Journal of Infectious Diseases, 185, 944–949.*

Greenwood BM. Greenwood AM. Bradley AK. Tulloch S. Hayes R. Oldfield FS. Deaths in infancy and early childhood in a well-vaccinated, rural, West African population. *Ann Trop Paediatr.* 1987;7:91–9.

Guerrant RL, Brush J, Ravdin JI, Sullivan JA, Mandell GL (1981). Interaction between *Entamoeba histolytica* and human polymorphonuclear neutrophils. *J Infect Dis* 143(1):83--93.

Guerrant RL, Oria R, Bushen OY, Patrick PD, Houpt E, Lima AA (2005). Global impact of diarrheal diseases that are sampled by travelers: the rest of the hippopotamus. *Clin Infect Dis* 1; 41 Suppl 8:S524-30.

Guerrant RL, Van Gilder T, Steiner TS, Thielman NM, Slutsker L, Tauxe RV, Hennessy T, Griffin PM, DuPont H, Sack RB, Tarr P, Neill M, Nachamkin I, Reller LB, Osterholm MT, Bennish ML, Pickering LK; Infectious Diseases Society of America (2001). Practice guidelines for the management of infectious diarrhea. *Clinical Infectious Diseases,* 32(3), 331-51.

Haghighi A, Kobayashi S, Takeuchi T, Thammapalerd N, Nozaki T (2003). Geographic diversity among genotypes of *Entamoeba histolytica* field isolates. *Journal of Clinical Microbiology,* 41, 3748-56.

Haque R, Ali IKM, Akther S, Petri JrWA (1998). Comparison of PCR, isoenzyme analysis, and antigen detection for diagnosis of *Entamoeba histolytica* infection. *Journal of Clinical Microbiology,* 36, 449–452.

Herikstad H, Yang S, Van Gilder TJ, Vugia D, Hadler J, Blake P, Deneen V, Shiferaw B, Angulo FJ (2002). A population-based estimate of the burden of diarrhoeal illness in the United States: FoodNet, 1996-7. Epidemiology and Infection, 129(1), 9-17.

Hou Y, Mortimer L, Chadee K (2010). Entamoeba histolytica cysteine proteinase 5 binds integrin on colonic cells and stimulates NFkappaB-mediated pro-inflammatory responses. *Journal of Biological Chemistry,* 285(46), 35497-504.

Houf K, Tutenel A, De Zutter L, Van Hoof J, Vandamme P (2000). Development of a multiplex PCR assay for the simultaneous detection and identification of *Arcobacter butzleri, Arcobacter cryaerophilus* and *Arcobacter skirrowii. FEMS Microbiol Lett* 193:89-94.

Houpt E, Bushen OY, Sa NE, Kohli A, Asgharpour A, Ng CT, Calfee DP, Guerrant RL, Maro V, Ole-Nguvaine S, Shao JF (2005). Short report: asymptomatic *Cryptosporidium hominis* infection among human immunodeficiency virus-infected patients in Tanzania. *American Journal of Tropical Medicine and Hygiene,* 73, 520–522.

Huang DB, Jiang ZD, Dupont HL (2003). Association of virulence factor-positive and -negative enteroaggregative Escherichia coli and occurrence of clinical illness in travelers from the United States to Mexico. *American Journal of Tropical Medicine and Hygiene,* 69(5), 506-8.

Humphreys EH, Smith NA, Azman H, McLeod D, Rutherford GW. Prevention of diarrhoea in children with HIV infection or exposure to maternal HIV infection. *Cochrane Database of Systematic Reviews*, 16(6), CD008563.

Hung CC, Deng HY, Hsiao WH, Hsieh SM, Hsiao CF, Chen MY, Chang SC, Su KE (2005). Invasive amebiasis as an emerging parasitic disease in patients with human immunodeficiency virus type 1 infection in Taiwan. *Archives of Internal Medicine,* 165, 409-15.

Hutin Y, Molina JM, Casin I, Daix V, Sednaoui P, Welker Y, Lagrange P, Decazes JM, Modai J (1993). Risk factors for *Clostridium difficile*-associated Diarrhea in HIV-infected patients. *AIDS* 7, 1441-7.

Idris NS, Dwipoerwantoro PG, Kurniawan A, Said M. Intestinal parasitic infection of immunocompromised children with diarrhoea: clinical profile and therapeutic response. *The Journal of Infection in Developing Countries,* 4(5), 309-17.

Javier-Enriquez F, Avila CR, Ignacio-Santos J, Tanaka-Kido J, Vallejo O, Sterling CR (1997). *Cryptosporidium* infections in Mexican children: clinical, nutritional, enteropathogenic, and diagnostic evaluations. *American Journal of Tropical Medicine and Hygiene,* 56, 254–257.

Jenkins C, Chart H, Willshaw GA, Cheasty T, Smith HR, (2006). Genotyping of enteroaggregative *Escherichia coli* and identification of target genes for the detection of both typical and atypical strains. *Diagnostic Microbiology and Infectious Disease, 55*(1), 13-19.

Jiang ZD, DuPont HL, La Rocco M, Garey KW (2010). In vitro susceptibility of *Clostridium difficile* to rifaximin and rifampin in 359 consecutive isolates at a university hospital in Houston, Texas. *Journal of Clinical Pathology,* 63(4), 355-8.

Kalischuk LD, Buret AG. A role for *Campylobacter jejuni*-induced enteritis in inflammatory bowel disease? *The American Journal of Physiology: Gastrointestinal and Liver Physiology*, 298(1), G1-9.

Kar S, Gawlowska S, Daugschies A, Bangoura B (2011). Quantitative comparison of different purification and detection methods for *Cryptosporidium parvum* oocysts. *Veterinary Parasitology,* 177(3-4), 366-70.

Karch H, Friedrich AW, Gerber A, Zimmerhackl LB, Schmidt MA, Bielaszewska M, (2006). New aspects in the pathogenesis of enteropathic hemolytic uremic syndrome. *Seminars in Thrombosis and Hemostasis,* 32, 105-12.

Karlström O, Fryklund B, Tullus K, Burman LG (1998). A prospective nationwide study of *Clostridium difficile*-associated diarrhea in Sweden. The Swedish *C. difficile* Study Group. *Clinical Infectious Diseases,* 26,141-5.

Kassi RR, Kouassi RA, Yavo W, Barro-Kiki CP, Bamba A, Menan HI, Kone M (2004). Cryptosporidiosis and isosporiasis in children suffering from diarrhoea in Abidjan]. Bull Soc Pathol Exot. 97(4):280-2.

Katsumata T, Hosea D, Ranuh IG, Uga S, Yanagi T, Kohno S (2000). Short report: possible *Cryptosporidium muris* infection in humans. *American Journal of Tropical Medicine and Hygiene,* 62, 70–72.

Kebede A, Verweij JJ, Endeshaw T, Messele T, Tasew G, Petros B, Polderman AM (2004). The use of real-time PCR to identify *Entamoeba histolytica* and *E. dispar* infections in prisoners and primary-school children in Ethiopia. *Annals of Tropical Medicine and Parasitology,* 98(1), 43--48.

Kelly P, Hicks S, Oloya J, Mwansa J, Sikakwa L, Zulu I, Phillips A (2003). Escherichia coli enterovirulent phenotypes in Zambians with AIDS-related diarrhoea. *Transactions of the Royal Society of Tropical Medicine and Hygiene,* 97(5), 573-6.

Kelly P, Hicks S, Oloya J, Mwansa J, Sikakwa L, Zulu I, Phillips A, (2003). *Escherichia coli* enterovirulent phenotypes in Zambians with AIDS-related Diarrhea. *Transactions of the Royal Society of Tropical Medicine and Hygiene,* 97, 573-6.

Kfir R, Hilner C, du Preez M, Bateman B (1995). Studies on the prevalence of giardia cysts and *Cryptosporidium* oocysts in South African water. *Water Science and Technology,* 31, 435–438.

Kirkpatrick BD, Daniels MM, Jean SS, Pape JW, Karp C, Littenberg B, Fitzgerald DW, Lederman HM, Nataro JP, Sears CL (2002). Cryptosporidiosis stimulates an inflammatory intestinal response in malnourished Haitian children. *J Infect Dis* 186, 94–101.

Kirkwood BR. *In: Feachem RG, Jamison DT, editors. Disease and mortality in sub-Saharan Africa.* New York, NY: Oxford University Press; 1991. Diarrhoea; pp. 134–57.

Kotler DP, Reka S, Chow K, Orenstein JM (1993). Effects of enteric parasitoses and HIV infection upon small intestinal structure and function in patients with AIDS. *Journal of Clinical Gastroenterology,* 16, 10-5.

Kuijper EJ, Coignard B, Tull P; the ESCMID Study Group for *Clostridium difficile* (ESGCD)* (2006). EU Member States and the European Centre for Disease Prevention and Control (ECDC) Emergence of *Clostridium difficile*-associated disease in North America and Europe. *Clinical Microbiology and Infections,* 6, 2-18.

Kurniawan A, Karyadi T, Dwintasari SW, Sari IP, Yunihastuti E, Djauzi S, Smith HV (2009) Intestinal parasitic infections in HIV/AIDS patients presenting with diarrhoea in Jakarta, Indonesia. *Transactions of the Royal Society of Tropical Medicine and Hygiene,* doi: 10.1016/j.trstmh.2009.02.017.

Larsen IK, Gradel KO, Helms M, Hornstrup MK, Jürgens G, Mens H, Rosager CL, Clausen TH, Kronborg G, Nielsen H (2011). Non-typhoidal *Salmonella* and *Campylobacter* infections among HIV-positive patients in Denmark. Scand J Infect Dis. 43(1):3-7.

Lashley FR (2006). Emerging infectious diseases at the beginning of the 21st century. Online J Issues Nurs. 31;11(1):2.

Lastovica AJ, Le Roux E (2000). Efficient isolation of campylobacteria from stools. *Journal of Clinical Microbiology,* 38, 2798–9.

Lastovica AJ, Skirrow MB (2000). Clinical significance of *Campylobacter* and related species other than *C. jejuni* and *C. coli,* p 89-120. *In* I. Nachamkin and M. J. Blaser (ed.), *Campylobacter,* 2nd ed. American Society for Microbiology, Washington, D.C. 2000.

Lebbad M, Svard SG (2005). PCR differentiation of *Entamoeba histolytica* and *Entamoeba dispar* from patients with amoeba infection initially diagnosed by microscopy. *Scandinavian Journal of Infectious Diseases,* 37(9), 680-685.

Lee JK, Song HJ, Yu JR (2005). Prevalence of diarrhea caused by *Cryptosporidium parvum* in non-HIV patients in Jeollanam-do, Korea. *Korean Journal of Parasitology,* 43, 111–114.

Lemee L, Dhalluin A, Testelin S, Mattrat MA, Maillard K, Lemeland JF, Pons JL (2004). Multiplex PCR targeting tpi (triose phosphate isomerase), tcdA (Toxin A), and tcdB (Toxin B) genes for toxigenic culture of *Clostridium difficile. Journal of Clinical Microbiology,* 42, 5710-4.

Liguory O, David F, Sarfati C, Schuitema AR, Hartskeerl RA, Derouin F, Modai J, Molina JM (1997). Diagnosis of infections caused by *Enterocytozoon bieneusi* and *Encephalitozoon intestinalis* using polymerase chain reaction in stool specimens. *AIDS*. 11, 723-726.

Limor JR, Lal AA, Xiao L (2002). Detection and differentiation of *Cryptosporidium* parasites that are pathogenic for humans by real-time PCR. *Journal of Clinical Microbiology,* 40(7), 2335-8.

Linton D, Lawson AJ, Owen RJ, Stanley J (1997). PCR detection, identification to species level, and fingerprinting of *Campylobacter jejuni* and *Campylobacter coli* direct from diarrheic samples. *Journal of Clinical Microbiology,* 35, 2568–2572.

Lu SS, Schwartz JM, Simon DM, Brandt LJ (1994). *Clostridium difficile*-associated diarrhea in patients with HIV positivity and AIDS: a prospective controlled study. *Americal Journal of Gastroenterology,* 89, 1226-9.

Maingat F, Halloran B, Acharjee S, van Marle G, Church D, Gill MJ, Uwiera RR, Cohen EA, Meddings J, Madsen K, Power C. Inflammation and epithelial cell injury in AIDS enteropathy: involvement of endoplasmic reticulum stress. FASEB Journal, 2011 Mar 22.

Mandomando IM, Macete EV, Ruiz J, Sanz S, Abacassamo F, Vallès X, Sacarlal J, Navia MM, Vila J, Alonso PL, Gascon J (2007). Etiology of diarrhea in children younger than 5 years of age admitted in a rural hospital of southern Mozambique. *American Journal of Tropical Medicine and Hygiene,* 76(3), 522-7.

Marshall SM, Melito PL, Woodward DL, Johnson WM, Rodgers FG, Mulvey MR (1999). Rapid identification of *Campylobacter, Arcobacter,* and *Helicobacter* isolates by PCR-restriction fragment length polymorphism analysis of the 16S rRNA gene. *J Clin Microbiol* 37:4158-60.

Matsheka MI, Lastovica AJ, Elisha BG (2001). Molecular identification of *Campylobacter concisus. Journal of Clinical Microbiology,* 39, 3684-9.

Medina AM, Rivera FP, Romero LM, Kolevic LA, Castillo ME, Verne E, Hernandez R, Mayor YE, Barletta F, Mercado E, Ochoa TJ. Diarrheagenic Escherichia coli in human immunodeficiency virus (HIV) pediatric patients in Lima, Peru. *American Journal of Tropical Medicine and Hygiene,* 83(1), 158-63.

Mercado EH, Ochoa TJ, Ecker L, Cabello M, Durand D, Barletta F, Molina M, Gil AI, Huicho L, Lanata CF, Cleary TG (2011). Fecal Leukocytes in Children Infected with Diarrheagenic Escherichia coli. *Journal of Clinical Microbiology,* 49(4), 1376-81.

Moodley D, Jackson TFHG, Gathiram V, van den Ende J (1991). *Cryptosporidium* infections in children in Durban. *South African Medical Journal,* 79, 295–297.

Moran AP (2010). The role of endotoxin in infection: Helicobacter pylori and *Campylobacter* jejuni. *Subcellular Biochemistry,* 53, 209-40.

Moran P, Ramos F, Ramiro M, Curiel O, Gonzalez E, Valadez A, Gomez A, Garcia G, Melendro EI, Ximenez C (2005). *Entamoeba histolytica* and/or *Entamoeba dispar*: infection frequency in HIV+/AIDS patients in Mexico city. *Experimental Parasitology,* 110, 331-4.

Moyo SJ, Gro N, Matee MI, Kitundu J, Myrmel H, Mylvaganam H, Maselle SY, Langeland N (2011). Age specific aetiological agents of diarrhoea in hospitalized children aged less than five years in Dar es Salaam, Tanzania. BMC Pediatrics, 23; 11:19.

Nagamani K, Pavuluri PR, Gyaneshwari M, Prasanthi K, Rao MI, Saxena NK (2007). Molecular characterisation of *Cryptosporidium*: an emerging parasite. *Indian Journal of Medical Microbiology*, 25(2),133-6.

Nataro JP, Mai V, Johnson J, Blackwelder WC, Heimer R, Tirrell S, Edberg SC, Braden CR, Glenn Morris J Jr, Hirshon JM, (2006). Diarrheagenic *Escherichia coli* infection in Baltimore, Maryland, and New Haven, Connecticut. *Clinical Infectious Diseases*, 43, 402-407.

Nel ED, Rabie H, Goodway J, Cotton MF. A Retrospecive Study of Cryptosporidial Diarrhea in a Region with High HIV Prevalence. Journal of Tropical Pediatrics, 2010 Oct 14.

Nesbitt RA, Mosha FW, Katki HA, Ashraf M, Assenga C, Lee CM (2004). Amebiasis and comparison of microscopy to ELISA technique in detection of *Entamoeba histolytica* and Entamoeba dispar. *Journal of the National Medical Association*, 96(5), 671--677.

Newman RD, Sears CL, Moore SR, Nataro JP, Wuhib T, Agnew DA, Guerrant RL, Lima AAM (1999). Longitudinal study of *Cryptosporidium* infection in children in Northeastern Brazil. *Journal of Infectious Diseases*, 18 (1), 167–175.

Nguyen AM, Engstrand L, Genta RM, Graham DY, El-Zaatari FA (1993). Detection of *Helicobacter pylori* in dental plaque by reverse transcription polymerase chain reaction. *Journal of Clinical Microbiology*, 3 1, 783-787.

Nurtaev KhS, Badalova NS, Zalialieva MV, Osipova SO (2005). [Intestinal parasitic diseases in HIV-infected patients in Uzbekistan]. *Med parazitol parazit bol* 3, 45-9.

Obi CL, Bessong PO (2002). Diarrheagenic bacterial pathogens in HIV-positive patients with Diarrhea in rural communities of Limpopo province, South Africa. *Journal of Health Population and Nutrition*, 20, 230–234.

Obi CL, Green E, Bessong PO, de Villiers B, Hoosen AA, Igumbor EO and Potgieter N, (2004). Gene encoding virulence markers among *Escherichia coli* isolates from diarrhoeic stool samples and river sources in rural Venda communities of South Africa. *Water SA* 30: 515-519.

Obi CL, Momba MNB, Samie A, Igumbor JO, Green E and Musie E (2007). Microbiological, physico-chemical and management parameters impinging on the efficiency of small water treatment plants in the Limpopo and Mpumalanga Provinces of South Africa Water SA Vol. 33 No. 2 :229 - 237.

Okamoto M, Kawabe T, Ohata K, Togo G, Hada T, Katamoto T, Tanno M, Matsumura M, Yamaji Y, Watabe H, Ikenoue T, Yoshida H, Omata M (2005). Amebic colitis in asymptomatic subjects with positive fecal occult blood test results: clinical features different from symptomatic cases. *American Journal of Tropical Medicine and Hygiene*, 73(5),934--935.

Olivier BJ, Bond RP, van Zyl WB, Delport M, Slavik T, Ziady C, Terhaar sive Droste JS, Lastovica A, van der Merwe SW (2006). Absence of *Helicobacter pylori* within the Oral Cavities of Members of a Healthy South African Community. *J Clin Microbiol* 44: 635–636.

Opintan JA, Newman MJ, Ayeh-Kumi PF, Affrim R, Gepi-Attee R, Sevilleja JE, Roche JK, Nataro JP, Warren CA, Guerrant RL (2010). Pediatric diarrhea in southern Ghana:

etiology and association with intestinal inflammation and malnutrition. *American Journal of Tropical Medicine and Hygiene,* 83(4), 936-43.

Orenstein JM (2003). Diagnostic pathology of microsporidiosis. *Ultrastruct Pathol* 27, 141-9.

Orenstein JM, Benator D, Kotler DP (1994). Microsporidia and HIV-related diarrhea. *Ann Intern Med* 120, 973-4.

Orenstein JM, Tenner M, Cali A, Kotler DP (1992). A microsporidian previously undescribed in humans, infecting enterocytes and macrophages, and associated with diarrhea in an acquired immunodeficiency syndrome patient. *Hum Pathol* 23, 722-8.

Pituch H, Obuch-Woszczatynski P, Luczak M, Meisel-Mikolajczyk F (2003). *Clostridium difficile* and enterotoxigenic *Bacteroides fragilis* strains isolated from patients with antibiotic associated Diarrhea. *Anaerobe* 9:161-3.

Potgieter N, Obi CL, Bessong PO, Igumbor EO, Samie A, Nengobela R (2005). Bacterial contamination of Vhuswa–a local weaning food and stored drinking-water in impoverished households in the Vhembe district of South Africa. Journal of Health, Population, and Nutrition, 23, 150–155.

Pulvirenti JJ, Mehra T, Hafiz I, DeMarais P, Marsh D, Kocka F, Meyer PM, Fischer SA, Goodman L, Gerding DN, Weinstein RA (2002). Epidemiology and outcome of *Clostridium difficile* infection and diarrhea in HIV infected inpatients. *Diagnostic Microbiology and Infectious Disease,* 44, 325-30.

Qadri F, Das SK, Faruque AS, Fuchs GJ, Albert MJ, Sack RB and Svennerholm AM, (2000). Prevalence of toxin types and colonization factors in enterotoxigenic *Escherichia coli* isolated during a 2-year period from Diarrheal patients in Bangladesh. *Journal of Clinical Microbiology,* 38, 27–31.

Quinn TC, Stamm WE, Goodell SE, Mkrtichian E, Benedetti J, Corey L, Schuffler MD, Holmes KK (1983). The polymicrobial origin of intestinal infections in homosexual men. N Engl J Med. 309(10):576-82.

Ramos F, Moran P, Gonzalez F, Garcia G, Ramiro M, Gomez A de Leon Mdel C, Melendro EI, Valadez A, Ximenez C (2005). *Entamoeba histolytica* and *Entamoeba dispar*: prevalence infection in a rural Mexican community. *Experimental Parasitology,* 110(3), 327--330.

Rappelli P,Maddau G, Mannu F,ColomboMM, Fiori PL,Cappuccinelli P (2001). Development of a set of multiplex PCR assays for the simultaneous identification of enterotoxigenic, enteropathogenic, enterohemorrhagic and enteroinvasive *Escherichia coli*. *New Microbiologica,* 24, 77–83.

Raymond J, Nguyen VB, Vidal-Trecan G, Kalach N (2005). *Helicobacter pylori* infection in children of developing countries. *Médecine tropicale,* 65, 383-8.

Reichardt C, Chaberny IF, Kola A, Mattner F, Vonberg RP, Gastmeier P (2007). [Dramatic increase of diarrhea associated with *Clostridium difficile* in Germany: has the new strain PCR-ribotype 027 reached us?] *Deutsche Medizinische Wochenschrift,* 132, 223-8.

Rivera WL, Santos SR, Kanbara H (2006). Prevalence and genetic diversity of *Entamoeba histolytica* in an institution for the mentally retarded in the Philippines. *Parasitology Research,* 98, 106-10.

Samie A, Barrett LJ, Bessong PO, Ramalivhana JN, Mavhandu LG, Njayou M, Guerrant RL (2010). Seroprevalence of *Entamoeba histolytica* in the context of HIV and AIDS: Case of the Vhembe district, Limpopo Province. *Annals of Tropical Medicine & Parasitology*, 104 (1), 55–63.

Samie A, Bessong PO, Obi CL, Sevilleja JEAD, Stroup S, Houpt E, Guerrant RL (2006) *Cryptosporidium species:* Preliminary descriptions of the prevalence and genotype distribution among school children and hospital patients in the Venda region, Limpopo Province, South Africa. *Experimental Parasitology*, 114, 314 - 322.

Samie A, Njayou M, Bessong PO, Obi CL, Mouchili F, Tuikue Ndam NG, Sabeta CT, and Mduluza T. (2006). Use of an immuno-peroxidase staining method for the detection of *Entamoeba histolytica* in stool samples in endemic areas. Journal of Tropical *Microbiology and Biotechnolology* 2: 10 – 18.

Samie A, Obi CL, Barrett LJ, Powell SM, Guerrant RL (2006) Prevalence of *Campylobacter* species, *Helicobacter pylori* and *Arcobacter* species in stool samples from the Vhembe district, Limpopo, South Africa: Studies using molecular diagnostic methods. *Journal of Infection,* 54(6), 558-66.

Samie A, Obi CL, Bessong PO, Stroup S, Houpt E, Guerrant RL (2006b). Prevalence and Species Distribution of *E. Histolytica* and *E. Dispar* In the Vhembe district, Limpopo, South Africa. *American Journal of Tropical Medicine and Hygiene*, 75, 565-71.

Samie A, Obi CL, Dillingham R, Pinkerton RC, Guerrant RL. (2007) Enteroaggregative *Escherichia Coli* in Venda, South Africa: Distribution of Virulence-Related Genes by Multiplex PCR in Stool Samples of HIV Positive and HIV Negative Individuals and Primary School Children. *American Journal of Tropical Medicine and Hygiene,* 77(1), 142-150.

Samie A, Obi CL, Franaziak J, Archbald-Pannone L, Bessong PO, Alcantara-Warren C, Guerrant RL (2008). PCR detection of *Clostridium difficile* triose phosphate isomerase (tpi), toxin A (tcdA), toxin B (tcdB), binary toxin (cdtA, cdtB) and tcdC genes in Vhembe district, South Africa: *American Journal Of Tropical Medicine and Hygiene.* 78, 577-585.

Samie A, Obi CL, Stroup S, Houpt E, Njayou M, Sabeta CT, Mduluza T, Guerrant RL (2008). Genetic diversity of *Entamoeba histolytica* from Africa based on the serine- rich gene polymorphism. *Experimental Parasitology,* 118(3), 354-61 .

Samie A, Obi CL, Tzipori S, Weiss LM, Guerrant RL. (2007). Microsporidiosis in South Africa: PCR detection in stool samples of HIV positive and HIV negative individuals and school children in the Vhembe district, Limpopo Province. *Transactions of the Royal Society of Tropical Medicine and Hygiene,* 101(6), 547-54.

Samie A, Obi LC, Bessong PO, Stroup S, Houpt E, Guerrant RL (2006) Prevalence And Species Distribution of *E. Histolytica* And *E. dispar* In The Venda Region, Limpopo, South Africa. *American Journal of Tropical Medicine and Hygiene*, 75(3), 565-71.

Samie A, Obi LC, Bessong PO, Stroup S, Houpt E, Guerrant RL (2006). Prevalence and Species Distribution of *E. Histolytica* and *E. Dispar* in the Vhembe district, Limpopo, South Africa. *American Journal of Tropical Medicine and Hygiene,* 75, 565-71.

Samie A, Ramalivhana J, Igumbor EO, Obi CL. (2007). Prevalence, Hemolytic and Hemagglutination Activities and Antibiotic Susceptibility Profiles of *Campylobacter spp* Isolated from Human Diarrheal Stools in the Vhembe District, South Africa. *Journal of Health Population and Nutrition,* 25 (4), 406 - 413.

Samie A., Obi CL, Barrett LJ, Powell SM, Guerrant RL (2007). Prevalence of *Campylobacter* species, *Helicobacter pylori* and *Arcobacter* species in stool samples from the Venda region, Limpopo, South Africa: Studies using molecular diagnostic methods. *Journal of Infection*, 54(6), 558-66.

Sarfati C, Bourgeois A, Menotti J, Liegeois F, Moyou-Somo R, Delaporte E, Derouin F, Ngole EM, Molina JM (2006). Prevalence of intestinal parasites including microsporidia in human immunodeficiency virus-infected adults in Cameroon: a cross-sectional study. *American Journal of Tropical Medicine and Hygiene*, 74, 162-4.

Scaletsky ICA, Fabbricotti SH, Aranda KR, Morais MB, and Fagundes-Neto U (2002). Comparison of DNA Hybridization and PCR Assays for Detection of Putative Pathogenic Enteroadherent *Escherichia coli Journal of Clinical Microbiology*, 40, 1254–1258.

Siddiqui U, Bini EJ, Chandarana K, et al. Prevalence and impact of diarrhea on health-related quality of life in HIV-infected patients in the era of highly active antiretroviral therapy. J Clin Gastroenterol 2007; 41:484.

Silva RC, Benati FJ, Pena GP, Santos N (2010). Molecular characterization of viruses associated with gastrointestinal infection in HIV-positive patients. Braz J Infect Dis. 14(6):549-52.

Simango C, Mutikani S (2004). Cryptosporidiosis in Harare, Zimbabwe. *Centl Afr J Med* 50, 52–54.

Snelling WJ, McKenna JP, Hack CJ, Moore JE, Dooley JS (2006). An examination of the diversity of a novel *Campylobacter* reservoir. *Arch Microbiol*. 186:31- 40.

Snijders F, van Deventer SJ, Bartelsman JF, den Otter P, Jansen J, Mevissen ML, van Gool T, Danner SA, Reiss P (1995). Diarrhea in HIV-infected patients: no evidence of cytokine-mediated inflammation in jejunal mucosa. *AIDS* 9, 367-73.

Speelman P, I Kabir and M Islam (1984). Distribution and spread of colonic lesion in Shigellosis: a colonoscopic study. *Journal of Infectious Diseases,* 50, 899-903.

Spigaglia P, and Mastrantonio P (2002). Molecular analysis of the pathogenicity locus and polymorphism in the putative negative regulator of toxin production (TcdC) among *Clostridium difficile* clinical isolates. *Journal of Clinical Microbiology,* 40, 3470-3475.

Stark D, Barratt JL, van Hal S, Marriott D, Harkness J, Ellis JT. Clinical significance of enteric protozoa in the immunosuppressed human population. *Clinical Microbiology Reviews*, 22(4), 634-50.

Steiner TS, Lima AAM, Nataro JP, Guerrant RL (1998). Enteroaggregative *Escherichia coli* produce intestinal inflammation and growth impairment and cause interleukin-8 release from intestinal epithelial cells. *Journal of Infectious Diseases,* 177, 88–96.

Steiner TS, Samie A, Guerrant RL (2006). Infectious diarrhea: new pathogens and new challenges in developed and developing areas. *Clinical infectious Diseases*, 43(4), 408-10.

Stubbs S, Rupnik M, Gibert M, Brazier J, Duerden B, Popoff M (2000). Production of actin-specific ADP-ribosyltransferase (binary toxin) by strains of *Clostridium difficile*. *FEMS Microbiology Letters,* 186, 307-12.

Sturbaum GD, Reed C, Hoover PJ, Jost BH, Marshall MM, Sterling CR (2001). Species-specific, nested PCR-restriction fragment length polymorphism detection of single

Cryptosporidium parvum oocysts. Applied Environmental Microbiology, 67(6), 2665-8.

Sulaiman IM, Hira PR, Zhou L, Al-Ali FM, Al-Shelahi FA, Shweiki HM, Iqbal J, Khalid N, Xiao L (2005). Unique endemicity of cryptosporidiosis in children in Kuwait. *Journal of Clinical Microbiology*, 43, 2805–2809.

Tadesse A, Kassu A (2005). Intestinal parasite isolates in AIDS patients with chronic diarrhea in Gondar Teaching Hospital, North West Ethiopia. *Ethiopian Medical Journal*, 43(2), 93--96.

Taniuchi M, Verweij JJ, Noor Z, Sobuz SU, Lieshout L, Petri WA Jr, Haque R, Houpt ER. High throughput multiplex PCR and probe-based detection with Luminex beads for seven intestinal parasites. *American Journal Of Tropical Medicine and Hygiene*, 84(2), 332-7.

Taylor AD, Ladd J, Yu Q, Chen S, Homola J, Jiang S (2006). Quantitative and simultaneous detection of four foodborne bacterial pathogens with a multi-channel SPR sensor. *Biosens Bioelectron* 22:752- 8.

Thielman NM, Guerrant RL (2004). Clinical practice. Acute infectious diarrhea. The New England Journal of Medicine, 350(1), 38-47.

Thomas JE, Gibson JR, Darboe MK (1992). Isolation of *Helicobacter pylori* from feces. *Lancet* 340: 1194- 1195.

Turner SM, Scott-Tucker A, Cooper LM, Henderson IR (2006). Weapons of mass destruction: virulence factors of the global killer enterotoxigenic *Escherichia coli*. *FEMS Microbiology Letters*, 263, 10-20.

Valenstein P, Pfaller M, Yungbluth M (1996). The use and abuse of routine stool microbiology: a College of American Pathologists Q-probes study of 601 institutions. *Archives of Pathology & Laboratory Medicine*, 120(2), 206-11.

Van Der Hulst RW, Keller JJ, Rauws EA, Tytgat GN (1996). Treatment of *Helicobacter pylori* infection: *a* review of the world literature. *Helicobacter* 1:6- 19.

Verweij JJ, Oostvogel F, Brienen EA, Nang-Beifubah A, Ziem J, Polderman AM, (2003). Short communication: Prevalence of *Entamoeba histolytica* and *Entamoeba dispar* in northern Ghana. *Tropical Medicine and International Health*, 8(12), 1153--1156.

Victora CG, Bryce J, Fontaine O, Monasch R (2000). Reducing deaths from diarrhoea through oral rehydration therapy. Bulletin of the World Health Organization, 78 (10), 1246-55.

Wang L, Calderon J, Stanley SL Jr (1997). Short report: identification of B-cell epitopes in the serine-rich *Entamoeba histolytica* protein. *American Journal Of Tropical Medicine and Hygiene*, 57, 723-6.

Wanke CA, Gerrior J, Blais V, Mayer H, Acheson D (1998b). Successful treatment of diarrheal disease associated with enteroaggregative *Escherichia coli* in adults infected with human immunodeficiency virus. *Journal of Infectious Diseases*, 178:1369-72.

Wanke CA, Mayer H, Weber R, Zbinden R, Watson DA, Acheson D (1998a). Enteroaggregative *Escherichia coli* as a potential cause of diarrheal disease in adults infected with human immunodeficiency virus. *Journal of Infectious Diseases*, 178, 185-190.

Wilcox MH (1996). Cleaning up *Clostridium difficile* infection. *Lancet* 348:767–8.

World Health Organization. World health report 2004: changing history. Geneva: World Health Organization, 2004. 200.

Wultanska D, Pituch H, Obuch-Woszczatynski P, Meisel-Mikolajczyk F, Luczak M (2005). [Profile of toxigenicity of *Clostridium difficile* strains isolated from paediatric patients with clinical diagnosis of antibiotic associated diarrhea (AAD)] *Medycyna Doswiadczalna I Mikrobiologia,* 57, 377-82.

Zaki M, Reddy SG, Jackson TF, Ravdin JI, Clark CG (2003). Genotyping of *Entamoeba* species in South Africa: diversity, stability, and transmission patterns within families. *Journal of Infectious Diseases,* 187, 1860-9.

9

Reducing Urogenital Infections Including HIV in Sub-Saharan Africa - Can Probiotics Be a Viable Paradigm?

Kingsley C. Anukam[1,2], Enya B. Bassey[3] and Emmanuel O. Osazuwa[2]
[1]*TWAS Research Unit on Probiotic Genomics, Department of Medical Laboratory Science, School of Basic Medical Sciences, College of Medical Sciences, University of Benin,*
[2]*Department of Pharmaceutical Microbiology, Faculty of Pharmacy, University of Benin,*
[3]*World Health Organization (WHO), Ministry of Health, Uyo, Akwa Ibom State, Nigeria*

1. Introduction

The economic burden, albeit low quality of life of people in sub-Saharan Africa with non-sexually transmitted recurrent urogenital tract infections is not the desired state of health. Associations exist between abnormal vaginal/penile microbiota and HIV. Excluding sexually transmitted diseases, microorganisms that originate from the gastrointestinal tract cause almost all infections of the vagina and bladder. There is a strong correlation between presence of the normal microbiota, particularly lactobacilli in the vagina with health, and an absence of these microorganisms in patients with urogenital infections. Disruption of the normal vaginal microbiota is caused by the use of broad-spectrum antibiotics, spermicides, hormones, dietary substances and factors not, as yet, fully understood. There is increasing body of evidence that probiotic microorganisms delivered in food such as yogurt or milk based foods and capsular preparations do have a role in preventing urogenital tract infections and in ameliorating diarrhea [Walker et al., 2006].

The use of probiotics defined as "live microorganisms which when administered in adequate amounts, confer health benefits on the host" (WHO/FAO, 2001), for the maintenance of health is already in use in developed countries. Probiotics are yet to be adopted in sub-Saharan Africa by health care providers. There are clinical evidence to show that probiotics can play a significant role in resolving diarrhea, boost immune system and prevent recurrent urogenital infections including bacterial vaginosis, which is a risk factor in HIV acquisition. The aim of this chapter is to highlight the burden of urogenital infections in Africa, impact of abnormal vaginal microbiota, clinical evidence on the use of probiotics for urogenital health care and last but not the least, the rationale for suggesting the use of probiotics in the management of HIV infection in sub-Saharan Africa.

2. Burden of urogenital infections in Africa

Non-sexually transmitted urogenital infections such as bacterial vaginosis (BV), yeast vaginitis, urinary tract infections (UTI) afflict more than one billion women around the world annually [Hay, 2000]. However, it is worthwhile to briefly explain what BV is.

BV is a syndrome defined by symptoms and signs of a white, homogenous, malodorous discharge, vaginal itching, increase in vaginal pH above 4.5, development of a fishy odor when 10% KOH reacts with an altered organic acid pattern (including increases in putrescine, cadaverine, and trimethylamine), and vaginal epithelial cells observed on wet mount spotted with adherent small rods or cocci ("clue cells"). Three of 4 (discharge, pH, odor, clue cells) clinical or laboratory signs are required for BV diagnosis by the Amsel criteria [Amsel et al., 1983]. The relative changes in bacterial concentrations have been tracked by Nugent scoring, which uses staining and microscopy to grade the predominance of 3 morphotypes: lactobacilli, small gram-variable rods or Gram-negative rods (*G. vaginalis, Bacteroides*), and curved gram-variable rods [Nugent et al 1991]. Currently, molecular techniques are providing new ways to categorize the change in composition of the vaginal microbiota [Verhelst et al 2005]. The predominance of *G. vaginalis, Bacteroides* spp., and *A. vaginae* in BV is also accompanied by increases in other anaerobes, such as prevotella, mobiluncus, genital mycoplasmas, and an unfolding community of unculturable bacteria but not necessarily a decrease in the geometric mean concentration of lactobacilli [Fredricks et al 2007]

Although the estimate for non-sexually transmitted urogenital infections in women in sub-Saharan Africa is difficult to get, but statistics may be grim due to the rising trend in HIV/AIDS in the region. The infection process is not a hygiene issue. Anatomically, the proximity of the vagina and the anus predisposes women to these infections. Most cases of BV, UTI, and yeast vaginitis arise from the host's gastrointestinal tract, as microbes ascend 4 to 5 cm from the anus, thereby showing that the intestine and urogenital tracts are 'connected' and that intestinal health can influence the vagina and bladder. The process is mediated by bacterial adherence and is not altered by antibiotic use. Studies have shown that the host's cells remain susceptible to pathogen adhesion before, during and after antibiotic administrations [Reid et al 1988]. Since the discovery of the 'magic bullet', the therapeutic approaches to treatment and prevention of urogenital infections in Africa and in the rest of the world have remained constant for more than half of a century. Antibiotics and antifungals still remain the armaments of therapy, despite their well-known side effects chronicled in Pharmaceutical compendia, ranging from super infections, diarrhea, depression, to renal failure. The emergence of 'superbugs' as a result of antimicrobial resistance is not only an economic burden to the health sector, but also constitute a treat to the survival of the human species.

The burden of urogenital infections is becoming more worrisome in that most women are not aware that they have particularly, bacterial vaginosis. Klebanoff et al [2004], recently revealed that women not detecting odor or discharge do not realize that their vaginal microbiota is abnormal and a 14.2% prevalence of BV have been found in healthy Nigerian women [Anukam et al 2006]. Consequently the quality of life of the women with these acute and chronic infections has been found to be adversely affected significantly [Ellis &Verma, 2000). There is an association between BV and preterm delivery [Hay, 1994] and also between BV and early spontaneous miscarriage prior to 16 weeks gestation [Oakeshott et al., 2002]. Associations between BV and urinary tract infections (UTI) [Hillebrand et al., 2002] as well as between BV and history of infertility caused by tubal factors [Wilson et al., 2002] have been reported in other studies. There is also an association between smoking and BV (Smart et al., 2004).

A previous longitudinal study of women in the United Kingdom showed that at any given time during the menstrual cycle, the vaginal microbiota may be "abnormal" [Keane et al 1997]. When symptoms of pain, discharge, and itching occur, many women diagnose these symptoms as yeast infections and self-treat with over-the-counter antifungals, when in fact they have BV. This misdiagnosis and mistreatment can result in adverse consequences [Ferris et al 1996]. Antimicrobial treatment for BV is suboptimal, with some cure rates as low as 60% 1 month after treatment, and subsequent overgrowth of pathogenic bacteria in the vagina often occurs [Livengood et al 1999].

3. Abnormal vaginal/penile microbiota and HIV

Studies have found a significant association between BV and human immunodeficiency virus (HIV) infection (Sewankambo et al., 1997). In a prospective study of Kenyan sex workers, the absence of lactobacilli in vaginal cultures was associated with a 2.0-fold increase in HIV acquisition and a 1.7-fold greater risk of developing gonorrhea (Martin et al., 1999). Similar studies have also documented evidence indicating that human immunodeficiency virus infection have a strong association with abnormal vaginal microbiotia particularly, bacterial vaginosis [Taha, 1999]. Studies have also shown that the absence or depletion of lactobacilli in the vagina associated with overgrowth of anaerobic pathogens causing BV results in significantly increased risk for HIV (as well as gonorrhea, chlamydia, and herpes simplex virus infections) [Wiesenfeld, 2003]. By mechanisms yet to be elucidated, BV displaces lactobacilli, elevating vaginal pH and creating an environment within which the pathogens survive and can infect the host. It is important to note also that penile microbiota may contribute significantly to susceptibility to HIV infection. Several randomized trials demonstrated decreased risk of trichomoniasis and bacterial vaginosis (BV) in the female sexual partners of circumcised men (Gray et al 2009). It is very pertinent to better understand the biological mechanisms by which male circumcision reduces the risk of HIV infection as this may lead to the development of novel, non-surgical prevention strategies. It has been asserted that male and female genital microbial communities may play an important role in modulating HIV risk [Galvin & Cohen, 2004]. Genital mucosal inflammation induced by microbes leads to the activation of HIV target cells and an increase in HIV susceptibility [de Jong & Geijtenbeek, 2009]. The dominant HIV target cells in the genital mucosa are two dendritic cell types, langerin+ Langerhans' cells and DC-SIGN+ dendritic cells. The biological mechanism underlying circumcision-conferred protection against HIV is likely to be multifactorial. Post- circumcision anatomical, immunological, and microbiological changes have all been hypothesized to contribute to the reduction in HIV risk. From the anatomical and immunological perspective, the inner surface of the foreskin is lightly keratinized and contains abundant Langerhans cells close to the mucosal surface resulting in a large number of exposed HIV target cells in the erect uncircumcised penis (Patterson et al., 2002; McCoombe & Short, 2006). From a microbiological perspective, the intact foreskin may support the survival of genital microbes associated with increased foreskin mucosal inflammation and Langerhans' cell activation. Of note, the protection against sexually transmitted infections and BV conferred to the female partners of circumcised men [Bailey et al., 2007;Auvert et al., 2005;Gray et al., 2009] strongly suggests circumcision-associated microbiological changes in the male genital mucosa.

In a study that assessed the penile (coronal sulci) microbiota in 12 HIV-negative Ugandan men before and after circumcision revealed a total of 42 unique bacterial families in the coronal sulci microbiota, with 38 bacterial families among pre-circumci- sion samples versus 36 detected among post-circumcision samples. Pseudomonadaceae was the most abundant family irrespective of circumcision status, constituting over 50% of the coronal sulci microbiota, followed by Clostridiales Family XI, Oxalobacteraceae, and Prevotellaceae for pre-circumcision and Corynebacteriaceae, Oxalobacteraceae, and Staphylococcaceae for post-circumcision (Price et al 2010). The study suggests that anoxic microenvironment of the subpreputial space may support pro-inflammatory anaerobes that can activate Langerhans cells to present HIV to CD4 cells in draining lymph nodes. Thus, the reduction in putative anaerobic bacteria after circumcision may play a role in protection from HIV and other sexually transmitted diseases.

4. The role of normal vaginal microbiota

It has been reported previously that more than 60 different bacterial species colonize the healthy vagina (Reid et al 1990). A recent study sampled the vaginal bacterial communities of 396 asymptomatic North American women who represented four ethnic groups (White, Black, Hispanic and Asian) and the species composition was characterized by pyro-sequencing of barcoded 16S rRNA genes. The study revealed that the bacterial communities clustered into five groups: four were dominated by *Lactobacillus iners, L. crispatus, L. gasseri,* or *L. jensenii,* whereas the fifth had lower proportions of lactic acid bacteria and higher proportions of strictly anaerobic organisms, indicating that a potential key ecological function, the production of lactic acid, seems to be conserved in all communities. The proportions of each community group varied among the four ethnic groups, and these differences were statistically significant (Ravel et al. 2011). This shows that different vaginal bacterial ecosystems varies in people but conferring the same protective role as the human vaginal microbiota seem to play a key role in preventing a number of urogenital diseases, such as bacterial vaginosis, yeast infections, sexually transmitted infections, urinary tract infections and HIV infections (Taha, 1999). Studies have shown that urogenital cells are covered by dense bacterial biofilms, whose composition changes constantly, but in which lactobacilli predominate, at least until menopause. Vaginal lactobacilli have been shown to inhibit the growth of *Gardnerella vaginalis* and mobiluncus in vitro, with the greatest inhibition observed in the presence of lactobacilli producing lactic acid. Hydrogen peroxide-producing lactobacilli have been recovered from the vagina of 96% of 28 non-pregnant women without bacterial vaginosis, compared with 6% of 67 women with bacterial vaginosis (Eschenbach et al. 1989). The presence of lactobacilli on vaginal epithelial cells seems to act, not only as a barrier to infection, by blocking adherence of pathogens, but their capability of producing such antibacterial materials as hydrogen peroxide to limit pathogen growth, production of biosurfactants that inhibit pathogen adherence, and their ability to prime macrophages, leukocytes, cytokines, and other host defenses also contribute to the protection of the vagina against uropathogens (Reid, 1999). Full genome sequencing of *Lactobacillus plantarum* KCA1 isolated from the vagina of a healthy Nigerian woman has revealed the presence of several novel phage defense genes encoding clustered regularly interspaced short pallindromic repeats (CRISPR)-associated proteins and abortive infection systems (Anukam et al. 2011). One of the fastest evolving genetic elements in bacterial genomes are clustered regularly interspaced short palindromic repeats (CRISPRs) (Sorek et al., 2008). CRISPRs have been identified within the genomes of many archaeal and bacterial species especially in some vaginal lactobacilli such *L. plantarum* KCA-1, the only plantarum strain know to date with CRISPR. The Spacers are derived from foreign nucleic acids, such as those from phage or plasmids and can protect bacteria from subsequent infection by homologous phage and plasmids. As a bacterial immune system against foreign DNA,

CRISPRs evolve rapidly in response to changing phage pools (Vale & Little, 2010) that is usually encountered in the vaginal niche as a result of changes occasioned by the menstrual cycle.

5. The impact of HIV/AIDS in Africa

Recently, the United Nations AIDS program (UNAIDS) estimated that around 25 million people around the world have died from AIDS in the past 30 years since it was recognized, and about 40 million more are currently infected with the virus. It is astonishing that 14,000 new infections occur per day, which means that in every six seconds someone in the world will be infected with the HIV virus. Sub-Saharan Africa has been hit hardest by the pandemic: about 83% (18.26 million) of AIDS deaths and 71% (28.4million) of HIV infections have occurred in this war-ravaged, poverty stricken part of the continent probably due to political instability and global climate changes. African region holds just over 10% of the world's population, but is home to more than 60% of all people living with HIV and more than two-third of all women living with HIV. In some African nations, over 30% of the adult population is HIV-positive. (UNAIDS, 2002). In Nigeria, with about 25% of the African population, a recent national HIV prevalence sentinel survey by the Federal Ministry of health showed that the number of people living with HIV/AIDS in 2009 was between 3.2 and 3.8 million (Report, 2009). According to the report, the age group 20-24 years had the highest national prevalence of 5.6 per cent, and the HIV prevalence for women aged 15-24 years remains 5.2 per cent. The statistics are very grim all over Africa, in that in 2000, of the 1.4 million children world-wide living with HIV/AIDS, 1.1 million were in sub-Saharan Africa alone (Sengupta and Somini, 2002). By 2002, about 11 million children in Africa had lost one or both parents to AIDS. If the disease remains unchecked, the number of African children orphaned by AIDS will jump to 20 million by 2010 and most will be old enough to watch their parents die from the disease. (Altman and Lawrence, 2002).

In Africa alone, AIDS has surpassed armed conflict as the leading cause of death (Van Niekerk, 2001). With the increasing number of people living and dying of AIDS, only a few people have easy access to life-prolonging antiretroviral drug therapy. According to UNAIDS, in a press release in July 2, 2002 "In high-income countries, where an estimated 500,000 people were receiving antiretroviral treatment, 25,000 people died of AIDS in 2001. In Africa, however, where only 30,000 of the 28.4 million people infected, were receiving antiretroviral treatment, AIDS killed 2.2 million people". In Nigeria, if not for PEPFAR, the situation is harrowing in terms of provision of antiretroviral drugs to people living with HIV/AIDS. According to Dr. Peter Piot, executive director of UNAIDS, "The devastating impact of HIV/AIDS is rolling back decades of development progress in Africa, and has caused economic growth to plummet as much as 4% in sub- Saharan Africa". HIV/AIDS will prevent many sub-Saharan African countries from achieving the Millennium Development Goals (MDGs). In high-prevalence countries (those with more than 10% of adults infected: Botswana, Lesotho, Malawi, Mozambique, Namibia, South Africa, Swaziland, Swaziland, Zambia and Zimbabwe), AIDS is the leading cause of death (MSF, 2009).

Over 7,000 women become infected each day. In sub-Saharan Africa, around one quarter of females under the age of 30 have HIV and an estimated half billion are at risk of acquiring the virus through sexual contact. Although efforts to provide condoms, develop a vaccine, use spermicides or anti-retrovirals, have contributed significantly to stem the epidemic due to massive investment by International organizations, such as the Joint United Nations Programme on HIV/AIDS (UNAIDS), the Global Fund to Fight AIDS, Tuberculosis and Malaria (the Global Fund) and the US President's Emergency Plan for AIDS Relief (PEPFAR). These organizations were formed to specifically address HIV/AIDS. The United Nations estimated that at least US $1.5 billion a year could make it possible to achieve massively higher levels of implementation of all major components of successful prevention programs for the whole of sub-Saharan Africa.

Having HIV/AIDS is especially devastating among children from the developing countries such as sub-Saharan Africa. To comprehend the reality of the vulnerability of children affected by the condition, it is important that health care professionals and national policy makers understand the global magnitude of the problem. More than 90% of HIV infection occurs among the children of southern Africa. Seventy-five percent of those children reportedly die before the age of 5 years (DeBaets et al., 2007). Children with HIV/AIDS in developing countries continue to be underrepresented among recipients of antiretroviral therapy or supportive care, including palliative care (Kline, 2006). A significant number of children infected with HIV are also orphans of parents who died of HIV, and they suffer from complications including extreme malnutrition. Children who receive professional care are often hospitalized for many months at the end of life. The need for prevention and alternative management is very obvious

Meanwhile, more than half of those in need still do not have access to treatment, and treatment is posing new challenges for sustainable funding. Most countries with mid to high prevalence cannot afford the cost of treatment without international aid; as aid is reduced or cancelled, treatment programmes are threatened, drug resistance develops and large numbers of people living with HIV may die. In countries like Uganda, patients are being turned away from treatment clinics due to lack of resources; 300,000 Ugandans in need of treatment are denied their right to health (McNeil, 2010). These numbers will continue to grow if both effective prevention and sustainably funded treatment programmes are not maintained. Nigeria may not be able to sustain the free anti-retroviral drug program from PEPFAR and the future of new infected person may be grim. In 2009, UNAIDS and WHO predicted that the $25.1 million needed for HIV/AIDS programmes in 2010 would not be forthcoming (UNAIDS, 2009). The total amount of Global Fund grants recommended for funding in 2009 was 35% lower than in 2008 (MSF, 2009).

The programs by all these agencies are planned to cover sexual, mother-to- child and transfusion-related HIV transmissions, and would involve approaches ranging from awareness campaigns through media to voluntary HIV counseling and testing and the promotion and supply of condoms.

No doubt these programs are laudable, but other alternative measures, such as nutrition fortification and probiotics, have not been included as one of the UNAIDS intervention programs. Death from AIDS is often precipitated by gastrointestinal infections and diarrhea, and indeed, many non-AIDS deaths are due to these infections. It has been estimated that a child dies every 15 seconds from diarrheal diseases. While sanitation and early hydration based interventions can reduce this death rate, probiotics too could play a role.

6. Probiotics with clinical evidence against urogenital infections

During the early periods of probiotics, Scientists paid more attention to gastrointestinal effects, but in recent times probiotics are now useful for more than just gastrointestinal health. In fact, there are specific probiotic products that can help prevent and treat female urogenital conditions like bacterial vaginosis, vulvovaginal candidiasis, urinary tract infections. It should be noted that the vaginal tract is not internally connected to the alimentary canal, however the two are intimately related. Bacteria that pass through the digestive system can ascend via the perineum to the vagina. So it's almost a no-brainer to expect what promotes gastrointestinal health to have relevance for urogenital health.

In the late 1980s, human studies were carried out in which *L. rhamnosus* GR-1 in a douche suspension was instilled into the vagina (Bruce and Reid, 1988). This was followed by studies using a gelatin capsule containing freeze-dried lactobacilli inserted into the vagina (Reid et al 2001). In both cases, the process did not result in any adverse events but did show a potential to reduce the risk of recurrence of UTI. The use of orally administered lactobacilli was more recently tested, on the basis that if pathogens infect the host from the anal skin, why couldn't lactobacilli also ascend from the anus to the vagina and repopulate the area? This concept was verified in several labs (Reid et al, 2001;Antonio et al 2005), and *Lactobacillus* strains GR-1 and RC-14 were shown to reduce UTI, BV and yeast pathogens as well as infections (Reid et al 2001; Reid et al. 2003]. The mechanism of action is likely multifactorial and could include the ingested lactobacilli ascending from the rectal skin to the vagina, or causing a reduced pathogen ascension, or influencing the immune or host system in a way that reduces infectivity.

As this approach to restoration and maintenance of women's health has become more recognized, other groups have undertaken studies using different strains. A prospective clinical pilot study was performed to confirm the safety and effectiveness of *Lactobacillus* vaginal suppositories against the recurrence of UTI. The patients enrolled in the study were instructed to administer vaginal suppositories containing the strain *L. crispatus* GAI 98322. A significant reduction in the number of recurrences was noted, without any adverse complication (P=0.0007). The administration of vaginal suppositories containing *L. crispatus* GAI 98332 seemed to be a safe and promising treatment for the prevention of recurrent UTI (Uehara 2006). Delai et al., (2006) demonstrated the effectiveness of the contemporary oral administration of *L. paracasei* subsp *paracasei* F19 in association with vaginal suppositories containing an unnamed *L. acidophilus* in the treatment of BV. The study had a potentially fatal flaw in that not all the 60 subjects had confirmed diagnosis of BV. The subjects were randomized in 2 groups: Group A treated with vaginal suppositories containing *L. acidophilus;* Group B treated with the same vaginal suppositories + *L. paracasei* subsp *paracasei* F 19 for oral administration. There was a significant reduction of vaginal pH, an improvement in the amine sniff test and in subjective symptomatology after 3 months of treatment and follow-up (3 months). This study needs to be repeated with larger sample size, but nevertheless, reviews of the evidence from microbiological and clinical studies have indicated that probiotics can be beneficial for preventing recurrent UTI in women in a safe manner (Falagas 2006;Reid and Bruce 2006; Hoesl and Altwein 2005).

The usefulness of orally administered lactobacilli for urogenital health has been demonstrated in several other important studies. In a randomized, double-blind, placebo controlled trial, 106 women with BV were given a single oral dose of metronidazole (500mg) twice daily from days 1-7, plus oral *L. rhamnosus* GR-1 and *L. reuteri* RC-14 or placebo twice daily from days 1-30. The cure rate in the antibiotic/probiotic group was 88% compared to 40% in the antibiotic/placebo group ($p<0.001$). High counts of *Lactobacillus* sp.

(>10^5CFU/ml) were recovered from the vagina of 96% of probiotic treated subjects compared to 53% controls at day 30 (Anukam et al 2006a). In another study using the same probiotics, there was a 90% cure of BV following intravaginal administration of the probiotic alone, compared to 33% cure with intravaginal metronidazole treatment. In the study, 40 women diagnosed with BV were randomized to receive either two dried capsules containing *L. rhamnosus* GR-1 and *L. reuteri* RC-14 each night for five days, or 0.75% metronidazole gel, applied vaginally twice a day (in the morning and evening). Follow-up at day 6, 15 and 30 showed cure of BV in significantly more probiotic treated subjects (16, 17 and 18/20 respectively) compared to metronidazole treatment (9, 9 and 11/20: P= 0.016 at day 6, P= 0.002 at day 15 and P= 0.056 at day 30) [Anukam et al 2006b]. This is the first proven cure of BV using probiotics and provides hope that alternative remedies to antibiotics can be found.

7. Mechanisms of action

Probiotics apparently fulfills the definition as "live microorganisms which, when administered in adequate amounts, confer a health benefit on the host" through a variety of somewhat disparate, somewhat overlapping mechanisms. These include the regulation of intestinal microbial homeostasis, the interference with the ability of pathogens to colonize and infect the mucosa, the modulation of local and systemic immune responses, the stabilization or maintenance of the gastrointestinal barrier function, the inhibition of procarcinogenic enzymatic activity and the induction of enzymatic activity that favors good nutrition. For example, with respect to epithelial barrier function, probiotics can conceivably act through general antimicrobial effects, effects on intestinal permeability in the absence of invasive bacteria, effects on epithelial cell inflammatory responses and effects on epithelial cell survival. One important effect of probiotics on barrier function is the ability of commensal organisms to act through Toll-like Receptors (TLR) on epithelial cells (such as TLR2 and TLR4). In particular, it has been shown that such interactions induce the production of protective cytokines such as IL-6 that mediate epithelial cell regeneration and inhibit epithelial cell apoptosis in the face of agents that otherwise result in epithelial cell ulceration (Rakoff-Nahoum et al., 2004). It should be noted, however, that probiotics do not affect expression of all TLRs in the same manner. Thus, as shown by Ewaschuk *et al.*, (2007) whereas exposure of HT-29 epithelial cells to DNA from pathogenic organisms resulted in increased TLR9 expression, exposure to a probiotic did not have this effect. This is in keeping with the lesser ability of commensal organisms to induce TLR expression as compared with pathogenic organisms. Probiotics may also have effects on epithelial barrier function via cellular mechanisms that have little to do with TLR signaling. Thus, in a study by Zyrek *et al.*, (2007) it was shown that the probiotic, *E. coli* Nissle 1917 (EcN) counteracts the disruptive effects of enteropathic *E. coli* (EPEC) on T-84 epithelial cell monolayers by altering protein kinase C signaling and causing the redistribution and increased expression of zonula-occludens-2 (ZO-2), an important factor in maintaining epithelial tight junction function. Along similar lines, Yan *et al.*, (2007) showed that proteins isolated from broths of the probiotic *Lactobacillus rhamnosus* activated mouse epithelial cell Akt and inhibited TNF-α-mediated apoptosis and promoted growth of both human and mouse colon epithelial cells or cultured mouse colon explants.

Production of antimicrobial substances, such as organic acids or bacteriocins
Upregulate immune response (eg, secretory IgA) to possible pathogens or to vaccines
Downregulate inflammatory response
Assist in early programming of the immune system to result in a better balanced immune response and reducing risk of development of allergy
Improvement of gut mucosal barrier function
Enhance stability or promote recovery of commensal microbiota when perturbed
Modulate host gene expression
Deliver functional proteins (eg, lactase) or enzymes (natural and cloned)
Decrease pathogen adhesion

Table 1. Some proposed probiotics mechanisms of actions

From the accumulated information on the relation of regulatory T cells and their associated cytokines to the function of probiotics, it can be said with some certainty that probiotic administration does lead to the increased elaboration of regulatory cytokines and these cytokines play a major role in the protective effect of the probiotics. It seems likely that probiotics bring about these effects via their interactions with mucosal dendritic cells which then produce regulatory cytokines themselves or induce T cells with these properties. There is the possibility that probiotics act through the induction of regulatory T cells that suppress inflammation-inducing effector cells. This emphasis is based on a rising tide of evidence that probiotics have properties that allow them to interact with the mucosal immune system that does not arouse an inflammation inducing innate response and the consequent induction of master inflammatory cytokines such as IL-12. For example human circulating dendritic cells or lamina propria mononuclear cell populations were cultured with cell wall preparations from each of the probiotic species in VSL#3 and then assessed cytokine production. It was found that bifidobacteria components were generally the most potent in up-regulating IL-10 by both CD11+ and CD11− dendritic cells whereas components of all VSL#3 strains decreased IL-12 production (Mohamadzadeh et al., 2005). While studies on vaginal lactobacilli with respect to their probiotic potential are increasing, significant basic research studies have only been performed on strains GR-1 and RC-14, particularly looking at modes of action. It is clear that these organisms are multifunctional and may affect each host differently. The GR-1 strain does not produce hydrogen peroxide but does produce anti-candida activity as well as bacteriocins and other components, including AI-2 inducers that influence the growth and biofilm development of uropathogens. The organism can down-regulate inflammatory processes, using IL-10 dependent and independent pathways, as shown in macrophages studies (Kim et al. 2006). A human genome array study has shown that a single intravaginal insertion of Lactobacillus GR-1 can up-regulate host defense factors known to be important in fighting infection (Kirjavainen et al., 2008). Meanwhile, studies with Lactobacillus RC-14 strain have shown that it can up-regulate mucin production which may act as a barrier to infection (unpublished data), and down-regulate virulence factor expression in pathogens such as staphylococci [Laughton et al 2006]. The organism also affects cell membrane components in E. coli and produces biosurfactants that inhibit their adhesion to surfaces.

8. The rationale for the use probiotics in reducing the risk associated with HIV

Tremendous efforts are being made to develop effective microbicides for the prevention of HIV-1 sexual transmission and in clear terms it should represents a primary goal for the control of AIDS epidemics worldwide. A promising strategy is the use of bacteria belonging to the vaginal microbiota as live microbicides for the topical production of HIV-1 inhibitors. A recent review has chronicled the potentials of probiotics to prevent HIV (Bolton et al., 2008) and some of the points are lighted in line with the objectives of this section. A study engineered a human vaginal isolate of *Lactobacillus jensenii* to secrete the anti-HIV-1 chemokine RANTES, as well as C1C5 RANTES, a mutated analogue that acts as a CCR5 antagonist and therefore is devoid of proinflammatory activity. Full-length wild-type RANTES and C1C5 RANTES secreted by *L. jensenii* were purified to homogeneity and shown to adopt a correctly folded conformation. Both RANTES variants were shown to inhibit HIV-1 infection in CD4□ T cells and macrophages, displaying strong activity against HIV-1 isolates of different genetic subtypes. The work provides proof of principle for the use of some Lactobacilli, notably *L. jensenii*-produced C1C5 RANTES to block HIV-1 infection of CD4□ T cells and macrophages, setting the basis for the development of a live anti-HIV-1 microbicide targeting CCR5 in an antagonistic manner [Luca et al 2010]

Other studies have previously used Lactobacilli and other probiotic genetically modified bacteria to produce specific HIV inhibitory proteins, both membrane-bound and secreted. A strain of *L. jensenii* was engineered to produce functional CD4, the primary receptor for HIV [Chang et al, 2003]. There are several classes of proteins that bind to the mannose residues of HIV, including a unique 11 kd protein from cyanobacteria (*Nostoc ellipsosporum*) called cyanovirin-N and mannose-binding lectins which also bind to *Neisseria gonorrhoeae* [Botos & Wlodawer, 2005].The human commensal bacterium *Streptococcus gordonii, L. lactis, L. plantarum,* and *L. jensenii* have been genetically engineered to express functional, HIV-binding cyanovirin-N [Pusch et al 2005; Liu et al 2006].An *E. coli* strain which colonizes the colon and rectum, and may thus potentially prevent anal transmission, has been modified to secrete peptides hybridized with hemolysin A, a protein that can complex with the HIV fusion protein gp41 [Rao et al 2005]. FI-1, FI-2, and FI-3 are also peptides that can interfere with gp41 and were cloned into *L. plantarum* and *L. gasseri* [Pusch et al 2006]. *L. reuteri* RC-14, which has been studied as a potential probiotic, was modified to produce 3 HIV entry and fusion inhibitors: CD4D1D2IgKLC, MIP-1□, and T-1249 [Liu et al 2006] Antibody to the cellular adhesion molecule intercellular adhesion molecule has been shown to inhibit cell-mediated trans- epithelial HIV-1 transmission in vitro and was functionally excreted by a bioengineered strain of *L. casei* [Chancey et al 2006]. Some of these products have been used in rodent models, but none has been tested in humans.

By their production of lactic acid, lactobacilli may help maintain a low vaginal pH that can inhibit other bacteria and viruses. Among postmenopausal women receiving estrogen replacement therapy, those who were lactobacilli-positive had low pH 4.4 compared with the lactobacilli-negative women pH 5.2 (Ginkel et al 1993). In 55 menarchal women, colonization with hemolytic streptococci, *G. vaginalis,* or mixed organisms was associated with higher vaginal pH than colonization with normal microbiota and yeast (Caillouette et al. 1997). As previously mentioned, BV is associated with a lack of hydrogen peroxide-producing lactobacilli. Colonization with hydrogen peroxide producers is associated with lower frequency of gonorrhea (Antonio et al 1999). Compared with women colonized with hydrogen peroxide-producing lactobacilli, women colonized with hydrogen peroxide nonproducers or without lactobacilli had unadjusted odds ratios of HSV-2 seroconversion of 2.4 and 2.6, respectively (Cherpes et al 2003). The difference in seroconversion rates may be due to a direct antiviral effect of hydrogen peroxide or due to an increased risk of HSV infection in women with BV.

Several mammalian peroxidases, including myeloperoxidase, eosinophil peroxidase, and lactoperoxidase can combine with hydrogen peroxide and a halide (chloride, iodide, bromide, thiocyanate) to form "a powerful antimicrobial system" effective against many pathogens (Klebanoff et al 1991). Lactobacilli, streptococci, and pneumococci can release hydrogen peroxide and in vitro, in mixed cultures, their toxicity against other bacteria, fungi, viruses, spermatozoa, and tumor cells can be boosted by addition of a peroxidase and a halide. This system was found to inhibit cell-free HIV replication in culture in the presence of hydrogen peroxide-producing, but not nonproducing, lactobacilli (Klebanoff et al 1991a, Klebanoff et al 1991b). *L. crispatus* and *L. jensenii* inhibit gonococci at both acidic and neutral pH. This inhibition is susceptible to bovine catalase, suggesting that hydrogen peroxide is the primary mediator (St Amant et al 2002). Lactobacilli have been found to produce many other bacteriocins, enzymes, and antimicrobial peptides that may make them more competitive in the vaginal microbiota (Silva et al 1987;Naidu et al 1999).

Another potentially beneficial characteristic of probiotic bacteria studied in the gastrointestinal tract is their pleomorphic effect on host mucosal immunity that could affect the vaginal mucosa's defense against HIV and other STIs or resistance to BV (Sheih et al 2001). Evidence for enhancement of humoral responses to rotavirus and *Salmonella typhi* has been shown through IgA levels in probiotic treated children and adults (Kaila et al., 1992). Animal and human data suggest that probiotic use is associated with induction of innate and cell-mediated immune responses (Cross 2002), including increased macrophage phagocytic activity (Miettinen et al 2000), complement and reticuloendothelial activation (Gill et al 2000), stimulation of interferon-gamma, interleukin (IL)-12, and IL-18 (Hessle et al., 1999) and increased natural killer cell activity (Matsuzaki and Chin, 2000). However, the major cell wall component of lactobacilli, muramyldipeptide, can be pyrogenic, and there is concern that lactobacillus enhancement of the T-helper-1 proinflammatory pathway could have negative health consequences (Perdigon and Holgado, 2000). Also, there is concern that the dosage and duration of therapy must be considered so as to optimally enhance and not suppress immunity (Perdigon et al., 1991). Fortunately, probiotic strains have not been found to cause a systemic antibody response (Sheen et al 1995).

Modification of intestinal mucosal immunity by orally administered probiotics may also affect vaginal mucosal immunity to specific pathogens (de Vrese and Schrezenmeir, 2002). In fact, genetic engineering of probiotic bacteria to express pathogen antigens and serve as oral vaccines is being explored (Reveneau et al 2002). In other mucosal vaccine trials, introduction of antigens from HPV and HIV has been accomplished in *S. gordonii* (an oral commensal) and *L. casei*. Local and systemic immune responses were detected in BALB/c mice and Cynomolgus monkeys after vaginal colonization with these strains (Medaglini, 1998). However, there is not yet a good understanding of the relationship between mucosal immunity and BV. In a study of adolescents, BV was found to be inversely associated with lactobacilli counts but was independent of lactobacilli-specific immune responses in isolated peripheral blood leucocytes, and independent of local immune responses measured by antibodies and cytokines measured in cervicovaginal lavages (Alvarez-Olmos et al 2004). In a study of pregnant women, carriage of a variant of the toll-like receptor-4 gene compared with carriage of the dominant genotype was associated with higher vaginal pH and a 10-fold increase in vaginal *G. vaginalis* levels. Colonization with *G. vaginalis* or anaerobic Gram-negative rods in the dominant allele carriers was associated with elevated vaginal IL-1 and IL-1ra but not in the variant homozygotes (Genc 2004). Probiotic modulation of mucosal immunity may help prevent BV and other STIs including HIV, but it is difficult to predict which strains might do this without knowing the immune correlates of protection and how specific strains will affect these factors. More studies are needed in these areas of scientific enquiry.

9. Some clinical evidence of probiotics in helping to reduce the impact of HIV/AIDS

The increased searchlight on HIV/AIDS care in Africa has been rekindled following financial donations from spirited organizations and individuals on increasing access to antiretroviral (ARV) medication. Nevertheless this is cardinal, efforts are also needed to provide safe and affordable interventions for those without access to ARVs or with CD4 counts too high to initiate ARV therapy, yet whose quality of life is diminished by micronutrient deficiencies, gut infections such as diarrhea, and other complicated conditions associated with HIV infection. The use of micronutrients, most notably vitamin B-complex in combination with C and E, appears to be an effective intervention that have been associated with reduced mortality and in most cases it results in increasing the CD4 counts of the infected person.(Kanter et al., 1991; Kaiser et al., 2006;Jiamton et al., 2003) The WHO/FAO has recommended that an "increased micronutrient intake can be best achieved through an adequate diet,"(WHO, 2003) favoring food-based interventions.

It should be noted that the gastrointestinal tract is one of the most severely affected organ by HIV (Kotler et al., 1984;Sharpstone et al., 1999). Inflammation results in damage to the epithelial barrier, leading to an increased leakage of microbial products into the bloodstream. Recently, it was theorized that this may be an ongoing source of systematic immune activation that fuels HIV (Brenchley, 2006) although this association was less clear in an African population (Redd et al., 2009). Capsule proteins of HIV may further facilitate viral replication by eliciting a profound Th-2 activation that inhibits an effective immune response against the virus (Kanter et al., 1991).

Probiotic bacteria can potentially restore an effective gut barrier (Luyer et al., 2005;Yan et al., 2007) thereby reducing systemic immune activation. Furthermore, probiotics have been shown to upregulate T-regulatory lymphocytes (Baroja et al., 2007;Foligne et al., 2008) potentially skewing the immune system away from a Th-2-dominant state (Mohamadzadeh et al., 2005). Probiotic usage has been shown to be safe among people living with HIV (Wolf et al., 1998;Salminen et al., 2004) and recent randomized trials in Brazil (Trois et al., 2008) and Nigeria (Anukam et al., 2006) suggest that probiotic use can increase the CD4 count. In the Nigerian study, conventional yogurt fermented with Lactobacillus delbruekii var bulgaricus and Streptococcus thermophilus was supplemented with probiotic Lactobacillus rhamnosus GR-1 and L. reuteri RC-14. Twenty-four HIV/AIDS adult female patients (18 to 44years) with clinical signs of moderate diarrhea, CD4 counts over 200, and not receiving antiretrovirals or dietary supplements, consumed either 100 mL supplemented or unsupplemented yogurt per day for 15 days. Hematologic profiles, CD4 cell counts, and quality of life was evaluated at baseline, 15 and 30 days postprobiotic-yogurt feeding. There was no significant alteration in the hematologic parameters of both groups before and after the probiotic-yogurt feeding, with the probiotic yogurt group at baseline, 15 and 30 days had a mean WBC count of 5.8 ± 0.76 $X10^9/L$, 6.0 ± 1.02 $X10^9/L$, and 5.4 ± 0.14 $X10^9/L$, respectively. However, the mean CD4 cell count remained the same or increased at 15 and 30 days in 11/12 probiotic-treated subjects compared to 3/12 in the control. Diarrhea, flatulence, and nausea resolved in 12/12 probiotic-treated subjects within 2 days, compared to 2/12 receiving yogurt for 15 days. This is the first study to show the benefits of probiotic yogurt on quality of life of women in Nigeria with HIV/AIDS, and suggests that perhaps a simple fermented food can provide some relief in the management of the AIDS epidemic in Africa.

The most commonly used vehicle for supplying probiotics; yogurt, is a significant source of vitamin A, B-complex, zinc, and high-biologic-quality protein (Sattler et al., 2008) and is therefore, an excellent food-based intervention to improve micronutrient intake among people living with HIV/AIDS. On the basis of these notions, a community kitchen in Mwanza, Tanzania, was established in 2004 to produce yogurt supplemented with Lactobacillus rhamnosus GR-1 (Fiti) to be distributed as an adjunct to the diet of people living with HIV. Irvine et al., (2010) carried out an observational retrospective study over a period of 3 years, with longitudinal comparison of the CD4 count within participants (n=68) before and during probiotic yogurt consumption, and compared with a control group of participants not consuming the yogurt (n=82). Among the yogurt consumers before use and the nonconsumers, an average increase in CD4 count was seen of 0.13 cells/mL/day (95% CI; 0.07-0.20, P=<0.001). After commencing consumption, yogurt consumers experienced an additional increase of 0.28 cells/mL/day (95% CI; 0.10-0.46, P=0.003). When adjusting for length of time using antiretroviral medication, the additional increase explained by yogurt consumption remained 0.17cells/mL/day (95% CI; 0.01-0.34, P=0.04). Treatment with antiretroviral medication was associated with an increase of 0.27 cells/mL/day (95% CI; 0.17-0.38, P=<0.001). The study concluded that introduction of probiotic yogurt, made by local women in a low-income community in Tanzania, was significantly associated with an increase in CD4 count among consumers living with HIV. Another similar study assessed among women with HIV, whether long-term oral Lactobacillus rhamnosus GR-1 and Lactobacillus reuteri RC-14 supplementation can prevent bacterial vaginosis (BV) and enhance the cure rate of metronidazole among those with BV. It involved a randomized, double-blind, placebo-controlled trial conducted among 65 HIV-infected women with an aberrant microbiota (Nugent score 4–10) were selected to receive daily probiotics or placebo for 6 months. Those with BV (Nugent score 7–10) additionally received metronidazole for 10 days (400 mg twice daily). Although there was no enhanced cure rate of BV among women with HIV treated with adjuvant probiotics to metronidazole treatment. However, among women with an intermediate vaginal flora, probiotics tended to increase the probability of a normal vaginal flora (odds ratio 2.4; P=0.1) and significantly increased the probability of a beneficial vaginal pH (odds ratio 3.8; P=0.02) at follow-up (Hummelen et al., 2010)

10. Beware of some probiotic claims

While we suggest the potential use of probiotics may be important in ameliorating the impact of urogenital infections in Africa, however there must be caution in terms of controlling the importation of probiotic products. National agencies in Africa in charge of natural products should be prepared to know the probiotic products there are really called probiotics. There are numerous probiotic claims over the internet which may mislead people in buying useless products.

A number of so-called probiotic products claim to be useful for UTI management. Sadly, their marketing hype is not supported by properly performed human studies. US based Natren, makers of probiotic face cream, claim that oral and vaginal GyNaTren helps 'balance the intestinal and vaginal ecology' and should be used to treat vaginitis. No peer-reviewed studies validate this claim. Other products available in Europe, namely Lactovaginal, Gynoflor, Fermalac, Florgynal, Ecovag, Culturelle VC, SymbioFem Plus and Yeast- guard all suffer from lack of appropriate clinical sub- stantiation, and cannot be recommended to prevent UTI. Clearly, companies marketing such products have an obligation to provide evidence of clinical efficacy. This is predicated on the fact that some products may contain different genera, different species, or even different strains of the same species, and not all products should be expected to work the same. Therefore, claims of efficacy should be target specific and should be made only for products that have been found efficacious in carefully designed studies. The marketplace has many examples of different strains of the same species: Lactobacillus acidophilus NCFM and La-1; L. rhamnosus GR-1 and L. rhamnosus GG; Lactobacillus casei Shirota and DN-114 001; Lactobacillus reuteri RC-14 and ATCC 55730; and Bifidobacterium lactis HN019 and BB-12; *Lactobacillus plantarum* WCFS1, *Lactobacillus plantarum* KCA-1. Each of these strains has a unique dossier to document individual health benefits. It is noteworthy, however, that among dozens of European commercial products, the same biotype (based on pulsed-field gel electrophoresis of chromosomal DNA) was predominant among Bifidobacterium- containing products (Masco et al., 2005), suggesting that Bifidobacterium strains used commercially may not be so diverse. The fact that consumers buy such products suggests that the current management of urogenital infections is not sufficiently well handled by the sole use of antimicrobials. In addition, patients, particularly those suffering from recurrent infections, are well aware of the side effects of antibiotic therapy and the ever-increasing problem of bacterial resistance.

11. Can the use of probiotics make an impact in Africa?

The presence of bacterial vaginosis-causing organisms that are perhaps more prevalent in Africa provokes the loss of normal vaginal bacterial flora, and causes vaginal inflammation and increased pH levels. The resulting altered vaginal environment increases the risk of transmission of HIV. In addition diarrhoeal diseases, HIV/AIDS complications, and other infectious diseases are major contributors to morbidity and mortality in sub-Saharan Africa. Morbidity from these illnesses causes economic hardship and mortality results in the loss of the next generation and destruction of the present adult leadership. Several studies have pointed out that the use of probiotics can significantly improve the wellbeing of individuals infected with HIV/AIDS (Anukam, 2007). For example, studies conducted in Africa have estimated the average annual increase in CD4 count of 90cells/mL with ARV treatment (Lawn et al., 2006) and an average decline of 20 to 50 cells/mL/year without ARV treatment (Holmes et al., 2006;Urassa et al., 2004). In the Tanzanian study, (Irvine et al., 2010), a similar rate of increase was observed of 99 cells/mL with ARV treatment (0.27 cells/mL/d), whereas no significant decrease was observed without ARV treatment. The results of this study indicate that probiotic yogurt consumption is associated with an overall increase in CD4 count of 62 cells/mL/year (0.17 cells/mL/d). This could be due to an accelerated immune reconstitution after initiation of ARV treatment, thus shortening the time of severe immune deficiency, or may be due to an increase in CD4 count among those not yet eligible for ARV treatment, which may potentially delay the need for ARV medication. However, this study is yet to be replicated in other African sites with similar burden of HIV infections.

Indication	Probiotic Genus, Species and Strain	Source and Product format
Vaginal application	*Lactobacillus rhamnosus* GR-1 and *Lactobacillus reuteri* RC-14	Fem-Dophilus (capsules) www.urexbiotech.com; www.jarrow.com
Antibiotic associated diarrhea; *Clostridium difficile*	*Saccharomyces cerevisiae* (*S. boulardii*)	Florastor (powder) www.florastor.com Lalflor (capsule) www.institut-rosell.com
	L rhamnosus GG	Culturelle (capsule) www.culturelle.com Danimals (drinkable yogurt) www.danimals.com
	L casei DN114001	DanActive (fermented milk) www.danactive.com
	L acidophilus CL1285 plus L casei	BioK□CL1285 (fermented milk, capsule) www.biokplus.com
Gut transit time	*B animalis* DN173 010 (Bifidus regularis)	Activia (yogurt) www.activia.com
Infant diarrhea	*L rhamnosus* GG (LGG)	Culturelle (capsule) www.culturelle.com Danimals (drinkable yogurt) www.danimals.com
	L casei DN114001 (Immunitas)	DanActive (fermented milk) www.danactive.com
Inflammatory bowel conditions (primary evidence in pouchitis)	8-strain combination of 3 *Bifidobacterium* strains, 4 *Lactobacillus* strains and *S. thermophilus*	VSL#3 (powder) www.vsl3.com
Keeping healthy	*L reuteri* ATCC 55730	BioGaia Chewable Gut Health Tablets, BioGaia Gut Health Probiotic Straws, www.everidis.com
Lactose intolerance	Most strains *L bulgaricus* and/or *S thermophilus*	All yogurts with live, active cultures
Immune support	*B lactis* HN019 (HOWARU or DR10)	Strain sold as an ingredient for dairy and supplement products—contact Danisco www.danisco.com
	B lactis Bb-12	Good Start Natural Cultures (infant formula) www.verybestbaby.com/GoodStart/Overview.aspx Yo-Plus (yogurt) www.yo-plus.com
	L casei DN114001	DanActive (fermented milk) www.danactive.com

Table 2. Some probiotic products with published clinical studies

12. Conclusions

Several studies have shown that probiotics could enhance the health and well-being of individuals in sub-Saharan Africa, but sadly the use of probiotics has not become popular for several reasons outlined by Anukam and Reid (2005). First, pharmaceutical companies that manufacture probiotics would be forced to lower prices, which would adversely affect their revenues. Secondly, storage and distribution problems make the allocation of probiotics difficult. Dairy versions of probiotics require refrigeration, and other forms incorporated in tablets, capsules, and powders must be retained in proper vials with appropriate dessicants. Accordingly, storage and distribution issues present major challenges to the effective implementation of probiotic treatment since domestic technology is frequently insufficient for proper maintenance. Finally, cultural acceptance presents a major challenge for probiotic use. For example, if local customs call for a diet free of dairy products, it could be difficult to convince these people to consume a fermented milk drink.

The lack of any probiotic fermented food products in Africa at present, with the exception of a grass roots community kitchen in Tanzania where probiotic *Lactobacillus rhamnosus* GR-1 is used (www.westernheadseast.ca), makes it difficult to perform studies and provide benefits to the population. Until this happens, hopefully with clinically proven products and not simply ones where the term probiotic is used or bacteria are added as an ingredient without testing, indigenous fermented foods may be explored further as a source of health benefits.

While many fermented foods are eaten in Africa soon after being produced, the lack of refrigerated distribution networks makes it difficult to reach a large population. In this context, McMaster et al., (2005), developed a microencapsulation delivery system for *Bifidobacterium lactis* DSM 10140, which if successfully applied to foods might overcome some of the shelf-life problems faced by lack of refrigeration. The study used two existing traditional fermented foods, "amasi" and "mahewu." The gellan/xanthan microcapsules containing viable *B. lactis* were tested under simulated physiological conditions and added to pasteurized beverages. The results showed protection of the organism in low pH and against the biocidal activity of pancreatic and bile acids. For "mahewu," microencapsulation of *B. lactis* with storage aerobically at 4oC and 22oC enhanced survival over a 21-day period compared to free cells. This is still not reflective of extreme temperatures found in Africa, so further studies are needed to confirm if this method will lead to making 'mahewu' available to people.

In confirming the validity of evidence on probiotics, the United Nations Food and Agriculture Organization and the World Health Organization (WHO/FAO, 2001) sponsored an Expert Consultation in 2001. The resulting Report stressed that "Efforts should be made to make probiotic products more widely available, especially for relief work and populations at high risk of morbidity and mortality". Eleven years later, this clarion call to the healthcare community and to the food industries in providing probiotics to the people of sub-Saharan Africa has yet to be answered.

With the increasing number of people living and dying of AIDS, only a few people have easy access to life-prolonging antiretroviral drug therapy. The HIV/AIDS pandemic is propelled by social, cultural and economic gender inequalities that limit children and women's ability to protect themselves from infection. The main strategies by UNAIDS for HIV prevention are promotion of condoms, reducing the number of sexual partners, and treatment of reproductive tract infections. These strategies are laudable but not feasible for many women. Occasionally, it may seem appropriate to provide perspective and to verbalize concerns and disquietude anytime the UN publishes the life expectancy of the people from developing countries. No one has taken the pain to ask the question why the Japanese, coincidently with a long history of probiotic consumption, have the highest life expectancy in the world today and low HIV prevalence (<0.1%, contributed through contaminated blood products) (Oelrichs, 2004), while the people from sub-Saharan Africa, coincidently with no classically defined probiotic consumption, have the lowest life expectancy in the world, and the highest HIV prevalence. Besides, there are no available probiotics to boost the immune system (Gill et al., 2002), treat diarrhea and prevent urogenital infections.

More studies and interest are needed to expand our understanding of this approach to healthcare in sub-Saharan Africa, to knowing their limitations and understanding their mechanisms of action, and examining economic, social, political and behavioral changes for more expansive introduction of probiotic concepts. Hopefully, concerted research efforts will stimulate other scientists, students, and physicians to explore this area. The development of recombinant strains expressing potent anti-HIV microbicides may provide a more specific preventive approach in future years.

Making probiotic products available to both the uninfected and infected persons, gives them opportunity to choose among other health promoting products. Probiotics may be a viable paradigm towards reducing the risk associated with acquisition of HIV mostly in women by restoring the vaginal microbiota and help relieve the suffering of AIDS patients, most of who suffer from chronic diarrhea.

13. Acknowledgement

Dr. Kingsley C Anukam research on probiotic genomics is funded by the Academy of Sciences for the Developing World (TWAS).

14. References

Altman, L (2002) 'By 2010, AIDS May Leave 20 Million African Orphans'. *New York Times;* 11:A-10.

Alvarez-Olmos MI, Barousse MM, Rajan L, et al., (2004).Vaginal lactobacilli in adolescents: Presence and relationship to local and systemic immunity, and to bacterial vaginosis. *Sex Transm Dis,* 31:393–400.

Amsel R, Totten PA, Spiegel CA, et al., (1983). Nonspecific vaginitis. Diagnostic criteria and microbial and epidemiologic associations. *Am J Med,* 74:14–22

Antonio MA, Rabe LK, Hillier SL. (2005).Colonization of the rectum by Lactobacillus species and decreased risk of bacterial vaginosis. *J Infect Dis.* 192(3):394-8.

Antonio MA, Hawes SE, Hillier SL. (1999). The identification of vaginal *Lactobacillus* species and the demographic and microbiologic char- acteristics of women colonized by these species. *J Infect Dis* 180:1950 -1956.

Anukam KC, Macklaim JM, Gloor GB, Reid G, Seizen R (2011). Genome sequencing of Lactobacillus plantarum KCA-1, a potential probiotic lactica bacterium isolated from the vagina of a healthy Nigerian woman. *Joint International Conference of the African and South African Societies of Human Genetics,* Cape Town, South Africa, 6-9 March 2011. Poster 013.

Anukam KC, Osazuwa EO, Ahonkhai I, Reid G. (2006). Lactobacillus vaginal microbiota of women attending a reproductive health care service in Benin City, Nigeria. *Sex Trans Dis.* 33(1): 59-62

Anukam KC, Osazuwa EO, Ahonkhai I, Ngwu M, Osemene G, Bruce AW and Reid G (2006a). Augmentation of antimicrobial metronidazole therapy of bacterial vaginosis with oral probiotic *Lactobacillus rhamnosus* GR-1 and *Lactobacillus reuteri* RC-14: randomized, double-blind, placebo controlled trial. *Microbes Infect*, 8 (6):1450-1454

Anukam KC, Osazuwa E, Osemene GI, Ehigiagbe F, Bruce AW, Reid G (2006b). Clinical study comparing probiotic *Lactobacillus* GR-1 and RC-14 with metronidazole vaginal gel to treat symptomatic bacterial vaginosis. *Microbes Infect*, 8 (12-13):2772-2776.

Anukam KC, Osazuwa EO, Osadolor HB, et al. (2008). Yogurt containing probiotic *Lactobacillus rhamnosus* GR-1 and *L. reuteri* RC-14 helps resolve moderate diarrhea and increases CD4 count in HIV/AIDS patients. *J Clin Gastroenterol.* 42:239–243.

Anukam KC (2007). The potential role of probiotics in reducing poverty-associated infections in developing countries. *J Infect Developing Countries,* 1(2):81-83.

Anukam K, Reid G (2005). Providing probiotics to sub-Saharan Africa: ethical principles to consider. *J Complementary and Integrative Med,* 2: Article 10.

Auvert B, Taljaard D, Lagarde E, Sobngwi-Tambekou J, Sitta R, et al. (2005) Randomized, controlled intervention trial of male circumcision for reduction of HIV infection risk: The ANRS 1265 trial. *PLoS Med* 2(11): e298.

Bailey RC, Moses S, Parker CB, Agot K, Maclean I, et al. (2007). Male circumcision for HIV prevention in young men in kisumu, kenya: A randomised controlled trial. *Lancet*, 369(9562): 643–656.

Baroja ML, Kirjavainen PV, Hekmat S, et al., (2007). Anti-inflammatory effects of probiotic yogurt in inflammatory bowel disease patients. *Clinical Experimental Immunol*, 149:470–479

Bolton M, Straten AV, Cohen CR (2008). Probiotics: potential to prevent HIV and sexually transmitted infections in women. *Sex Trans Dis*, 35(3):214-225.

Botos I, Wlodawer A (2005). Proteins that bind high-mannose sugars of the HIV envelope. *Prog Biophys Mol Biol,* 88:233–282.

Brenchley JM, Price DA, Schacker TW, et al., (2006). Microbial translocation is a cause of systemic immune activation in chronic HIV infection. *Nat Med.*12:1365–1371.

Bruce AW, Reid G (1988). Intravaginal instillation of lactobacilli for prevention of recurrent urinary tract infections. *Can J Microbiol.* 34:339–343.

Caillouette JC, Sharp CF Jr, Zimmerman GJ, et al. , (1997). Vaginal pH as a marker for bacterial pathogens and menopausal status. *Am J Obstet Gynecol*, 176:1270–1275; discussion 5–7.

Chancey CJ, Khanna KV, Seegers JF, et al., (2006). Lactobacilli-expressed single-chain variable fragment (scFv) specific for intercellular ad- hesion molecule 1 (ICAM-1) blocks cell-associated HIV-1 trans- mission across a cervical epithelial monolayer. *J Immunol.* 176:5627–5636.

Chang TL, Chang CH, Simpson DA, et al., (2003). Inhibition of HIV infec- tivity by a natural human isolate of *Lactobacillus jensenii* engi- neered to express functional two-domain CD4. *Proc Natl Acad Sci U S A*, 100:11672–11677.

Cherpes TL, Meyn LA, Krohn MA, et al., (2003). Association between acquisition of herpes simplex virus type 2 in women and bacterial vaginosis. *Clin Infect Dis*, 37:319–325

Cross ML (2002). Microbes versus microbes: Immune signals generated by probiotic lactobacilli and their role in protection against microbial pathogens. *FEMS Immunol Med Microbiol*, 34:245–253

DeBaets AJ, Bulterys M, Abrams EJ, Kankassa C, Pazvakavambwa IE (2007). Care and treatment of HIV-infected children in Africa: issues and challenges at the district hospital level. *Pediatr Infect Dis J*, 26(2):163-173

de Jong MA, Geijtenbeek TB (2009). Human immunodeficiency virus-1 acquisition in genital mucosa: Langerhans cells as key-players. *J Intern Med*, 265(1): 18–28.

Delia A, Morgante G, Rago G, Musacchio MC, Petraglia F, De Leo V (2006). Effectiveness of oral administration of *Lactobacillus paracasei* subsp. *paracasei* F19 in association with vaginal suppositories of *Lactobacillus acidofilus* in the treatment of vaginosis and in the prevention of recurrent vaginitis. Minerva Ginecol. 58(3):227-31.

de Vrese M, Schrezenmeir J (2002). Probiotics and non-intestinal infectious conditions. *Br J Nutr*, 88(suppl 1):S59–S66.

Ellis AK, Verma S. (2000). Quality of life in women with urinary tract infections: is benign disease a misnomer? *J Am Board Fam Pract*, 13:392-397.

Eschenbach DA, Davick PR, William BL, et al. (1989). Prevalence of hydrogen peroxide-producing Lactobacillus species in normal women and women with bacterial vaginosis. *J Clin Microbiol*, 27:251-256.

Ewaschuk JB, Backer JL, Churchill TA, *et al., (2007)*. Surface expression of Toll-like receptor 9 is upregulated on intestinal epithelial cells in response to pathogenic bacterial DNA. *Infect Immun*, 75:2572–2579.

Falagas ME, Betsi GI, Tokas T, Athanasiou S (2006). Probiotics for prevention of recurrent urinary tract infections in women: a review of the evidence from microbiological and clinical studies. Drugs. 66(9):1253-61

Ferris DG, Dekle C, Litaker MS (1996). Women's use of over-the-counter antifungal medications for gynecologic symptoms. *J Fam Pract*, 42:595-600.

Foligne B, Zoumpopoulou G, Dewulf J, et al., (2007). A key role of dendritic cells in probiotic functionality. PLoS ONE, 2:e313.

Fredricks DN, Fiedler TL, Thomas KK, et al.,(2007). Targeted polymerase- chain-reaction for the detection of vaginal bacteria associated with bacterial vaginosis. *J Clin Microbiol*, 45:3270–3276.

Galvin SR, Cohen MS (2004). The role of sexually transmitted diseases in HIV transmission. *Nat Rev Microbiol*, 2(1): 33–42.

Genc MR, Vardhana S, Delaney ML, et al., (2004). Relationship between a toll-like receptor-4 gene polymorphism, bacterial vaginosis-related flora and vaginal cytokine responses in pregnant women. *Eur J Obstet Gynecol Reprod Biol*, 116:152–156

Gill HS, Rutherfurd KJ, Prasad J, et al., (2002). Enhancement of natural and acquired immunity by *Lactobacillus rhamnosus* (HN001), *Lacto- bacillus acidophilus* (HN017) and *Bifidobacterium lactis* (HN019) *Br J Nutr*, 83:167–176.

Ginkel PD, Soper DE, Bump RC, et al., (1993). The vaginal flora in post-menopausal women: The effect of estrogen replacement. *Infect Dis Obstet Gynecol*, 1:94.

Gray RH, Kigozi G, Serwadda D, Makumbi F, Nalugoda F, et al. (2009). The effects of male circumcision on female partners' genital tract symptoms and vaginal infections in a randomized trial in rakai, uganda. *Am J Obstet Gynecol*, 200(1): 42.e1–42.e7.

Hay PE, Lamont RF, Taylor-Robinson D, Morgan DJ, Ison C, Pearson J (1994). Abnormal bacterial colonisation of the genital tract and subsequent preterm delivery and late miscarriage. *Bmj,* 308(6924):295-298

Hay P. (2000). Recurrent bacterial vaginosis. *Curr Infect Dis Rep,* 2: 506-512.

Hessle C, Hanson LA, Wold AE (1999). Lactobacilli from human gastrointestinal mucosa are strong stimulators of IL-12 production. *Clin Exp Immunol,* 116:276–282.

Hillebrand L, Harmanli OH, Whiteman V, Khandelwal M (2002). Urinary tract infections in pregnant women with bacterial vaginosis. *Am J Obstet Gynecol,* 186(5):916-917

Hoesl CE, Altwein JE (2005). The probiotic approach: an alternative treatment option in urology. *Eur Urol.,* 47(3):288-96

Hummelen R, Changalucha J, Butamanya NL, Cook A, Habbema JDF, Reid G (2010). *Lactobacillus rhamnosus* GR-1 and L.*reuteri* RC-14 to prevent or cure bacterial vaginosis among women with HIV, *Int J Gynecol Obstet,* doi:10.1016/j.ijgo.2010.07.008

Irvine SL, Hummelen R, Hekmat S, Looman CWN, Habbema JDF, Reid G (2010). Probiotic yogurt consumption is associated with an increase of CD4 count among people living with HIV/AIDS. *J Clin Gastroenterol,* 44:e201–e205.

Holmes C, Wood R, Badri M, et al., (2006). CD4 decline and incidence of opportunistic infections in Cape Town, South Africa: implications for prophylaxis and treatment. *J Acquired Immune Deficiency Syndromes,* 42:464–469.

Jiamton S, Pepin J, Suttent R (2003). A randomized trial of the impact of multiple micronutrient supplementation on mortality among HIV-infected individuals living in Bangkok. AIDS (London, England), 17:2461–2469.

Kaila M, Isolauri E, Soppi E, et al., (1992). Enhancement of the circulating antibody secreting cell response in human diarrhea by a human *Lactobacillus* strain. *Pediatr* Res, 32:141–144.

Kanter AS, Spencer DC, Steinberg MH, et al., (1999). Supplemental vitamin B and progression to AIDS and death in black South African patients infected with HIV. *J Acquir Immune Defic Syndr,* 21:252–253.

Kaiser JD, Adriana MC, Ondercin JP, et al. Micronutrient supplementation increases CD4 count in HIV-infected indivi- duals on highly active antiretroviral therapy: a prospective, double-blinded, placebo-controlled trial. J Acquired Immune Deficiency Syndromes (1999). 2006;42:523–528.

Keane FE, Ison CA, Taylor-Robinson D (1997). A longitudinal study of the vaginal flora over a menstrual cycle. *Int J STD AIDS* 8:489-494.

Kim SO, Sheikh HI, Ha S, Martins A, Reid G (2006). G-CSF-mediated inhibition of JNK is a key mechanism for *Lactobacillus rhamnosus*-induced suppression of TNF production in macrophages. *Cell Microbiol,* 8(12), 1958–1971.

Kirjavainen P K, Laine RM, Carter D, Hammond JA, Reid G. 2008. Expression of anti-microbial defense factors in vaginal mucosa following exposure to *Lactobacillus rhamnosus* GR-1. *Int. J. Probiotics.* 3: 99-106.

Klebanoff SJ, Coombs RW (1991a). Viricidal effect of *Lactobacillus acidophilus* on human immunodeficiency virus type 1: Possible role in heterosexual transmission. *J Exp Med,* 174:289–292.

Klebanoff SJ, Hillier SL, Eschenbach DA, et al (1991b). Control of the microbial flora of the vagina by H2O2-generating lactobacilli. *J Infect Dis,* 164:94–100

Klebanoff MA, Schwebke JR, Zhang J, Nansel TR, Yu KF, Andrews WW (2004). Vulvovaginal symptoms in women with bacterial vaginosis. *Obstet Gynecol,* 104(2):267-72

Kline MW (2006). Perspectives on the pediatric HIV/AIDS pandemic: catalyzing access of children to care and treatment. *Pediatrics,* 117(4):1388-1393.

Kotler DP, Gaetz HP, Lange M, et al., (1984). Enteropathy associated with the acquired immunodeficiency syndrome. *Ann Intern Med,* 101:421–428.

Laughton J, Devillard E, Heinrichs D, Reid G, McCormick J. (2006). Inhibition of expression of a staphylococcal superantigen-like protein by a secreted signaling factor from *Lactobacillus reuteri. Microbiology,* 152: 1155-1167

Lawn SD, Myer L, Bekker LG, et al., (2006). CD4 cell count recovery among HIV-infected patients with very advanced immuno- deficiency commencing antiretroviral treatment in sub-Saharan Africa. *BMC Infectious Diseases,* 6:59.

Liu X, Lagenaur LA, Simpson DA, et al., (2006). Engineered vaginal *Lactobacillus* strain for mucosal delivery of the human immunodeficiency virus inhibitor cyanovirin-N. *Antimicrob Agents Chemother,* 50:3250–3259.

Liu JJ, Reid G, Jiang Y, et al., (2006). Activity of HIV entry and fusion inhibitors expressed by the human vaginal colonizing probiotic *Lactobacillus reuteri* RC-14. *Cell Microbiol,* 31:31.

Livengood CH, Soper DE, Sheehan KL, et al. (1999). Comparison of once-daily and twice-daily dosing of 0.75% metronidazole gel in the treatment of bacterial vaginosis. *Sex Transm Dis,* 26:137-142.

Luyer MD, Buurman WA, Hadfoune M, et al. (2005). Strain-specific effects of probiotics on gut barrier integrity following hemorrhagic shock. *Infection Immunity,* 73:3686–3692.

Martin HL, Richardson BA, Nyange PM, et al., (1999). Vaginal lactobacilli, microbial flora, and risk of human immunodeficiency virus type 1 and sexually transmitted disease acquisition. *J Infect Dis.* 180:1863-1868.

Masco L, Huys G, De Brandt E, et al., (2005). Culture-dependent and culture-independent qualitative analysis of probiotic products claimed to contain bifidobacteria. *Int J Food Microbiol,* 102:221–30.

Matsuzaki T, Chin J (2000). Modulating immune responses with probiotic bacteria. *Immunol Cell Biol,* 78:67–73.

McCoombe SG, Short RV (2006) Potential HIV-1 target cells in the human penis. *AIDS,* 20(11): 1491–1495.

McMaster LD, Kokott SA, Reid SJ, Abratt VR (2005). Use of traditional African fermented beverages as delivery vehicles for *Bifidobacterium lactis* DSM 10140. *Int J Food Microbiol,* 102:231–237.

McNeil D (2010). At Front Lines: AIDS War is Falling Apart. *New York Time,* May 8.

Medaglini D, Oggioni MR, Pozzi G (1998). Vaginal immunization with recombinant gram-positive bacteria. *Am J Reprod Immunol* 39:199 -208

Miettinen M, Lehtonen A, Julkunen I, et al., (2000). Lactobacilli and Streptococci activate NF-kappa B and STAT signaling pathways in human macrophages. *J Immunol,* 164:3733–3740

Mohamadzadeh M, Olson S, Kalina WV, et al (2005). Lactobacilli activate human dendritic cells that skew T cells toward T helper 1 polarization. *Proc Natl Aca Sci USA.*102:2880–2885

MSF (2009). *HIV/AIDS treatment in developing countries: The battle for long-term survival has just begun.* Geneva: Médicins Sans Frontières

Naidu AS, Bidlack WR, Clemens RA (1999). Probiotic spectra of lactic acid bacteria (LAB). *Crit Rev Food Sci Nutr*, 39:13–126

Nugent RP, Krohn MA, Hillier SL (1991). Reliability of diagnosing bacterial vaginosis is improved by a standardized method of gram stain interpretation. *J Clin Microbiol*, 29:297–301.

Oakeshott P, Hay P, Hay S, Steinke F, Rink E, Kerry S (2002). Association between bacterial vaginosis or chlamydial infection and miscarriage before 16 weeks' gestation: prospective community based cohort study. *Bmj*, 325(7376):1334

Oelrichs R, (2004). The subtypes of human immunodeficiency virus in Australia and Asia. *Sexual Health* 1:1-11.

Patterson BK, Landay A, Siegel JN, Flener Z, Pessis D, et al. (2002) Susceptibility to human immunodeficiency virus-1 infection of human foreskin and cervical tissue grown in explant culture. *Am J Pathol*, 161(3): 867–873.

Perdigon G, Alvarez S, Pesce de Ruiz Holgado A (1991). Immunoadjuvant activity of oral *Lactobacillus casei*: Influence of dose on the secretory immune response and protective capacity in intestinal infections. *J Dairy Res*, 58:485–496

Perdigon G, Holgado APdR (2000). Mechanisms involved in the immunos- timulation by lactic acid bacteria. In: Perdigon G, Fuller R, eds. *Probiotics*. Amsterdam, The Netherlands: Kluwer Academic, 213–233.

Price LB, Liu CM, Johnson KE, Aziz M, Lau MK, et al. (2010) The Effects of Circumcision on the Penis Microbiome. *PLoS ONE* 5(1): e8422. doi:10.1371/ journal.pone.0008422.

Pusch O, Boden D, Hannify S, et al., (2005). Bioengineering lactic acid bacteria to secrete the HIV-1 virucide cyanovirin. *J Acquir Immune Defic Syndr*, 40:512–520.

Pusch O, Kalyanaraman R, Tucker LD, et al., (2006). An anti-HIV microbicide engineered in commensal bacteria: Secretion of HIV-1 fusion inhibitors by lactobacilli. *AIDS*, 20:1917-1922.

Rakoff-Nahoum S, Paglino J, Eslami-Varzaneh F, *et al.*, (2004). Recognition of commensal microflora by toll-like receptors is required for intestinal homeostasis. *Cell*, 118:229–241.

Rao S, Hu S, McHugh L, et al., (2005). Toward a live microbial microbicide for HIV: Commensal bacteria secreting an HIV fusion inhibitor peptide. *Proc Natl Acad Sci U S A*, 102:11993–11998.

Ravel J, Gajer P, Abdo Z, Schneider GM, Koenig SK, McCulle SL, Karlebach S, Gorle R, Russell J, Tacket CO, Brotman RM,

Davis CC, Ault K, Peralta L, Forney LJ (2011). Vaginal microbiome of reproductive-age women. Proc Natl Acad Sci USA, 108: 4680–4687.

Redd AD, Dabitao D, Bream JH, et al., (2009). Microbial translo- cation, the innate cytokine response, and HIV-1 disease progression in Africa. *Proc Natl Aca Sci USA*, 106:6718–6723

Reid G, Bruce AW, Cook RL, Llano M.(1990). Effect on the urogenital flora of antibiotic therapy for urinary tract infection. *Scand J Infect Dis*, 22:43–7

Reid G, Bruce AW, Taylor M (1995). Instillation of Lactobacillus and stimulation of indigenous organisms to prevent recurrence of urinary tract infections. *Microecol. Ther*. 23:32–45.

Reid G. (1999). The scientific basis for probiotic strains of Lactobacillus. *Appl Environ Microbiol*, 65:3763-3766.

Reid G, Beuerman D, Heinemann C, Bruce AW (2001). Probiotic *Lactobacillus* dose required to restore and maintain a normal vaginal flora. *FEMS Immunol. Med. Microbiol*, 32: 37-41

Reid G, Bruce AW, Fraser N, et al., (2001). Oral probiotics can resolve urogenital infections. *FEMS Microbiol Immunol.* 30:49–52.

Reid G, Bruce AW (2006). Probiotics to prevent urinary tract infections: the rationale and evidence. *World J Urol.* 24(1):28-32.

Reid G, Charbonneau D, Erb J, et al. (2003). Oral use of Lactobacillus rhamnosus GR-1 and L. fermentum RC-14 significantly alters vaginal flora: randomized, placebo-controlled trial. *FEMS Immunol Med Microbiol*, 35:131–134.

Report (2009). National HIV/AIDS Sentinel Seroprevalence Survey. Federal Ministry of Health (FMOH), Abuja, Nigeria. 20

Reveneau N, Geoffroy MC, Locht C, et al., (2002). Comparison of the immune responses induced by local immunizations with recombinant *Lactobacillus plantarum* producing tetanus toxin fragment C in different cellular locations. *Vaccine,* 20(13–14): 1769 -1777.

Salminen MK, Tynkkynen S, Rautelin H, et al., (2004). The efficacy and safety of probiotic Lactobacillus rhamnosus GG on prolonged, noninfectious diarrhea in HIV patients on anti- retroviral therapy: a randomized, placebo-controlled, cross- over study. *HIV Clinical Trials*, 5:183–191.

Sattler FR, Rajicic N, Mulligan K, et al., (2008). Evaluation of high-protein supplementation in weight-stable HIV-positive subjects with a history of weight loss: a randomized, double- blind, multicenter trial. *American J Clinical Nutr.* 88: 1313–1321.

Sengupta, (2002). "U.N. Session Begins to Tally the Perils of Being Young". *New York Times,* 9:A- 14.

Sewankambo N, Gray RH, Wawer MJ, et al., (1997). HIV- 1 infection associated with abnormal vaginal flora morphology and bacterial vaginosis. Lancet, 350:546-550

Sharpstone D, Neild P, Crane R, et al., (1999). Small intestinal transit, absorption, and permeability in patients with AIDS with and without diarrhoea. *Gut*, 45:70–76.

Sheen P, Oberhelman RA, Gilman RH, et al., (1995). Short report: A placebo-controlled study of *Lactobacillus* GG colonization in one-to-three-year-old Peruvian children. *Am J Trop Med Hyg*, 52:389–392.

Sheih YH, Chiang BL, Wang LH, et al., (2001). Systemic immunity-enhancing effects in healthy subjects following dietary consumption of the lactic acid bacterium *Lactobacillus rhamnosus* HN001. *J Am Coll Nutr* 20(2 suppl):149–156

Silva M, Jacobus NV, Deneke C, et al., (1987). Antimicrobial substance from a human *Lactobacillus* strain. *Antimicrob Agents Chemother* , 31:1231–1233.

Smart S, Singal A, Mindel A (2004). Social and sexual risk factors for bacterial vaginosis. *Sex Transm Infect*, 80(1):58-62.

Sorek R, Kunin V, Hugenholtz P (2008). CRISPR—a widespread system that provides acquired resistance against phage in bacteria and archaea. *Nat. Rev. Microbiol.* 6:181–186

St Amant DC, Valentin-Bon IE, Jerse AE (2002). Inhibition of *Neisseria gonorrhoeae* by *Lactobacillus* species that are commonly isolated from the female genital tract. *Infect Immun*, 70:7169–7171

Taha TE, Hoover DR, Dallabetta GA, et al. (1999). Bacterial vaginosis and disturbances of vaginal flora: association with increased acquisition of HIV. *AIDS.* 12:1699-706.

UNAIDS (2009). *Report on the Global AIDS Epidemic.* Geneva.

UNAIDS (2002).Press release. "UNAIDS Releases New Data Highlighting the Devastating Impact of AIDS in Africa."

http:/www.unaids/whatsnew/press/eng/pressarc02/G8_250602.html (accessed 4 July 2010)

Urassa W, Bakari M, Sandstrom E, et al. , (2004). Rate of decline of absolute number and percentage of CD4T lymphocytes among HIV-1-infected adults in Dar es Salaam, Tanzania. *AIDS*, 18:433–438.

Vale PF, Little TJ. (2010). CRISPR-mediated phage resistance and the ghost of coevolution past. *Proc. R. Soc. Lond. B Biol. Sci.* 277:2097–2103

Van Niekerk A(2001). 'Moral and Social Complexities of AIDS in Africa'. Journal of Medicine and Philosophy, 27;2: 144

Verhelst R, Verstraelen H, Claeys G, et al., (2005). Comparison between Gram stain and culture for the characterization of vaginal microflora: Definition of a distinct grade that resembles grade I microflora and revised categorization of grade I microflora. *BMC Microbiol*, 5:61.

Walker WA, Goulet O, Morelli L, Antoine JM(2006). Progress in the science of probiotics: from cellular microbiology and applied immunology to clinical nutrition. *Eur J Nutr.* 45 Suppl 9:1-18

Wiesenfeld HC, Hillier SL, Krohn MA, Lander DV, Swet RL (2003). Bacterial vaginosis is a strong predictor of *Neisseria gonorrhoeae* and *Chlamydia trachomatis* infection. *Clin Infect Dis*, 36:663-668.

Wilson JD, Ralph SG, Rutherford AJ (2002). Rates of bacterial vaginosis in women undergoing in vitro fertilisation for different types of infertility. *Bjog*, 109(6):714-717

WHO/FAO (2001). Health and nutritional properties of probiotics in food including powder milk with live lactic acid bacteria, a joint FAO/WHO expert consultation. [WHO website] October 1–4. Available at:
www.who.int/foodsafety/publications/fs_management/en/probiotics.pdf
Accessed March 30, 2011.

WHO (2003). Technical Consultation on Nutrient Requirements for People Living with HIV/AIDS. Available at:
http://www.who.int/nutrition/publications/
Content_nutrient_requirements.pdf. Accessed March 30, 2011.

Wolf BW, Wheeler KB, Ataya DG, et al., (1998). Safety and tolerance of Lactobacillus reuteri supplementation to a population infected with the human immunodeficiency virus. *Food Chem Toxicol.* 36:1085–1094.

Yan F, Cao H, Cover TL, et al., (2007). Soluble proteins produced by probiotic bacteria regulate intestinal epithelial cell survival and growth. *Gastroenterology*, 132:562–575.

Zyrek AA, Cichon C, Helms S, *et al.*, (2007). Molecular mechanisms underlying the probiotic effects of Escherischia coli Nissie 1917 involve ZO-2 and PKCzeta redistribution resulting in tight junction and epithelial barrier repair. *Cell Microbiol*, 9:804–816

10

Poverty, Parasitosis and HIV/AIDS - Major Health Concerns in Tanzania

Kennedy Daniel Mwambete and Mary Justin-Temu
Muhimbili University of Health and Allied Sciences, Tanzania

1. Introduction

Poverty, parasitosis and HIV/AIDS are closely interlinked and co-circulate in many populations. HIV/AIDS, parasitic infections like malaria and other opportunistic infections, and in a few are by far the commonest causes of ill-health and death in the poorest countries of the world, that happen to be in the tropics and temperate countries in Africa, Asia, and South America. Parasitic infections remain an important cause of morbidity and mortality in developing countries especially among HIV-infected persons.

There are indications that HIV-1 (the most prevalent in Tanzania) interacts significantly with many other parasitic infections within individual hosts, but the population-level impacts of co-infection are not well-characterized. Among those parasitic opportunistic infections, *Cryptosporidum parvum, Isospora belli, Cyclospora cayetanensis* and *Microspordia* species frequent causes of diarrhea. Likewise, *Pneumocystis jiroveci* pneumonia and *Candida* species infections have been implicated in life threatening fungal infections among people living with HIV/AIDS.

In this chapter, poverty is defined as a state of having little or no money and few or no material possessions. Poverty can be caused by unemployment, low education, deprivation and homelessness. Lack of health facilities and low-cost healthy foods, along with public space for physical activities, may be among the factors that contribute to poor health and even higher risk of death due to curable diseases among patients who live in poverty.

HIV/AIDS deepens poverty and increases inequalities at every level, household, community, regional and sectoral. The HIV/AIDS epidemic undermines efforts at poverty reduction, income and asset distribution, productivity and economic growth resulting in reverse progress of development targets. Certainly, there is relationship between poverty and the development of epidemics of communicable diseases and at the same time epidemic diseases, like any illness, have the potential to increase poverty.

The impact of HIV/AIDS and poverty on children has different dimensions that include children being deprived of education to care for sick adults, thus compromising their basic right to education, placing the household at further long-term risk for poverty that may take decades to reverse. Illiteracy and/or lack of skills also appear to influence vulnerability to HIV infection. A correlation between educational qualifications and HIV infection exists, which indicates that people with formal educational qualifications acquire economic independence and threfore do not engage in risky behaviors as compared to those without it.

Financial constrains or budgetary deficits in government expenditure on health in Tanzania, like most African countries translate into an increase in a number of untreated disease conditions, including sexually transmitted diseases that are known to facilitate the rapid transmission of HIV. HIV/AIDS appears to interact strongly with poverty and has increased the depth of vulnerability of the affected families/households because of being in needs (caring ill relatives, death and decreased manpower to seek for daily bread). The relation between poverty and HIV/AIDS is bidirectional. However, there is conceptual confusion about the nature of the relationship, probably because of lack of rigorous scientific researches on the links between poverty, HIV/AIDS and parasitosis.

There is strong evidence that socio-economic and gender inequalities exacerbate the spread of HIV while AIDS-related diseases and death increases these inequalities, a potentially vicious cycle. Poverty per se may not be the most important factor conditioning the risk of being exposed to HIV, but undoubtedly, it is the poor in these countries, and especially poor women, who are suffering the most with the subsequent impacts of AIDS. Given that malnutrition is a function of poverty, there is thus a good reason to assume that poverty helped to hasten the spread of HIV in sub-Saharan Africa.

However, when examining HIV vulnerability at the level of households and communities, the evidence appears to be mixed. Since the richer and better educated are likely to have better access to reproductive health care, condom use is generally low in Africa and other resources-limited countries. It is also postulated that poverty is placing individuals from poor households at greater risk of exposure to HIV through the economically-driven adoption of risky behaviors. Moreover, poverty and food insecurity (malnutrition) seem to increase sexual risk taking, particularly among women who may engage in transactional sex to procure food for themselves and their children.

Consequently, combating malnutrition, including worm infestation, requires more than providing treatment. It requires multisector approaches to address the broader causes such as poor water and sanitation provision and lack of food security. The approaches should also focus on HIV/AIDS control involving but not be limited to mainstreaming of HIV implications into the policy and practice of many sectors.

Although HIV prevalence has fallen in Tanzania over the past decade, thousands of people become infected with HIV every year and 86,000 Tanzanians died from AIDS in 2009 alone. While the poor are undoubtedly hit harder by the downstream impacts of AIDS, in a variety of ways, their chances of being exposed to HIV in the first place are not necessarily greater than wealthier individuals or households. Poverty, in a nutshell includes illiteracy, parasitosis/diseases, food insecurity plus HIV/AIDS are the major problem currently facing Tanzanians. Therefore, a joint effort is urgently required to combat them in their totality, with that approach, the victory is evident.

2. Poverty, parasitosis and HIV/AIDS

2.1 HIV/AIDS

2.1.1 A brief history and Trends of HIV and AIDS in Tanzania

The first cases of AIDS were reported in the Kagera region (north western of Tanzania) in 1983 and by 1987 every region in the country had reported AIDS cases. In 1985, the government set up the National AIDS Control Programme (NACP) to coordinate the response and established AIDS coordinators in each district in the country, Tanzania Commission for AIDS (TACAIDS). In order to confront the growing epidemic, the NACP developed a medium term plan for the period 1987-1991 which was then followed by two more medium term plans covering 1992-1996 and 1998-2002. These plans had three main aims: the decentralization of the health sector responses, reducing HIV transmission and relieving the social consequences of HIV/AIDS through care and assistance. However, according to Tanzania's first National Multisectoral Framework (2003-2007) the three medium term plans did not halt the spread of HIV. By the time the third medium term plan came into being HIV prevalence had reached 8 percent.

A national policy, which had been under development since 1991, was finalized in 2001, following the declaration of 'war' on HIV/AIDS by former His Excellency President Mkapa. TACAIDS was then established in 2002 to coordinate the multisectoral response, bringing together all stakeholders including government, business and civil societies to provide strategic guidance to HIV/AIDS programmes, projects and interventions.

A study published in 2005, using evidence drawn from the past 20 years exposed some findings which challenged some widely held assumptions about the effects of HIV and AIDS. The study found that generally the highest prevalence of HIV was found amongst the well off individuals/households, particularly affecting rich women, as opposed to poorer and rural households (Shelton et al., 2005). The findings pointed out that wealthier people tend to have the resources which lead to greater and more frequent mobility and expose them to wider sexual networks, encouraging multiple and concurrent relationships. But it was also observed that the wealthier people tend to have greater access to HIV medications that prolong their lives and are more likely to live in urban areas, which have the highest prevalence.

However, HIV prevalence gap between poor urban groups and poorer rural communities is slowly closing. A 2008 study found that knowledge of sexually transmitted infections (STI) was 'alarmingly low' in rural Tanzania and associated with low condom use and HIV infection. Reduced prevalence has mainly been noted among the most educated (those who attended secondary school) while among those with no formal education, prevalence has not decreased and the number of new infections has risen (Hargreaves et al., 2010). Because access to health care and knowledge of HIV and AIDS is typically lower in rural areas. This led to adoption of more aggressive measures towards educating the rural people on preventive efforts and thus further spread of the epidemic.

In a nut shell, some contextual factors shaping the HIV/AIDS epidemic in the country include:

- Poverty and transactional sex with increasing numbers of commercial sex workers
- Men's irresponsible sexual behaviour due to cultural patterns of virility
- Social, economic and political gender inequalities including violence against women
- Substance abuse such as alcohol consumption
- Local cultural practices e.g. widow cleansing
- Mobility in all its forms which leads to separation of spouses and increased establishment of temporary sexual relationships
- Lack of male circumcision

2.1.2 Immigration and rural-urban migration of people

HIV infection is unevenly distributed across geographic area, gender, age, groups and social economic classes in the country. The prevalence rates of HIV/AIDS range from less than 1%

to more than 15% in certain regions. Nevertheless, the epidemic has struck more the most economically active group of adults, those aged 15-45, which is also the productive age-group of individuals. Population movement is common in Tanzania, especially among the youths (18-45 years old). Growth and/or expansion of the mining sector and education have led to greater urbanization and mobility between rural and urban areas. This created an avenue for young and sexually active persons to interact socially and forming 'high risk sexual networks', which include sex workers, women at truck stops and miners, whom most of them are HIV seropositive.

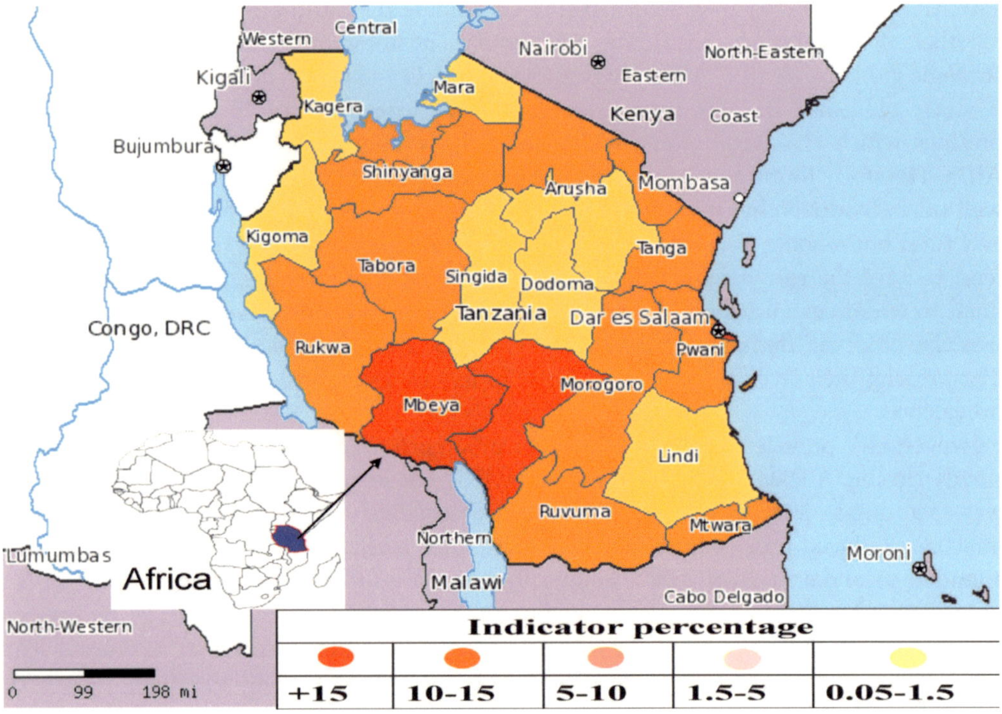

Fig. 1. Prevalence of HIV/AIDS among adults in Tanzania

Tanzania is also well known for its hospitality. Since the era of the Former President Late Mwalimu Nyerere, founder of the nation, our country has been hosting a myriad of refugees from all over the continent, who definitely had established close ties with citizens. This relationship could also have brought some "exogenous and detrimental effects".

2.1.3 Dependence on foreign aids on combating HIV infections and stigma

On the other hand, Tanzania's coastal trade as well as its border with eight countries exposes its vulnerable populations to HIV. In border and lake areas, 1 in 5 people are HIV positive. A study conducted by International Organization of Migration in 2010, revealed that transport workers, fishermen, border personnel, and seafarers were more likely to have multiple sexual partners and less likely to use condoms than the general population. Worse still, access to treatment and prevention initiatives in these areas was also minimal; underlining the regional variation in access to HIV services.

About only 8 years ago, the National Policy on HIV/AIDS recognized antiretroviral therapy as a right for all people living with HIV, at a time when no Tanzanians were receiving antiretroviral treatment. In 2003, the William J. Clinton Foundation and a group of Tanzanian experts created a Care and Treatment Plan (2003-2008), which was then adopted by the Tanzanian Government. The five-year plan proposed the roll out of antiretroviral therapy aiming at providing antiretroviral drugs free of charge to all people living with HIV by 2008. However, by 2004, only about 0.5% of those with advanced HIV were receiving treatment. Presumably, one of the major reasons is the Tanzanian HIV/AIDS response being heavily dependent on foreign funding sources. Because about 95% of the funding for HIV/AIDS programmes comes from foreign donors of whom more than two thirds is from the Global Fund and the U.S. President's Emergency Plan for AIDS Relief (PEPFAR). HIV/AIDS funding makes up one third of all aid coming to Tanzania.

Discrimination leads to an unwillingness to take an HIV test and to disclose results to family, friends or sexual partners. One study conducted in Dar es Salaam in 2005, found that only half of HIV positive respondents had disclosed their status to intimate partners. Time lapse from receiving results to disclosing them was 2.5 years for men and 4 years for women. Stigma, specifically fear of abandonment, job or property loss and violence were reasons for this delay. Contradictory perceptions exist among Tanzanians in respect of contracting STI, some believe that is a symbol of being sexually active and potent while other think it is ungodly and is a shame. However, when it comes to seeking for medical attentions, both groups find it uneasy. Such mixed notions ascribe to fear and hesitancy to disclose their status thus that increasing the chance of transmitting the STI, HIV inclusive to a partner, by avoidance of preventative measures and thus delay of timely of treatment (Mshana et al., 2006; Roura, 2009). In most regions/communities lack of knowledge about HIV/AIDS is a major cause of stigma and discrimination. Four out of ten women and a third of men surveyed in the 2007-2009 HIV and Malaria Indicator Survey reported that they would not buy fresh vegetables from a shopkeeper who has HIV, and half of all women and 40% of men said they would feel it necessary to keep it a secret if a family member was infected with HIV.

2.2 Poverty and HIV/AIDS

2.2.1 Economy overview

Tanzania is one of the world's poorest economies in terms of per capita income, however, Tanzania average 7% gross domestic product (GDP) growth per year between 2000 and 2010 on strong gold production and tourism. The economy depends heavily on agriculture, which accounts for more than one-fourth of GDP, provides 85% of exports, and employs about 60% of the work force. The World Bank, the IMF, and bilateral donors have provided funds to rehabilitate Tanzania's aging economic infrastructure, including rail and port infrastructure that are important trade links for inland countries.

"Hunger is the first obstacle to ending poverty. Hungry is poverty. A person who is always hungry is always poor. We can talk about the eradication of poverty all we want. We can never achieve it, if we don't first end hunger. The hungry live in rural areas and urban slums, in refugee camps and on farming homesteads. Wherever they are, hungry families live in the grey area between crisis and normality. Their poverty keeps them vulnerable to hunger. And hunger keeps them poor. Investments in infrastructure need to place more emphasis on ensuring that the assets truly are for the poor like community-based ponds, woodlots, roads and the like. Yet physical infrastructure alone cannot lead to less poverty or better food security. A bridge may make the local market half an hour away rather than half a day. But when you have no education, poor health, and no energy, all the opportunities the market holds are beyond your reach," Statement by the Executive Director World Food Programme.

Therefore, defining poverty is a great challenge to researchers because of its complex nature. Poverty is the state of having little or no money and few or no material possessions. Poverty can be caused by unemployment, low education, deprivation and homelessness. Lack of local health clinics and low-cost healthy foods, along with public space for physical activities, may be among the factors that contribute to poor health and even higher risk of death due to curable diseases among patients who live in poverty. East Africans are some of the poorest people in the world ranking in this order: Kenya-Uganda-Tanzania. Therefore, Tanzania being one of the poorest countries, her citizens face several socio-economic problems, especially for unemployed, elders and orphans. The World Bank defines poverty as "the inability to attain a minimum standard of living" and produced a "universal poverty line", which was "consumption-based" and comprised of two elements: "the expenditure necessary to buy a minimum standard of nutrition and other basic necessities and a further amount that varies from country to country, reflecting the cost of participating in everyday life of society. The World Bank uses this definition largely for inter-country comparisons, and is not necessarily depicting what happens in households.

Poverty is also about more than income and economics. There are many types of poverty:

- Service poverty, where people are unable to access or are not provided with services such as health and education;
- Resource poverty, where though they have sufficient incomes people are unable to access resources because they may be poor in terms of their rights, representation or governance.

However, for reasons of space and scope of this theme, we focus on types of poverty outlined above centering on income and social capital, which seem to apply in Tanzania.

2.2.2 Decomposition changes in poverty

Most of the tools used in the analysis of poverty can be similarly used for the analysis of inequality. One could draw a profile of inequality, which would look at the extent of inequality among certain groups of households. This informs on the 'homogeneity' of the various groups, an important element to take into account when designing interventions. Gini-coefficient of inequality: This is the most commonly used measure of inequality. The coefficient varies between 0, which reflects complete equality and 1, which indicates complete inequality (one person has all the income or consumption, all others have none). Using 1993 as a baseline for Tanzania, **Table 1** below shows how per capita growth rates and changes in inequality would translate into changes in poverty over a 20-year period. With a zero real per capita growth rate and no change of inequality, the poverty rate would

Poverty rate with	1993	2005	2015
0 % growth , no growth in Gini	50	50	50
1.5% growth, no change in Gini	50	35	18
1.5% growth, Gini reduction by 0.5%/year	50	30	3
3.0% growth, no change in Gini	50	25	5

Table 1. Poverty, Inequity, and Growth in Tanzania.

remain unchanged. A 1.5 percent sustained per capita growth rate with no change in the distribution of income (all household get a 1.5 percent income gain per year) would yield a substantial reduction in poverty. If inequality were to improve at the same time, the poverty reduction would be greatly accelerated, even with a similar growth level.
Equally, the impact of economic growth can be analyzed by various ways viz. by comparing inequality between different groups, by decomposing inequality to assess the major contributors to inequality, by analyzing inequality, growth and poverty and their relationship and finally, by decomposing changes in inequality over time as shown in **Table 1**.
Therefore, it is occasionally feasible to elucidate how much of the observed changes in poverty over time can be attributed to changes in distribution and to changes in mean income or consumption. For example, lower poverty could result either from a general increase in the income of all households (without change in the income distribution) or from a decrease in inequality (redistribution from the rich to the poor without change in mean income or consumption). A change in poverty can always be decomposed into a growth component, a redistribution component, and a 'residual' component. An example can be taken from rural Tanzania, which experienced a decrease in poverty but an increase in inequality. Decomposing changes in poverty incidence (headcount) and depth (poverty gap) reveals that while the poor benefited from growth over the period, the rich captured a much greater share of economic improvement. In fact, if the distribution of income hadn't changed, the reduction in poverty incidence would have been much larger and the poverty gap would have also decreased. **Table 2** below presents the results of the analysis and show that, using a high poverty line, the head count would have decreased by 38% and the poverty gap by 24%. The changes in distribution (and interaction factors) resulted in a decrease in the head count of only 14% and in the poverty gap of only 2%.

Poverty line	**Growth component**	**Redistribution component**	**Residual**	**Total change in poverty**
		Head count index		
High	-38.5	11.8	12.6	-14.1
Low	-34.4	16.7	5.7	-12.0
		Poverty gap index		
High	-23.7	20.5	1.6	-1.6
Low	-19.0	22.9	-1.9	2.0

Table 2. Decomposition in changes in Poverty in Rural Tanzania (1983-1991). Source (Ferreira, 1996)

Tanzania suffers widespread and severe poverty, with nearly 60% of the population living on less than $2 per day and an estimated 20% living on less than $1 per day. As a result, Tanzania is ranked 164th out of 177 countries in the U.N. Human Development Index. As it also suffers a heavy disease burden, Tanzania exemplifies the intimate link between poverty and health. Lacking funds and infrastructure lead to difficulties in accessing primary health care for more than two-thirds of the population, with 39.9% lacking the money needed for treatment and 37.6% unable to travel the necessary distance for treatment.
Consequently, HIV/AIDS may deepen poverty and exacerbates inequalities at every level, household, community, regional and sectoral. The epidemic undermines efforts at poverty reduction, income and asset distribution, productivity and economic growth. HIV/AIDS

has reversed progress towards international development goals because of the influence it has on all development targets. There is an undoubted relationship between poverty and the development of epidemics of communicable diseases and at the same time epidemic diseases, like any illness, have the potential to increase poverty.
It has been suggested that illness and poverty affect household resources and income, as consequence of rising costs of medical care/treatment, and an increased need for nutritious foods. When adults/parents are stricken by HIV/AIDS or any other illness, with the progression of the illness, the demand for care also rises. Children are often withdrawn from schools to care for sick adults, compromising their basic right to education. The deprivation of education could place the household at further long-term risk for poverty, lack of skills and disempowerment. Consequently, this results in a cycle of household impoverishment that may take decades to reverse. Illiteracy and/or lack of skills also appear to influence vulnerability to HIV infection. One previous study in South Africa found that those with tertiary educational qualifications had lower rates of HIV infection than those with only school level qualifications. This implies that people with the necessary educational qualifications, thus acquiring economic independence for survival do not engage in risky behaviors than those with limited education.
Financial constrains or budgetary deficits in government expenditure on health in most African countries translate into an increase in a number of untreated STIs that are known to facilitate the rapid transmission of HIV. This could have serious long-term health implications resulting from the rapid spread of HIV. Apparently, HIV/AIDS appears to interact strongly with poverty and has increased the depth of vulnerability of those households already vulnerable to shocks. HIV/AIDS has acted to intensify the disadvantages imposed on the poor households and communities. HIV/AIDS leads to financial, resource and income impoverishment as households become poorer as a result of the illness and death of members, and in many cases it is the income-earning adults who are lost. Ultimately the high cost of care and burials leave heavy burden on the already overburdened households, orphans and dependants, people living with HIV/AIDS (PLHAs) and vulnerability to HIV infection (Ngalula et al., 2002). Therefore the 'poverty factor' at the household level has to be addressed simultaneously with the National efforts to combat the HIV/AIDS epidemic.
However, the impact is more than financial. Illness and death leads to an erosion of social capital and socially reproductive forces. In other words, the term social capital refers to the effort that goes into the reproduction of social and economic infrastructures. Therefore, at the social level, there are variety of relationships such as physical infrastructures, beliefs about trust, rituals of bargaining and price setting, mechanisms for regulating weights and measures, means of resolving disputes, and repeated activities which ensure that all these things continue to exist. These are not only matters of economic activity but also the maintenance and development of institutions, the reinforcement of community daily activities that also become negatively affected as consequence of the HIV/AIDS. Ultimately, the human capital loss has serious social and economic development in all sectors and at all levels. Hence, raising living standards of households and communities over the long-run through productivity-enhancing investments in agricultural technology generation and diffusion, improved crop marketing systems, basic education, infrastructure, and governance could improve their ability to withstand the social and economic stresses caused by HIV/AIDS.

It is now recognized that poverty significantly influences the spread and impact of HIV/AIDS. In many ways it creates vulnerability to HIV infection, causes rapid progression of the infection in the individual due to malnutrition and limits access to social and health care services. Poverty causes impoverishment as it leads to death of the economically active segments of the society and bread winners leading to reduction in income or production. Impacts of HIV/AIDS in most developing countries, Tanzania inclusive, have been visualized with poor resolution microscopes and thus studies of the effects of AIDS on households and most focus on economic impacts of death rather than illness. These show a distorted image. In Northern Tanzania (Kagera), a study conducted by the World Bank with Tanzanian co-investigators found that households stricken by deaths of their beloved ones especially adults, spent more on medical care and number of working time was significantly reduced. Similarly, it was revealed that even in well off families/households (for African standards) 29% of non-orphaned children were stunted while 50% of orphaned children were wasted. In poorer households 39% of non-orphaned children were stunted while 51% of orphaned children were wasted. These figures point to the effects on all children of growing up in a poor society.

Most African countries were performing poorly even before HIV/AIDS began to spread, largely due to their government's start-stop approach to economic reform. With the HIV/AIDS epidemic now at full force, these countries can only begin counteracting the effects of the epidemic if they undertake far more dramatic restructuring than they were prepared to previously. However, HIV/AIDS has worsened the situation as school-going age children born from HIV victimized families suffer both long-and short term consequences. Some of the effects are poor physical conditions, compromised immune systems and mental functioning is negatively affected by stunted growth, which is their long term effect. Hence, it may affect the ability of children to benefit from education and to function socially and economically later in their lives. Usually, orphans are unlikely to have proper schooling as the death of a parent or both parents in a family reduces a child's school attendance or just being unable to pay for schooling. This may automatically force the child to engage into "adults' duties". Sick adults may have reduced expectations of the returns to investing in children's education, as they do not expect to live long enough to recoup the investment. When a child goes to another household after its parents' deaths, the obstacles become greater as the child is not their own, particularly when even their own children are not guaranteed with all basic needs: food, clothing and school fees. These are some of the results of poverty (under-resourcing of public education) as consequence of the HIV/AIDS epidemic. AIDS increases teacher deaths and they may be difficult to replace, particularly in deprived, rural or otherwise remote communities. On the other hand, teachers' illness can lead to pupils being untaught for extended periods and replacement is difficult while staff members are on sick leave.

Therefore, the relationship between HIV/AIDS and poverty is synergistic and symmetrical. HIV/AIDS impacts households on two main levels, namely the social and economic levels. On a social level, households have to deal with issues around stigmatization, social exclusion and disintegration of family structure and social support networks. On the economic level, households and the surviving members have to pay for medical costs and funeral expenses and, if the deceased was a breadwinner, there will be further financial impacts in a form of a loss of income. Thus HIV/AIDS can directly contribute to poverty.

As much as HIV/AIDS exacerbates poverty through morbidity and mortality of productive adults, poverty facilitates the transmission of HIV. In developing countries, especially those in Sub-Saharan region, HIV/AIDS is reaching a stage at which AIDS morbidity and mortality are increasing rapidly (Dorrington et al., 2001). Once adults are sick and some are bedridden, then the young and elderly are forced to care for them. The situation can exert unbearable pressure on households in their struggle for survival. Poor households are usually the worst hit and more vulnerable to the long-term effects of HIV/AIDS and poverty. In some regions of Tanzania, more than half of hospital beds are occupied by patients with HIV/AIDS related conditions. The treatment costs related to these admissions may lead to further impoverishment especially at household level. Poverty is associated with vulnerability to severe diseases like HIV, through its effects on delaying access to health care and inhibiting treatment adherence. The costs incurred while seeking diagnosis and treatment for HIV/AIDS are common causes of delays in accessing health care especially for the poor. To a certain extent, this forces some families to seek medical attentions from traditional healers, due to their easy accessibility and affordability. Poor households may not necessarily have the financial resources to seek help from health facilities, nor food security to enable members to adhere to their treatment. The lack of these resources is significant cause of the delays in accessing health services by poor households. Food security here is concerned with physical and economic access to food of sufficient quality and quantity. Food security is necessary, but by itself insufficient, for ensuring nutrition security. Nutrition security is achieved for a household when secure access to food is coupled with a sanitary environment, adequate health services, and adequate care to ensure a healthy life for all household members.

Poverty limits the options for treating infectious diseases like HIV. Infection with other STI is an important co-factor of HIV, and it provides a point of entry for HIV. Poor households become even more vulnerable when unable to raise the necessary funds to pay for treatment as they largely depend on the state to provide these services. Women in Tanzania also have severely limited access to education, employment, credit, and transportation. As a result, northern coastal women—married and unmarried, young and old—are increasingly turning to sex work, exposing them to a high risk of HIV infection. "We accept that it is now the female burden to provide for our children," says a woman from Mkwaja village. "We risk dying from AIDS for the sake of our children''. The true scope of HIV prevalence in the coastal region is not known because of low diagnostic and testing rates. (Fifty-eight percent of all Tanzanian adults living with HIV/AIDS are women). A barmaid with a 3-years old baby in Mbeya says '' I do sell myself in order to safeguard my child/daughter and guarantee that she has something to eat. If I don't do that right now, for sure she will die in my arms. Then what is the point seeing my kid dying or me dying in the next ten or so years?''. Mbeya is one the two badly HIV/AIDS stricken regions in the country with prevalence rate of 15-20%; another region is Iringa. Mbeya has boarders with Malawi and Zambia. This kind of despair and total lack of hope of improving wellbeing at household, drive this woman and several other into ''problem''.

Contradictory evidences exist with regard to HIV vulnerability at the level of households and communities (Wojciki 2005; Giraldo, 1997). Early studies had demonstrated positive correlations between household economic resources, education, and HIV infection, as the epidemic progressed; however currently, this relationship is somehow slightly changing. Generally, in Tanzania and most African countries, relatively rich and better educated men and women have higher rates of partner change because they have greater personal autonomy and spatial mobility. The richer and better educated are likely to have better access to reproductive health care, condom use is generally low in Africa and other parts of the developing world. At a later stage, however, it has been argued that individuals with higher socioeconomic status tend to adopt safer sexual practices, once the effects of AIDS-related morbidity and mortality become more apparent. It is also postulated that poverty (possibly itself fuelled by AIDS) is placing individuals from poor households at greater risk of exposure to HIV via the economically-driven adoption of risky behaviors. Poverty and food insecurity are thought to increase sexual risk taking, particularly among women who may engage in transactional sex to procure food for themselves and their children.

For that reason, HIV/AIDS mortality can change the demographic structure of the household, reverse the roles of the members, exacerbate poverty, rob children of their parents thereby creating more orphans, infringe on the basic rights of the child in areas such as education, food, nutrition, health and others. Unless households are strengthened and empowered through focused interventions, poor households are likely to fall deeper into poverty for the generations to come. For PLHA and poor, it will be harder for them to sustainably access antiretroviral therapy, since some may not afford transport costs, regardless that they may be willing to go for the ART. But also some may be unable to afford to buy nutritious food, which is actually part and parcel of ART. At the household level, poverty will worsen the impacts of other livelihood stresses and shocks, and close down options for effectively dealing with hardships and challenges of life.

Therefore, food security is an important element for the survival of any household across the spectrum of wealth. Households affected by HIV and poor may find it difficult to maintain their food security. Both HIV and poverty exert tremendous pressure on the household's ability to provide for the basic needs like food. Let alone that poor nutrition is often linked with adverse outcomes in HIV/AIDS. Poor nutritional status is linked to vulnerability to progression from HIV infection to mortality. Poor nutrition weakens the body's defense against infection, and infection in turn weakens the efficiency of absorption of nutrients. Micronutrient deficiencies undermine the body's natural defenses against infections, thus contributing further to the vulnerability to HIV infection. Households experiencing food shortages as a result of poverty and effects of HIV/AIDS increase the chances of fast progression of HIV infection to AIDS and inevitable death of the ill person. Given that malnutrition is a function of poverty, therefore there is a substantial reason to assume that poverty helped hasten the spread of HIV in sub-Saharan Africa.

2.3 Poverty, malnutrition and HIV/AIDS

The term malnutrition was previously regarded as synonymous with undernutrition. This was before the emergence of the nutrition transition. Nowadays, a broader and more comprehensive definition of malnutrition is necessary since in actual sense, the term refers to the entire spectrum of deviant nutritional status, from short stature and below normal weight. There is considerable information describing the nutrition situation in different parts of Tanzania, based on spot surveys, child growth monitoring systems or research work. Most of this information is not nationally representative and is focused more on children under-fives than other population groups. Only scanty serial national information is available making it possible to discern trends over time in only a few indicators and in specific areas of the country. Tanzania's main problems of nutrition are similar to those of other countries in Sub-Saharan Africa. They are related to undernourishment, and these are protein-energy-deficiency (PED), iron deficiency anaemia (IDA), iodine deficiency disorders (IDD) and vitamin A deficiency (VAD).

Apart from these deficiency disorders, there are two nutrient excess disorders represented by fluorosis in the northern and north-western and central parts of mainland; and the problem of overweight, obesity and diet-related non-communicable diseases which seem to be increasing especially in the urban elite and business sections of the community emulating unhealthy food habits and lifestyles. Compared to Sub-Saharan Africa; Tanzania is just slightly better than the average of 30% for underweight. For developing countries, excluding China, Tanzania is worse off for stunting but better off in wasting and underweight. Since the young population depends on a small adult population to sustain the economy and to provide the resources needed for adequate food, care and health; malnutrition in adults is of serious consequence. In such a situation, malnutrition becomes both a result and a cause of poverty. Malnourished adults cannot respond well to the challenges of economic and even political reforms which need both physical and mental energy. Maternal malnutrition is of even more severe consequence, as malnourished women produce malnourished children who will grow into malnourished adults creating a vicious cycle.

The nutritional status of adults is anthropometrically measured by using the Body Mass Index (BMI) which is a number derived from dividing the subject's weight in kilograms by the square of the height in meters (W/H^2). The distribution of Body Mass Index (BMI) in a few regions surprisingly show that more than a third of adults have low BMIs with rural areas having higher prevalence rates of undesirable BMIs than urban areas. Nonetheless, economic and historical analysis, epidemiological evidence, and common sense indicate that widespread childhood malnutrition will undermine investments in health, education, and ultimately economic development. Investments in cost effective treatments combined with broader nutrition based interventions must get higher priority.

Demographics, food supply and epidemiological transitions determine the specific relevance of the malnutrition-infection interaction in individual circumstances. Until the advent of the AIDS pandemic, average life-expectancies were rising in Tanzania and everywhere in the world; this was largely as a consequence of a reduction in early deaths from infectious childhood diseases. Today, HIV/AIDS is a world-wide calamity, though its impact is heavily felt in Africa. All of the poverty-related poor health and poor health care factors that go into increased susceptibility to HIV also affect the speed with which it progresses to full-blown AIDS and to death by opportunistic infections (Barnett et al. 2001). In particular, poverty-related lack of access to medical treatment, either to reduce viral load or to prevent and treat opportunistic infections, results in a lower quality of life, more rapid development of AIDS, and more rapid demise for poor PLHA. For example, people infected with HIV, who also have latent tuberculosis, are 30-50 times more likely to develop active TB. Similarly, ten percent of HIV infected persons develop cryptococcal meningitis, a fungal infection which leads inexorably to an extremely painful death within 30 days unless treated with powerful fungicides.

Proper nutrition is required to ensure optimal health. Consumption of a wide variety of foods, with adequate vitamins and minerals intake, is the basis of a healthy diet. Nutritionists outline that no single nutrient is the key to good health, but that optimum nutrition is derived from eating a diverse diet, including a variety of fruits and vegetables. Because foods such as fruits and vegetables provide many more nutrients than vitamin supplements, food is the best source for acquiring vitamins and minerals.

2.3.1 Nutrition, immune system and infection/parasitosis

Nutrition (also called nourishment or aliment) is the provision, to living cells, tissues and organisms, of the materials necessary (in the form of food) to support life. Many common health problems can be prevented or alleviated with a healthy diet. One of the most innovative researches in the past 40 years is the increased knowledge on how the immune system operates; from a point of view of cellular biology and humoral responses, which formed the so-called immunobiology that encompasses other field of studies like the nutritional community (Maclean and Lucas, 2008). Recognizing the magnitude of nutritional problem in the country, the government established the Tanzania food and nutrition centre (TFNC) that deal with nutrition-related issues. Some of the main responsibilities of TFNC are:

- Reduction of all forms of malnutrition to acceptable levels
- Effective coordination of nutrition activities in the country
- Promote nutrition of the socio-economical deprived and nutritionally vulnerable groups

Tanzania, like other developing countries, her citizens faces a huge problem of malnutrition (undernutrition and/or over-nutrition), and this could greatly contribute to progression of HIV to AIDS. Until recently, obesity (overweight) was regarded as symbol of wealth and being healthy by majority of Tanzanians. Obese individuals demanded respect among the societies. On the other hand, skinny or slim persons were regarded as underfed/nourished, synonymous with being poor (unable to feed oneself adequately. With advent of HIV/AIDS, skinny 'slim" individuals were thought to be infected by HIV, from which the word "slim" was derived. However, when the government launched ART, and both slim and overweight individuals enrolled in the therapy, this perception has drastically changed. Though, the extent of knowledge between the urban and rural living people could still significantly differ. This to some extent is a product of illiteracy among the population. To date, overweight/over nutrition is not a major health concern to majority of Tanzanians.

Notwithstanding, over nutrition may result into accumulation/deposit of unused/excess of nutrients: excess of carbohydrates into fatty acids and proteins being converted to fatty acids and then stored as lipids as well. This kind of nutrients accumulation has detrimental effects to the body. The quantity and nature of lipids are important factors in the process of immune system modulation. Several mechanisms have been involved in the modulation of the immune system by fatty acids:

- Membrane fluidity,
- Production of lipid peroxides,
- Eicosanoid synthesis and
- Effect on gene regulation.

Speculations exist that fatty acid immuno-modulation occurs not only singly, but also as a collective action of these factors.

A change in phospholipids' fatty acid compositions due to dietary lipid manipulation is ascribable to alterations in the membrane fluidity. Fatty acids from dietary lipids can be incorporated into any of the different phospholipids within the plasma membrane and they are clearly altered by the availability of dietary lipids. The changes in fatty acid composition of this structure have great importance because of the alteration of plasma membrane characteristics. This fact may be attributed to changes produced in the activity of proteins associated with the membrane, which act as receptors, form ion channels or are related to enzymatic functions (Liu et al., 2003). Therefore, the changes in the expression of surface proteins may be due to a vertical displacement of the membrane proteins by lipid action. While the expression of surface molecules such as adhesion and major histocompatibility molecules from human monocytes are inhibited by eicosapentaenoic acid. Instead, a significant increase in the expression of human lymphocyte antigen (HLA) is observed in monocytes incubated with docosahexaenoic acid (Maclean and Lucas, 2008).

Fatty acids play a major role in the production of eicosanoids, because they are key determinants of membrane-bound enzyme and receptor expression. The influence of fatty acids on gene expression is not well understood. Nevertheless, fatty acids released from membrane phospholipids are important second messengers or substitute for the classical second messengers, such as inositide phospholipid or adenoside monophosphate cyclic (AMPc) signal transduction pathways. These messengers act in a reversible manner at a precise intracellular location for a very short time in order to amplify, attenuate or deviate a signal in a direct or indirect (by conversion from arachidonic acid to eicosanoids) pathway (Riemersma et al. 1998).

The human body is greatly affected by nutritional status that in turn has been associated with alteration of the immune responses. Several dietary fatty acids or free fatty acids are involved in the modulation of the immune system through mechanisms that modify the immune response (Franchin et al., 2000). The immune parameters susceptible to modification by fatty acids supplied in the diet or free fatty acids added into cellular cultures are lymphocyte proliferation, cytokine production, activity of natural killer (NK) cells, phagocytosis, and expression of markers in the surface of the cells (Calder, 1995; Kelley et al., 1999; Roitt et al., 2001). The immune system modulation induced by fatty acids depends on several biological and methodological factors, such as the type and concentration of fatty acids, cell types, species of experimental animals, serum used in the *ex vivo* or *in vitro* cultures and so on (De Pablo and Alvarez de Cienfuegos, 2000).

Therefore, it seems that because of immunomodulation role associated with fatty acids, in future they may be applied to the amelioration and prevention of diseases characterized by an over-activation of the immune system, such as inflammatory or autoimmune disorders. In addition to these applications, unsaturated fatty acids may be used to reduce the susceptibility against bacterial infections due to the possibility of several lipids playing important roles in the efficient elimination of different micro-organisms or reducing host resistance against an infectious process due to the immunosuppression promoted by dietary unsaturated fatty acids. However, it should be noted that immunosuppression promoted by different dietary lipids has to be balanced, because this process may lead to an impairment of host response and increase the risk of infections.

2.3.2 Protein-energy- malnutrition

Protein-energy-malnutrition (PEM) also known as protein-energy deficiency (PED) is generally a nutritional problem that results from varying proportions of protein and calorie deficiency in infants and young children of developing countries (Nnakwe, 1995). It is a global public health problem, affecting children from African, Asian, Latin American and Caribbean regions (de Onis et al., 2000; Bisai et al., 2010). PEM is directly or indirectly responsible for about half of the 10.8 million deaths per year in under five children in developing countries. In Tanzania, it is estimated that 60% of deaths, among children under 5 years of ages, are associated with undernutrition (Villamor et al., 2005). The major risk factors that can predispose a child to having PEM include poverty, lack of access to quality food, cultural and religious food customs, poor maternal education, inadequate breast feeding, and lack of quality healthcare. In addition to macronutrient deficiency, there is clinical and/or sub-clinical deficiency of micronutrients (Jahoor et al., 2008).

Recent researches show that HIV prevalence is highly correlated with falling calorie consumption, falling protein consumption, unequal distribution of income (inequity) and other variables conventionally associated with susceptibility to infectious disease, however transmitted. "The causal chain runs from macro-factors that result in poverty: through the community, the household, the individual and into the resilience of the individual's immune system. Work in cell biology has shown the mechanisms which connect malnutrition and parasite infestation; depressing both specific and non-specific immune responses by weakening epithelial integrity and the effectiveness of cells in the immune system. PEM, IDA, VAD, all of these poverty related conditions decrease resistance to disease in general and to HIV in particular.

Trace elements are required by human body for proper functioning but unlike most vitamins and minerals that our body needs, trace elements are needed only in extremely low quantities. The human body needs about 72 trace elements for normal functioning. There are seven essential trace elements described in human body chromium, copper, cobalt, iodine, selenium and zinc. Iron is an important dietary mineral and involves in various body functions. In humans, iron is an essential component of proteins involved in oxygen transport. It is also essential for the regulation of cell growth and differentiation. Iron is main component of hemoglobin a protein molecule that carries oxygen and plays critical role to the whole respiration process of the total iron in the body 60-70% is stored in hemoglobin. The body contains between 3.5 and 4.5% of iron 2/3 of which is present in hemoglobin (Pradeep et al., 2010).

The ubiquitous iron is an essential nutrient for most tissue cells and deficiency brings about recognizable deleterious results affecting many organs. The lymphoid apparatus is no exception. Iron deficiency with or without anemia is associated with partial atrophy of various lymphoid organs and alteration in many molecular and cellular immune functions. Iron and its binding protein have immunoregulatory properties and shifting of immunoregulatory balances by iron excess or deficiency may produce severe deleterious physiological effects. People with low levels of iron tend to have low resistance to infections. Anemia in HIV infected patients can have serious implication which varies from functional and quality of life decrement to an association with decreased progression and decreased survival. The prevalence of anaemia in HIV disease varies considerably ranging from 1.3-95%. Anaemia is more prevalent in HIV positive women, children and injected drug users. Human with advance HIV infection present some evidence of iron accumulation, which is manifested with an increased ferritin concentration (Pradeep et al., 2010).

Moreover, trace metal overload suppress immune function and increase the morbidity and mortality. If the iron overload becomes severe (usually when the amount of iron in the body exceeds 15 g) the condition is diagnosed as hemochromatosis. This is an inherited blood disorder that causes the blood to retain excessive amount of iron, which lead to serious health consequences such as cirrhosis of the liver (Bullen *et al.*, 1991). Irons stored in the body become depleted and hemoglobin synthesis is inhibited. Iron is central to physiology in general and required for particular steps of the HIV replication life-cycle in cells.

HIV infection has therefore been associated with disturbances in host iron metabolism. Advanced HIV/AIDS disease condition, anemia can coincide with increase ferritin and bone marrow iron content and the anemia is commonly unresponsive to iron supplementation (Strauss, 2004). Increased bone marrow iron is associated with shortened survival and increased opportunistic infections. Iron could be playing an important role in the interaction between host and virus. Host homeostasis adapt during deficiency, overload and infection to balance requirement against toxicity and availability to potential pathogens. Knowledge of these interactions is necessary to predict morbility response to disturbance in host iron homeostasis (Pradeep et al., 2010). Because the progression of HIV infection towards its more advance stages is accompanied by increasing body iron stores there is urgent need for careful clinical studies to clarify the role of iron status on the course of HIV infection. Proper iron supplementation may provide sufficient iron to restore normal storage levels of iron and to replenish hemoglobin deficits thereby increase the survival of HIV sero-positives.

Nowadays it is well recognized that all infections have an adverse effect on nutritional status. However, the clinical and public health significance of the effect of a single infectious episode depends on the prior nutritional state of the individual. Recently, a clear synergistic relationship between nutrition and infection has been elucidated and thus most public health interventions for prevent infection focus on correction of malnutrition. With the ever increasing resistance of important pathogenic microorganisms to available chemotherapeutic agents, this area of study calls for further researches (Strauss, 2004; Villamor et al., 2005; Jahoor et al., 2008).

2.3.3 Impact of poverty on environment

The fact that HIV/AIDS affects people in their productive ages between ages 25 and 45 years, the poverty that the epidemic precipitates can have deleterious impacts on agricultural productivity and natural resources. These impacts can hit particularly hard in a country like Tanzania, where livelihoods are highly dependent on agriculture, mining and fishing. As men and women die or become too ill to work, family members are forced to find new ways to provide for their families. The loss of income from a male head-of-household puts additional burdens on his wife and children to find alternative sources of income, which can ultimately lead to more intense and less-sustainable resource use and extraction. Some regions in northern coastal Tanzania, such alternative practices often include unsustainable harvesting of forests and forest products such as wild foods and medicinal plants, which are then sold at local markets. Increased woodcutting to produce charcoal for sale is also common, especially when families face severe food shortages and must secure cash quickly to buy food. And the use of small-mesh nets for both marine and freshwater fishing has increased as widowed women and their children try desperately to make a living from declining shallow-water fish stocks.

Therefore, poverty and food insecurity increase sexual risk taking, particularly among women who may engage in transactional sex to procure food for themselves and their children. Women's economic dependence on their partners may also make it difficult for them to insist on safer sex like condom use. Several ethnographic studies have suggested that material poverty has increased the incidence of transactional sex. To some extent, this indicates that while the poor are undoubtedly hit harder by the downstream impacts of AIDS, in a variety of ways, their chances of being exposed to HIV in the first place are not necessarily greater than wealthier individuals or households. This brings a different school of thought that possibly poverty itself fuelled by AIDS, is placing individuals from poor households at greater risk of exposure to HIV via the economically-driven adoption of risky behaviors.

In Tanzania there are substantial urban-rural, regional and socio-economic divergences, which have driven youths to migrate to urban areas looking for jobs (better living) and some engaging themselves into risky activities like unsafe sex, prostitution and drug abuse just to mention a few. On the other hand, rural poor children are more likely than their urban counterparts to die, and when they survive, they are more likely to be malnourished as depicted in poverty and human development report (PHDR, 2005).

2.4 Parasitosis and HIV/AIDS

Since the first HIV/AIDS cases were described, a high prevalence of gastrointestinal alterations has been reported, especially diarrhea associated with parasitosis. This became more evident when the appearance of a syndrome named "Slim Disease", characterized by an intense weight loss accompanied by chronic diarrhea, prolonged fever and diffuse muscle weakness, was observed in Africa, especially in Uganda. However, the site and timing of the first reported cases suggest that the disease arose in Tanzania. Studies conducted in Tanzania, Uganda and other African countries have shown prevalence of 60 to 80% of parasitic organisms attributing to "Slim Disease", such as *Isospora spp., Cryptosporidium spp., Salmonella spp., Shigella spp.* and *Campylobacter* species, amounting to a prevalence of 60 to 80% (Tarimo et al., 1996; Brink et al., 2002). "Slim Disease" has been observed in advanced stages of HIV infection (Mhiri et al., 192). The expression "Wasting Syndrome" was adopted in substitution by WHO in 1987 on the basis of criteria laid down by the (Center for Disease Control [CDC, 1987]).

Opportunistic infections caused by intestinal parasites vary according to the geographical area and the endemic levels in each location. The progressive decline of immunological and mucous defense mechanisms predisposes patients to early, intermediary and late gastrointestinal manifestations of HIV infection. At later stages of the disease, the alterations in non-specific defense mechanisms in the production of immunoglobulin A and the reduction in local immune cell response also progress, thus increasing the susceptibility to a number of intestinal opportunistic pathogens, among which *Cryptosporidium parvum, Isospora belli* and Microsporidia species are the most prominent (Akinbo et al., 2010).

After the emergence of AIDS, these parasites, until then known solely in veterinary medicine, were no longer considered as commensal organisms and are nowadays recognized as opportunistic pathogens common to these patients. Infections by these agents constitute a major secondary aggravating factor of the disease, often responsible for worsening the general health conditions, due to manifestations of diarrhea which are difficult to control, sometimes resulting in the death of the patient. Thus, where as infections in the gastrointestinal tract play a critical role in AIDS pathogenesis and diarrheic diseases assume a prominent role, reaching a rate of up to 50% in developed countries, in developing countries there have been reports of incidence of up to 95%, as in Haiti and the African continent. Amongst the causes of diarrhea in developing countries, those of a parasitic origin are prominent in patients with HIV/AIDS (Akinbo et al., 2010).

The immune system can simplistically be divided into two components, namely, nonspecific immunity (skin, other mucosal barriers and soluble factors) and the adaptive immune system, which involve recognition of pathogens and subsequent production of antibodies as well as cell-mediated defense. The immune system is being challenged by the worldwide increment in immunological stressor agents of chemical, physical, biological, mental, and nutritional origin. However, the diversity and intensity of these risks or etiologic factors for HIV/AIDS vary from person to person, from group at risk to group at risk, from country to country, and from continent to continent. This is the principal reason why the frequency of AIDS is not homogeneous in all places and countries (Giraldo, 1998; Roitt et al., 2001).

The capabilities and possibilities of the immune system are neither infallible nor infinite. HIV/AIDS is the maximum state of deterioration that the human immune system can reach as result of HIV-infection. If the pathogenic process of AIDS is not stopped, eventually it will kill the person (Roitt et al., 2001). While the most important risk factor for HIV/AIDS in developed countries is the new epidemic of drugs abuse. The most important risk factor for

HIV/AIDS in underdeveloped countries is poverty, with all its consequences: malnutrition, unsanitary conditions, infections, parasites, and lack of hope for a better life, all of which have reached unprecedented high levels in the last few decades (Giraldo, 1998). Any component of the immune system can be functionally or genetically abnormal as a result of acquired, for instance through HIV infection, lymphomas, frequent use of high-dose steroids or other immune-suppressive medications) or congenital illnesses, with more than 120 congenital immunodeficiencies described to date that either affect humoral immunity or compromise T-cell function. Immunosuppression may also occur in malnourished persons, patients undergoing chemotherapy for malignancy, and those receiving immunosuppressive therapy. However, for parasitic infections, cell-mediated (T-cell) abnormalities predominate. Such persons tend to be susceptible to common pathogens with delayed clearance. With profound cell-mediated defects, reactivation of previously controlled pathogens may occur. Moreover, such individuals are at risk of infection by opportunistic "nonpathogenic" parasites (Cunningham and Fujinami, 2000). Nevertheless, with reconstitution of the cell-mediated immunity, the risk of parasitic infections reverts to that for a normal host.

The mechanisms, by which malnutrition, tuberculosis, STI, malaria, trypanosomiasis, schystosomiasis, leishmaniasis, systemic mycosis, as well as other infections and parasites weaken, destroy, and collapse the immune system will be briefly elucidated. These mechanisms should well understood for any attempt to design more effective interventions on the current occurrence of the HIV/AIDS epidemic in the poorest areas of the underdeveloped countries, where the poor have never before been so poor and so sick as they are now. Moreover, these poor countries, the levels of malnutrition, microbial and parasitic infections have reached very alarming levels (Cates, 1988).

Therefore, poverty, parasitosis and HIV/AIDS seem to be closely interlinked and co-circulate in many populations, particularly in underdeveloped countries. HIV/AIDS, parasitic infections like malaria and other opportunistic infections, and in a few are by far the commonest causes of ill-health and death in Tanzania and other poor countries of the world. Most of these countries happen to be in the tropics and temperate countries in Africa, Asia, and South America. Currently, parasitic infections are major health concerns attributed to high morbidity and mortality in developing countries especially among HIV-infected persons. Children aged 2 to 5 years are most at risk of severe morbidity (Chopra et al., 2006).

Programs to prevent HIV transmission are unlikely to succeed unless they address the underlying causes of its spread. HIV prevention must be based on scientific evidence regarding cofactor conditions, not, as they currently are, on unproven assumptions about the primacy of behavioral factors. In addition to food security, deworming, schistosomiasis prevention and treatment, and malaria control programs should thus be integrated as critical components of a broad-based approach to HIV prevention.

2.4.1 Protozoan infections and HIV/AIDS

Malaria is caused by an intracellular protozoan transmitted via the bite of an infected female *Anopheles* mosquito. Malaria is not an opportunistic infection for HIV-infected people, but the effect of HIV infection on the natural history of malaria has not been completely defined. HIV infection and malaria coexist in regions where the health surveillance systems are poorly performing so that the magnitude of any interaction is difficult to determine. Nevertheless, the evidence of such interaction has recently grown and is still increasing (Nkuo-Akenji et al., 2008). The incidence of symptomatic malaria episodes, severe or uncomplicated, and the corresponding parasite density is higher in HIV infected individuals with low CD4 count (Atzori et al., 1993; Sherman, 1998).

In Tanzania, malaria is the major killer of children under 5 years of age. Prevalence rates of malaria among children between 6-59 months old vary according to geographic positions and socio-economic activities in a particular area. The highest rate has been observed around Lake Zone regions, Kagera region taking a lead with prevalence of 41.1% followed by Lindi (35.5%) while Zanzibar and Arusha have lowest rates of 0.8% and 0.4% respectively. Malaria is the cause of more mortality and morbidity in Tanzania than any other disease, in large part due to growing resistance to antimalarial drugs. It is estimated that over 1% of GDP is devoted to the disease, representing US$2.2 per capita, and 39% of total health expenditure nationally. Government facilities devote almost one-third of their resources to the disease.

Due to poor living conditions, the majority of Tanzanians suffer from malaria -a preventable disease that can have a serious negative impact on pregnant women and young children. Mothers who contract malaria during pregnancy run the risk of having low birth weight babies, maternal anemia, impaired fetal growth, spontaneous abortions, stillbirths, and premature babies. Recently, the country introduced an anti malaria campaign " Malaria *Haikubaliki*" a Swahili slogan that means "Malaria is unacceptable" - which involves all sectors of the society including entertainment, business, sport and religion sectors in the battle against malaria across the country. "Africans think that malaria is inevitable; that there is nothing they can do about it. We are going to prove this wrong. We can eliminate malaria deaths," said the Minister for Health and Social Welfare, Prof. David Mwakyusa. This initiative is of paramount importance because of the presumed potential interaction between malaria and HIV/AIDS.

Researchers have demonstrated a potential role for the dual infection in fueling the spread of HIV/AIDS and malaria in endemic regions (Whitworth et al., 2000; Abu-Raddad et al., 2006; Nkuo-Akenji et al., 2008). Besides a direct effect, HIV infection may indirectly influence the malaria burden by increasing the malaria parasite biomass and consequently the probability of drug resistant parasites emerging. Antimalarial drug resistance, particularly for *Plasmodium falciparum*, is considered a major contributor to the global resurgence of malaria observed over the last three decades and one of the greatest obstacles for an effective malaria control (Marsh, 1998). The basis of resistance lies in one or several genetic mutations in the parasite genome. Malaria parasites with such mutations when in contact with a given drug survive the treatment and eventually spread (Van Geertruyden et al., 2008). Evidences collected from four longitudinal population-based studies in rural Uganda and Malawi, where malaria is highly endemic showed odds ratios of symptomatic malaria in HIV infected compared to uninfected adults of 6.0, 3.4 and 1.2 for CD4 counts <200/μl, 200–499/μl and ≥ 500/μl, respectively, in Uganda (Whitworth et al., 2000). In Malawi, incidence rates of symptomatic malaria in HIV-1 infected adults varied with CD 4 count; compared to individuals with CD4 count of ≥ 500, the malaria incidence was 3 fold higher with a CD4 count of 200–499/μL and a 4.4-fold higher with a CD4 count<200/μL (Borkow et al., 2001; Graham et al., 2006).

Additionally, it is purported that HIV infection contributes to the emergence and spread of antimalarial drugs resistance by increasing drug exposure and drug pressure. HIV infection increases the probability of a malaria infection progressing to symptomatic illness and to a higher parasite density, increasing the probabilities of treatment and contact between the parasites and the drug (Nkuo-Akenji et al., 2008). This can be explained by the fact that,

HIV-infected patients with already low immunity suffer frequently of non-malaria-attributable acute fevers that may be misdiagnosed as malaria and treated with antimalarials. This phenomenon can justify the observed increase in the parasite biomass in HIV symptomatic patients and asymptomatic carriers alike. Besides contributing to the emergence and spread of antimalarials drug resistance, HIV infection may influence and modify its expected geographical pattern as consequence of and influence of various malaria control intervention by exposing large number of Plasmodium parasites to antimalarials. A way out for this is an easy access, prompt diagnosis and appropriate combination therapy that can alleviate or halt the emergence and spread of antimalarial drug resistance (Van Geertruyden et al., 2008).

A study conducted in a rural area of Malenga Makali (Tanzania) involving 300 sexually-active adults selected at random among patients, who were attending a dispensary because of diarrhoea of at least 2 weeks' duration, revealed potential associations between the patient's health (in terms of the WHO's clinical definition of AIDS), HIV-1 seroprevalence and malaria and other parasitic infections. Although malaria infection was more common in HIV-1 seropositives than in the seronegatives, the intensity of the *Plasmodium falciparum* infections, intestinal amoebiasis and giardiasis did not appear to be correlated with HIV infection. In contrast, intestinal infections with *Cryptosporidium parvum* and *Isospora belli* were virtually restricted to HIV seropositive individuals who had had diarrhoea for a relatively long time (Atzori et al., 1993). Similarly, it was noticed that maternal weight and low CD8+ cell counts were inversely associated with low body weight (LBW). While advanced-stage HIV disease, previous history of preterm birth, *Plasmodium falciparum* malaria, and any helmintic infection are associated with higher risk of LBW (Dreyfusset al., 2001). The intestinal parasites *Entamoeba histolytica* and *Strongyloides stercoralis* seemed to be predictors of LBW despite their low prevalence in the cohort. Moreover, the newborns' body mass index, midupper arm circumference, CD4 cell count <200 x 10^6 cells/L (200 cells/mm^3), primiparity, maternal literacy, and infant HIV infection at birth are significantly associated with birth weight in addition to risk factors associated with the LBW.

Cryptosporidiasis in AIDS patients usually causes chronic, bulky and intermittent diarrhea, with liquid non-bloody stools, accompanied by pain and abdominal colic, and a noticeable loss of weight can be observed. Asymptomatic cases are rarely described, occurring mostly in developing countries, Tanzania inclusive with patients showing milder. Cryptosporidium spp are common opportunistic parasites that cause chronic diarrhoea and wasting in HIV/AIDS patients with CD4+ T-cell counts <100 cells/µL and antimicrobial agents have limited efficacy in preventing or eradicating infections with it. Although studies assessing reduction in the incidence of cryptosporidiosis are lacking, diarrhoea due to cryptosporidia are known to resolve spontaneously with immune restoration among HIV/AIDS patients on antiretroviral therapy. Extra-intestinal manifestations have been clearly described in the literature, especially in the gall bladder, biliary ducts and pancreas, leading to conditions such as papillary stenosis, sclerosing cholangitis and calculous cholecystitis as well as chronic bronchitis (McGowan et al., 1997).

Isospora belli is a coccidian parasite that has a global distribution limited to mainly tropical regions in developing countries where it is endemic (especially Africa, the Middle East, and South America). The parasite invades the intestinal epithelium, where it completes its life cycle in the cytoplasm of the enterocyst. Unsporulated oocysts are excreted in feces and mature outside the host, where they develop into infective sporulated oocysts. Infection is then acquired through ingestion of these infective oocysts. Immunodeficiency was shown to increase the susceptibility to infection with *Isospora belli*, which accounted for up to 20% of cases of diarrhea in HV/AIDS patients. The lower prevalence of isosporiasis may be ascribed to the secondary prophylaxis for pneumocystosis through administration of sulfamethoxazole-trimethoprim during the course of HV/AIDS, since *Isospora belli* is sensitive to this chemotherapeutic agent.

The diarrheic condition is also noteworthy and is accompanied by fever, intestinal colic, anorexia, abdominal pain, loss of weight and peripheral eosinophilia. Isosporiasis can also show extraintestinal dissemination features, affecting the mesenteric, periaortic, mediastinal and tracheobronchial lymph nodes. It may also be related to biliary disease, causing manifestations of acalculous cholecystitis. Despite this high prevalence, classical protozoa such as *Giardia lamblia* and *Entamoeba histolytica* are less frequent as causes of severe illnesses in HIV-infected patients, when compared with *Isospora belli*and *Cryptosporidium parvum* and they are not considered as opportunistic infections in HV/AIDS. Amebiasis may present with invasive characteristics, but this has rarely been reported in the literature (Angarano et al., 1997).

Parasite infections especially malaria, and intestinal parasites undermine the nutritional status and compromise the immune system yet further, effectively exhausting it. These parasite infections are endemic in Tanzania, but the situation is made worse by inadequate health care and infrastructure, which actually by itself a function of poverty and low levels of development that leaves most parasite infections untreated.

2.4.2 Intestinal helminthic infections and HIV/AIDS

Neglected tropical diseases (NTDs) are a devastating burden for the people of Tanzania and are prevalent throughout the country. The country is endemic with all seven of the most common NTDs: schistosomiasis, lymphatic filariasis, onchocerciasis, trachoma, and the soil-transmitted helminths (hookworm, ascariasis, and trichuriasis). Such high prevalence rates of multiple NTDs increase the risk for co-infection with two or more diseases, a phenomenon that leads to more severe health consequences (Bundy et al., 2000; Luong et al., 2003).

Intestinal helminths are ubiquitous in low-income countries with prevalence of, for example 50–80% for ascariasis, trichuriasis and hookworm infections in many populations. Intestinal helminths induce immunological alterations that favor the progression from HIV seroconversion to AIDS. After HIV has spread to the systemic circulation its replication is limited by the fact that usually few activated lymphocytes and differentiated macrophages are present in the blood stream and that resting T cells and undifferentiated monocytes are not susceptible to HIV infection. However, in patients infected with intestinal helminths the number of activated T cells expressing human leucocyte antigen (HLA)-DR and HIV coreceptors is elevated. This is followed by HIV replication, preferentially in T-helper cells (Th cells) of Th2 and Th0 type clones. While Th2 cells are usually abundant in individuals infected with helminthes. Similarly, peripheral blood mononuclear cells of patients with helminthic infection are significantly more susceptible to infection with HIV than those of uninfected controls. Finally, elevated IL-4 levels, characteristic of the Th2 type of immune response in helminthic infections, down-regulate Th1 differentiation and function.

Therefore, parasitic infection could be a primary contributing factor to HIV/AIDS in Africa where men and women alike are at risk. Parasites are also endemic in people who are also at higher risk for HIV/AIDS, and most of these countries are underdevelopment/third world.

Activation of T cells, macrophages and other antigen presenting cells is necessary for HIV replication. This fact alone, may explain why lymphotropic and monocyte-tropic viruses originated in parasite endemic regions where suitable hosts reside. Indeed, Human T-lymphotropic virus-1 (TLV-1), HIV and Epstein-Barr virus (EBV). These are lymphotropic viruses that are found in close geographical relationship with parasite endemic regions. Women, especially in these developing countries of the world, are also prone to harbor chronic vaginal infections such as trichomoniasis, or have other predisposing vaginal factors for HIV/AIDS.

Among the helminthes in association with AIDS, there is no doubt that the most important pathogen is *Strongyloides stercoralis,* which is geohelminth presents its major effects in immunodepressed patients, leading to the dissemination of the infection. This occurs in transplanted patients, individuals presenting malnutrition and patients submitted to prolonged use of corticosteroids, suffering from leukemia, lymphomas or AIDS (Cimerman et al., 1998). In immunosuppressed patients, self-infestation is speeded up and a large number of larvae are released, causing the dissemination of the infection. Nevertheless, data from a single source published in 2010; show that in Tanzania the prevalence of helminthic infections in HIV-positive patients is around 8.2%, in comparison with 15.8% in non-HIV infected population (Mwambete et al., 2010). Hookworm (*Ancylostoma duodenale* and *Necator americanus*) infections being the most prevalent among HIV patients (17.1%) followed by *S. stercoralis* (3.3%). Although, there was no significant difference in respect of prevalence rates of helminthic infections between HIV-infected and non-infected patients; the study revealed direct correlation between CD4+ counts (HIV status) with helminthic infections among the HIV-infected patients. Nevertheless, helminthic infections are a grave health problem in Tanzania particularly among children from poor households as indicated in the Table 3 below (Mwambete and Kalison, 2006).

CD+4 counts	Helminthiasis (%)				
	Trichuris	**Hookworm**	**Ascaris**	**None**	**Total**
< 100	5(1.4)	2(0.6)	2(0.5)	14(3.8)	**23(6.4)**
101 - 200	50(13.7)	31(8.5)	35(9.6)	125(34.3)	**241(66.2)**
201 - 400	21(5.8)	6(1.6)	8(2.2)	31(8.5)	**66(18.2)**
401 - 500	7(1.9)	0(0.0)	1(0.3)	13(3.6)	**21(5.8)**
501 - 600	2(0.5)	0(0.0)	0(0.0)	4(1.1)	**6(1.6)**
601- 700	1(0.3)	0(0.0)	0(0.0)	6(1.6)	**7(1.9)**
Total	**86(23.6)**	**39(10.7)**	**46(12.6)**	**193(53.0)**	**364**

Table 3. Prevalence of helminthiasis in relation to HIV/AIDS status (CD+4 counts)

The other most common helminthes in Tanzania include *Ascaris lumbricoides, Trichuris trichura, Enterobius vermicularis* just naming a few. These are ubiquitous parasites in tropical and subtropical areas associated with causing diarrhea and hyperinfection syndrome in individuals with immunosuppressive disorders, including HIV/AIDS. Unfortunately, there are scant data or unavailable at all that relate and indicate the magnitude of the problem of parasitic infections among HIV-infected patients. A study conducted in rural Tanzania in 1995, revealed the prevalence rate of 81.8% (n= 287) of intestinal parasites in HIV-negative than in HIV-positive patients. The prevalence of *Ascaris lumbricoides* was higher in HIV-negative than in HIV-positive patients ($p < 0.01$; $p < 0.04$) (10.5% and 3.7% for *A. lumbricoides*). On the other hand, *Strongyloides stercoralis* prevalence was higher in HIV-positive than in HIV-negative patients ($P < 0.01$).

Schistosomiasis is another systemic helminthic infection, which is the second most prevalent tropical disease after malaria and affects approximately 200 million people in Africa, Asia, South America and other temperate regions. Severity of the infection largely depends on the intensity of infection, the *Schistosome* species involved, the topographic site affected by sequestered eggs and the immune responsiveness of the host. Urinary schistosomiasis is more prevalent in school-aged children than in adults. A prevalence of 57.9% was revealed in a study conducted in Kilosa (a semi-arid central district in Tanzania) among school-age children, which somehow is an indication of probably having even higher prevalence in lake areas (Mkopi et al., 2005; Clement et al., 2006).

In women, genital schistosomiasis occurs in about 60% of individuals infected with *Schistosoma haematobium*. Genital manifestations involve the vulva, vagina and the cervix as well as upper genital organs and result in pathology similar to that observed in some STIs. The cervix is the site predominantly affected, followed by the vagina and vulva. Thinning, erosion and ulceration of the epithelium is a typical clinical finding of genital schistosomiasis (Kjetland et al., 1996). This is important, as breaks in the integrity of the mucosal barrier, due to either trauma or sexually transmitted genital ulcer diseases are associated with an increased risk of HIV transmission (Mabey 2000).

Likewise, Schistosome eggs stimulate a complex array of cellular and humoral immune responses. Inflammations/granulomata form around eggs with a radius 5–10 times larger than the size of the egg. These granulomata are composed among others of activated lymphocytes, macrophages and epitheloid cells as well as some Lagerhan's giant cells, cell types known to express the CD4+ T cell receptor. In the wall of the bladder a considerable proportion of these granulomata ulcerate into the lumen. Similarly, in genital schistosomiasis egg-induced ulcerative lesions could be the port of entry for HIV. In the cervix, peri-oval granulomata are frequently formed near the basal layer of the epithelium. Within the egg granulomata, and also in adjacent areas, T cells, macrophages and Lagerhans cells abound (Helling-Giese et al., 1996). In mice, CD4+ T cells amount to 8–10% of all granuloma cells. The abundance of CD4 receptor-bearing cells within the confines of the granulomata and in adjacent areas make a rapid binding of virus after penetration through the friable and eroded epithelium of the cervix very likely. Therefore, genital schistosomiasis in males also points at an increased risk of HIV transmission. *Schistosoma haematobium* infection in males induces a chronic inflammation in the pelvic genitals, which looks like bacterial urethritis, accompanied with an increased viral shedding in the semen in HIV co-infected individuals.

Dar es Salaam, which is the largest commercial city, has an extensive drain network, mostly with inadequate water flow, making *Anopheles* and *Culex* larvae common. However, the importance of drains as larval habitats was previously unknown. The researchers analyzed detailed surveys of both mosquito habitats and drain conditions in the city; their findings suggest that simple but well-organized environmental management interventions, aimed to restore and maintain the functionality of drains, may help reduce mosquito-borne disease transmission. Lymphatic filariasis (LF) is a leading cause of disability due to parasitic infections in Tanzania. As of 2004, all districts were endemic with the disease, and prevalence rates reached up to 45%. Onchocerciasis (river blindness) has been documented in five regions and 15 districts throughout Tanzania, with an estimated 4 million people at risk for infection overall. In certain focal endemic areas, prevalence rates reach up to 64%.

Lymphatic filariasis is widely distributed in the tropics. It particularly occurs in areas with a high HIV prevalence such as sub-Saharan Africa and south-east Asia. There is no data available to show an impact of HIV infection on the prevalence or on the natural history of the disease. However, lymphatic filariasis is an example for a harmful interaction in the other direction. Replicative capacity of HIV is significantly enhanced in peripheral blood mononuclear cells from patients with untreated lymphatic filariasis. Consequently, untreated patients with lymphatic filariasis and co-infected with HIV could be at risk for rapid progression to AIDS once infected with HIV. Furthermore, the chronic manifestations of filariasis can have significant, and often very negative, social impacts. The chronic disabling manifestations of this disease, including lymphoedema of the limbs, breasts and external genitalia, have a profoundly detrimental effect on the quality of life of affected individuals.

The degree of social disability varies between cultural settings, but the degree of stigmatization appears to be directly correlated with the severity of visible disease (Evans et al., 1993). In conservative contexts, affected individuals avoid seeking treatment for fear of drawing attention to their condition. Failure to treat the disease results in recurrent acute febrile attacks and progressive damage to the lymphatic system. Without access to simple hygiene advice, sufferers are unable to prevent further progression of the outwardly visible complications of LF.

Women bear a double burden in societies where much of their role and identity is dependent upon marriage and the ability to give birth to children. Young unmarried women with LF may be forced to lead a reclusive existence in an attempt to hide their illness or because their limited marriage prospects make them a burden to their families. In Thailand and in West Africa there is a general perception that children born to a woman affected by LF will be similarly affected. Shame and anxiety related to difficulties in conceiving children are common for LF patients around the world (Evans et al., 1993). Young females with LF are considered poor marriage prospects because the disease's recurrent debilitating acute episodes limit their ability to perform paid and unpaid work. The costs associated with long-term health care as the disease progresses result in perceptions of these women as financial burdens.

2.4.3 Ectoparasite infections and HIV/AIDS

Epidermal parasitic skin diseases (EPSD) occur worldwide and have been known since ancient times. Despite the considerable burden caused by EPSD, this category of parasitic diseases has been widely neglected by the scientific community and health-care providers. This is illustrated by the fact that in the 2006 edition of The Communicable disease control handbook, a reference manual for public health interventions, only one EPSD (scabies) is mentioned (Fieldmeier and Heukelbach, 2009). Epidermal parasitic skin diseases fulfill the criteria defined by Ehrenberg and Ault (2005) for neglected diseases of neglected populations, but are not listed on national or international agendas concerning disease

control priorities (Ehrenberg and Ault, 2005). This probably explains why efforts to control EPSD at the community level have very rarely been undertaken (Heukelbach et al., 2002).
Six EPSD are of particular importance: scabies, pediculosis (head lice, body lice and pubic lice infestation), tungiasis (sand flea disease) and hookworm-related cutaneous larva migrans. They are either prevalent in resource-poor settings or are associated with important morbidity. This chapter focuses on these diseases, summarize the existing knowledge on the epidemiology and the morbidity in resource-poor settings and focus on the interactions between EPSD and poverty. The distribution of EPSD is irregular, and incidence and prevalence vary in relation to area and population studied. A study in a resource-poor community in urban Bangladesh, for example, showed that virtually all children aged less than 6 years developed scabies within a period of 12 months (Stanton et al., 1987). In a rural village in Tanzania, the overall prevalence is 6% and in rural India 13%, while in Australian Aboriginal communities the prevalence in this age group approached 50% (Sharma et al., 1984; Currie and Carapetis, 2000). Situation is even worse in displaced communities, where of 5-9-year-olds children in Sierra Leone, 86% are infested with *Sarcoptes scabiei*.
Poverty influences the epidemiology of EPSD in several ways because it creates animal reservoirs, ensures ongoing transmission, facilitates atypical ways of spreading the infectious agent and increases the chances of exposure. This results in an extraordinarily high prevalence and intensity of infestation and significant morbidity of EPSD. Again, stigma, lack of access to health care and hesitancy in seeking health care are the reasons why EPSD frequently progress untreated.
Inequality and neglect seem to be the major driving forces that keep the disease burden at an intolerably high level. Health-care stakeholders and political decision-makers must acknowledge that EPSD are debilitating and merit much more attention from health professionals than hitherto given. The ongoing uncontrolled urbanization in Tanzania and other developing countries makes it likely that EPSD will remain the overriding parasitic diseases for people living in extreme poverty and remain indicators of neglect by societies and particularly public health policies.

3. Conclusion

There are plenty of ways to help prevent HIV/AIDS by changing the biological and economic context in which the epidemic is spreading. Behavioral interventions are necessary, but their effectiveness is often a matter of faith more than documented results. So far, neither preaching abstinence nor handing out condoms has had an appreciable impact on the epidemic because sexual behavior is not the most important difference between high-prevalence and low-prevalence populations. Governments can change customs regulations or deliver safe water supplies and multivitamins more easily than they can chase down every person having unprotected sex. It is not a coincidence that the countries with the highest rates of HIV have serious environmental, economic, and bureaucratic problems. Most of the worst affected countries like Tanzania have problems of border-breach, ineffective parasitic infections control programmes, risky environment for HIV infection that all together is HIV/AIDS related.
Researchers have shown that there is a common immunopathogenetic basis for the detrimental interaction between HIV and pathogens biologically as different as for example, plasmodia and helminthes. Chronic immune activation by parasitic infection could be one of the several causes of T cells depletion in HIV infection and could considerably contribute to

the progression of HIV disease. Infection with intestinal helminthes, parasitic organisms living in a compartment aside of the systemic immune system, induces a status of chronic immune activation. The prolonged and enhanced immune activation is even more prominent in systemic parasitic infections, whether protozoa or helminthes. Even before HIV infection supervenes, chronic immune activation induced by parasites is associated with several of the immunological features of HIV disease.

In principle, the fact that parasites preferentially activate a Th2 type of help, among other functions Th2 cells down-regulate the development of Th1 cells, inhibit macrophage activity and impair the cytotoxic T-lymphocyte response. They encourage entry of HIV through the CD4 receptors located on the Th2 cells surfaces. The early presence of IL-4 is the most potent stimulus for Th2 differentiation. The inducing effect of IL-4 dominates over other cytokines so that, if IL-4 levels reach a certain threshold, differentiation of the Th cell into the Th2 phenotype ensues, thus favoring proliferation of the HIV, and particularly because of the low levels of Th1 cells that are necessary for the containment of HIV infection via cell-mediated immunity, whereby intracellular pathogens like HIV could be removed.

In contrast to HIV infection, which in the tropics is mainly a sexually transmitted disease, parasitic infections usually abound in childhood and/or adolescence. Moreover, in endemic areas sensitization towards the respective antigens already occurs early during prenatal period (*in utero*) as mothers are likely to be infected with the parasites as well. Notwithstanding, exposure to antigens *in utero* results in generation of cytokine responses similar to those found in adults and the ability of primed T cells to react accordingly can persist into childhood. Such early exposure generate memory cells of Th2 type of help would be a considerable disadvantage when later in life the immune system of the affected individual encounters HIV. Consequently, not only is HIV infection acquired more easily but more rapid progression from asymptomatic HIV infection to AIDS disease.

Summarily, it seems evident that people living in the tropics not only face a health threat in view of still expanding HIV epidemic, they also have to fear that once infected with HIV this will alter the natural history of parasitic infections they are suffering from in an unfavorable way. Besides the parasites they harbor impair the immune response towards HIV. In this way makes rapid progression from HIV infection to AIDS rather likely. As the great majority of parasitic diseases can be treated and /or to some extent be prevented, it is now logical that the control of parasitic infections should be included as a tool in the combat of HIV infections.

Although HIV prevalence has fallen in Tanzania over the past decade, thousands of people become infected with HIV every year and 86,000 Tanzanians died from AIDS in 2009 alone. While the poor are undoubtedly hit harder by the downstream impacts of AIDS, in a variety of ways, their chances of being exposed to HIV in the first place are not necessarily greater than wealthier individuals or households. However, the poor are more prone to parasitic infections. Poverty (illiteracy, food insecurity, poor public services and inequality), parasitosis and HIV/AIDS are the major problem currently facing Tanzanians. Therefore, a joint effort is urgently required to combat them in their totality, with that approach, the victory is evident.

4. References

Abu-Raddad, LJ., Patnaik, P., and Kublin, JG. (2006). Dual infection with HIV and malaria fuels the spread of both diseases in sub-Saharan Africa. *Science* Vol. 314:1603-1606. ISSN: 113238

Akinbo, FO., Okaka, C E., and Omoregie, R. (2010). Prevalence of intestinal parasitic infections among HIV patients in Benin City, Nigeria. *Libyan J Med* Vol. 5: 5506. ISSN:1993-2820

Angarano, G., Maggi, P., Di Bari, MA., Larocca, AM., Congedo, P., Di Bari, C., Brandonisio, O., and Chiodo, F. (1997). Giardiasis in HIV: a possible role in patients with severe immune deficiency. *Eur J Epidemiol* Vol.13(4): 485-7. ISSN: 0393-2990

Atzori, C., Bruno, A., Chichino, G., Bernuzzi, AM., Gatti, S., Comolli G., and Scaglia, M. (1993). HIV-1 and parasitic infections in rural Tanzania. *Ann Trop Med Parasitol* 87:585–93. ISSN: 0003-4983

Barnett, T., Whiteside, A., and Desmond, C. (2001) "The Social and Economic Impact of HIV/AIDS in Poor Countries: a Review of Studies and Lessons" in *Progress in Development Studies* Vol. 1(2), pp. 151–170.ISSN:1464-9934

Bisai, S., Ghosh, T., and Bose, K. (2010). Prevalence of underweight, stunting and wasting among urban poor children aged 1- 5 years of West Bengal, India. *Int J Current Res* Vol. 6: 39-44. ISSN: 0975-833X

Borkow, G., Weisman, Z., Leng, Q., Stein, M., Kalinkovich, A., Wolday, D., Bentwich, Z. Helminths, human immunodeficiency virus and tuberculosis. *Scandinavian Journal of Infectious Diseases* 33, 568–571. PMID: 11525348. ISSN: 0036-5548

Brink, AK., Mahé, C., Watera, C., Lugada, E., Gilks, C., Whitworth, J., and French, N. (2002)."Diarrhea, CD4 counts and enteric infections in a community-based cohort of HIV-infected adults in Uganda." *J Infec* Vol. 45(2):99-106. PMID: 12217712. ISSN: 0163-4453

Bullen, JJ., Spalding, PB., Ward, CG., and Gutteridge, JMC. (1991). Hemochromatosis iron and septicemia caused by *Vibrio vulnificus*. *Arch Inter Med* Vol. 151: 1606-1609. ISSN 0022-2615. ISSN: 0300-5127

Bundy, D., Sher, A., and Michael, E. (2000). Good worms or bad worms: do worm infections affect the epidemiological patterns of other diseases? *Parasitology Today* Vol. 16:273–274. ISSN: 0169-4758

Calder, PC. (1995). Fatty acids, dietary lipids and lymphocyte functions. *Biochem Soc Trans* Vol. 23: 302–9. ISSN: 0300-5127

Cates, W Jr. (1988). The "Other STD's" Do They Really Matter? *JAMA* Vol. 259: 3606-36-08. ISSN: 0098-7484

CDC (1987). Revision of the CDC surveillance case definition for acquired immunodeficiency syndrome. *MMWR*. Vol. 36(Suppl 1):1S-15S. ISSN: 0149-2195

Chopra, M. (2006). Mass deworming in Ugandan children. *BMJ* Vol. 333 : 105. Doi: 10.1136/BMJ.333.7559.ISSN: 09598138

Cimerman, S., Cimerman, B., and Lew, SD. (1999). Enteric parasites and Aids. *Sao Paulo Med* J Vol.117 (6): 226-273. ISSN 1516-3180

Clements, AC., Lwambo, N., Blair, L., Nyandindi, U., Kaatano, G., Kinunghi, S., Webster, J., Fenwick, A., and Brooker, S. (2006). Bayesian spatial analysis and disease mapping: tools to enhance planning and implementation of a schistosomiasis control programme in Tanzania. *Trop Med Int Health* Vol. 11:490–503. ISSN:1360-2276

Cunningham, MW., Fujinami, RS. (2000). Effects of Microbes on the Immune System. Philadelphia: Lippincott Williams and Wilkins; 2000: 662. ISBN: 1555811949

Cunningham Rundles S, McNeeley DF and Moon A (2005) Mechanisms of nutrient modulation of the immune response. J *Allergy Clin Immunol* 115, 1119-1128. ISSN: 0091-6749

Currie, BJ., and Carapetis, JR. (2000). Skin infections and infestations in Aboriginal communities in northern Australia. *Australas J Dermatol* Vol. 41:139-43. ISSN: OOO4 8380

De Onis, M., and Blössner, M. (2000). Prevalence and trends of overweight among preschool children in developing countries. *Am J Clin Nut Vol.* 72: 1032–9. Accesed on 21 February 2011, Available from: http://www.ajcn.org/content/72/4/1032.full.pdf. ISSN: 00029165

De Pablo, MA., and Alvarez de Cienfuegos, G. (2000). Modulatory effects of dietary lipids on immune system functions. *Immuno Cell Biol* Vol. 78, 31–39. ISSN: 0818-9641 ISSN: 0002-9165

Dorrington, R., Bourne, R., Bradshaw, D., Laubscher, R. and Timaeus, IM. (2001). The impact of HIV/AIDS on adult mortality in South Africa. ISBN 1-919809-14-7.

Dreyfuss ML, Msamanga GI, Spiegelman D, Hunter DJ, Urassa EJN, Hertzmark E and Fawzi WW. Determinants of low birth weight among HIV-infected pregnant women in Tanzania. *Am J Clin Nutrition* Vol. 74(6): 814-826, December 2001. ISSN 0002-9165

Ehrenberg, JP., and Ault, SK. (2005). Neglected diseases of neglected populations: thinking to reshape the determinants of health in Latin America and the Caribbean. *BMC Public Health* Vol.5:119. ISSN: 1471-2458

Evans, DB., Gelband, H., and Vlassoff, C. (1993). Social and economic factors and the control of lymphatic filariasis: a review. *Acta Trop* Vol. 53: 1-26. ISSN: 0001-706X

Feldmeier, H., and Heukelbach, J. (2009). Epidermal parasitic skin diseases: a neglected category of poverty-associated plagues. *Bull World Health Organ* Vol.87 (2), Genebra. ISSN: 0042-9686

Ferreira, ML. (1996). In: Handbook on Poverty and Inequality. "Poverty and Inequality during Structural Adjustment in Rural Tanzania." Policy Research Working Paper No. 1641, World Bank, Washington, DC. ISBN: 9780821376133

Franchin, G., Zybarth, G., Dai, WW., Dubrovsky, L., Reiling, N., Schmidtmayerova, H., Bukrinsky, M., and Sherry, B. (2000). Lipopolysaccharide inhibits HIV-1 infection of monocyte- derived macrophages through direct and sustained down-regulation of CC chemokine receptor 5. *J Immunol* Vol. 164:2592–2601. ISSN: 0022-1767

Giraldo, RA. (1997). AIDS and Stressors III: A Proposal for the Natural History of AIDS. In: AIDS and Stressors, Medellín-Colombia. Impresos Begón. pp. 97-131. ISBN: 9589458033

Graham, SM., Taylor, TE., and Plowe, CV. (2006). Impact of HIV-associated immunosuppression on malaria infection and disease in Malawi. *J Infect Dis* Vol.193:872-878. ISSN: 00221899

Hargreaves, J. and Howes, LD. (2010). 'Changes in HIV prevalence among differently educated groups in Tanzania between 2003 and 2007. *AIDS* Vol. 24(5) 755-761. ISSN: 0269-9370

Helling-Giese, G., Sjaastad, A., Poggensee, G., Kjetland, E,. Richter, J., Chitsulo, L., Kumwenda, N., and Racz, P. (1996). Female genital schistosomiasis (FGS): relationship between gynecological and histopathological findings. *Acta Tropica* Vol.62: 257–267. ISSN: 0001-706X

Heukelbach, J., Mencke, N., and Feldmeier, H. (2002). Cutaneous larva migrans and tungiasis: the challenge to control zoonotic ectoparasitoses associated with poverty. *Trop Med Int Health* Vol. 7:907-10. ISSN:1360-2276

Jahoor, F., Badaloo, A., Reid, M., and Forrester, T. (2008). Protein metabolism in severe childhood malnutrition. *Ann Trop Paediatr* Vol. 28: 87-101. ISSN:0272-4936

Kelley, DS., Taylor, PC., Nelson, GJ., Branch LB., Taylor, PC., Rivera, YM., and Schmidt, PC. (1991). Docosahexaenoic acid ingestion inhibits natural killer cell activity and production of inflammatory mediators in young healthy men. *Lipids* Vol. 34: 317-24. ISSN: 0269-1205

Kjetland, EF., Poggensee, G., Helling-Giese, G., Richter, J., Sjaastad, A., Chitsulo, L., Kumwenda, N., Gundersen, SG., Krantz, I., and Feldmeier, H. (1996). Female genital schistosomiasis due to *Schistosoma haematobium* Clinical and parasitological findings in women in rural Malawi. *Acta Tropica* Vol.62: 239-255. ISSN: 0001-706X

Liu, Z., Wang, D., Xue, Q., Chen, J., Li, Y., Xiaoli, B., and Chang, L. (2003). Determination of Fatty Acid Levels in Erythrocyte Membranes of Patients with Chronic Fatigue Syndrome. *Nutritional Neuroscience* Vol.6 (6): 389-392. ISSN: 1028-415X

Luong, TV. (2003). De-worming school children and hygiene intervention. *Inter J Environ Health Res* Vol. 13: S153 - S159. ISSN 0960-3123

Mabey, D. (2000). Interaction between HIV infection and other sexually transmitted diseases. *Tropical Med Interl Health* Vol. 5 (Suppl.):A32–A36. ISSN:1360-2276

Maclean, WC. Jr and Lucas, A. (2008). Peadric nutrition: A distinct subspecialityIn: . In Duggan C, Watkins JB and Walker WA. Nutrition in peadiatric 4. Basic Science-Clinical applications. International Print-O-Pac Ltd. India. ISBN 978-1-55009-361-2

Marsh, K. (1998). Malaria disaster in Africa. *Lancet* Vol. 352:924. ISSN: 0140-6736

McGowan, I., Chalmers, A., Smith, GR., and Jewell, D. (1997). Advances in Mucosal Immunology. *Gastroenterol Clin North Am* Vol. 26:145-173. ISSN: 0889-8553

Mhiri, C., Bélec, L., Di Constanzo, B., Georges, A., and Gherardi, R. (1992). The slim disease in African patients with AIDS. *Trans R Soc Trop Med Hyg* Vol. 86:303-6. ISSN: 0035-9203

Mkopi, A., Urassa, H., Mapunjo, E., Mushi, F., and Mshinda, H. (2005). Impact of school health programme on urinary schistosomiasis control in school children in Kilosa, Tanzania. *Tanzania Health Research Bulletin* Vol.7. ISSN: 0035-9203

Mshana, GH., Wamoyi, J., Busza, J., Zaba, B., Changalucha, J., Kaluvya, S., and Urassa, M. (2006). 'Barriers to accessing antiretroviral therapy in Kisesa, Tanzania: a qualitative study of early rural referrals to the national program.' *AIDS Patient Care STDS* Vol. 20(9):649-57. ISSN: 1087-2914

Mwambete, KD., and Kalison, N. (2006). Prevalence of Intestinal Helminthic Infections Among Under fives and Knowledge on Helminthiases Among Mothers of Under fives in Dar es Salaam, Tanzania. *East Afr J Public Heath* Vol. 3(1):8-11. ISSN: 0856-8960.

Mwambete, KD., Justin-Temu, M., and Peter, S. (2010). Prevalence and management of intestinal helminthiasis among HIV-infected patients at MNH. *J Inter Asso Physicians AIDS Care* Vol. 9(3):150-156. ISSN: 1545-1097

Ngalula, J., Urassa, M., Mwaluko, G., Isingo, R. and Boerma, JT. (2002). Health service use and household expenditure during terminal illness due to AIDS in rural Tanzania. *Trop Med Int Health.* Vol. 7(10):873-7. ISSN:1360-2276

Nkuo-Akenji, T., Tevoufouet, EE., Nzang, F., Ngufor, N., and Fon, E. (2008). High prevalence of HIV and malaria co-infection in urban Douala, Cameroon. *African J AIDS* Res Vol. 7 (2):229 - 235 ISSN: 1608-5906

Nnakwe, N. (1995). The effect and causes protein-energy malnutrition in Nigerian children. *Nutr Res* Vol. 15:785-794. ISSN: 0300-9831

PHDR. (2005). Poverty and Human Development.Report-2005. The research and analysis working group. Published by Mkuki na Nyota Publisher. Dar es Salaam, Tanzania. ISBN 9987-686-72-9

Pradeep, MA., Thiruvalluvan, M,. Aarthy, K. and Mary Stella J. (2010). Determination of Iron Deficiency among Human Immunodeficiency Virus Sero Positives. *Am Medical J* Vol.1 (2): 77-79. ISSN 1949-0070

Riemersma, RA., Armstrong, R., Kelly, RW.,and Wilson, R. (1998). Essential oils and Eicosanoids-invited papers from the 4th International congress. AOCS Press. USA. ISBN: 0-935315-96-9.

Roitt, I., Brostoff J., and Male, D. (2001). Immunology. 6th Edtion. Mosby. London. ISBN: 0723432422.

Roura, M., Busza, J., Wringe, A., Mbata, D., Urassa, M., and Zaba, B. (2009). Barriers to sustaining antiretroviral treatment in Kisesa, Tanzania: a follow-up study to understand attrition from the antiretroviral program. *AIDS Patient Care STDS* Vol. 23(3):203-10. ISSN: 1087-2914

Scrimshaw, NS., and SanGiovanni, JP. (1997). Synergism of nutrition, infection and immunity: an overview. *Am J Clin Nutr* Vol. 66:464S–477S. Online ISSN: 1938-3207

Sharma, RS., Mishra, RS., Pal, D., Gupta, JP., Dutta, M., and Datta, KK. (1984). An epidemiological study of scabies in a rural community in India. *Ann Trop Med Parasitol Vol.*78:157-64. ISSN: 0003-4983

Shelton, JD., Cassell, M., and Adetunji, A. (2005). 'Is poverty or wealth at the root of HIV?'. *Lancet* Vol. 366 (9491): 1057-8. ISSN: 0140-6736

Sherman, IW. (1998). Malaria: Parasite biology, pathogenesis and protection. Washington DC. American Society of Microbioogy Press. ISBN:1-55581-131-0

Stanton, B., Khanam, S., Nazrul, H., Nurani, S., and Khair, T. (1987). Scabies in urban Bangladesh. *J Trop Med Hyg* Vol.90:219-26. ISSN: 0022-5304

Strauss, RG. (2004). Iron deficiency, infections and immune function: a reassessment. *Am J Clinical Nutrition* Vol. 79(3):516-521. ISSN: 0002-9165

Tarimo, DS., Killewo, JZ., Minjas, JN., and Msamanga, GI. (1996). Prevalence of intestinal parasites in adult patients with enteropathic AIDS in north-eastern Tanzania. *East Afr Med J* Vol.73(6):397-9. ISSN: 0012-835X

Van Geertruyden J, Menten J, Colebunders R, Korenromp E, and D'AlessandroU. (2008).The impact of HIV-1 on the malaria parasite biomass in adults in sub-Saharan Africa contributes to the emergence of antimalarials drug resistance. *Malaria Journal* Vol. 7:134-147. ISSN: 0043-3144

Villamor, E., Misegades, L., Fatak,i MR., Mbise, RL., and Fawzi, WW. (2005). "Child mortality in relation to HIV infection, nutritional status, and socio-economic background." *Inter J Epidemiol* Vol 34(1) 61-8. ISSN: 0300-5751

Wojciki, JM. (2005). Socio-economic status as a risk factor for HIV infection in women in East, Central and Southern Africa: a systematic review. *J Biosocial Sci* Vol. 37:1-36. ISSN: 0021-9320

11

Collaborative Approach to Prevent Leprosy and HIV Coinfection in Abia, Ebonyi and Oyo States of Nigeria - Best Practices for a Healthier Population

Ezinne E. Enwereji[1], Chukwunenye I. Okereke[2] and Kelechi O. Enwereji[3]
[1]*Department of Community Medicine, College of Medicine, Abia State University,Uturu, Abia State,*
[2]*Department of Sociology, University of Port-Harcourt, Rivers State,*
[3]*Nnamdi Azikiwe University Teaching Hospital, Nnewi, Anambra State, Nigeria*

1. Introduction

The human immunodeficiency virus (HIV) pandemic has disproportionately affected many developing countries including Nigeria especially where dermatoses like leprosy is endemic. Though leprosy is an infectious disease, the risk of developing it is low. It is estimated that about 16,000 people are infected with leprosy annually. Early in the HIV epidemic, researchers feared that HIV infection would threaten leprosy control programmes, as have occurred with tuberculosis. It was suspected that patients with leprosy and HIV infection would have increased risk of lepromatous disease as well as clinical advancement. Moreover, that treatment for leprosy with HIV coinfection would be very difficult. Incidentally, reports on these concerns are to the contrary unlike what was noted with HIV and tuberculosis interaction. This paper, which will be organized in four sections, describes the various public health disease control programmes for leprosy and HIV infections in Nigeria. It details interaction between leprosy and HIV infection by evaluating and presenting the current situations. The paper will review the risks patients with leprosy and HIV coinfection face in clinical evolution, and likely difficulties encountered during treatment. Strengths and weaknesses in the entire programmes will be emphasized.

The potent effects of leprosy and HIV infections on the human immune system, and the dearth of current information on the prevalence of co-infected patients make this area of investigation necessary. The review of the epidemiological, clinical, and pathological data relating to leprosy and HIV coinfection will provide information on the interaction between leprosy and HIV in developing countries. This will give insight to the problem by providing proper understanding of the classification system of the interaction which includes (1) leprosy and HIV true coinfection, (2) opportunistic leprosy disease, and (3) leprosy related to highly active antiretroviral therapy. Therefore, research on clinical, and management aspects of this coinfection is reviewed.

In this review, some studies confirmed that in developing countries, there exists large cohort of patients concurrently infected with HIV and M. leprae. Sparse but provoking evidence exists that infection with HIV may increase the incidence of leprosy among individuals with sub-clinical infection with M. leprae. Similarly, it was postulated that concurrent infections with certain other viral and bacterial pathogens in HIV-positive patients may aggravate mycobacterial leprae disease and accelerate the progress of HIV infection to AIDS. The interplay between HIV and leprosy infection and the impact on the lives of the cases is highlighted. Possible effects of HIV epidemic on leprosy control programmes and few guidelines for the clinical care of co-infected patients as outlined by the World Health Organization (WHO) are emphasized. Also the WHO responses to conventional therapeutic regimens which appear to be excellent, though, no follow-up data were observed even in larger reported field studies are indicated. The introduction of highly active antiretroviral therapy (HAART) for HIV has been lifesaving, but few patients undergoing HAART are reported to experience clinical deterioration caused by immune reconstitution inflammatory syndrome (IRIS). For leprosy, it can be easily treated with 6–12-months course of multi-drug therapy (MTD). This treatment has been highly effective with few side effects; low relapse rates and no known drug resistance was noted. Although some researchers argue that treating leprosy patients with HIV coinfection may not affect public health services but the true effect remains to be clarified because leprosy has a wide range of clinical manifestations, which sometimes impose a clinical challenge that leads to misdiagnosis. If coinfection is properly documented it may help to unmask the true scenario of leprosy and HIV co-infection, particularly in areas where these disease conditions are highly endemic.

Further the paper describes significant contributions made by the government, stakeholders and International organizations of Anti-Leprosy Associations (ILEP) like, Damien Foundation of Belgium (DFB), German Leprosy and Tuberculosis Relief Association (GLRA), Netherlands Leprosy Relief (NLR) and others towards the well-being of those affected by leprosy and HIV.

Although awareness of the relevance of leprosy and human immunodeficiency virus (HIV) coinfection is increasing worldwide, there is need for research on leprosy and HIV coinfection in a developing country like Nigeria because several aspects of this coinfection is yet to be understood. This means that co-infection with human immunodeficiency virus (HIV) and *Mycobacterium leprae* represent unique opportunities for more investigation on the interaction between both pathogens.

In this paper, report of 3 leprosy patients who were diagnosed HIV-positive patients and were on HAART initiation as well as on multidrug therapy (MTD), will be reported. The 3 patients were among the sample studied in three leprosy settlements who were infected with leprosy and HIV co-infection. During the study, there were misconceptions that HIV could be transmitted through casual social contact and saliva. This was influenced by the patients' behavior as they reported that they avoided interactions with some family members. For instance, one of the patients commented that: "because of the fear that her daughter will get HIV, she stopped cooking, bathing and drinking from same cup with her daughter."

This paper includes counseling as an important technique in improving HIV related knowledge among the sample. The paper further highlights the beneficial effects of peer counseling as an intervention. Leprosy has now been reported as presenting immune reconstitution disease among patients commencing highly active antiretroviral treatment (HAART). Little or no studies in interactions between leprosy and HIV are available. Therefore, further research on all aspects of the coinfection especially the clinical and management aspects are warranted.

Assessment of leprosy and HIV control programmes is an essential component of intervention research effort aimed at addressing the strengths and limitations of the programmes for optimum benefit of the patients. Assessing available services is part of Public Health intervention that fills an important gap in the literature for public health researchers, practitioners, scholars, trainers, donors and students. This study is necessary because the well-being of those with leprosy and HIV should attract attention in research. The study will help in generating resources for academic contributions.

For the purposes of organizing this work, there will be four sections. The first section provides background information on leprosy and HIV work in Nigeria. It will emphasize the design and implementation of public health disease control programmes by examining the strengths and weaknesses of the programmes.

The paper details interaction between leprosy and HIV infection by evaluating and presenting the current situations. The second section will review the risks patients with leprosy and HIV coinfection face in clinical evolution, and likely difficulties encountered during treatment. It will include the roles of international bodies, stakeholders and others in care and support of the patients. Highlight of the guidelines of the clinical care of co-infected patients will be emphasized. The third section contains interventions needed to improve HIV related knowledge among HIV positive individuals. Theoretical and practical bases for planning rehabilitation and other activities for patients will be highlighted. This section also contains information on how materials and financial supports are obtained for intervention services. Strategies for continuing the intervention beyond its initial phase will be noted. The true effects of public health services would be clarified because leprosy has a wide range of clinical manifestations. The final section examines current work and problems encountered by the patients as well as projecting future trends and/or activities useful in meeting the needs of the patients.

2. Background information on leprosy and HIV prevention programmes in Nigeria

This section gives some historical information on leprosy and HIV work in Nigeria. It outlines various prevention programmes and the organizations that supported these programmes. It gives account of how each disease prevention programme was conducted and highlights the progresses made. It starts with giving vivid account of how leprosy prevention programmes were conducted.

3. Leprosy prevention programmes

Leprosy work started in 1920s with the establishment of leprosy colonies where Christian Missionaries provided care and support to those infected. In other to assist these Missionaries and the Nigerian government to provide quality leprosy control programmes, International Federation of Anti-Leprosy Association (ILEP) Partners like Damien

Foundation of Belgium (DFB), German Leprosy and Tuberculosis Relief Association (GLRA) and Netherlands Leprosy Relief (NLR) volunteered material and human resources. Four events characterized this period. These are the establishment of high standard medical intervention for detecting and treating cases, building of leprosaria, working as advocates for those affected with leprosy, and providing personal and professional staff development to meet the needs of patients. These international organizations that pioneered these services during the Nigerian civil war(1966-1970) left to their respective countries and handed over the management of these services as well as the affairs of the leprosaria to the government and other interested stakeholders. The unstable nature of the social and economic well-being of Nigeria during the civil war affected the smooth running of leprosy programmes as well as that of the leprosaria. Most inmates took to the streets to beg for alms for survival.

4. Types of leprosy programmes carried out

Leprosy work in Nigeria concentrated on reducing the incidence of leprosy through early case detection and ensuring that Multi-drug Therapy and hospital services were widely available. A vital part of this work includes Prevention of Disability and rehabilitation of people affected by leprosy. The followings are the main leprosy control programmes conducted:

5. Orthopaedic project

Workshops for producing protective footwear and other orthopaedic gadgets were established. In these workshops protective footwear like sandals and other orthopaedic appliances to improve the quality of life of people affected by leprosy were produced and shared to those in need.

5.1 Training

Health workers were trained to detect and provide leprosy care. Also some inmates in the leprosaria were trained in crafts like weaving, tailoring, sewing, and others so as to enable them live a life of fulfillment. In addition, health education was used to create awareness at the grassroots on the cause and prevention of leprosy.

Also through training, discharged patients and their family members learnt how to protect themselves from injury and further disability using long term self care routines. This was considered very important because the patients were equipped with how to avoid ulcers, infections, as well as the benefits of strengthening exercises, and wearing protective footwear on anaesthetic feet.

5.2 Socio-Economic Rehabilitation (SER)

Through SER programmes, people affected by leprosy were empowered and enabled to become economically independent. Those who completed vocational training were allowed micro-credit schemes to enable them form cooperative where making and marketing of their local crafts and souvenirs were organized.

5.3 Leprosy referral hospital

A good number of the religious groups assisted with financial and professional support in the provision of services to people affected by leprosy. For instance, Church of Scotland Mission in 1927, Qua Iboe Church in 1932, and Methodist Church in 1937 established hospitals where healthcare services were provided to people affected by leprosy as well as to the local population. These hospitals accepted leprosy referrals from all over Nigeria. Patients self-help groups were formed after treatment. These groups were encouraged to regularly meet in their respective communities so as to support each other in self-care routines.

5.4 Advocacy

The Missionaries, in partnership with leprosy organizations, hospitals, governments and communities worked to reduce the negative attitudes surrounding leprosy. International networking and advocacy organizations served as a powerful voice for those stigmatized by leprosy. These organizations worked hard to eliminate leprosy as a public health problem. The activities they carried out in order to realize their aims laid solid foundations in attaining the goal of World Health Assembly proposal of 1991 in which leprosy as a public health problem was estimated to achieve a global level of leprosy prevalence of less than one case per 10 000 population in the year 2000. Consequently, the Strategic Plan for Leprosy Elimination for 2000-2005 was initiated to mobilize support by encouraging leprosy-endemic countries to ensure that leprosy services would be available and accessible to all persons affected by leprosy at their nearest health facility. Leprosy campaigns during this period centered on increased coverage through mass campaigns and a widespread reduction of the global prevalence of cases registered for treatment.

6. Community rehabilitation services

While much of the leprosy services concentrated on the medical by detecting , treating and curing those affected by leprosy, some aspects of holistic and integrated rehabilitation approaches like counseling, advocacy, distribution of mobility gadgets, micro-credit loan to cater for the needs of those affected by leprosy were undertaken. To ensure livelihoods and economic independence for these patients, they were encouraged to take up their traditional occupations, start new vocations or set up small businesses. This means that individuals were empowered to live productive and dignified lives, through improving mobility and creating opportunities to earn a living. By this method, beneficiaries became powerful advocates for reducing the stigma of leprosy in their respective communities. Also for those with disabilities, physiotherapy and mobility aids were provided.

7. Background information on HIV prevention programmes in Nigeria

HIV and AIDS were first noted in Nigeria in 1985. In 1987 the Nigerian health sector established the National AIDS Advisory Committee (NAAC) and the National Expert Advisory Committee on AIDS (NEACA). These two committees were charged with matters connected with HIV and AIDS prevention. In 1991, exactly four years after forming the two committees, the Federal Ministry of Health on assessing Nigeria's AIDS situation, noted that the government was slow in responding to the increasing rates of HIV transmission. The results of the Federal Ministry of Health's assessment showed that HIV prevalence rose from 3.8% in 1993 to 4.5% in 1998 indicating urgent intervention to slow the trend.

In 1999, when Olusegun Obasanjo became the president of Nigeria, meaningful progress in the activities of HIV prevention, treatment and care in Nigeria was noticed. During this period, HIV and AIDS prevention and control became one of the government's primary concerns. To assist him realize the goal of increasing HIV prevention to reduce HIV prevalence in Nigeria, the President formed Presidential Committee on AIDS (PCA) as well as the National Action Committee on AIDS (NACA) . Subsequently, the government formed the corresponding Committees on HIV and AIDS at State level, State Action Committee on AIDS (SACA) and at Local Government level, Local Action Committee on AIDS (LACA). Consequently, the government in 2001 set up strategies for achieving these goals by outlining a three-year HIV and AIDS Emergency Action Plan (HEAP) .

Despite the government's efforts to control HIV epidemic, by 2006 it was noted that only 10 percent of HIV-infected individuals were receiving antiretroviral therapy while 7 percent of pregnant women were receiving treatment to reduce the risk of mother -to -child transmission of HIV.

Ten years after establishing NACA, precisely in 2010, NACA launched its comprehensive National Strategic Framework to cover 2010 to 2015 implementation of HIV prevention. The aims of this framework are to:

- reach 80 percent of sexually active adults and most at-risk populations with HIV counselling and testing by 2015;
- ensure that 80 percent of eligible adults and 100 percent of eligible children are receiving anti-retroviral therapy (ART) by 2015 and,
- to improve access to quality care and support services to at least 50 percent of people living with HIV by 2015.

Despite the laudable aims of National Strategic Framework as itemized, Nigeria being the largest oil producing country in Africa, and the 12th largest in the world, is still faced with huge financial challenges in fighting its HIV and AIDS epidemic. It has been estimated that the Nigerian government is contributing only 5 percent of the funds for the antiretroviral treatment programmes. The majority of the funding comes from development partners like, in 2002, the World Bank alone loaned US$90.3 million to Nigeria to support her 5-year HIV/AIDS Programme Development Project. In 2008 PEPFAR provided US$448 million to Nigeria for HIV/AIDS prevention, treatment and care while Global Fund offered US$95 million to expand treatment, prevention, and prevention of mother-to-child transmission programmes.

8. How HIV is transmitted in Nigeria

It has been documented that in Nigeria, HIV is transmitted by three main routes such as:

- **Heterosexual sex,** this accounts for approximately 80-95 percent of HIV infections in Nigeria. Factors that contribute to this mode of HIV transmission include lack of information about sexual health, low levels of condom use, and high prevalence of sexually transmitted diseases among adolescents. Reports have shown that females are more affected by HIV infection than males. For instance, in 2009 females accounted for 56 percent of all adults aged 15 and above living with HIV virus.
- **Blood transfusions,** this second mode of HIV transmission accounts for the second largest source of HIV infection in Nigeria. It is disheartening to note that some Nigerian

hospitals do not have the technology to effectively screen blood and thereby exposing individuals to the risk of using unsafe or contaminated blood. To check this ugly trend, the Nigerian Federal Ministry of Health have sponsored a legislation that requires hospitals to only use blood from the National Blood Transfusion Service, which is assumed has far more advanced blood-screening technology than other hospitals. However, it has been noted that not all hospitals use blood from the National Blood Transfusion Service.

- **Mother-to-child transmission**, this is the third mode of HIV transmission. It is estimated that 360,000 children are living with HIV in Nigeria. Most of these children were infected from their mothers.

A number of studies have indicated a rise in HIV prevalence among injecting drug users. Although HIV transmission through injecting drug is not among the main HIV transmission routes, there is need to mention it because reports show that HIV transmission through injecting drug use now account for an increasing number of new HIV infections.

HIV treatment and care in Nigeria

In early 1990s when antiretroviral drugs (ARVs) were introduced in Nigeria, the drugs were only available to those who paid for them. The drugs were unaffordable because the overwhelming majority of Nigerians were living on less than $2 a day. That is, only the wealthy minority was able to afford the treatment.

In 2002 the Nigerian government introduced antiretroviral treatment programme, which was aimed at providing treatment to 10,000 adults and 5,000 children yearly. To realize this aim, $3.5 million worth of ARVs were imported from India. This was to be delivered at a subsidized monthly cost of $7 per person. At this time the programme was applauded because it was regarded as 'Africa's largest antiretroviral treatment programme. Two years later, precisely in 2004, the programme suffered a major setback. There was an expanding waiting list of patients because of lack of drugs to meet the high demands. Some patients waited for more than three months before receiving more drugs. The result was that patients who were on treatment had to wait for three to four months before more drugs were supplied. This caused severe reverse to the progress the drugs had already made thereby increased the risk of HIV resistance to the ARVs.

To this end, the Nigerian government had to set 2010 as the year of providing universal access to HIV prevention, care, and treatment. The government outlined and implemented a number of strategies to scale up HIV prevention as follows:

Sex education

The discussion of sex with teenagers in Nigeria is often seen as a taboo. Attempts to provide sex education to young people are usually hindered by religious and cultural objections. In 2009, only 23 percent of schools provided HIV education, and just 25 percent of men and women between the ages of 15 and 24 could correctly identify ways to prevent sexual transmission of HIV without any misconceptions about HIV transmission.

In most regions of Nigeria, girls marry relatively young, and most times, to much older men. For instance, in North Western Nigeria, half of the girls marry between the ages of 15 to 18 years. Studies have confirmed that women who marry at a younger age lack correct knowledge about HIV and AIDS than those who marry later in life. To this group of women,it is assumed that they were not exposed to sex education especially HIV and AIDS before marriage. Studies have recommended that HIV and AIDS education initiatives should center on this class of young married women, because of their limited knowledge of health information.

9. Condom use

Restrictions on condom promotion by individuals especially religious leaders hampered HIV prevention efforts in Nigeria. Religious leaders saw condom as a taboo and therefore condemned its use. As a result, most adolescents use condom clandestinely. In 2001, a radio advertisement by the Advertising Practitioners Council of Nigeria (APCON) was suspended because they promoted messages suggesting that it is safe to engage in premarital sex as long as a condom is used. Members of the religious bodies frowned at this and cautioned the advertising company to desist from such advertisement in the interest of youths. In 2006 APCON also started another advertisement on condom and this time it enforced stricter regulations on condom advertisements that encouraged 'indecency in the use of condom. By APCON's advertisement, youths were advised to ensure that they carry with them condom always.

10. Media campaigns and public awareness

Several people in different parts of Nigeria were reached using media campaigns. Media campaigns are useful because they are the practical ways of reaching many people to raise HIV awareness. For instance, "Future Dreams", radio campaign programmes created by the Society for Family Health in 2001 have recorded tremendous success in increasing knowledge and changing behaviour of many individuals on HIV and AIDS. "Future Dreams" are serial broadcast made in nine different languages on 42 different radio channels which focused on encouraging consistent condom use, increasing knowledge and skills for condom negotiation among sexually active individuals between the ages of 18 and 34.

In 2005, another campaign, which raised more public awareness of HIV/AIDS than others, was launched in Nigeria. This campaign sent text messages with information about HIV/AIDS to at least 9 million owners of mobile phones.

Further, a high profile media campaign to create more HIV awareness was fronted by Femi Kuti, the son of Fela Kuti, the famous Afrobeat musician who died of AIDS in 1997. Fela Kuti's pictures were put on billboards alongside the roads throughout Nigeria with the slogan 'AIDS: No dey show for face', which means you can not identify someone who has AIDS by looking at the face. This message was very popular and had a lot of impression on youths who desired to prevent HIV infection.

11. Prevention of mother-to-child transmission of HIV

The programme to prevent the transmission of HIV from mother to child (PMTCT) started in Nigeria in July 2002. Initially, this programme of strengthening PMTCT interventions, suffered a major setback due to inaccessibility and un-affordability of anti-retroviral drugs. Records in 2007 show that only 5.3 percent of HIV positive women are on antiretroviral drugs to reduce the risk of mother-to-child transmission. However, by 2010, the percentage of HIV positive women on antiretroviral drugs rose to 22 percent , but still this falls far short of the recommended universal access targets.

12. HIV testing programmes

In 2007, only 3 percent of the health facilities in Nigeria had functional HIV testing and counselling services. Also 11.7 percent of women and men aged 15-49 had received an HIV test to find their sero-prevalence.

In 2009 HIV counseling services translated to merely one HIV testing and counselling facility for approximately every 53,000 Nigerian adults. This shows the extent to which the government desperately needs to scale up HIV testing and counseling services. There is evidence to show that in Nigeria, health care facilities that offer HIV testing scarcely follow the international standards on confidentiality and ethics. For instance, a survey carried out on HIV testing showed that half of the people interviewed reported that they were not aware that they were being tested for HIV virus. Also one in six health care professionals interviewed admitted that they do not receive informed consent for HIV tests before they test their clients.

The government's National HIV and AIDS Strategic Framework for 2005 to 2009 planned to provide ARVs to 80 percent of individuals with advanced HIV infection as well as 80 percent of HIV-positive pregnant women by 2010 . However, out of this goal, only 31 percent of people who needed treatment for advanced HIV infection received it. There is need to beef up HIV counseling and testing services to meet the needs of clients.

13. Constraints in providing disease control programmes

In Nigeria, several constraints are encountered in the process of carrying out disease control programmes. For instance, there is a distinct lack of political will among some of the leaders. Disease prevention programmes on both leprosy and HIV are poorly funded by government. These leaders, by their actions lack the intention to ensure sustainability of disease control programmes. They do not promote integration within the general health system. This results to lack of focus on issues that encourage quality services, especially to the underserved communities. There is no effective partnerships that would further reduce the disease burden. Another constraint is government's poor implementation of the country's specific strategies and plans of action aimed to sustain and provide high quality services to individuals and their families affected by leprosy and/or HIV. Therefore, there should be activities based on current evidence, professional knowledge and best practices for the implementation of leprosy and HIV coinfection control. This will ensure that laws and policies that would encourage the mitigation of HIV and institutionalization of best practices in care and support for people living with HIV and AIDS are maintained.

Nigeria's public health care system has deteriorated because of lack of resources and more especially, a "brain drain" of Nigerian doctors and nurses to other countries. Because Nigeria is yet to fully recognize the gravity of the epidemic of leprosy and HIV, provision of care, treatment, and prevention services to those with coinfection remains inadequate and the level of unmet need continues to increase.

The fact is that resources needed to provide sufficient treatment and care for those affected by leprosy and HIV in Nigeria are seriously lacking. Health workers lack sufficient training on treatment and disease prevention techniques especially on leprosy and HIV. Also a good number of the health facilities lack enough medications, equipment and materials for disease control activities.

Leprosy and HIV coinfection

The current situation concerning leprosy endemicity and HIV prevalence in Nigeria as well as in other developing countries emphasizes the importance of monitoring co-infections. Leprosy takes a long time to develop and patients may die from other causes resulting from HIV infection before leprosy becomes clinically apparent. The effect of this is a lowering of resistance to a wide range of opportunistic and other infections. Lepromatous leprosy may make the patient more susceptible to HIV, since leprosy also presents with a depression in the cell-mediated immunity (CMI) to M. leprae. Therefore, it is essential to detect HIV infection in areas where leprosy is endemic for a better understanding of the risk of spreading the mycobacterial disease in the community. Co-infections with human immunodeficiency virus (HIV) and *Mycobacterium leprae* represent unique opportunities for investigating the interaction between both pathogens.

The present study was undertaken to find out the prevalence of HIV infection in the population of those affected by leprosy. The low percentage of HIV infection among these leprosy patients suggests that HIV does not pose a serious problem in already M. leprae-specific subjects. The clinical presentation and disability grade of HIV infected leprosy patients were similar to that of leprosy patients without HIV infection. Our results indicate that HIV infection does not contribute to a more serious clinical presentation of leprosy among leprosy patients in leprosy settlements.

Although many studies reported more seropositivity in lepromatous patients than in tuberculoid patients, in our study no clear association between these groups was noted. Various other studies have also noted a similar non-association between BL/LL leprosy and HIV. Further, some authors stressed that leprosy could develop with HIV infection. However, in the present study, none of the leprosy patients reported being infected with HIV before leprosy infection.

Three case reports of leprosy patients who developed human immunodeficiency virus (HIV) infection are presented. The three co-infected leprosy patients were among the 227 leprosy patients studied in the three settlements in Nigeria. The coinfected patients were on highly active antiretroviral therapy (HAART). The result indicates low prevalence of leprosy and HIV coinfection. However, the reports from the three patients suggest that they had leprosy acute inflammatory episodes which probably were triggered off by HAART immune reconstitution.

Therefore, coinfection is possible because during the study, a good number of the patients were seen either pregnant or nursing babies without being properly married. This suggests that multiple sexual relationships were common among the leprosy patients in the settlements. The leprosy patients studied showed poor knowledge of HIV modes of transmission. For instance, during the study, there were misconceptions that HIV could be transmitted through casual social contact and saliva. This was influenced by the patients' behavior as they reported that they avoided interactions with some family members so as to protect them from being infected. For example, one of the patients commented that: "because of the fear that her daughter will get HIV, she stopped cooking, bathing and drinking from same cup with her daughter." To further show scanty knowledge about HIV transmission among the patients, the study noted that scarcely could 20% of the patients give two correct modes of HIV transmission during counselling. This suggests that national HIV prevention programmes may not be available to the leprosy patients. These observations suggest the need to include leprosy patients in national HIV prevention programmes.

The present study was considered necessary because understandably, leprosy and HIV infections are both greatly feared in developing countries because of the stigma, rejection and ostracism individuals affected by the two attract in the society.

In conclusion, the prevalence of HIV and leprosy coinfection in leprosy settlements in Nigeria is low . It can be said that HIV related knowledge among the patients was very low and positively influenced by HIV counseling. In addition, counseling by peers was effective in improving the knowledge of HIV among the patients. Hence, HIV related knowledge of these subjects should be assessed periodically and counseled.

14. References

Breton, G., X. Duval, C. Estellat, et al. 2004. Determinants of immune reconstitution inflammatory syndrome in HIV type 1-infected patients with tuberculosis after initiation of antiretroviral therapy. Clin. Infect. Dis. 39:1709-1712

Couppie P, Abel S, Voinchet H, Roussel M, Helenon R, Huerre M, et al. Immune reconstitution inflammatory syndrome associated with HIV and leprosy. Arch Dermatol 2004;140:997-1000.

Lawn SD, Wood C, Lockwood DN. Borderline tuberculoid leprosy: an immune reconstitution phenomenon in a human immunodeficiency virus-infected person. Clin Infect Dis 2003;36:e5-6.

Lawn SD, Bekker LG, Miller RF. Immune reconstitution disease associated with mycobacterial infections in HIV-infected individuals receiving antiretrovirals. Lancet Infect Dis *2005;5:361*-73.

Leonard G, Sangare A, Verdier M, Sassou-Guesseau E, Petit G, Milan J, M'Boup S, Rey JL, Dumas JL, Hugon J, N'Gaporo I, Denis F, 1990. Prevalence of HIV infection among patients with leprosy in African countries and Yemen. *J Acquir Immune Defic Syndr 3:* 1109–1113.

Lawn SD, 2004. AIDS in Africa: the impact of coinfections on the pathogenesis of HIV-1 infection. *J Infect 48:* 1–12.

Lienhardt C, Kamate B, Jamet P, Tounkara A, Faye OC, Sow SO, Bobin P, 1996. Effect of HIV infection on leprosy: a threeyear survey in Bamako, Mali. *Int J Lepr Other Mycobact Dis 64:* 383–391.

Pignataro, P., A. S. Rocha, J. A. Nery, et al. 2004. Leprosy and AIDS: two cases of increasing inflammatory reactions at the start of highly active antiretroviral therapy. Eur. J. Clin. Microbiol. Infect. Dis. 23:408-411.

Shelburne, S. A., III, and R. J. Hamill. 2003. The immune reconstitution inflammatory syndrome. AIDS Rev. 5:67-79.

Trindade, M. A., N. Y. Valente, M. I. Manini, M. D. Takahashi, C. F. Anjos, G. Benard, and B. Naafs. 2006. Two patients coinfected with *Mycobacterium leprae* and human immunodeficiency virus type 1 and naive for antiretroviral therapy who exhibited type 1 leprosy reactions mimicking the immune reconstitution inflammatory syndrome. J. Clin. Microbiol. 44:4616-4618

Ustianowski AP, Lawn SD, Lockwood DN. Interactions between HIV infection and leprosy: a paradox. Lancet Infect Dis 2006;6:350-60.

World Health Organization. 22 December 2006, last update. Leprosy tools and guidelines. World Health Organization, Geneva, Switzerland.

12

The Impact Water, Sanitation and Hygiene Infrastructures Have on People Living with HIV and AIDS in Zimbabwe

Natasha Potgieter[1], Tendayi B. Mpofu[1] and Tobias G. Barnard[2]
[1]*Department of Microbiology, University of Venda,*
[2]*Water and Health Research Unit, University of Johannesburg,*
South Africa

1. Introduction

Acquired Immune Deficiency Syndrome (AIDS) emerged in the 1980s as the most terrifying epidemic of modern times. AIDS as a disease is caused by a virus called the Human Immunodeficiency Virus (HIV). The total number of people living with HIV worldwide in 2009 was 33.3 million (UNAIDS, 2009). Sub-Saharan Africa continues to be the hardest hit by the global HIV and AIDS epidemic with an estimated 22.5 million infected people in 2009. AIDS was first reported in Zimbabwe in 1985 and by the beginning of the 1990s, around 10% of the adult population were thought to be infected with HIV (UNAIDS 2005). The estimated adult HIV prevalence rate (aged 15-49) during 2009 in Zimbabwe was reported to be 14.3% (UNICEF webpage).

Presently very little data is available on how water, sanitation and hygiene infrastructures are affecting the lives of people living with HIV and AIDS (PLWHA) in Zimbabwe. Literature has identified a series of linkages between water, sanitation and hygiene and HIV and AIDS (USAID/WSP, 2007). According to UNICEF (2005), a hygienic environment, clean water and adequate sanitation are key factors in preventing opportunistic infections associated with HIV and AIDS, and in the quality of life of people living with the disease. PLWHA are more susceptible to water-related diseases than healthy individuals, and they become sicker from these infections than people with healthy immune systems (UNICEF, 2005).

The urban areas of the Bulawayo metropolitan province of Zimbabwe consist primarily of high-density sub-urban areas and peri-urban settlements with municipal treated water supplies. Some peri-urban areas have unprotected water sources (rivers) and limited or totally inadequate sanitation. Although communal taps serve most peri-urban settlements, critical water shortages force these communities to rely on water from boreholes, unprotected wells and rivers for domestic use. Most of these households use pit latrines and some use the bush. Households in the rural areas mainly rely on boreholes as water sources, with a few households having piped water supply from Zimbabwe National Water Authority (ZINWA). This made the Bulawayo metropolitan the ideal study area to obtain representative data about the possible impact water, sanitation and hygiene infrastructures can have on the health of PLWHA in Zimbabwe.

Diarrhoeal diseases are the most common opportunistic infections experienced by PLWHA in Africa and elsewhere. Most of these diarrhoeal infections are either water borne or water washed. Patients with HIV infection or AIDS are commonly affected by gastrointestinal infections, with diarrhoea as the most common presentation (Janoff and Smith, 1988). Diarrhoea occurs in 30-60% of AIDS patients in developed countries and in about 90% of AIDS patients in developing countries (Framm and Soave, 1997). Enteric pathogens that cause diarrhoea include bacteria, parasites, fungi and viruses (Mitra et al., 2001). *Escherichia coli* (*E. coli*) are commonly used as an indicator of faecal pollution in water, indicating the possible presence of other bacterial pathogens that could have been shed into the water source.
Although *E. coli* is used as an indicator it also has the capability of contriburting to the diarrheal load in an area. Five classes of *E. coli* bacteria that cause diarrhoeal diseases are now recognised: enterotoxigenic *E. coli* (ETEC), enteroinvasive *E. coli* (EIEC), enterohaemorrhagic *E. coli* (EHEC), enteropathogenic *E. coli* (EPEC) and enteroaggregative *E. coli* (EAEC). Each class falls within a serological subgroup and manifests distinct features in pathogenesis and subsequent diarrhoea (Todar, 2002). The importance of *E. coli,* both as an indicator organism and as a diarrhoeagenic pathogen is well documented. The aim of this study is therefore to determine the impact water, sanitation and hygiene infrastructures and their associated health risks facing people living with HIV and AIDS through detection of pathogenic *E. coli* in domestic drinking water and on sanitation facilities in the and around Bulawayo in Zimbabwe.

2. Materials and methods

2.1 Ethical consent

Registration of the project and ethical clearance was obtained from the University of Venda's Health, Safety and Research Ethics Committee. The Medical Research Council of Zimbabwe and the City of Bulawayo, through the Director of Health Services provided the necessary authority to proceed with the study.
Staff at Opportunistic Infections Clinics (OICs) was used to identify the HIV and AIDS patients and only those that volunteered and signed consent forms were included in the study. The consent forms were translated into the vernacular language of the patient.

2.2 Data collection using questionnaires

Structured questionnaires were used to obtain information regarding household demographics, water sources used, water collection practices; time spent collecting water, water storage practices, costs involved in water and sanitation services, hygiene practices associated with sanitation and the level of hygiene understanding in each household.

2.3 Study area

The Bulawayo metropolitan in Zimbabwe was chosen as the study site for the project. A total of 414 households with individuals living with HIV and AIDS from high density sub-urban areas (n=150 households), peri-urban areas (n=121 households) and rural villages (n=142 households) in and around Bulawayo were included in this study.

2.4 Sample collection

Samples were collected aseptically from household water storage containers in sterile 1 litre plastic bottles and transported on ice to the laboratory for further analysis. Toilet seats were

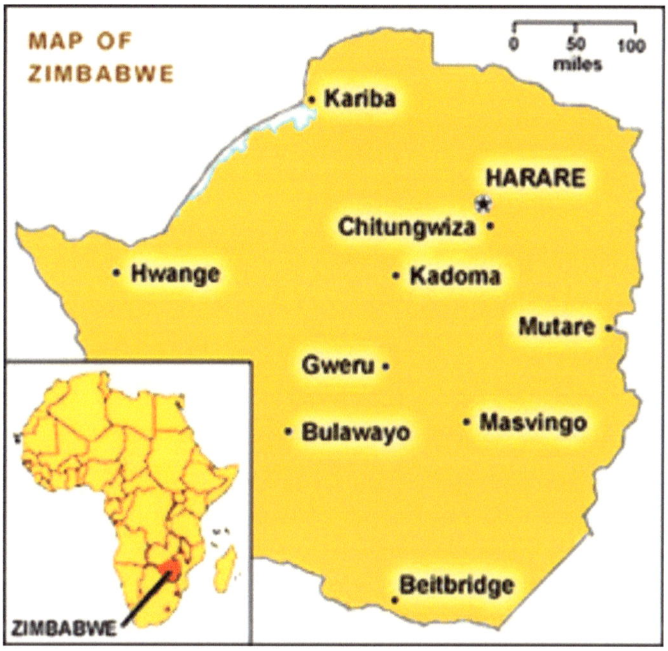

Fig. 1. Map of Zimbabwe showing the location of the study area

swabbed using sterile methods and the swab placed into sterile containers with 100 ml phosphate buffered saline (pH 7.4) (PBS) and transported on ice to the laboratory for further analysis. Hands of 20% of the people living with HIV and AIDS in each of the three areas included in the study, were swabbed and the swabs placed into sterile containers with 100 ml PBS and transported on ice to the laboratory for further analysis.

2.5 Determination of total coliform bacteria and *Escherichia coli*

Total coliforms and *E. coli* were detected using the Colilert® Quanti-Tray/2000 System manufactured by IDEXX and supplied by DEHTEQ. Appropriate dilutions of the samples were made according to the procedures described by the manufacturers (IDEXX). The trays were incubated at 35°C for 18 to 22 hours and the positive (yellow and fluorescing) wells and *E. coli* bacteria were counted and converted into the most probable number of total coliforms and *E. coli* present in samples, using tables and formulae provided by the manufacturer. Included in the experiment were positive and negative controls (distilled water, *E. coli, Klebsiella* and *Pseudomonas*).

Selection of potential *E. coli* bacteria was made of fluorescing wells that could clearly be counted as the actual indicator in the selective growth media. The contents of positively identified *E. coli* wells were collected using 1 ml syringes and kept in clearly marked cryotubes at -70°C. A multiplex PCR method was performed according to Omar et al., (2010). The five diarrhoeagenic strains of *E. coli* and a commensal *E. coli* strain that were employed in the study are shown in Table 1.

All strains were obtained from the South African National Health Laboratory Services (NHLS) (2010), and stored at -70°C in a mixture of Plate Count Agar (PCA) with 10% (v/v) glycerol. The strains were routinely cultured on PCA and incubated under aerobic conditions at 37°C. Liquid cultures of the bacteria were obtained by inoculating 5 ml Luria-

Bacterial strain	Reference number	Genes targeted
Enterotoxigenic *Escherichia coli* (ETEC)	H10407	*Mdh, Lt, St*
Enteropathogenic *E. coli* (EPEC)	B170	*Mdh, eaeA*
Enteroaggregative *E. coli* (EAEC)	3591-178	*Mdh, Eagg*
Enterohaemorrhagic *E. coli* (EHEC)	C4193-1	*Mdh, eaeA, stx1, stx2*
Enteroinvasive *E. coli* (EIEC)	C316-58	*Mdh, lal*
Commensal *E. Coli*	Field isolate, API20E confirmed	*Mdh*

Table 1. Bacterial strains used for the experimental work

Bertani (LB) media in test tubes for 16 hours while rotating at 200 rpm at 37°C. Genomic DNA isolation was performed on 2ml of each sample using an adapted protocol as described in Omar et al., (2010). All buffers used, were prepared as described by Omar et al (2010).

2.6 DNA extraction and multiplex polymerase chain reactions (PCR)

The samples were centrifuged at 12,000xg for 2 minutes at room temperature to pellet any bacterial cells present. After removing the supernatant, each pellet was dissolved in 700 µl extraction buffer and left for 10 min at 37°C, after which 250 µl of 99% ethanol was added and thoroughly mixed. This was left for 10 minutes at 56°C, after which 40 µl celite suspension was added, mixed and left for 10 minutes with occasional mixing. Pellets were again collected by centrifugation at 12,000xg for 30 seconds at room temperature (the supernatant removed). The pellets were washed twice with 500 µl washing buffer. This was followed by two 70% (v/v) ethanol wash steps. The pellets were dried at 56°C for 10 minutes, mixed with 100 µl TE buffer (10 mM Tris-HCl, 1 mM EDTA, pH 8.0), heated for 10 minutes at 56°C and briefly centrifuged to pellet the celite. The DNA containing supernatant was removed and the elution repeated once as described. All PCR reactions were performed in BIORAD Mycycler™ Thermal cycler as described by Omar et al., (2010).

DNA was analysed on a horizontal agarose slab gel [1% (w/v)] with ethidium bromide (0.5µg/ml) in TAE buffer (40 mM Tris acetate; 2 mM EDTA, pH 8.3). Electrophoresis was done for one hour in an electrical field strength of 5.9 $V.cm^{-1}$ gel and DNA was visualised with UV light (Gene Genius Bio Imaging system, Vacutec). The relative sizes of the DNA fragments were estimated by comparing their electrophoretic mobility with that of the standards run with the samples on each gel. Gene ruler (Fermentas) was used as standards.

2.7 Data analysis

The data from the questionnaires and microbiological data on commensal and pathogenic *E. coli* strains was coded and collated before being entered into an MS Excel spread sheet. The data was imported into the Stata Release 8.0 statistical software package for cleaning and editing. For categorical data, frequencies of occurrence of response were calculated. For numerical variables the data was summarised using the arithmetic, geometric and harmonic means and a corresponding 95% confidence interval. Testing was done at the 0.05 level of significance. All statistical analyses were done by Professor Piet Bekker from the Medical Research Council Statistical Unit in Pretoria, South Africa.

3. Results and discussion

3.1 Age and gender distribution of study population

As indicated in Table 2, the average family size of the urban household was 5.2 people, with females constituting 57% and males 43% of the urban study population. There was an average of 2.2 males and 3 females in the urban households. The peri-urban household average family size was 4.7 people, with females being 54% and males 46% of the peri-urban study population. There was an average of 2.5 females and 2.2 males in the peri-urban households. In rural areas the average family size was 5.3 people; females formed 54% and males 46% of the household composition. There was an average of 2.9 females and 2.4 males in the rural household. The urban and rural family sizes were the same, with the peri-urban family size being slightly smaller, due to a number of single member families found in peri-urban areas. In all areas there were more females than males in the households; the peri-urban and rural household composition was the same, whilst the urban household composition had a larger difference between the female and male members of households.

In all areas the children aged between 5 years and 12 years were the largest age-group. There were significantly less men in the age group 41 to 50 years (15.5%) in rural areas compared to peri-urban (23.1%) and urban (25.3%) areas. This may be due to rural to urban migration of this age group in search of employment. In the age group 61 to 70 years there was a significantly higher percentage of males in rural areas (10.6%) compare to urban and peri-urban areas (3.3% in both areas). This again may be related to migrant work, with this age group having returned from urban areas where they had been working.

3.2 Age and gender distribution of PLWHA

Most of the PLWHA were in the age groups 31 to 40 years and 41 to 50 years. These results agree with household surveys in 28 sub-Saharan Africa which revealed that in all but five countries peak HIV prevalence occurs between the ages 30 and 34 for women and in the late 30s and early 40s or men (Macro International, 2008). These are the sexually active members of society and the results of this study showed that the HIV in Bulawayo could be predominantly sexually transmitted.

Of the one hundred and fifty PLWHA from urban areas one hundred and nine (73%) were female and forty-one (27%) were male. One of the participants was in the age group 16 to 22 years (0.7%); twelve were in the age group 21 to 30 years (8%); sixty-one were in the age group 31 to 40 years (40.7%); fifty-six were in the age group 41 to 50 years (37.3%); fifteen were in the age group 51 to 60 years (10%); three were in the age group 61 to 70 years (2%) and two were above 70 years of age (1.3%).

In peri-urban areas, twelve (9.3%) of the one hundred and twenty-two participants were in the age group 21 to 30 years; fifty-two (42.6%) were in the age group 31 to 40 years; forty-three (35.2%) were in the age group 41 to 50 years; eleven (9%) were in the age group 51 to 60 years and two (1.6%) were in each of the age groups 61 to 70 years and above seventy years of age.

Age in years	Urban Average family size = 5.2 Female = 57% Male = 43%			Peri-urban Average family size = 4.7 Female = 54% Male = 46%			Rural Average family size = 5.2 Female = 54% Male = 46%		
	F (n)	**M (n)**	**Per age (%)**	**F (n)**	**M (n)**	**Per age (%)**	**F (n)**	**M (n)**	**Per age (%)**
Infant 0 -1	5	6	11 (2%)	10	6	16 (3%)	13	7	20 (3%)
Toddler >1 -5	31	40	71(9%)	27	24	51 (9%)	39	31	70 (9%)
Child >5 -12	71	69	140 (18%)	65	67	132 (23%)	59	90	149 (20%)
Adolescent >12 -16	60	40	100 (13%)	26	17	43 (8%)	34	36	70 (10%)
Adolescent >16 - 20	57	38	95 (12%)	21	25	46 (8%)	39	33	72 (10%)
Adult 21- 30	58	43	101 (13%)	40	33	73 (13%)	50	43	93 (13%)
Adult 31 - 40	75	33	108 (14%)	49	38	87 (15%)	55	31	86 (12%)
Adult 41 - 50	50	38	88 (11%)	40	28	68 (12%)	46	22	68 (9%)
Adult 51 - 60	23	13	36 (5%)	11	12	23 (4%)	24	25	49 (7%)
Adult 61 - 70	13	5	18 (2%)	8	4	12 (2%)	15	15	30 (4%)
Adult >70	4	6	10 (1%)	8	7	15 (3%)	16	8	24 (3%)
Total	**447**	**331**	**684 (100%)**	**305**	**261**	**566 (100%)**	**390**	**341**	**731 (100%)**

Table 2. Demographics of study population

In rural areas, six (4.3%) of the one hundred and forty-two participants were in the age group 16 to 20 years; twenty-five (17.7%) were in the age group 21 to 30 years; forty-six (32.6%) were in the age group 31 to 40 years; thirty-nine (27.7%) were in the age group 41 to 50 years; twenty-one (14.9%) were in the age group 51 to 60 years and four (2.8%) were in the age group 61 to 70 years.

3.3 CD4 counts of PLWHA

The cells mostly affected by HIV when it infects humans are the CD4 cells. After having been affected for a long time the number of CD4 cells decreases indicating that the immune system is being weakened. Normal CD4 counts are usually between 500 and 1 600 (AIDS InfoNet , 2010). An HIV positive person with CD4 count of less than 200 is considered to have AIDS, and preventive therapy should be started even if the person has no symptoms

(Lab Test Online, 2009). Of late most health care providers begin antiretroviral therapy (ART) when the CD4 count goes below 350 (AIDS InfoNet, 2010).
The CD4 count results of all the 150 people living with HIV and AIDS in urban areas were obtained (Table 3). The geometric mean for the CD4 count results was 221. In peri-urban

HIV and CD4 count tests	Urban	Peri-urban	Rural
Where first HIV test was done	**n = 150**	**n = 121**	**n = 142**
New Start Centre	70 (46.7%)	59 (48.8%)	64 (45.1%)
Local clinic	49 (32.7%)	48 (39.7%)	51 (35.9%)
Hospital	26 (17.3%)	13 (10.7%)	27 (19.0%)
Private Doctor	1 (0.7%)	1 (0.8%)	0 (0%)
Other	4 (2.6%)	0 (0%)	0 (0%)
Where first CD4 count test was done	**n = 149**	**n = 121**	**n = 142**
Not done	0 (0%)	0 (0%)	1 (0.7%)
New Start Centre	8 (5.4%)	5 (4.1%)	7 (4.9%)
Local clinic	78 (52.4%)	49 (40.5%)	17 (12%)
Hospital	47 (31.5%)	20 (16.5%)	90 (63.4%)
Private Doctor	13 (8.7%)	0 (0%)	1 (0.7%)
Other	3 (2%)	47 (38.9%)	26 (18.3%)
Frequency of follow-up tests	**n = 150**	**n = 121**	**n = 133**
Not done	0 (0%)	3 (2.5%)	0 (0%)
Once a year	57 (38%)	16 (13.2%)	41 (30.8%)
Every 6 months	21 (14%)	5 (4.1%)	8 (6%)
Every 3 months	6 (4%)	3 (2.5%)	6 (4.5%)
Not done	43 (28.7%)	92 (76%)	77 (57.9%)
Other	23 (15.3%)	2 (1.7%)	1 (0.8%)
Last CD4 count test	**n = 149**	**n = 121**	**n = 114**
Not done	2 (1.34%)	47 (38.84%)	0 (0%)
Within last month	38 (25.5%)	72 (59.5%)	21 (18.4%)
>1 month, <3 months	13 (8.7%)	13 (10.7%)	23 (20.2%)
3 to 6 months	10 (6.7%)	4 (3.3%)	13 (11.4%)
6 to 12 months	32 (21.5%)	14 (11.6%)	24 (21.1%)
>12 months	56 (37.6%)	18 (14.9%)	33 (28.9%)

Table 3. Details of places of testing and or frequency for HIV and CD4 tests

areas 119 PLWHA out of 121 in the study had their CD4 count results recorded and the mean was 224. All the 141 PLWHA in rural areas had their CD4 count results obtained and the mean was 235. The mean CD4 count in all the areas was below the normal CD4 count of between 500 and 1 600, however it was above 200, at which one is said to have AIDS (AIDS InfoNet, 2010).
PLWHA that had taken their first test for HIV at a New Start Centre were 47% in urban areas, 49% in peri-urban and 45% in rural areas. Those that were first tested for HIV at their local clinic were 33% in urban areas, compared to 40% in peri-urban areas and 36% in rural areas. Those that had their first test for HIV done at a hospital were 17% in urban areas, 11% in peri-urban areas and 19% in rural areas. The rest (3% in urban areas and 1% in peri-urban areas) had been first tested for HIV at a private doctor or some other testing facility.
The first CD4 count tests were done at the local clinic for 52% of PLWHA in urban areas, 41% of those in peri-urban areas and 12% of those in rural areas. Those that had the first CD4 count test done at a hospital were 32% in urban areas, 17% in peri-urban areas and 63% in rural areas. CD4 tests done by private doctors were 9% in urban areas and 1% in rural areas. Some PLWHA (2% in urban areas, 39% in peri-urban areas and 18% in rural areas) had their first CD4 count test done as special request because they had been commenced on treatment using the WHO staging without the CD4 count test.
After the initial CD4 count test getting a follow-up test was not easy, and most of the PLWHA had not had regular follow-up CD4 count tests. In urban areas 29% had not done a follow-up CD4 count test, compared to 76% in peri-urban areas and 58% in rural areas.
Those that had a CD4 count test done once every year were 38% in urban areas, 13% in peri-urban areas and 31% in rural areas. Those that had a follow-up test every 6 months were 14% in urban areas, 4% in peri-urban areas and 6% in rural areas. Those that a follow-up test every 3 months were 4% in urban areas, 2.5% in peri-urban areas and 6% in rural areas. In urban areas 15% had not had regular follow-up CD4 count tests, compared to 1% in peri-urban and rural areas.

3.4 Sanitation in study population

The Urban Councils Act and the municipal bylaws require all houses to have a flush toilet before being occupied. These provisions by and large complied with in the urban areas. Problems arose during periods of water unavailability when the households had to resort to pouring water to flush these toilets. Being situated in a water scarce region, Bulawayo needs a relook into the appropriate toilet technology for the city. A technology that would not be dependent on water would best suit the city. There is no specific policy on sanitation for peri-urban areas due to their semi-formal and in some cases informal nature. However, as in rural areas, the ventilated improved pit (VIP) latrine offers an appropriate option. The guidelines for rural sanitation recommend a VIP latrine for each household.
In urban areas 98% of the households had a water closet connected to a public sewer, the rest did not have toilet facilities and used the bush. In peri-urban areas 48% of the households had a VIP latrine, 2% had a water closet connected to a septic tank and 1% had a substandard pit latrine. The remaining 49% of the households had no toilet facilities and used the bush. In rural areas 66% of the households had VIP latrines, 15% had pit latrines with a slab and 4% had pit latrines without a slab. One household had a water closet connected to a septic tank. The remaining 14% of the households had no toilet facilities and used the bush.
Approximately 98% of households in the urban areas had access to improved sanitation; however, 49% of households in peri-urban areas and 34% in rural areas did not have access to an improved sanitation facility. The need for access to improved sanitation is critical for

HIV and AIDS patients. Nearby latrines are necessary for weak patients. In some patients, diarrhoea is chronic, further weakening them. In order for HIV infected people to remain healthy as long as possible and for people with AIDS to reduce their chances of getting diarrhoea, adequate sanitary facilities are of the utmost importance (Kamminga and Wegelin-Schuringa, 2003). The hygiene infrastructures were generally inadequate, especially with regards to hand washing facilities.

3.5 Water in study population

Zimbabwe does not have national standards for water accessibility; the SPHERE project recommended standard of 500m to a water point was therefore used (World Vision, 2006). Whenever water was available it was easily accessible from taps within the house (67%) or within the yard (33%) in urban areas. In peri-urban areas most of the households collected water from communal standpipes (70%) and boreholes (5%) to their homes over distances that varied from less than 500m to more than 2km. Up to 25% of the households collected water from unprotected wells or springs. Those that collected water from a water source more than 500m away from their homes were 9% of the households in peri-urban areas and 27.5% in rural areas. Table 4 summarises information on water availability. Travelling more than 500m to a water source is likely to be tedious especially to young children, the elderly and those weakened by illness. In peri-urban and rural areas containers of up to 25 litres were used to collect water and were mainly carried on the heads. This was a considerable strain especially for the vulnerable people. Whilst water sources were accessible to most households in all the three areas, the unavailability of water was a major constraint, especially in urban areas where 60% of the households reported that water was not always available. In peri-urban areas 36% of the households and 13% in rural areas said water was not always available. During the period August to September 2008, in urban areas and peri-urban areas supplied with municipal piped water was available only two days a week and in some cases only for a few hours. Some of these communities had gone for more than a month with intermittent water supplies. The intermittent water supply meant that even though water was piped to the house it had to be collected and stored for those periods when it was not available from the tap.

This resulted in increased water handling with a subsequent increase in opportunities for contamination (USAID, 2006). Unsanitary and inadequately protected water containers could contribute to the contamination of water at the point-of-use (Dunker, 2001). Inadequate storage conditions have been shown to result in the increase in the number of some microorganisms such as heterotrophic bacteria and total coliform bacteria over time (Reiff et al., 1996). Potable water is critical for PLWHA; they need it for taking antiretroviral (ARV) medication, bathing, washing soiled linen and clothing and for essential hygiene, which reduces exposure to opportunistic infections (WRC, 2005).

Various factors affected the availability of water in urban and peri-urban areas during different periods of the study. At one point the major supply dams had dried up resulting in water shortages. There was also a time when the municipality was reported to have run out of water treatment chemicals, and were unwilling to distribute water that had not been fully treated. In all the areas solving the water problems being experienced was taking quite long, with 39% in urban areas, 83% in peri-urban areas and 77% in rural areas having reported that it took more than a month to have the problems fixed. During these periods of water being unavailable from the usual sources 5% of households in urban areas collected water from unprotected wells, compared to 26.5% in urban areas and 10.5% in rural areas. Resorting to unsafe water sources puts the PLWHA at a risk of contracting water-borne diseases.

Water supplies	Urban % (n=150)	Peri-urban % (n=121)	Rural % (n =142)
Source			
Piped water into dwelling	66.67	0	2.82
Piped water to yard	32.67	0	11.97
Public tap/standpipe	0	70.25	23.94
Tubewell/borehole	0	4.96	50
Protected well	0	0	4.23
Unprotected dug well	0.67	23.97	6.34
Protected spring	0	0	0
Unprotected spring	0	0.83	0
Distance from home			
0 - 50m	99.33	23.97	21.83
>50 -100m	0	32.23	21.13
>100 - 200m	0.67	16.53	16.2
>200 - 300m	0	7.44	6.34
>300 - 400m	0	2.48	1.41
>400 - 500m	0	8.26	5.63
>500m - 1km	0	4.13	15.49
>1km - 2km	0	3.31	10.56
>2km	0	1.65	1.41
Time taken to water source and back			
<30 min	0.67	73.55	51.41
30 min - 1hr	0	16.53	27.46
>1hr	0	9.92	4.23
Water on premises	99.33	0	16.9
Frequency of unavailability			
	n=148	n=44	n=18
Always available	39.19	0	0
Everyday	5.41	11.36	38.89
Every other day	3.38	4.55	11.11
Twice a week	19.59	13.64	38.89
More than twice a week	25	47.73	5.56
Other	7.43	22.73	5.56
Time taken to fix problem			
	n=148	n=36	n=13
No problem	38.51	0	0
On the same day	8.11	2.78	0
1 day - 3 days	8.73	2.78	0
>3 days - 5 days	0	2.78	7.69
>5 days - 1 week	0	0	0
>1 week - 2 weeks	0	2.78	0
>2 weeks - 1 month	2.7	5.56	15.38
>1 month	39.19	83.33	76.92

Table 4. Details of sources of water supplies, water accessibility and availability

In urban areas under normal circumstances water was available on the premises and no collection times were applicable. However during periods of water shortages water had to be collected from alternative sources such as boreholes (31%) or water tankers supplied by the municipality (61%). During these time 79% of the respondents said they collected water in the morning, 23% at midday, 35% in the afternoon and 48% said they collected water in the evening.

In 3% of the households it was the responsibility of girls to collect water. Women were responsible for water collection in 30% of the household whilst men were responsible for water collection in 4% of the household. In 10% of the households women and girls were responsible for water collection. Women and boys collected water in 1% of the households and in another 1% it was women and children. The PLWHA collected water in 76% of the households. The main reasons why the PLWHA did not collect water were because they were too weak to do so (67%) or as men they did not consider it their chore (28%).

In peri-urban areas water was collected in the morning in 92% of the households, at midday in 6%, in the afternoon in 20% and in the evening in 36% of the households. Collection was done more than once a day in several households. Women were responsible for water collection in 42% of the households compared to 14% of the households where men were responsible. In 15% of the households women and girls were responsible for water collection. In 8% of the households all family members collected water. In 3% of the households it was women and children who collected water. Women and boys collected water in 2% of the households. The PLWHA collected water in 87% of the households. Where they did not collect water it was mainly because they were too weak to do so (56%) or they were ill at that moment (19%) or as men they did not consider water collection as their chore (19%).

In rural areas water was collected in the morning in 99% of the households, at midday in 17%, in the afternoon in 26% and in the evening in 45% of the households. In most households water was collected more than once a day. Women were responsible for collecting water in 54% of the households. In 10% of the households it was women and girls who collected water. Men were responsible for collecting water in 6% of the households. In 3% of the households all family members collected whilst in another 3% it was women and boys who collected water. Boys collected water in 2% of the households, and in another 2% of the household it was children who collected water. Women and children collected water in 1% of the households. In 81% of the households the PLWHA collected water. The reasons for not colleting water were that they were too weak to do so (46%) or they were ill at that moment (31%) or being men they did not consider it their chore to collect water. In all the areas more women than men were responsible for water collection, and 28% of men who did not collect water considered collecting water not to be one of their chores. This indicated that water collection to some extent remains a gender issue. Even though the majority of the PLWHA in all areas collected water, the fact that some did not do so because they were too weak to do so or they were ill at the time shows their vulnerability if water is not easily accessible.

In urban areas in 29% of the households water for drinking was boiled before it was consumed, compared to 18% in peri-urban areas and 17% in rural areas. The households where drinking water was disinfected with chlorine before consumption were 24% in urban areas, 21.5 in peri-urban areas and 23% in rural areas (Table 5). The disinfectant, in the form of *Aquatabs* (167mg sodium dichloroisocyanurate) was supplied either by the municipality or by some NGO supporting the PLWHA. Allowing the water to stand and settle was used by 8.3% of the peri-urban households, 4.9% of rural households and 0.7% of urban households.

Although the water was kept for long periods of time under sub-optimal conditions, the majority of households did not treat the water before consuming it. Water stored in the home tends to be more contaminated that water at the collection point, suggesting that substantial contamination takes place during transport, storage and use. Those households collecting water from communal supplies must, of necessity transport water to their homes and store it. Those households with water on the premises may have intermittent or poor quality water.

Proper handling and storage and household-level disinfection is therefore necessary to maintain the quality of water (USAID, 2006). It has been observed in a wide variety of settings that water quality improvements at the point-of-use are likely to have a positive impact on health at all levels of the water supply system (USAID, 2006). There are physical and chemical treatments available as interventions to improve the quality of water at the point of use (Sobsey, 2002).

Treatment method	Urban % (n=150)	Peri-urban % (n=121)	Rural % (n=142)
Boiling	29	18	17
Bleach/chlorine	24	21.5	23
Straining with cloth	4	0	0
Filter (sand, ceramic etc)	0	0	1.4
Solar disinfection	0	0	0
Stand and settle	0.7	8.3	4.9

Table 5. Domestic pre-treatment of drinking water

3.6 Total coliform and *Escherichia coli* counts

In urban areas 77% of the hands swabs from PLWHA were positive for total coliforms, compared to 83% and 72% in peri-urban and rural areas respectively. A total of 3% of the hand swabs in urban areas, 10% in peri-urban areas and 17% in rural areas were positive for *E. coli*. In 88% of the urban toilets, 83% of the peri-urban toilets and 73% of the rural toilets the toilet seat swabs were positive for total coliforms. *E. coli* was found in 41% of the urban, 58% of the peri-urban and 42% of the rural toilet seat swabs. The unsatisfactory cleaning of the toilets and the lack of use of disinfectants could be the reason for these results. Toilet seats can be classified as disease transfer points because they are regularly touched by the bare skin of more than one person. The spread of bacteria such as *E. coli* can not be controlled unless a disinfecting process is performed on these surfaces (CDC, 2008).

The results from the study indicated that the water collected from household storage containers was positive for total coliform bacteria in 93% of urban households, 98% of peri-urban households and 89% of rural households. The water samples positive for *E. coli* were 33% in urban areas, 67% in peri-urban and 41% in rural areas. The microbial quality of water did not meet the standards set out in the WHO guidelines which Zimbabwe uses. In all water intended for drinking, treated water entering the distribution system or treated water in the distribution system, total coliform bacteria and *E. coli* must not be detectable in any 100 ml sample (WHO, 2008). These results indicated contamination of the water from a faecal source, indicating indicating that the water might potentially be contaminated with pathogenic microorganisms. This is likely to expose the PLWHA to infection with diarrhoeal diseases and other opportunistic infections (Kamminga and Wegelin-Schuringa, 2003). The quality of drinking water is a well-recognised factor in the transmission route for infectious diarrhoea and other diseases (WHO, 2003).

Sample type	Urban	Peri-urban	Rural
	Number (%)	Number (%)	Number (%)
Hand swabs	24 (77%) n=31	25 (83%) n=30	21 (72%) n=29
Toilet seats	132 (88%) n=150	47 (83%) n=57	88 (73%) n=120
Water storage container	140 (93%) n=150	118 (98%) n=121	127 (89%) n=142

Table 6. Total coliform counts given as colony forming units per 100 ml (cfu/100 ml)

Sample type	Urban	Peri-urban	Rural
	Number (%)	Number (%)	Number (%)
Hand swabs	1 (3%) n=31	3 (10%) n=30	5 (17%) n=29
Toilet seats	61 (41%) n=150	33 (58%) n=57	50 (42%) n=120
Water storage container	50 (33%) n=150	81 (67%) n=121	58 (41%) n=142

Table 7. *E. coli* counts given as colony forming units per 100 ml (cfu/100 ml)

Contamination of water at household levels has been shown to be a risk factor in the transmission of the Hepatitis E virus (DREF, 2008). More than half of the hospital beds in the developing countries are estimated to be occupied by patients suffering from ailments associated with water of poor quality (UNDP, 2006). Improving the quality of water at household level would go a long way in addressing diarrhoeal diseases, particularly amongst PLWHA. The storage conditions and the unhygienic maintenance of containers could have contributed to the poor results.

3.7 Prevalence of pathogenic *Escherichia coli* strains

The one *E. coli* positive sample found from the hand swab samples in urban areas and all three isolates from the peri-urban areas did not test positive for virulence genes virulence genes. In rural areas one of the three *E. coli* positive hand swab samples tested positive for atypical EPEC. The presence of atypical EPEC (which is more frequently isolated from diarrhoea cases than typical EPEC) on the hands of PLWHA indicates the potential risk of contracting diarrhoea.

In toilet seat samples, atypical EPEC was the most prevalent pathogenic *E. coli* strain found in urban areas at 25%, followed by typical EPEC at 24%. EAEC was also fairly prevalent at 18%, with ETEC following at 10%. Almost 83% of *E. coli* strains identified in urban areas were pathogenic, compared to 40% in peri-urban areas and 69% in rural areas. The higher presence of pathogenic *E. coli* strains in urban areas could contribute to higher diarrhoea prevalence.

In household water storage container samples from the urban areas, the most prevalent pathogenic strain was typical EPEC (25.5%), followed by atypical EPEC (11%), EAEC (9.1%), ETEC (0.8%), EHEC (1.8%) and EIEC (1.8%). The remaining 49% of the samples had commensal *E. coli.* In peri-urban water storage samples ETEC was 4.9%, atypical EPEC was 3.7% and EHEC was 2.5%. EAEC was the least prevalent at 1.2%. The rest of the *E. coli* positive samples (87.7%) only had commensal *E. coli* present. In rural areas the most prevalent pathogenic *E. coli* strain detected in water samples was EAEC (14%), followed by atypical EPEC and EHEC (5% each). ETEC was 3.4% and the least prevalent was EIEC at 1.7%.

E. coli from toilet seats could be transferred to water during storage and handling resulting in these poor results, especially with inadequate hand-washing after using the toilet. The presence of pathogenic strains of *E. coli* in water at household level indicated the risk that the PLWHA were exposed to diarrhoeagenic bacteria, reinforcing the need for appropriate household level water supply and storage. Most of the households in all the areas had to store water in their dwellings. In urban areas 99.3% of the households had water stored inside the house, 96% in peri-urban areas and 99.3% in rural areas also stored water inside the house. Those that stored water outside the house were 3.3% in urban areas, 9% in peri-urban areas and 2% in rural areas. A few households stored water both inside the house as well as outside the house. The same containers used for water collection were also used for storage. In most households in the urban and peri-urban areas the same room that was used for water storage was also used for various other uses such as sleeping, cooking and in some cases, even bathing. In general water was not adequately protected from contamination.

Though in most of the households water containers were found clean, both inside and outside of the container, quite a number of household containers were found with either loose particles of dirt inside (27% in urban areas, 40% in peri-urban areas and 43% in rural areas) or with a biofilm (3% in urban areas, 7% in peri-urban areas and 9% in rural areas). The external conditions of containers were found to be unsatisfactory in more than half of the households in all the three areas. In about half of the households in all areas (51% in urban areas, 54% in urban areas and 48% in rural areas) both wide-mouthed containers and those with screw-type mouths were used. In 41% of the urban households, 22% of the peri-urban households and 21% of the rural households, only containers with screw tops were

used. Wide mouth bucket type containers were used in 8% of the urban households, 24% of the peri-urban households and 31% of the rural households.
The main water uses mentioned by the respondents in all the areas were cooking, drinking, bathing and laundry, dishwashing and cleaning. Some households in urban areas mentioned toilet flushing as a use whilst some peri-urban households mentioned drinking water for animals as a use. The largest volume of water was used for laundry in most households, however in most cases laundry was done only once or twice a week and in some rural households laundry was done at the water source. Bathing used the second largest amount of water in most of the households in all the areas.
The average total volume of water containers in each urban household was 95 litres. The average actual volume of water found in each household was 87 litres. The average volume used by each urban household was 127 litres per day. Considering that the average family size of an urban household was 5, the per capita per day volume of water used was 25.4 litres, which is satisfactory if the SPHERE project recommended volume of 15 litres per capita per day is used. Even if the average actual volume of water found in each household is used, the volume per capita per day of 17.4 litres is still above the SPHERE recommended standard.
In peri-urban areas the average total volume of water containers in each household was 79 litres and the average actual volume found was 61 litres. The average total volume of water used in each household was 121 litres. The per capita per day volume of water used was 25.7 litres. Based on the actual volume of water found in each household the per capita per day water available was 13 litres, which is below the SPHERE recommended volume.
Each rural household had an average total volume of containers of 70 litres. There was an average of 48 litres of water found in each household. According to the respondents, an

E. coli strain	Hand swab samples			Toilet seat samples			Water storage container samples		
	Urban	Peri-urban	Rural	Urban	Peri-urban	Rural	Urban	Peri-urban	Rural
Commensal *E. coli*	1 (100%)	3 (100%)	2 (40%)	13 (16.4%)	18 (60%)	16 (31.3%)	27 (49%)	71 (87.7%)	41 (70.7%)
Atypical Enteropathogenic *E. coli*	0 (0%)	0 (0%)	1 (20%)	19 (24.0%)	2 (6.6%)	7 (13.7%)	6 (11%)	3 (3.7%)	3 (5.2%)
Typical enteropathogenic *E. coli* (bfp and eae)	0 (0%)	0 (0%)	0 (0%)	20 (25.3%)	0 (0%)	0 (0%)	14 (25.5%)	0 (0%)	0 (0%)
Enterohaemorrhagic *E. coli*	0 (0%)	0 (0%)	0 (0%)	2 (2.5%)	0 (0%)	1 (1.9%)	1 (1.8%)	2 (2.5%)	3 (5.2%)
Enterotoxigenic *E. coli*	0 (0%)	0 (0%)	0 (0%)	8 (10.1%)	6 (20%)	3 (5.8%)	1 (1.8%)	4 (4.9%)	2 (3.4%)
Enteroaggregative *E. coli*	0 (0%)	0 (0%)	2 (40%)	14 (17.7%)	4 (13.3%)	22 (43.1%)	5 (9.1%)	1 (1.2%)	8 (13.8%)
Enteroinvasive *E. coli*	0 (0%)	0 (0%)	0 (0%)	3 (3.8%)	0 (0%)	2 (3.9%)	1 (1.8%)	0 (0%)	1 (1.7%)

Table 8. Pathogenic *E. coli* strains detected in hand swabs, toilet seat and water storage container samples

average of 157 litres of water was used in each house every day. Based on this, the per capita per day volume of water used is 30 litres, however based on the average volume of water found in each household, the figure drops to 9.2 litres, far below the SPHERE project recommendation. The water volumes found in the rural house households were the lowest compared to the other areas.

In urban areas in 29% of the households water for drinking was boiled before it was consumed, compared to 18% in peri-urban areas and 17% in rural areas. The households where drinking water was disinfected with chlorine before consumption were 24% in urban areas, 21.5% in peri-urban areas and 23% in rural areas. The disinfectant, in the form of *Aquatabs* (167mg sodium dichloroisocyanurate) was supplied either by the municipality or by some NGO supporting the PLWHA. Allowing the water to stand and settle was used by 8.3% of the peri-urban households, 4.9% of rural households and 0.7% of urban households.

Proper handling and storage and household-level disinfection is therefore necessary to maintain the quality of water (USAID, 2006). It has been observed in a wide variety of settings that water quality improvements at the point-of-use are likely to have a positive impact on health at all levels of the water supply system (USAID, 2006). There are physical and chemical treatments available as interventions to improve the quality of water at the point of use (Sobsey, 2002).

4. Conclusions

The presence of total coliforms and *E. coli* in water, toilet seat and hand swab samples was determined using the Colilert® Quanti-Tray/2000 System. Multiplex PCR was used to identify pathogenic strains of *E. coli*. The technique was found to be appropriate in detection of virulence genes to identify various pathogenic *E. coli* strains from water, sanitation and hygiene samples. The presence of total coliforms and *E. coli* in household samples, especially in water samples and hand swabs indicated the potential risk of enteric diseases that the PLWHA are exposed to. Pathogenic *E. coli* strains found in household samples indicated the risks to which PLWHA are exposed to, more so in view of their compromised immune status.

There is therefore need for hygiene education at the household level on the importance of household water storage to prevent contamination. Appropriate household water treatment systems, such as filters or disinfectants are needed, especially in households where there are PLWHA, to ensure that the water is safe for human consumption. The presence of total coliforms in hand swabs was indicative of inadequate hand washing, especially non-use of soap and disinfectants. This increases the potential of faecal-oral transmission of enteric pathogens. Hygiene education on appropriate and effective hand washing needs to be reinforced in all the communities. Adequate cleaning and disinfection of toilets seats, which can be disease transfer points, is needed to reduce the potential of disease transmission.

5. References

AIDS infoNet (2010). AIDS InfoNet Fact Sheet Number 124; CD4 CELL TESTS http://www.aidsinfonet.org/ (accessed 2010-06-02)

CDC (2008) Guideline for Disinfection and Sterilization in Healthcare Facilities, 2008 http://www.cdc.gov/hicpac/pdf/guidelines/Disinfection_Nov_2008.pdf (accessed 2010/06/02)

DREF (2008). Uganda: Hepatitis E Virus (HEV). DREF operation n o MDGRUG009. International Federation of Red Cross and Red Crescent Societies.

Dunker L (2001) The KAP tool for Hygiene. A manual on: knowledge, attitudes and practices in rural areas of South Africa. Water Research Commission Report TT144/00. Water Research Commission, Pretoria, South Africa.

Framm SR and Soave R. (1997). Agents of diarrhea. *Med Clin North Am* 1997; *81:* 427-47.

Janoff EN and Smith PD. (1998) Prospectives on gastrointestinal infections in AIDS. *Gastroenterology Clinics of North America* 1988; *17:* 451-63.

Kamminga E and Wegelin/Schuringa M. (2003) HIV/AIDS and water, sanitation and hygiene. Thematic Overview Paper. Delft: IRC International Water and Sanitation Centre. http://www.irc.nl/page.php/111

Mitra AK, Hernandez CD, Hernandez CA and Siddiq Z. (2001) Management of diarrhea in HIV infected patients. *International Journal of STD & AIDS* 2001; *12:* 630/9.

Omar KB, Potgieter N and Barnard TG (2010) Development of a rapid screening method for the detection of pathogenic Escherichia coli using a combination of Colilert ® Quanti/Trays/2000 and PCR. *Water Science & Technology: Water Supply.* 10.1: 7/13.

Reiff F M, Roses M, Venczel L, Quick R and Witt VM (1996) Low cost safe water for the world: A practical interim solution. *Journal of Public Health Policy* 17, 398-408

Sobsey MD (2002) Managing water in the home: Accelerated health gains from improved water supply. World Health Organization Sustainable Development and Healthy Environments. World Health Organization, Geneva. WHO/SDE/WSH/02.07.

Todar K (2002) Pathogenic *E. coli.* University of Wisconsin/Madison Department of Bacteriology, USA

UNDP (2006) Sharing Innovative Experiences; Examples of Successful Experiences in Providing Safe Drinking Water, United Nations Development Programme, New York, USA

UNICEF (2009). UNICEF - Children and HIV and AIDS - Statistics.http;//www.unicef.org. Accessed March 2011

UNAIDS (2005) Evidence for HIV decline in Zimbabwe: A comprehensive review of the epidemiological data. November 2005.

UNICEF (2005) Water, Sanitation and Hygiene: Common water and sanitation-related diseases. http://www.unicef.org/wash/index_wes_related.html (accessed 2010-03-23)

USAID (2006) Environmental Health, Technical Areas, Hygiene Improvement for Diarrhoeal Disease Prevention, Point-of-use (POU) Water Quality, November 2006.

USAID/WSP (2007) Analysis of Research on the Effects of Improved Water, Sanitation, and Hygiene on the Health of People Living with HIV and AIDS and Programmatic Implications; Prepared by the USAID /Hygiene Improvement Project with the Water and Sanitation Program/World Bank. October 2007.

World Vision (2006) Zimbabwe Emergency Water and Sanitation Program (ZEWSP) Baseline Survey Report: Mangwe, Gwanda and Beitbridge District (Matabeleland South Province)

WHO (2003) Domestic Water Quantity, Service Level and Health. World Health Organisation, Geneva, Switzerland

WHO (2008) Guidelines for Drinking/water Quality THIRD EDITION INCORPORATING THE FIRST AND SECOND ADDENDA Volume 1 Recommendations; ISBN 978 92 4 154761 1; World Health Organisation, Switzerland

WRC (2005). Human rights project workbook 2. WRC report TT 296/07. Water Research Commission, Pretoria, South Africa.

13

Mycotic Leukonychia in HIV Patients

Patricia Chang[1], Gabriela Moreno-Coutiño[2] and Roberto Arenas[2]
[1]*Hospital General Enfermedades IGSS,*
[2]*Mycology Section "Dr Manuel Gea González" General Hospital, Mexico City*
[1]*Guatemala*
[2]*Mexico*

1. Introduction

Onychomycosis is the fungal infection of the nail, that can be caused by dermatophytes, *Candida* sp. or non-dermatophyte moulds (NDM). The term *tinea unguium* is a specific form of onychomycosis caused only by dermatophytes and thus, should not be regarded as synonymous. (Odds *et al.*, 1992)

On the other hand, the term leukonychia or white nails has a varied etiology, it can be congenital or acquired, infectious and non-infectious. In the case of onychomycosis, the diseased nail plate has an external origin, which is the fungal invasion that affects secondarily the normally formed nail. This is also known as fungal or mycotic leukonychia (Baran *et al.* 1994).

Onychomycosis, with all the different clinical presentations, is responsible for about 50% of all dystrophic nails and has a prevalence of 3-10% in the general population. Frequency also depends, on geographic conditions and age groups, with an increase in the prevalence in the elderly. It is now becoming more evident that immunosuppressed patients, particularly those living with HIV infection, are at a higher risk of presenting this nail fungal infection, and any clinical presentation is higher compared to the same age group of the general population (Denning *et al.* 1995; Moreno-Coutiño *et al.*, 2011; Winberg *et al.* 2003).

The first classification of onychomycosis was proposed by Zaias, and is based on the clinical appearance of the nails (Zaias, 1972). He described four clinical types: [1] distal subungual onychomycosis (DSO), [2] white superficial onychomycosis (WSO), [3] proximal subungual onychomycosis (PSO) and [4] *Candida* sp. onychomycosis. Since the publication of this paper, some modifications have been added. In 1998, Baran *et al.* proposed [I] distal and lateral subungual onychomycosis (DLSO), [II] superficial onychomycosis, [III] proximal subungual onychomycosis (PSO), [IV] endonyx onychomycosis and [V] total dystrophic onychomycosis (TDO). The most used these days is the following: DLSO, white superficial onychomycosis (WSO), PSO, *Candida* onychomycosis (paronychia) and TDO (Table 1) , (Baran *et al* 1998). WSO and PSO are also known as mycotic leukonychia. Further subdivisions are included in almost all the categories, and will be discussed further when necessary (Gupta & Summerbell, 1999).

In 1976, English described a classification based on etiology, instead of the clinical aspect of the fungal invasion. The categories are: (a) dermatophytes causing *tinea unguium*, (b) moulds (Non-dermatophyte moulds [NDM]) and (c) yeasts (Crozier *et al.* 1979). At this moment, the

Distal and lateral subungual onychomycosis (DLSO)
Proximal white subungual onychomycosis (PWSO)
Superficial white onychomycosis (SWO)
Total dystrophic onychomycosis (TDO)
Candida paronychia

Table 1. Current clinical classification

current classifications are not being specific enough to describe the clinical picture, etiology or prognostic factors regarding response to treatment (Grossman & Scher, 1990). Fungal or mycotic leukonychia was rather infrequent until the AIDS pandemia. PWSO is the least common form of onychomycosis in the HIV negative population, and DLSO is the most prevalent form of onychomycosis in patients living with HIV/AIDS. Since the identification of this disease in the 1980´s, many case reports and studies have been done. Although onychomycosis is not considered an AIDS-defining illness, and its presence is not useful for clinical classification, the presence of fungal leukonychia should alert the physician about possible immunosuppression. However, PSWO heralds advanced HIV disease and can be an early clinical marker of HIV infection (Chang & Arenas, 1995).
For some patients and even some physicians, onychomycosis is not a relevant medical condition. Nonetheless, it can have an important impact on the quality of life, particularly in patients living with HIV/AIDS. This group of patients commonly presents fingernail involvement as well as toenail infection more frequently than the non-immunosuppressed. This fact has negative effect on the quality of life because, unlike feet, hands are exposed all the time (Millikan *et al.,* 1999). Embarrassment, problems in the work area, including unemployment, reduction in social activities, alienation, fear of spreading the disease to others and pain, are the most common complaints (Drake *et al.,* 1999).
In the WHO clinical classification of HIV-associated disease is designed to be used in patients with confirmed HIV infection, the fungal nail infections are considered in clinical stage 2 (mild disease) that usually present with >450 CD4 cell count.

2. Epidemiology

According to the WHO, in 2009 the number of people living with HIV was 33.3 million worldwide. During 2009, 2.6 million were infected, and these numbers continue to rise (World Health Organization [WHO], 2009).
The incidence of all clinical forms of onychomycosis in HIV infected patients has slight variations in different countries, as has been noted in several reports. For instance, in Canada as well as in India, the incidence is 24%, 30% in France, and 20 % in Mexico.
Onychomycosis in open population in the USA is between 2-3%, 8.4% in Finland, 2.7% in the UK and 2.6% in Spain. Nonetheless, the Achilles project, the largest study on the prevalence of foot diseases in Europe found a much higher number, of 29.6%. In México, the incidence reported is 30%, but a recent national survey has showed a suspected frequency of 48% (Arenas, Bonifaz, et al. 2010). These reports include all age groups, and the numbers are similar to those reported in the HIV infected population, but if we separate the data by age group, the HIV group is younger for such an incidence compared to open population.
Specific epidemiologic data about mycotic leukonychia (WSO and PWSO) is scarce. It was only after the HIV pandemia developed that case reports were published, in the late 80´s. Before that time, the clinical presentation of fungal leukonychia was infrequent and the

fungi isolated were mostly NDM. WSO in general population has a prevalence of 1-2% and PWSO 8.3%.

For HIV positive population in 1998, Cribier *et al.* reported a prevalence of 8.5% for fungal leukonychias, Piraccini *et al.* of 9.5%, and Dompmartin *et al.* of 8%. This small numbers, contrast with other series such as the one published by Ravnborg et al. where 90% of their cases of onychomycosis, were clinically classified as PWSO (Ravnborg *et al.,* 1998). In a report of patients from Canada and Brazil, WSO had prevalence of 3.3% and 5% and for PWSO of 1.5% and 3% respectively. The overall prevalence for onychomycosis in HIV infected patients was reported of 23.2% (Arenas *et al.,* 2010; Cribier *et al.,* 1998; Dompmartin *et al.,* 1990; Gupta *et al.* 2000; Noppakun & Head, 1986; Weismann *et al.* 1988).

Among patients living with HIV/AIDS, onychomycosis is the fourth most common dermatological manifestation, with an incidence of 10-44%, and an estimated prevalence 15-40%. They are clinically more aggressive with rapid spread in finger or toenails (Herranz *et al.,* 1997) particularly in those with a cell count of 450 CD4 or lower. Some authors even report below 370 CD4. This finding suggests that the degree of immunosuppression plays an important role in the development of the disease. On the other hand, a Spanish study on prevalence and characteristics of dermatological diseases in HIV infected patients reported onychomycosis as the third most common dermatoses, particularly the DLSO clinical form, and found no statistical difference in the incidence between patients with <200 CD4 or ≥200 CD4 (Blanes *et al.,* 2010; Piraccini & Tosti, 2004; Singh *et al.,* 2009).

The age group most affected is the one of young adults, between 30 and 40 years of age (mean 36.6), because they are the majority of the HIV infected patients. As the HIV infection in many countries still predominates in the male gender, these comprise the majority of the patients with diagnosis of onychomycosis, with a sex ratio of 9:1 compared to females. However, the male:female ratio varies between countries. Where the infection rates are almost equal between genders, the ratio has been reported of 2:1.

Children in general, are a very low risk group for onychomycosis. The highest prevalence is reported in Latin American Countries as Mexico and Guatemala. In the former country is mainly observed in adolescents of both genders (Gupta *et al.* 1997; Vásquez del Mercado & Arenas, 2008).

The incidence reported varies from 0% in Wales, Finland and USA, 0.16% in Canada and 2.6% in Guatemala. This is thought to be because children have a reduced exposure to fungus, they have spent less time in contaminated environments, their nails grow faster, the nail surface is smaller so it provides less space for invasion, and they also have lower prevalence of tinea pedis which has been acknowledged as an important risk factor. There are no published series of HIV infected children regarding leukonychia.

The multiple studies published in adult population prove that the causative agents of fungal leukonychia, that include dermatophytes, *Candida* spp. and NDM remain the same despite the globalization of infectious diseases and that the worldwide prevalence of all superficial mycotic infections has been rising during the last decade, reaching up to 20-25% of the general population. They have a worldwide distribution, predominate in toenails, particularly caused by moulds. In fingernails, the association of constant contact with water and detergent damages the cuticle, facilitating fungal invasion of the nail plate and the main etiological agent is *Candida* sp. This is frequently seen in women involved in household activities (Arenas, 1990).

The most reported dermatophytes isolated are *Trichophyton rubrum, T. mentagrophytes.* Among the isolated NDM were: *Aspergillus niger, Cladoaporium* spp, *Scytalidium hyalinum, Penicillium* spp and *Gymnoascus dankaliensis,* and *Candida* spp. (Sujushe *et al.,* 2007).

The fungi capable of causing nail plate infection are ubiquitous. Tropical climate, heat and local humidity favor their development (between 25-28°C), as well as personal factors such as occlusive footwear, excessive sweating of feet, nail trauma, nail growth rate and in these particular cases, immunosuppression (table 2) (Elewski, 1998). The poor prognostic factors are: nail plate involvement of more than 50%, matrix area involvement, significant lateral disease, subungual hyperkeratosis >2mm, the presence of longitudinal streaks in the nail, NDM documented infection as well as diminished peripheral circulation. These infections have low tendency to self limitation (Scher *et al.*, 2007; Havlickova *et al.*, 2008).

<450 CD4/µL cell count
No ARV therapy
Occlusive footwear
Repeated trauma in nail apparatus
Tinea pedis, tinea cruris or corporis
Direct family members with onychomycosis

Table 2. Risk factors

3. Etiology and pathogenesis

Traditionally it is thought that the route of infection for fungal leukonychia is the dorsal aspect of the nail plate in the case of WSO and the PWSO is believed to originate from invasion through the proximal nail fold. However, controversy exists in both cases and will be further discussed.

The classic presentation of WSO initiates as white superficial patches without distinct edges that may gradually coalesce and invade the entire nail plate. At this point, the surface of the nail becomes uneven, porous and crumbles. *Trichophyton mentagrophytes* var. *interdigitale* is responsible for 90 % of the infections, associated or not to tinea pedis.

Other common pathogens that cause WSO are *T. rubrum* and non dermatophyte moulds (NDM) such as *Aspergillus* spp., *Fusarium* spp., and *Acremonium* spp. (Baran *et al.* 2007; Baran *et al.*, 2004)

According to Baran et al, WSO can be subdivided into:

1. Classical WSO with superficial invasion of the visible portion of the nail plate. Leukonychia presents as patches or striate superficial bands, alternated with normal color and appearance of the nail plate.
2. Clinically similar to the first form described, the difference is that this one originates beneath the proximal nail fold due to invasion of the ventral aspect of its eponiquial segment. Usually involves several toenails simultaneously. This form may be confused with PSWO and is frequently seen in the context of HIV infection.
3. WSO with deep invasion of the nail plate that progressed to deep penetration from the superficial aspect of the nail plate with possible extension beneath the nail fold.
4. Mixed forms, where WSO and other forms of onychomycosis coexist independently.

Several factors are involved in the development of SWO. The fungus must possess keratinolytic enzymes that enable it to penetrate the hard keratins of the nail plate. The invasion starts as superficial, but depending on host's and parasites characteristics, the entire depth and/or length of the nail plate may be involved. One of the most important host factors that influence the evolution of the disease is the decreased immune function against the fungus mainly because of the HIV infection, although chemotherapy and systemic steroid therapy may also be accounted responsible in other group of patients. It has been proposed that the low CD4 count affects the resistance to ordinary pathogens even in the avascular nail plate.

Another factor is the genetic background. By genetic predisposition, the nail surface is poorly resistant to the fungal penetration and invasion, so WSO can be considered an autosomal dominant disease. And, of course, as in any other type of onychomycosis, local humidity by occlusive shoes, nail plate thickness and nail plate growth rate, influence the development of the disease (Piraccini & Tosti, 2004).

PWSO is generally caused by dermatophytes, and is seen mainly in immunocompromised patients, especially when many nails are involved. When associated to paronychia, the infectious agent is generally a NMD. The dermatophyte *Trichophyton rubrum* is the most common isolated infectious agent. Other dermatophytes that have been reported to cause PWSO are *T. mentagrophytes* and even *Microsporum canis*. Among the NDM reported are *Aspergillus niger, A. sclerotiorum*, and *A. flavus*. (Table 3) (Weinberg, *et al.,* 1999).

T. rubrum	PWSO
T. mentagrophytes var. *interdigitale*	SWO
Microsporum canis	PWSO
Aspergillus spp	SWO
Fusarium spp.	SWO
Acremonium spp.	SWO
Candida spp	PWSO

Table 3. Most frequently isolated fungus

The most accepted theory for the route of infection in PWSO is the one that states that apparently, the stratum corneum on the ventral aspect of the proximal nail fold is the primary site of fungal invasion. When the fungus reaches the matrix, it mainly spreads to the lower part of the nail plate. However, Baran et al. have proposed a new theory. The fungal infection that initiates in the lunula region could be secondary to endogenous reactivation or auto-reinfection from a deeper site instead than from an external source. Based on evidence that dermatophyte antigenemia exists in patients with foot infections, they mention the possibility of reactivation after initial spread and sequestration with systemic dissemination either through retrograde lymphatic or hematogenous spread into the nail matrix and nail bed. Despite the known fact that dermatophytes are normally confined to the keratinous components of the skin and its appendages, some studies have proven that dermatophytes can survive in the bloodstream and lymphatic tissues and this, has led to think that this could explain the peculiar clinical manifestation and evolution of HIV-infected patients that present with PWSO.

This systemic spread theory is supported by the observation of multiple leukonychial transversal bands frequently seen in patients living with HIV/AIDS and PWSO. These bands are separated by histologically normal and micologically negative nail (Baran *et al.*, 2005).

Although poorly understood, as with any other infectious agent, it is clear that the immunological state of the patient plays an important role in the development and evolution of the onychomycosis. Immunological defects other than those affecting T-lymphocyte function, such as defective neutrophil chemotaxis, have also been associated with the appearance of PWSO.

It has been established that patients with HIV and dermatophytic infection are predisposed to suffer a chronic course and even, although very rare, to evolve to invasive disease. The impairment of cell-mediated immunity has been related with these conditions. Changes in the balance between TH1 and TH2 immune responses have been implicated in the progression of dermatophytosis associated to HIV infection (Woodfolk, 2005).

Diverse fungal species as dermatophytes and opportunistic fungi, are frequently cultured from the samples obtained from these patients. The most common remain *T. rubrum* and *T. mentagrophytes* despite their immunocompromised state and the globalization of infections.

This population frequently presents in the same nail plate PSWO associated to WSO. This may be initiated from the distal surface and the proximal nail fold independent one from the other. This is difficult to assess. Regardless of how or where the infection started, the fungus may spread to affect either or both the dorsal and ventral nail surfaces. This may even result eventually in a modification of the clinical presentation. That is, PWSO may turn into a DLSO or TDO. The same is true for WSO, which may convert to PSWO or any other category (Baran *at al.*, 2007; Baran *at al.*, 2004; Hogan, 2006).

Regarding identified risk factors, trauma was the major predisposing factor, followed by diabetes mellitus and peripheral vascular disease. Strong association to *tinea pedis* exists, as toenails are more commonly affected (Surjushe *et al.*, 2007).

4. Clinical signs

The clinical characteristics of onychomycosis in patients living with HIV are commonly recognized because of the extension, rapid evolution and limited response to treatment. (Table 4 & 5).

Usually more than 3 nails involved
Rapid evolution
Mostly toenails
Leukonychia or DLSO
<450 CD4/μL cell count
T. rubrum

Table 4. Clinical presentation of onychomycosis in patients living with HIV/AIDS

	WSO	PWSO
Nail plate appearance	Crumbly	Normal
White patches	Ill defined, irregular shapes multifocal	Distinct border
Localization in nail plate	Any part	Starts at the lunula
Most frequent organism	*Trichophyton mentagrophytes*	*Trichophyton rubrum*

Table 5. Differences between WSO and PWSO

HIV seronegative population normally present onychomycosis in one or both first toenails, which differs from patients living with HIV, who present with an atypical number of nails involved, usually more than three, and the first toenails may not be involved. Another important difference with open population is of course, the age group involved that is much younger if they are living with HIV infection.

Another typical characteristic of these patients is that they report a very short evolution, even two or three weeks in which they witness the rapid change in the appearance of their nails. It is not rare to see involvement of both finger and toenails, adding up to 15 or more nails infected. Anyhow, toenail infection remains the main infected area.

Candida spp., being a frequent opportunistic infectious agent of immunosuppressed patients, one could expect that candidal paronychia should be a common finding, but it is seldomly found in finger or toenails.

WSO is mostly seen in toenails. The reason for the low incidence on fingernails could be that it is a relatively superficial infection that could easily be washed off. So, even in immunosuppressed patients, the finding of WSO in fingernails is rare (Figure 1).

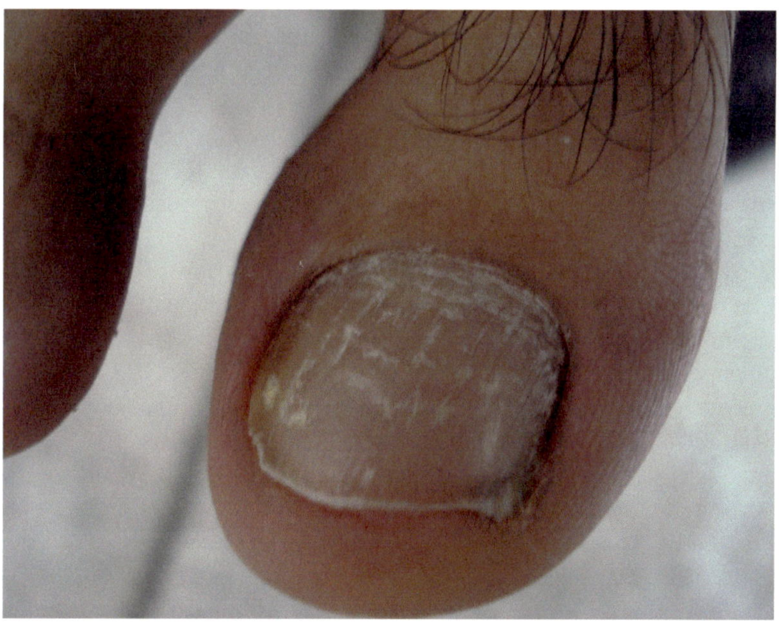

Fig. 1. White superficial onychomycosis

Clinically WSO is seen as opaque white scaly patches, ill defined, irregular and multifocal distributed along the dorsal surface of the nail plate. Each of these plaques corresponds to a fungal colony. Although this is a superficial infection, the nail plate surface looks affected. It is not smooth, but rather irregular and might even be porous and crumbly in some areas.

WSO usually affects toenails, more frequently seen in the first, second and/or third nails. The association to interdigital tinea pedis is common. This clinical form may rapidly evolve to a more deep form of onychomycosis, particularly if associated in that or any other nail to PWSO or DLSO (Figure 2).

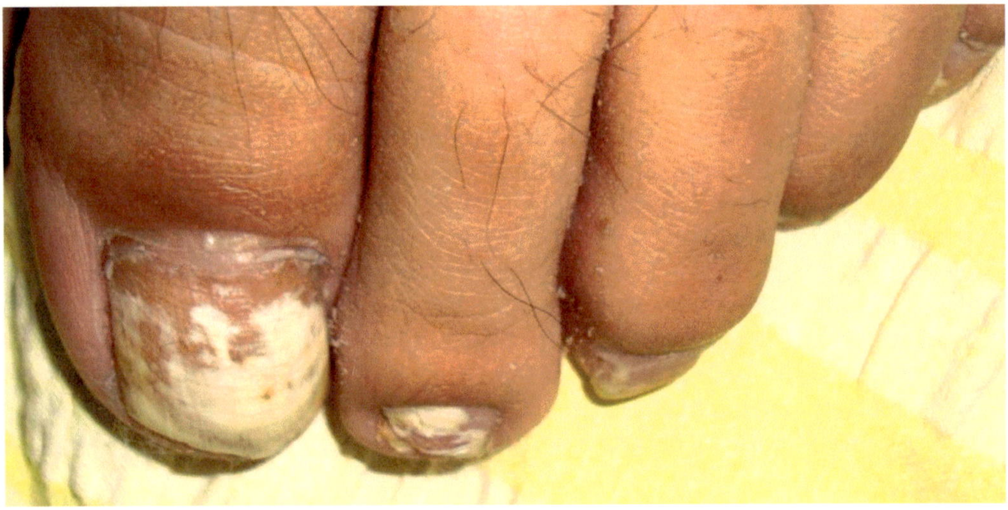

Fig. 2. White superficial onychomycosis and proximal white subungual onychomycosis

If paronychia is associated to WSO, it is generally due to infection of non-dermatophyte moulds (Piraccini & Tosti, 2004).

PWSO is considered by many physicians "the hallmark" of HIV infection. It is certainly true that this clinical form became widely known because of the AIDS pandemia, and although this still remains a rare form of onychomycosis, immunosuppression should be suspected when observed.

This clinical pattern initiates beneath the proximal nail fold, in the area of the lunula. A white, opaque and well defined macula is visible through the nail plate. The cuticle and other periungual tissues are unaffected. It may then continue to spread distally or may remain confined, although it will eventually grow out with the nail.

The most important clinical feature to differentiate it from other invasion patterns is that the nail plate is smooth and looks unaltered in consistency and thickness.

It is common to see different proportions of nail plates affected in the same individual. It can be seen either or in both finger and toenails.

Besides these "classic" characteristics, PWSO may present in a variety of other forms. They may be longitudinal bands of leukonychia of varying thickness, isolated or multiple transverse white bands that may even be a little curved, similar to the natural curvature of the lunula (Figure 3).

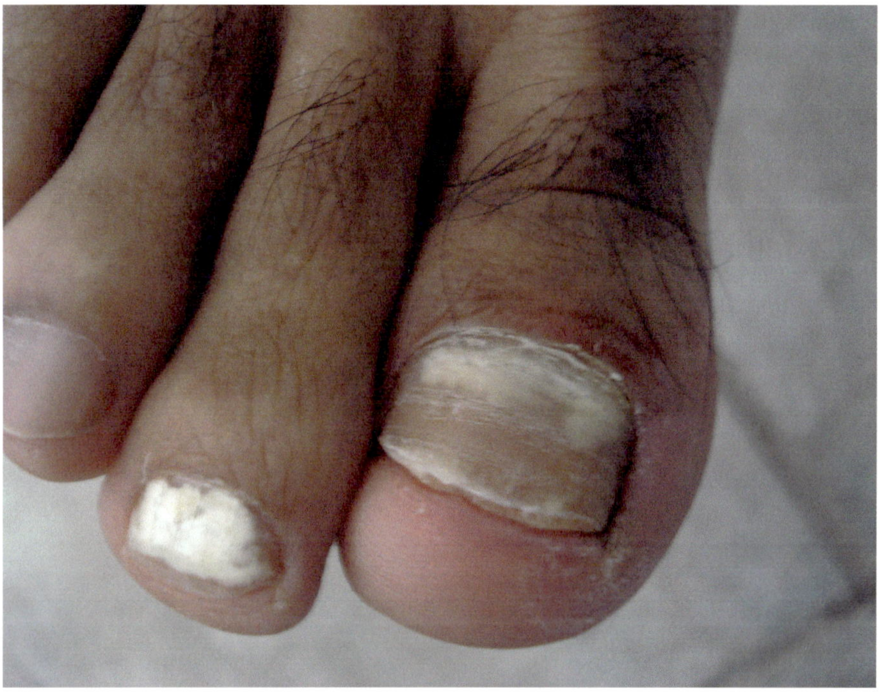

Fig. 3. Proximal white subungual onychomycosis

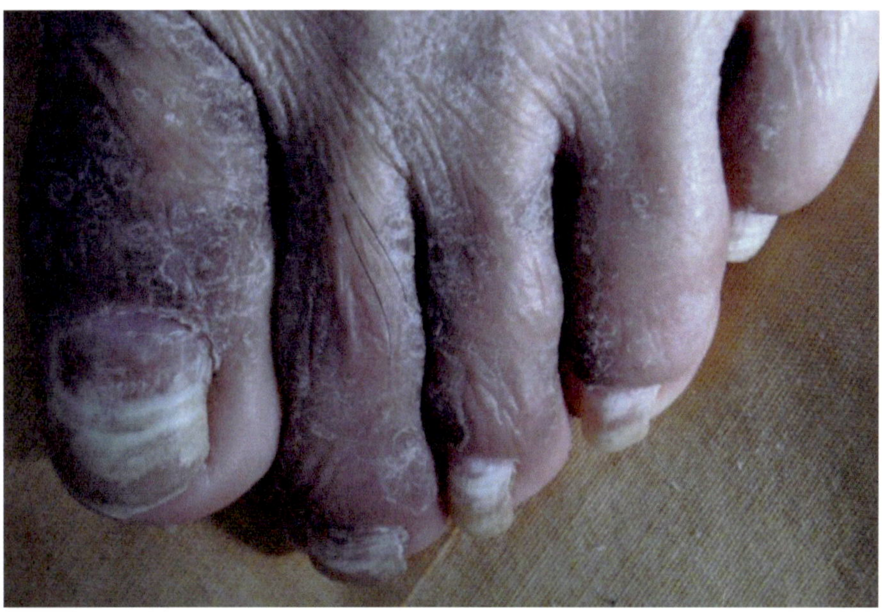

Fig. 4. Leukonychia in transversal bands

As confirmed by histopathology, these transverse bands are separated by normal nail plate, clinically and histologically (Figure 4). Immunosuppressed patients frequently present rapid

development in several digits simultaneously. A study found statistical differences in the incidence of onychomycosis correlated with the stage of AIDS reported. It was of 21% in patients with stage A, 30% with patients in stage B, compared to 54% of patients in stage C ($p<0.02$) (Baran *at al.,* 2005) .
With time, PWSO may evolve to cover the entire nail plate, the original macula may grow out (Figure 5), or DLSO or TDO may develop. These two last clinical presentations are common findings in longstanding onychomycosis infections.
Despite this clinical modification of the appearance of the nail plate and worsening in the appearance of the nail, these infections don´t disseminate systemically to other organs other than the nail apparatus, and therefore, are not life threatening infections (Havlickova, 2008).

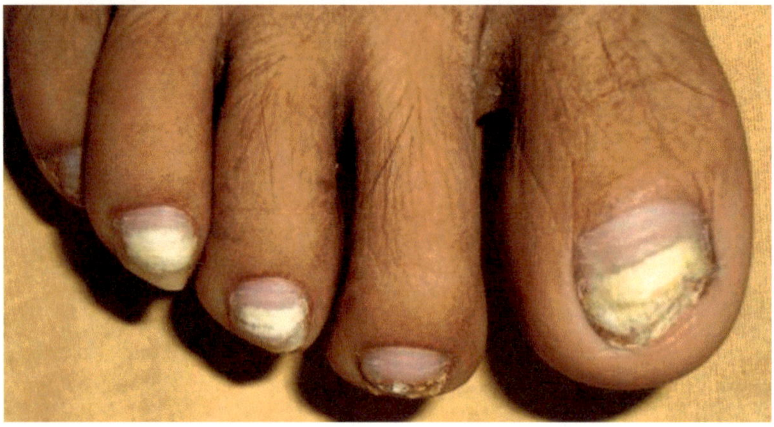

Fig. 5. Proximal white subungual onychomycosis growing out with the nail plate

5. Diagnosis

Clinical diagnosis is the many used method by most physicians, particularly non-dermatologists. However, we do not recommend this as the sole method because only 50% of nail dystrophies correspond to onychomycosis, and treatment with oral antifungals should be restricted to those patients where it has been widely justified.
The physical examination of the nails should be complemented with the medical history regarding sports habits such as swimming or running, because of the excessive humidity and repeated trauma to the nail apparatus respectively.
In immunosuppressed patients, complete physical exploration should be performed. Several reports have mentioned that tinea capitis or tinea inguinale can be precursors of onychomycosis by autoinoculation.

5.1 Laboratory tests

5.1.1 Direct mounts

Potassium hydroxide 10-20% (KOH) preparation and fungal culture in Sabouraud dextrose and/or Mycosel agar are the most known and used laboratory tests.
KOH mounts have the enormous advantage that one can obtain the result immediately, even during the office visit of the patient. It is painless, non-invasive and has very low cost. The downside to it is that only trained dermatologists, microbiologists or mycologists will be able to recognize the fungal structures in the nail scrapings, and one must have a light microscope at hand.

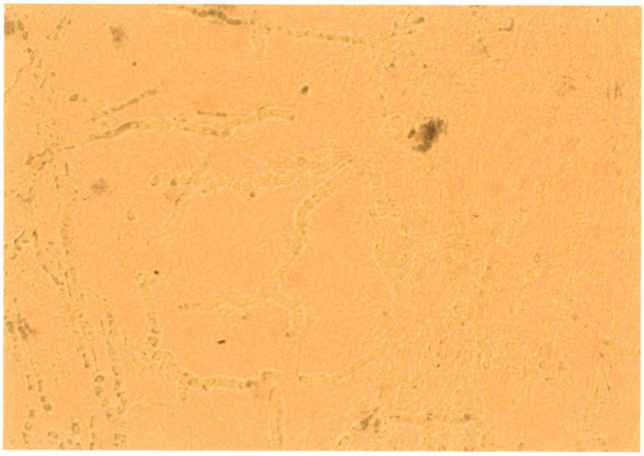

Fig. 6. KOH preparation 40X

The suggested technique for obtaining the sample for any type of onychomycosis is to clean the area with alcohol wipes, and scrape with a curette or a sterile scalpel blade the involved area of the nail. Part of the scale obtained is then placed in a slide with a drop of KOH and a coverslip. Slight heating of the slide's bottom with a match for a few seconds will accelerate the separation of the keratinocytes, facilitating the sample's observation. The rest of the scale will be used for culture. Of course, the clinical characteristics of the nail invasion will determine how the sample should be obtained.

For WSO, we recommend the use of a scalpel blade that should be used to scrape uniformly the affected area of the nail plate.

In the case of PWSO, the sampled area will depend on the localization of the white patch. When the leukonychia is proximal to the nail fold, a 15-scalpel blade is used to "drill" the dorsal area of the nail plate. We discard the first scales obtained, and save the ones from beneath. Much care should be placed in not perforating completely the nail plate's thickness. This would cause bleeding and pain. When the white area is already growing out of the nail, and has reached the distal border, or the leukonychia involves the totality of the nail plate, the sample can be obtained with a small curette, with the technique applied to DLSO, that is, scraping the ventral portion in the free border of the nail plate.

After the sample has been obtained and the mount prepared, the slide is placed in a light microscope and observed at 10X and 40X, where one can look for hyphae (Figure 6), arthroconidia or yeasts. In mycotic white nails fungal elements are usually abundant. After a few hours (3-4) the mount will no longer be useful.

Chlorazol black E is an aid for fungal structure identification. It is an acid stain that binds chitin found in the fungal structures, and not in the keratinocytes. The hyphae and or spores are stained green-blue, facilitating their identification under a light microscope. Studies have found that using Chlorazol black is more cost effective than KOH.

Clacofluor white is another stain employed for the identification of fungi in nail material. It binds to cellulose and chitin. It must be seen under a microscope with UV radiation (fluorescent) which are scarce and expensive. It is rarely used, but yields better results than KOH and Chlorazol black.

The sensibility of KOH mounts has been estimated of 80% (66-95%) and specificity of 72%. (47-72%). Positive and negative predictive values are 88 and 58% respectively. These results

rely mainly on the experience of the observer, and despite the previously described inconvenience, it is still considered the gold standard for the diagnosis of onychomycosis.
The sensibility for Chlorazol black has been reported of 94%, making it one of the most cost effective diagnostic tests for onychomycosis (Weinberg *et al.*, 2003; Lilly *et al.*, 2006).

5.1.2 Cultures

Culture is the gold standard for accurate identification of the pathogen involved but not for clinical diagnosis. It is routinely performed in mycology laboratories as well as the KOH examination.
In the selection of the culture media we must consider that Sabouraud agar enables growth of dermatophytes but also of opportunistic fungi, and even bacteria. This is useful particularly when non-dermatophyte mould infection is suspected. Sabouraud plus Chloramphenicol and Actidione (Mycosel®) is more specific for dermatophytes since the antibiotics added limit opportunistic and bacterial growth.
The sample is the same as for direct examination. The scales are placed with sterile technique in Sabouraud dextrose and/or Mycosel® agar. The media are incubated at 25°C and are checked for growth once a week during four weeks.
The growth in cultures is observed macro and microscopically. Macroscopically, the number of colonies, color, texture, rate of growth, pigment production and other and characteristics of the strain are noted (Figure 7).

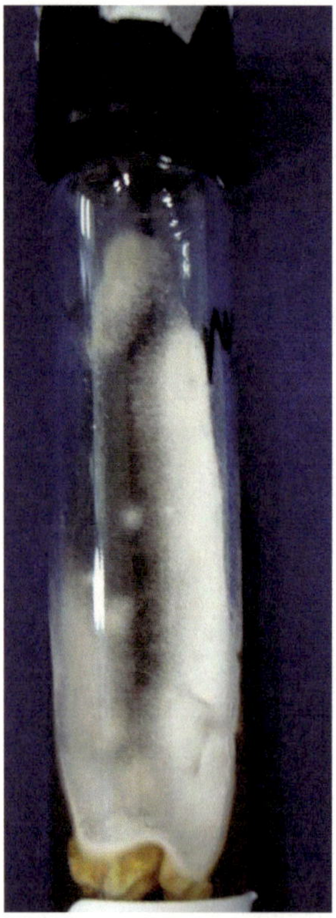

Fig. 7. *T. rubrum* culture

For microscopic identification, mounts are prepared with lactophenol-cotton blue and observed for microconida, macroconidia, hyphae or spores that will enable us to identify the etiological agent (Figure 8).

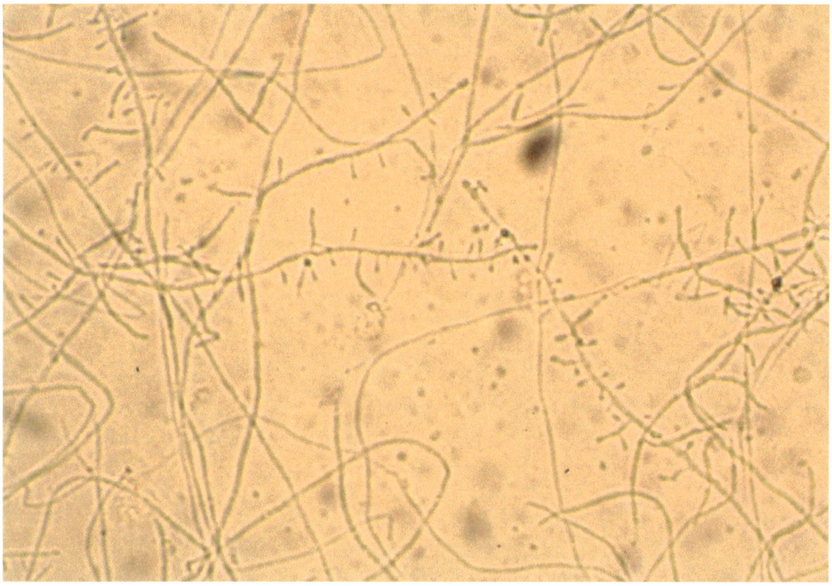

Fig. 8. *T. rubrum* 10X

The correct identification of the fungal species causing onychomycosis will allow the correct selection of the antifungal treatment.

The culture has a sensitivity of 59% (29-59%) and specificity of 82%. Between 30-50% of all cultures will grow, even with a positive direct examination, and it is important to recognize that this doesn't mean that there is no fungal infection. Many factors determine if a culture will grow, such as the sample site and amount of scale taken, viability of the dermatophytes, inoculation technique and storage temperature.

Correlation with KOH and clinical observations are fundamental for proper treatment and follow up.

5.1.3 Molecular biology

Some techniques such as polymerase chain reaction (PCR) are highly sensitive and specific for the identification of microorganisms such as fungi. The gene Chitin synthase 1 (CHS1) is shared by the three dermatophyte genera (*Trichophyton, Epidermophyton* and *Microsporum*) and can be evaluated in patients with onychomycosis.

This test not only allows the positive identification of fungal elements, it also identifies the fungal species, dermatophytes, non dermatophyte molds or yeasts, even in patients taking oral antifungal treatment.

PCR followed by restriction fragment length polymorphism (RFLP), real time PCR and multiplex PCR assay have been adapted for detection of dermatophytes in clinical specimens.

Maybe in the future at least one of these tests will be the gold standard for diagnosis and fungal species identification. For the moment, these techniques are inaccessible except for some select investigative laboratories (Garg *et al.,* 2009).

5.2 Histopathology

Nail plate or nail apparatus biopsy is rarely necessary for diagnosis, although it has been considered by some authors like the most sensitive and specific method for diagnosis. This could be true for those medical settings that lack a mycology laboratory.

The histopathological information that exists regarding the different clinical patterns of fungal invasion of the nail plate has been useful for the clinical classification of onychomycosis and hopefully will help understand more of the physiopathology of the disease.

Hematoxilin and eosin routine stain is performed, but the Peryodic Acid Schiff (PAS) staining technique is the most useful for this tissue (Figure 9). It easily enables the identification of the fungal structures where the hyphae and spores can be identified as eosinophillic structures mixed with the laminated keratinocytes that form the nail plate.

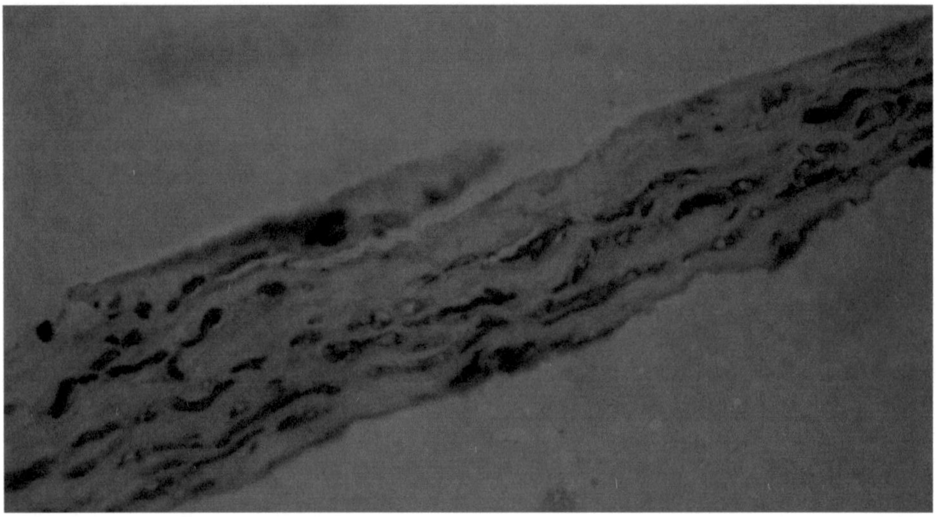

Fig. 9. Fungal structures in nail plate. PAS

The SWO has been identified as a superficial infection of the nail plate in most cases, and only rarely has been reported a "deep" SWO, involving as well the ventral aspect of the nail plate. The usual findings are hyphae and or spores in the dorsal aspect of the nail plate, generally confined to the upper half of the nail plate.

Some authors have suggested that SWO is not always caused by primary dorsal penetration, supported on the fact that sometimes the nail invasion is beneath the upper half that may even reach the ventral aspect of the nail plate. This may depend on the fungal agent involved and its affinity towards keratin and the enzymes required for its destruction.

The involvement in PWSO initiates and commonly remains localized to the ventral aspect of the nail, although progression to invasion of the entire nail plate thickness may also be seen.

Histology of leukonychia in transversal bands demonstrates that the nail is invaded intermittently, with spared areas of healthy nail that correlate to the band of healthy nail observed clinically. This suggests that re-activation may be episodic in these cases (Baran *et al.*, 2005; Moreno-Coutiño *et al.*, 2010; Nandedkar *et al.*, 2005).

Apparently, the etiological agent does not vary the infection pattern in the nail plate. Similar findings have been reported in *T. rubrum* and *M. canis* infected nails, where all the nail plate, from the matrix to the distal portion, shows invasion by numerous fungal elements, particularly in the ventral aspect of the nail plate.

Piraccini et al. evaluated the nail bed, searching for fungal invasion as well, since the principal amount of fungi are found in the part of the nail plate that is in direct contact with the nail bed. The histology showed that there is no fungal invasion of this tissue, and is also devoid of inflammatory changes (Piraccini *et al.*), .

Currently, the study of the nail plate by histology with PAS stain has been reported to have 92% (85-98.85) of sensibility and 72% of specificity, with a positive and negative predictive value of 89.7% and 77% respectively.

6. Treatment and outcome

The treatment of onychomycosis, that is a chronic and mostly asymptomatic disease, sometimes is postponed by many reasons, either from part of the physician or the patient.

However, immunocompromised patients such as those living with HIV, search for treatment due to psychosocial reasons. The burden of knowing themselves with the HIV infection, makes them extra-conscious of their appearance, beyond being esthetically acceptable, they seek a healthy appearance.

To choose the adequate antifungal drug, one must consider several factors. Of course, the clinical pattern of onychomycosis is probably the most determinant of all, as will be discussed further. The number of nails involved and the percentage of affection, previous treatments for the fungal infection and for other diseases, allergies, and finally, the socioeconomic status is a very important factor in this group of patients.

Recently, effective antimycotics, in particular terbinafine, was shown to enhance and restore cell-mediated immunity, which potentially improves the therapeutic outcome even for this group of patients

Currently, three main strategies apply: topical, oral and combination treatment. Amorolfine nail lacquer and oral terbinafine are the most effective drugs as monotherapy. However, the best cure rates are obtained with a combination of oral and local therapy (Lecha *et al.* 2005).

Clues to consider:

1. Clinical pattern of onychomycosis

As the name describes, WSO is superficial as the infection remains in the dorsal aspect of the nail plate. This is the only one that may be treated with topical medications such as a lacquer or by chemical avulsion of the nail plate. It is important to remember that transungual delivery of the drug is limited by the low permeability of the nail plate, so repeated dosing over a long period is required.

It is a common finding that WSO is combined with any other clinical form of onychomycosis. In this case, the patient must be treated according to the most sever pattern shown.

PWSO varies clinically depending on the time of the diagnosis. This onychomycosis initiates in the matrix area, and as the nail grows, the area involved may grow out too, or the disease may spread to affect the entire nail plate. For this clinical form, the recommended treatment approach is oral antimycotics, such as terbinafine or itraconazole.

General guidelines state that oral treatment is indicated if the matrix area is involved and/or more than 50% of the nail plate is affected.

2. Isolated fungi

Specific identification of the fungal pathogen is useful for adequate prescription. Dermatophytes are successfully treated with terbinafine or itraconazole. However, NDM have not shown a better cure rate if treated with oral anifungals. Terbinafine has no effect over *Candida* sp. infection, so in cases of paronychia, itraconazole is recommended Hogan, 2006).

3. Socioeconomic status

Antifungal medication, particularly oral and lacquer are very expensive, and should be administered continuously for several months. Before prescribing the antifungal, one must consider cost-benefit, availability and accessibility of the treatment.

4. Comorbidities and other prescription drugs

Most systemic antifungals potentially have interactions with other drugs.

6.1 Antifungals

6.1.1 Topical

Lacquer

Commercially three different antimycotics are available in lacquer. All of them show similar cure rates, but the continuous application is required for an average of 4 months (Sidou *et al.* 2004; Sigurgeisson Ket al. 2010; Subissi *et al.* 2010).

Amorolfine 5%

Is a morpholine derivative with broad spectrum as antifungal agent, including dermatophytes, NDM, and yeasts. It is fungicidal for most species. It rapidly penetrates the nail, and the clearance is slow because it is applied in a non-water soluble film that remains in the nail for a week. This drug is well tolerated and minor local adverse reactions are observed rarely. In vitro, apparently amorolfine synergizes with ketoconazole, griseofulvin and terbinafine.

It is indicated once a week, approximately 6 months. This is the most recommended drug, since it has shown longer remanence on the nail surface, more resistance to chemical trauma from soaps and mechanical aggressions to the nail apparatus, and is the most cost-effective of the lacquers. It is safe and effective as prophylaxis of recurrence in these patients that relapse frequently.

Ciclopirox 8%

It has a broad spectrum drug including almost all of the clinically relevant dermatophytes, yeasts and moulds. It is active against azole-resistant *Candida* and even some bacteria. The main antimicrobial activity apparently is by inhibition of the metal dependent enzymes that are responsible for degradation of peroxides within the fungal cell. The fungal resistance to this drug is extremely low and shows a mild anti-inflammatory effect in biochemical and pharmacological models. It is considered to have high affinity to keratin and good nail permeation. As a topical drug, it is devoid of systemic adverse reactions. Mild erythema has seldom been reported (<5% treated patients). This lacquer must be applied every other day the first month, twice a week the second and once a week for one or two more months.

Tioconazole 28%

It is an imidazole with activity against moulds and yeasts. This is the least recommended because of its posology and limited effectiveness. The suggested dosage is twice a day during 6-12 months .

Chemical avulsion

Chemical destruction of the nail plate with occlusive 40% urea and bifonazole 1% is recommended for patients that have very thickened nail plate, dermatophytoma or when

oral therapy is contraindicated. It is also an effective and low cost adyuvant to oral therapy, particularly in cases of NMD infection or pediatric patients.
Urea is a keratolytic that destroys hydrogen unions. This destruction allows the antifungal to penetrate deeply in the nail plate for better results. Bifonazole is a wide spectrum azolic derivate with activity against yeasts, dermatophytes and NDM, lipophilic and hydrophobic that allows long cutaneous retention of the drug. It is applied under occlusion once a day and the softened nail plate must be removed before reapplying the medication. The most common side effects are local erosion and pain that remit when the treatment is suspended (Arenas, 2001¸Carrillo-Muñoz *et al.* 2010).

6.1.2 Systemic (oral)

Terbinafine

This antimycotic is by far the most widely prescribed oral medication because of its low incidence of drug interactions compared to azoles. Terbinafine is an allylamine that reaches steady-state in the nail matrix and bed in one week, and plasma levels in 10-14 days. Because of its keratinophilic and lipophilic characteristics, this dug persists in the nail apparatus for 24-156 days.
It is fungicidal and fungistatic, with broad spectrum for moulds. Its absorption is not affected by food, is metabolized extensively in the liver and excreted principally in urine. The terminal half life is of 16-22 hr. that may be prolonged in patients with liver or renal impairment, particularly those with <50 mL/min of creatinine clearance or >300 µMol/ of serum creatinine. The most recognized drug interactions are with cimetidine and rifampin. Terbinafine also inhibits the cytochrome P4502D6 (CYP2D6) so caution is recommended when administering CYP2D6 substrates.
The mycological cure rate has been reported 48-90% on different trials, and has always been superior in comparison to placebo, itraconazole, griseofulvin and fluconazole. Only one case of *T. rubrum* resistant to terbinafine has been published.
It can be administered daily 250 mg/3-4 months, or in pulses, 250 mg twice a day for one week each month at least during four months.
No drug interactions have been observed in patients living with HIV/AIDS in several reports (Elewski & Tavakkol, 2005; Osborne *et al.* 2006).

Itraconazole

This is a fungistatic drug that diffuses through the matrix and nail bed 3-12 weeks, but then these levels are sustained in the nail plate for several months. It is well tolerated, and less than 3% of the patients report adverse effects. The most common are headache and gastrointestinal symptoms. In skin, rash and pruritus have been seldomly reported.
It is better absorbed if taken with food. It´s absorption is reduced by antacids as omeprazole, cimetidine and ranitidine. Because this drug is metabolized in the liver by CYP3A4, the potential for interaction with other drugs is important to consider. Its prescription is contraindicated with antidysrhymics, antimalarials, benzodiapines, antipsychotic and statins. Serum levels of warfarin, cisapride and cyclosporine should be monitored in concomitant therapy. Concurrent administration with antidiabetic drugs may cause hypoglycemia. Liver enzyme elevations are reported in 0.3-0.5%.
Specifically in patients living with HIV/AIDS, is important to remember that rifampin and other antituberculous drug may vary serum levels of itraconazole. Protease inhibitors also inhibit CYP3A4, and a dose reduction of itraconazole may be required.

However, despite all the contraindications and precautions, itraconazole is effective in clearing onychomycosis as well as systemic fungal infections commonly seen in this group of patients, so in clinical practice, itraconazole dosage is frequently adjusted to cure both fungal diseases.

The recommended dose for onychomycosis is 200 mg/day or 200 mg twice a day for one week during four months.

Fluconazole

This is another azole, with similar mode of action and drug interactions than itraconazole. It is widely prescribed as prophylaxis for opportunistic fungal infections in immunosuppressed patients Nonetheless, it is not recommended for onychomycosis treatment, since terbinafine and itraconazole have better cure rates in shorter periods.

6.2 Combination therapy

The combination of topical and systemic treatment increases antifungal spectrum, fungicidal activity and safety. It also reduces treatment duration.

Any lacquer or urea may be combined with systemic antifungals such as terbinafine or itraconazole. The decision must be made considering the clinical pattern, number of nails involved, general health status of the patient and accessibility to the drugs.

Many trials have reported the outcome of combination therapy. The most successful ones are those that include terbinafine or itraconazole. One of them reported that the combination of amorolfine and terbinafine had a 59% success rate compared to 45% in the group of oral terbinafine only. Treatment cost was lower in the combination group. Other combinations find similar results.

Another approach is the combination of oral antifungal with surgical avulsion of the infected nail. One of us has reported a better response rate, combining with terbinafine in pulses. However, we do not recommend this technique as first line of treatment, because it is invasive, painful, and must be preformed by a nail surgery expert (Baran *et al.* 2007; Domínguez-Cherit *et al.* 1999).

6.3 Observation

For patients that recently initiated antiretroviral therapy (ARV) we recommend observation for approximately six months. This obeys to several reasons. First of all, because they must accept and tolerate the ARV medications and its side effects which almost all patients refer. Even though most are mild and transient they must adequate their life style to them and wait for the majority of adverse effects to disappear. Another reason is that in our clinical practice, we have observed several times that these patients clinically improve, that is, the area of onychomycosis is reduced, or even cure completely by allowing the immune system restoration with ARV therapy (Tachikawa, *et al.*1999).

7. Differential diagnosis

Differential diagnosis should be done with any other cause of leukonychia. The list is long and includes congenital and acquired diseases. Among the most common causes in the HIV/AIDS infected patients include frequent skin diseases as dyshidrosis or erythema multiforme, systemic acute infections such as pneumonia, herpes zoster, or even intoxication with lead, antimony, fluoride, androgen therapy, cirrhosis, hyperalbuminemia, gout, protein deficiency, kidney transplant and renal failure either acute or chronic, parathyroid insufficiency, Hodgkin´s disease and intra-abdominal malignancies, cachectic state, peripheral neuropathy, shock, surgery and drugs such as hydroxyurea.

8. Conclusions

Fungal leukonychia is common in patients living with HIV/AIDS or those that have any other cause of immunosuppression. However, OSDL continues to be the most prevalent presentation of onychomycosis.

The findings of PWSO or SWO are not synonymous of HIV infection, but should alert the physician of that possibility.

Patients with HIV infection present onychomycosis in a more extensive manner, involving many nails simultaneously and with rapid evolution. This is apparently directly related to a decline in the immune system function.

An adequate approach to diagnosis will allow the best evaluation of each particular case, and on that basis, decide the best option of treatment for the patient. Ideally, every patient must be evaluated by a dermatologist who will take the scales for a KOH direct examination and a mycological culture.

The direct exam with KOH or Chlorazol Black is the best. test for diagnosis and most cost-effective. It should be complemented with a culture, although the possibility of a negative result is high. When the diagnosis is not clear after these tests, or a mycology laboratory is inaccessible, a biopsy of the nail plate, stained with PAS can be performed with high sensibility and specificity for diagnosis.

To determine the treatment, we must always keep in mind the general state and socioeconomic situation. This will allow us to choose the best option in each case.

9. References

Arenas R. 1990. Las onicomicosis. Aspectos clínico-epidemiológicos, micológicos y terapéuticos. *Gaceta Médica de México*;126:84-91, ISSN 00163813

Arenas R. Dermatophytosis In: Arenas R & Estrada R., 2001. *Tropical Dermatology*. Landes Bioscience, ISBN 1-57059-493-7 USA, pg 2-11

Arenas R, Bonifaz A, Arce M, Padilla MC, Atoche C, Barba J, Campos P, Fernández R, Mayorga J, Nazar D & Ocampo J. Onychomycosis. 2010. A Mexican survey. *Eur J Dermatol*; 20 (5)Sep-Oct 2010:611-614. ISSN 1167-1122

Baran R, & Dawber RPR. 1994 Physical signs, In: *Diseases of the nails and their management*. Baran R, & Dawber RPR, PP: 35-81;Blackwell Scientific Publications (2nd Edition), ISBN 0-632-03754-7, Spain.

Baran R, Hay R, & Perrin C. 2004. Superficial white onychomycosis revisited. *JEADV*; 18(5) Sep 2004: 569-571. ISSN 0926-9959

Baran R, McLoone N, & Hay RJ.2005. Could proximal white subungual onychomycosis be a complication of systemic spread? The lessons to be learned form maladie dermatophytique and other deep infections. *Br J Dermatol* 153(5)Nov 2005: 1023-1025 ISSN 0007-0963

Baran R, Faergemann J & Hay RJ. 2007. Superficial white onychomycosis-A syndrome with different fungal causes and paths of infection. *J Am Acad Dermatol* 57(5) Nov 2007: 879-882. ISSN 0190-9622

Baran R, Sigurgeirsson B, de Becker D, Kaufmann R, Lecha M, Faegemann J, Kerrouche N, & Sidou F. 2007. A multicentre, randomized, controlled study of the efficacy, safety and cost-effectiveness of a combination therapy with amorolfine nail lacquer and oral terbinafine compared with oral terbinafine alone for the treatment of onychomycosis with matrix involvement. *Br J Dermatol* 157(1)Jul 2007:149-157 ISSN 0007-0963

Blanes M, Belichón I, Merino E, Portilla J, Sánchez-Payá J, & Betlloch I. 2010. Prevalencia y características de las dermatosis relacionadas con la infección por VIH en la actualidad. *Actas Dermosifilogr* 101(8); Oct 2010: 702-709. ISSN 0001-7310

Carrillo-Muñoz AJ, Tur-Tur C, Hernández-Molina JM, Santos P, Cárdenes D, & Giusiano G. 2010. Antifúngicos disponibles para el tratamiento de las micosis ungueales. *Rev Iberam Micol* 27(2):Jun 2010:49-56 ISSN 1130-1406

Chang P, & Arenas R. 1995. Proximal white subungual onychomycosis in a kidney transplant patient. *Int J Dermatol* 34(8)Aug 1995: 591. ISSN 0011-9059

Cribier B, Leiva Mena M, Rey D, Partisani M, Fabien V, Lang JM, & Grosshans E.1998. Nail changes in patients infected with human immunodeficiency virus. *Arch Dermatol* 34(10) Oct 1998: 1216-1220.ISSN 0003-987X

Crozier WJ, & Lavrin LM.1979. An uncommon case of onychomycosis due to *Microsporum canis*. *Australasian Journal of Dermatology* 20(3):Dec 1979:144-146 ISSN 1440-0960

Denning DW, Evans EGV, Kibbler CC, Richardson MD, Roberts MM, Rogers TR, Warnock DW, & Warren RE. 1995.

Fungal nail diseases: a guide to good practice (report of a working group of the British Society for Medical Mycology) *BMJ* 311 (7015): Nov 1995: 1277-1281. ISSN 0959-8138

Drake LA, Patrick DL, Fleckman P, André J, Baran R, Haneke E, Sapéde C, & Tosti A. 1999. The impact of onychomycosis on quality of life: Development of an international onychomycosis-specific questionnaire to measure patient quality of life. *J Am Acad Dermatol* 41(2 Pt 1) Aug 1999: 189-196 ISSN 0190-9622

Domínguez-Cherit J, Teixeira F, & Arenas R. 1999. Combined surgical and systemic treatment of onychomycosis. *Br J Dermatol* 140(4): Apr 1999:778-780 ISSN 0007-0963

Dompmartin D, Dompmartin A, Deluol AM, Grosshans E, & Coulaud JP. 1990. Onychomycosis and AIDS clinical and laboratory findings in 62 patients. *Int J Dermatol* 29(5): Jun 1990:337-339. ISSN 0011-9059

Elewski, B.1998. Onychomycosis: pathogenesis, diagnosis and management. *Clin Microbiol Rev.* 11(3): Jul 1998:415–429. ISSN 0893-8512

Elewski B, & Tavakkol A. 2005. Safety and tolerability of oral antifungal agents in the treatment of fungal nail disease: a proven reality. *Ther Clin Risk Management* 1(4): Dec2005:299-306. ISSN 1176-6336

Garg J, Tilak R, Garg A, Prakash P, Gulati AK & Nath G. 2009. Rapid detection of dermatophytes from skin and hair. *BMC Res Notes* 2 ; Apr 2009:60. ISSN 1756-0500

Grossman M., & Scher RK. 1990. Leukonychia. Review and classification. *Int J Dermatol* 29(8), Oct 1990: 535-541. ISSN 0011-9059

Gupta AK, Sibbald RG, & Lynde ChW.1997. Onychomycosis in children: Prevalence and treatment strategies. *J Am Acad Dermatol* 36(3 pt 1); Mar 1997: 395-402 ISSN 01909622

Gupta AK, & Summerbell RC.1999. Combined distal and lateral subungual and white superficial onychomycosis in the toenails. *J Am Acad Dermatol* 41(6): Dec 1999:938-944 ISSN 0190-9622

Baran R, Hay RJ, Tosti A, & Haneke E. 1998. A new classification of onychomycosis. *Br J Dermatol* 139(4) Oct 1998:567-571 ISSN 0007-0963

Gupta AK, Taborda P, Taborda V, Gilmour J, Rachlis A, Salit I, Gupta MA, Mac Donald P, Cooper EA, & Summerbell RC.2000. Epidemiology and prevalence of onychomycosis in HIV-positive individuals. *Int J Dermatol* 39(10) Oct 2000: 746-753 ISSN 0011-9059

Havlickova B, Czaika VA, & Friedrich M. 2008. Epidemiological trends in skin mycoses worldwide. *Mycoses* 51 suppl 4; Sep 2008:2-15 ISSN 0933-7407

Herranz P, Garcia J, de Lucas R, Gonzalez J, Peña JM, Diaz R, & Casado M.1997. Toenail onychomycosis in patients with acquired immune deficiency syndrome: treatment with terbinafine. *Br J Dermatol* 137(4) Oct 1997:577-580 ISSN 0007-0963

Hogan M. 2006. Cutaneous infections associated with HIV/AIDS. *Dermatol Clin* 24(4) Oct 2006: 473-495 ISSN 0733-8635

Lecha M, Effendy I, Feullhade de Chauvin M, Di Chiacchio N, & Baran R. 2005.Treatment options-development of consensus guidelines. *J Eur Acad Dermatol Venereol* Suppl 1, 2005: 25-33.ISSN 1468-3083

Lilly KK, Koshnick RL, Grill JP, Khalil ZM, Nelson DB, Warshaw EM. Cost-effectiveness of diagnostic tests for toenail onychomycosis: a repeated-measure, single-blinded, cross-sectional evaluation of 7 diagnostic tests. *J Am Acad Dermatol* 55(4) Oct 2006: 620-626 ISSN 0190-9622

Millikan LE, Powell DW, & Drake LA. 1999. Quality of life for patients with onychomycosis. *Int J Dermatol* 38: suppl 2:Sep1999:13-16. ISSN 0011-9059

Moreno-Coutiño G, Toussaint-Caire S, & Arenas R. 2010. Clinical, mycological and histological aspects of white onychomycosis. *Mycoses* 53(2): Mar 2010:144-147 ISSN 0933-7407

Moreno-Coutiño G, Arenas R, & Reyes-Terán G. 2011. Clinical presentation of onychomycosis in HIV/AIDS: a review of 280 mexican cases. *Indian J Dermatol* 56(1) Jan-Feb 2011:120 ISSN 0019-5154

Nandedkar-Thomas MA, & Scher RK. 2005. An update in disorders of the nails. *J Am Acad Dermatol* 52(5) May 2005: 877-887 ISSN 0190-9622

Noppakun N, & Head E. 1986. Proximal white subungual onychomycosis in a patient with acquired immune deficiency syndrome. *Int J Dermatol* 25(9): Nov 1986:586-587 ISSN 0011-9059

Odds FC, Arai T, Disalvo AF, Evans EG, Hay RJ, Randhawa HS, Rinaldi MG, & Walsh TJ. 1992. Nomenclature of fungal diseases: a report and recommendations from a sub-committee of the international society for human and animal mycology (ISHAM) *J Med Vet Mycol* 30(1): 1992:1-10 ISSN 0268-1218

Osborne CS, Leitner I, Hofbauer B, Fielding CA, Favre B, & Ryder N. 2006. Biological, biochemical, and molecular characterization of a new clinical Trichophyton rubrum isolate resistant to terbinafine. *Antimicrob Agents Chemother* 50(6); Jun 2006: 2234-2236.ISSN 0066-4804

Piraccini BM, & Tosti A. 2004. White superficial onychomycosis: epidemiological, clinical and pathological study of 79 patients. *Arch Dermatol* 140(6): Jun 2004:696-701.ISSN 0003-987X

Piraccini BM, Morelli R, Stinchi C, Tosti A. Proximal subungual onychomycosis due to Microsporum canis. *Br J Dermatol* 134(1) Jan 1996: 175-177 ISSN 0007-0963

Ravnborg L, Baastrup N, & Svejgaard E. 1998. Onychomycosis in HIV-infected patients. Acta Derm Venereol 78(2):Mar 1998:151-152 ISSN 0001-5555 Scher RK, Tavakkol A, Sigurgeirsson B, Hay RJ, Joseph WS, Tosti A, Fleckman P, Ghannoum M, Armstrong DG,

Markinson BC, & Elewski B. 2007. Onychomycosis: diagnosis and definition of cure. *J Am Acad Dermatol* 56(6) Jun 2007:939-944 ISSN 0190-9622

Sidou F, & Soto P. 2004. A randomized comparison of nail surface remanence of three nail lacquers, containing amorolfine 5%, ciclopirox 8% or tioconazole 28% in healthy volunteers. *Int J Tissue React* 26(1-2) 2004:17-24. ISSN 0250-0868

Subissi A, Monti D, Togni G, & Mailland F. 2010. Ciclopirox: recent nonclinical and clinical data relevant to its use as a topical antimycotics agent. *Drugs* 70(16) Nov 2010: 2133-2152. ISSN 0968-7637

Sigurgeirsson B, Olafsson JH, Steinsson JT, Kerrouche N, & Sidou F. 2010. Efficacy of amorolfine nail lacquer for prophylaxis of onychomycosis over 3 years. *J Eur Acad Dermatol Venererol* 24 (8) Aug 2010: 910-915 ISSN 1468-3083

Singh H, Singh P, Tiwari P, Dey V, Dulhani N, & Singh A. 2009. Dermatological manifestations in HIV-infected patients at a tertiary care hospital in a tribal (Bastar) region of Chhattisgarh, *India. Indian J Dermatol* 54(4); 2009: 338-341 ISSN 0019-5154

Surjushe A, Kamath R, Oberai C, Saple D, Thakre M, Dharmshale S, & Gohil A. 2007. A clinical and mycological study of onychomycosis in HIV infection. *Indian J Dermatol Venereol Leprol* 73(6): Nov-Dec 2007: 397-401 ISSN 0019-5154

Tachikawa N, Yasuoka A, & Oka S. 1999. Improvement of Onychomycosis without AntifungalTherapy after Initiation of Highly Active Anti-Retroviral Therapy (HAART) in an HIV-Infected Patient. *Jpn J Infect Dis* 52(6); Dec1999: 245-46. ISSN 1344-6304

Vásquez del Mercado E, & Arenas R. 2008. Onicomicosis en niños. Estudio retrospectivo de 233 casos mexicanos. *Gac Med Mex* 144(1) Jan-Feb 2008: 7-9 ISSN 00163813

Weinberg JM, Koestenblatt EK, Don PC, White SM, Stein MN, & Bamji M. 1999. Proximal white subungual onychomycosis is the immunocompetent patient: report of two cases and review of the literature. *Acta Derm Venererol* 79(1) Jan1999: 81-95 ISSN 0001-5555

Weinberg JM, Koestenblatt EK, Tutrone WD, Tishler HR, & Najarian L. 2003. Comparison of diagnostic methods in the evaluation of onychomycosis. *J Am Acad Dermatol* 49(2); Aug 2003: 193-197 ISSN 0190-9622

Weismann K, Knudsen EA, & Pedersen C. 1988. White nails in AIDS/ARC due to Trichophyton rubrum infection. *Clin Exp Dermatol* 13(1) Jan1988: 24-25. ISSN 0307-6938

WHO case definitions of HIV for surveillance and revised clinical staging and immunological classification of HIV- related disease in adults and children, 2006 http://www.who.int/hiv/pub/guidelines/HIVstaging150307.pdf (April 11, 2011

Woodfolk JA. 2005. Allergy and dermatophytes. *Clin Microbiol Reviews* 18(1); Jan 2005:30-43. ISSN 0893-8512 www.who.int/hiv/data/2009_global_summary.png January 31st 2011

Zaias N. 1972. Onychomycosis. *Arch Dermatol.*105(2); Feb 197:263-74 ISSN 0003-987X

14

Cryptosporidiosis - From Epidemiology to Treatment

Anane Sonia
Faculty of Medicine, Tunis, Tunisia

1. Introduction

Cryptosporidiosis is a disease caused by *Cryptosporidium* spp, an obligate intracellular protozoan parasite.

It is a frequent cause of diarrheal disease in humans, and several groups of humans are particularly susceptible to cryptosporidiosis. In developing countries, *Cryptosporidium* infections occur mostly in children younger than 5 years (Newman et al, 1999; Bern et al, 2000; Bhattacharya et al, 1997; Gatei et al, 2006). In immunocompromised persons such as human immunodeficiency virus-positive (HIV) patients, the incidence and severity of cryptosporidiosis increases as the CD4 lymphocyte cell count falls (Navin et al, 1999; Pozio et al, 1997; Sorvillo et al, 1998).

Although cryptosporidiosis was initially described in mice in 1907 (Tyzzer, 1907), human disease was first identified almost three quarters of a century later. Two reports were published in 1976: one case in healthy child and one in an immunosuppressed adult (Meisel et al, 1976; Nime et al, 1976).

The next significant milestone was the emergence of chronic and life-threatening cryptosporidiosis with HIV/AIDS in the early 1980s. The association with AIDS and the appearance of early clinical and epidemiological reports implicating cryptosporidiosis as a frequent cause of acute diarrhea in the general population firmly established that the infection was serious and widespread in humans. The first case of cryptosporidiosis in a homosexual man with AIDS was reported in 1982 (Ma & Soave, 1983) and by mid-1983, some 50 cases had been reported (Ma, 1984). The link with AIDS was so strong that cryptosporidiosis became one of the defining features of the syndrome before the discovery of the causative virus.

Then, other immunocompromised patients and healthy people including veterinary workers and children were also diagnosed with cryptosporidiosis.

Cryptosporidiosis is an opportunistic parasitosis. It is characterised by self-limiting gastroenteritis in otherwise healthy people, while it is more severe in immunocompromised subjects in HIV-infected patients and constitutes a serious threat leading to chronic or fulminant disease, wasting and death (Hunter & Nichols, 2002; Chen et al, 2002).

While improved antiretroviral regimens have significantly reduced the prevalence of AIDS and AIDS-related opportunistic infections, cryptosporidiosis remains among the most common causes of diarrhoea in patients with AIDS (Hunter & Nichols, 2002; Morpeth & Thielman, 2006).

During the three last decades our knowledge about cryptosporidiosis has expanded remarkably.
The focus of this revue is to summarize current knowledge on taxonomy, epidemiology, diagnosis, treatment and prevention of cryptosporidiosis in AIDS patients.

2. Parasite

2.1 Taxonomy

Cryptosporidium species are apicomplexan parasites.
Over 100 years have passed since Ernest Edward Tyzzer first made his observations on the genus *Cryptosporidium*. *Cryptosporidium* was so named because of the absence of sporocysts within the oocysts, a characteristic of other coccidia. The first species described was *C. muris*, from the gastric glands of laboratory mice (Tyzzer, 1907). Tyzzer later published a more complete description of the life cycle and subsequently described a second species, also from laboratory mice. *C. parvum* differed from *C. muris* not only by infecting the small intestine rather than the stomach but also because the oocysts were smaller (Tyzzer, 1910, 1912).
Following the initial discovery of *Cryptosporidium*, over 50 years elapsed during which the parasite was commonly confused with other apicomplexan genera, especially members of the coccidian genus *Sarcocystis*.
After the recognition of true differences between *Cryptosporidium* and *Sarcocystis*, the erroneous concept of strict host specificity was applied to *Cryptosporidium* spp. This led to the creation of multiple new species including *C. agni* in sheep, *C. anserinum* in geese, *C. bovis* in calves, *C. cuniculus* in rabbits, *C. garnhami* in humans, and *C. rhesi* in monkeys (Levine, 1980; Barker & Carbonell, 1974).
Subsequent cross-transmission studies demonstrated that *Cryptosporidium* isolates from different animals can frequently be transmitted from one host species to another, which ended the practice of naming species based on host origin and the synonymization of many of these new *Cryptosporidium* species as *C. parvum*.
In recent years, molecular characterizations of *Cryptosporidium* have helped to clarify the confusion in *Cryptosporidium* taxonomy and validate the existence of multiple species in each vertebrate class.
As a result, several new species of *Cryptosporidium* have also been named, *C. andersoni* from cattle, *C. canis* from dogs, *C. molnari* from fish and *C. hominis* from humans (Xiao et al, 2004; Alvarez-Pellitero & Sitja-Bobadilla, 2002; Lindsay et al, 2000; Morgan-Ryan et al, 2002).
Human disease has been traditionally attributed to *C. parvum* but it was apparent from both the early epidemiological questions raised regarding the zoonotic status and transmission of the organism that variants occurred.
C. parvum, C. hominis were two confused species. The first observations of genetic heterogeneity among *C. parvum* (currently *C. parvum* and *C. hominis*) isolated from humans and livestock date back to 1992. Southern blotting of restriction enzyme-digested genomic DNA (Ortega et al, 1991), Western blotting (Nina et al, 1991) and isoenzyme profiles obtained from oocyst lysates (Ogunkolade et al, 1993) provided the first insights into the extent of heterogeneity in this species. Significantly, these studies showed for the first time that humans were infected with two subgroups *within C. parvum*, which were variously named "human" and "cattle", H and C or Type 1 and Type 2, respectively. These observations, subsequently confirmed in many laboratories, were significant in showing that humans are part of two distinct transmission cycles, one comprising ruminants and humans

ant the other exclusively comprising humans. It was a small step to the naming of a new species, *C. hominis*, proposed for *C.parvum* parasites exclusively infecting humans (Spano et al, 1998; Morgan-Ryan et al, 2002).

There are currently 16 recognized species of *Cryptosporidium*, which have been isolated from a large variety of hosts (Table 1), (Xiao et al, 2004) : *C. parvum, C. hominis, C. felis, C. canis, C. wrairi, C. varanii, C. suis, C. bovis, C. andersoni, C. muris, C. serpentis, C. galli, C. meleagridis, C. molnari, C. scophithalmi* and *C. baileyi.* The four basic requirements for the naming of *Cryptosporidium* species are (Xiao, 2010; Chalmers, 2008):

1. Morphometric study of oocysts and, if possible, sporozoites.
2. Multi-locus genetic characterisation by nucleotide sequence analysis of well studied genes or non-coding regions. The ssu rRNA gene is usually included.
3. Demonstration of natural and, if possible, experimental, host specificity.
4. Compliance with the International Code of Zoonotic Nomenclature.

Eight species are known to be infectious for man: *C. parvum, C. hominis, C. meleagridis, C.*

Species	Major host	Minor host	Location
C. muris	Rodents, bactrian camels	Humans, rock hyrax, mountain goat	Stomach
C. andersoni	Cattle, bactrian camels	Sheep	Abomasums
C. parvum	Cattle, sheep, goats, humans	Deer, mice, pigs	Stomach and intestine
C. hominis	Humans, monkeys	Dugongs, sheep	Small intestine
C. wrairi	Guinea, pigs		Small intestine
C. felis	Cats	Humans, cattle	Small intestine
C. canis	Dogs	Humans	Small intestine
C. meleagridis	Turkeys, humans	Parrots	Intestine
C. baileyi	Chicken, turkeys	Cockatiels, quails, ostriches, ducks	Cloacal, bursa, respiratory tract
C. galli	Finches, chicken, capercalles, grosbeaks		Proventriculus
C. serpentis	Snakes, lizards		Intestinal and cloacal mucosal
C. scophithalmi	Fish		Intestine
C. molnari	Fish		Stomach
C. varanii	Snakes, lizards		Intestinal and cloacal mucosal
C. suis	Pigs	humans	Stomach
C. bovis	Ruminants		Intestine

Table 1. Recorded species of *Cryptosporidium*

felis, *C. canis*, *C. suis*, *C. muris* and *C. andersoni*, although some are reported extremely rarely, particularly the latter three species, and the pathogenicity of some species for man has not been proven (Chalmers, 2008).

C. hominis and *C. parvum* are recognized globally as the most important *Cryptosporidium* species infecting humans (Dunand et al, 1997; Xiao & Ryan, 2004).

Muthusamy et al characterized cryptosporidial infections in 48 human immunodeficiency virus-infected individuals in india by multilocus genotyping. *C. hominis*, *C. parvum*, *C. felis*, *C. muris* and *C. meleagridis* were identified (Muthusamy et al, 2006).

2.2 Life-cycle

Sporulated oocysts, containing 4 sporozoites, are excreted by the infected host through feces and possibly other routes such as respiratory secretions. Following ingestion (and possibly inhalation) by a suitable host, excystation occurs. The sporozoites are released and parasitize epithelial cells of the gastrointestinal tract or other tissues such as the respiratory tract.

Cell invasion by sporozoites is followed by intracellular development to trophozoite.

In these cells, trophozoites undergo asexual multiplication (schizogony or merogony) to form schizonts or meronts.

Asexual replication occurs by re-infection of merozoites, released by type I meronts. Development of type II from type I meronts is the initial step of the asexual reproductive cycle. Merozoites are released from type II meronts and re-infect neighbouring cells where they develop into producing microgamonts (male) and macrogamonts (female) by sexual multiplication (gametogony). Upon fertilization of the macrogamont by the microgamont zygote develop, which undergoes further development into an oocyst.

Two different types of oocysts are produced, the thick-walled, which is commonly excreted from the host, and the thin-walled oocyst, which is primarily involved in autoinfection. Oocysts are infective upon excretion, thus permitting direct and immediate fecal-oral transmission.

3. Epidemiology

3.1 Risk factors

The risk of infection increases in more profoundly immunosuppressed persons, as measured by the CD4 T-lymphocyte counts (Houpt et al, 2005).

The incidence and severity of cryptosporidiosis increases as the CD4 T-lymphocyte cell count falls, especially when it falls to below 200 cells/l (Navin et al, 1999; Pozio et al, 1997; Sorvillo et al, 1999; Sara et al, 2008).

Various social and behavioral factors also increase the risk of infection. For example, in a large multicenter European study, the risk of cryptosporidiosis was significantly lower for intravenous drug users than for homosexual men and for women than for men, suggesting that sexual behaviour may be an important risk factor (Pedersen et al, 1996).

3.2 Modes of transmission

Transmission of the parasite is facilitated by a relatively low infectious dose and by the resistance of the parasite oocyst stage to commonly used disinfection techniques e.g chlorination of dinking water.

The infection is spread in a number of ways: from person to person, from animals, via food, and by water. Cryptosporidiosis is now the most common cause of waterborne disease in the world (Xiao & al, 2004).

Because *Cryptosporidium* spp. infects humans and a wide variety of animals and because of the ubiquitous presence of *Cryptosporidium* oocysts in the environment, humans can acquire *Cryptosporidium* infections through several transmission routes (Clark, 1999; Griffiths, 1998). In pediatric and elderly populations, especially in day care centers and nursing homes, person-to-person transmission probably plays a major role in the spread of *Cryptosporidium* infections (Xiao L et al, 2004; Neill et al, 1996; Tangermann, 1991). In rural areas, zoonotic infections via direct contact with farm animals have been reported many times, but the relative importance of direct zoonotic transmission of cryptosporidiosis is not entirely clear (Miron et al, 1991).

Numerous outbreaks of cryptosporidiosis due to contaminated food or water (drinking or recreational) have been reported in several industrialized nations, and studies have sometimes identified water as a major route of *Cryptosporidium* transmission in areas where the disease is endemic (Xiao et al, 2004; MacKenzie et al, 1991; Weinstein et al, 1993).

Many outbreaks in the United States have occurred in waterparks, community swimming pools, and day care centers.

Large outbreaks due to the contamination of water supplies have been documented in recent years (Richardson et al, 1991; Tzipori & Giovanni, 2008) and in one particular outbreak, contamination of a water-treatment plant in Milwaukee (USA) was estimated to result in infections in 403 000 people (Mac Kenzie et al, 1994). This outbreak was associated with municipal drinking water despite state-of-the art water treatment.

The magnitude of these outbreaks highlighted the significance of drinking contaminated water as a major risk factor for contracting cryptosporidiosis in the USA (Tzipori & Giovanni, 2008).

The sources and human infective potentials of *Cryptosporidium* oocysts in water, however, are largely unclear.

One major problem in understanding the transmission of *Cryptosporidium* infection is the lack of morphologic features that clearly differentiate one *Cryptosporidium* spp from many others (Mac Kenzie et al, 1994). Hence, one cannot be sure which *Cryptosporidium* spp is involved when one examines oocysts in clinical specimens under a microscope. Another major problem is the inability to grow the organisms in large numbers from contaminated sources. Adding to the diagnosis problem and technical difficulties is the confusion in the taxonomy of *Cryptosporidium* spp., which is partially caused by the lack of consistency in the classification of protozoan parasites in general.

C. hominis is believed to be transmitted exclusively between humans, whereas *C. parvum* is transmitted between humans as well as through a zoonotic cycle usually involving ruminants. Although calves are often implicated as the reservoir of *C. parvum*, the importance of animals in transmission of *C. parvum* has been brought into question by studies that found that humans are infected with subtypes that perpetuate almost exclusively among humans (Siobhan & Tzipori, 2008).

The study of *Cryptosporidium* transmission dynamics is made more complex when atypical species are considered. Human infections with *C. meleagridis*, *C. muris*, *C. felis*, *C. canis*, *C. andersoni* and *C. suis*, though uncommon, have been reported (Mor MS & Tzipori, 2008; Xiao & Ryan, 2004).

The natural reservoirs of these species are believed to be poultry, rodents, cats, dogs, cattle, and pigs, respectively; however the broad host ranges are not well characterized. Host factors may also increase the likelihood of infection following exposure to these species, because they are more frequently identified in HIV-positive persons. Two recent studies in East Africa have attempted to correlate species diversity with area of residence. In Malawi, *C. meleagridis* and *C. andersoni* were detected only in children from a rural district, although 70% of *C. parvum* cases were identified in urban areas and *C. hominis* predominated in both settings (Mor & Tzipori, 2008; Mersha & Tiruneh, 1992). In Kenyan children, 4% of cases were due to *C. canis*, *C. felis*, *C. meleagridis* and *C. muris*, and there was no discernible difference by region (Gatei et al, 2006).

4. Clinical features

4.1 Gastrointestinal diseases

Cryptosporidium species infect the microvillus border of the gastrointestinal epithelium of a wide range of vertebrate hosts, including humans. Infected individuals show a wide spectrum of clinical presentations. The pathogenicity of *Cryptosporidium* varies with the species of parasites involved and the type, age and immune status of the hosts.

In immunocompetent subjects, cryptosporidiosis is characterized by watery or mucoid diarrhoea and abdominal pain with spontaneous recovery following several days or weeks of symptoms (Mersha & Tiruneh, 1992).

Immunocompetent hosts control and eliminate the infection, which typically causes acute, self-limited watery diarrhea lasting 5 to 10 days. However, in patients with defects in cellular immune responses (e.g. AIDS), *Cryptosporidium* spp frequently causes persistent or chronic diarrhea which can lead to death and can also involve the hepatobiliary and the respiratory tract. It is an opportunistic infection.

The risk of infection increases in more profoundly immunosuppressed persons, as measured by the CD4-T-lymphocyte counts (Houpt et al, 2005; Morpeth & Thielman, 2006).

Various presentations of cryptosporidiosis in HIV-positive patients were described (Blanshard et al, 1992; Mc Gowan et al, 1993; Manabe et al, 1998).

U.S. workers described four clinical syndromes: chronic diarrhea (affecting 36% of patients), cholera-like disease (33%), transient diarrhea (15%), and relapsing illness (15%) (Blanshard et al, 1992, Manabe et al, 1998). Infected patients had a significantly shorter duration of survival from the time of diagnosis than did *Cryptosporidium*-negative AIDS patients (240 and 666 days, respectively; $P = 0.0004$).

One aspect of chronic cryptosporidiosis in patients with AIDS is the large weight loss that many experience (Blanshard et al, 1992). One study from France reported that the severity of weight loss in such patients is independently associated with levels of nutrient intake ($P < 0.005$) and high stool frequency ($P < 0.01$) but not with nutrient malabsorption (Beaugerie et al, 1998).

As well as developing a more severe form of typical gastrointestinal disease, people with HIV infection can develop atypical disease presentations, affecting body systems not usually affected in immunocompetent individuals. Some of these unusual presentations are discussed below.

4.2 Atypical gastrointestinal disease

Many cases of gastritis were described. One particularly problematic complication of gastric involvement is antral narrowing and gastric outlet obstruction (Iribarren et al, 1997; Moon et al, 1999). Such gastric outlet obstruction can lead to nausea and vomiting and eventually may cause a severe reduction in nutrient intake.

A further unusual complication of cryptosporidiosis in AIDS patients is pneumatosis cystoides intestinalis (Samson & Brown, 1996; Sidhu et al, 1994). This disease is characterized by the presence of thin-walled, gas-containing cysts in the intestinal wall. Sometimes these cysts can rupture, resulting in a pneumoretroperitoneum and pneumomediastinum.

There is a case report of cryptosporidiosis affecting the oesophagus in a 2-year-old child and resulting in vomiting and dysphagia (Kazlow et al, 1986). Finally, there is also a case report of *Cryptosporidium* infection causing appendicitis (Oberhuber et al, 1991). The diagnosis was confirmed histologically after an appendectomy was performed.

4.3 Biliary tract disease

Cholangitis, and particularly sclerosing cholangitis, is an important complication of AIDS. Although not appearing to adversely affect survival, the disease can be a cause of significant pain (Forbes et al, 1993). In a Spanish study of 43 AIDS patients with chronic diarrhea due to *Cryptosporidium* infection, 8 patients (18.6%) were reported to have *Cryptosporidium* infection of the common bile duct (Lopez-Velez et al, 1995).

4.4 Pancreatitis

A series of 15 autopsies on patients with AIDS and cryptosporidiosis showed that five had evidence of infection of the pancreas (Godwin et al, 1991). Histological changes were generally mild and were limited to hyperplastic squamous metaplasia.

Three people with AIDS presented with acute or chronic pancreatitis related to cryptosporidiosis (Calzetti et al, 1997). All three patients had abdominal pain resistant to analgesics, increased serum amylase levels, and abnormalities at both sonography and computed tomography. Endoscopic retrograde cholangiopancreotography revealed papillary stenosis in all three patients. It is difficult to assess the impact of cryptosporidiosis-related pancreatic disease. Certainly, the first study does not suggest significant morbidity due to *Cryptosporidium* in the pancreas (Hunter & Nichols, 2002).

4.5 Respiratory tract disease

In a study from Spain, 7 of 43 patients (16.3%) with chronic diarrhea due to *Cryptosporidium* had *Cryptosporidium* oocysts detectable in the sputum (Lopez-Velez et al, 1995). Of these seven patients, five had respiratory symptoms and an abnormal chest radiograph; *Mycobacterium tuberculosis* was isolated in two of the five, and *M. avium* was isolated in another two. The remaining two patients had no respiratory symptoms and normal chest radiographs.

Other case series of patients with respiratory cryptosporidiosis were reported (Clavel et al, 1996; Hunter & Nichols, 2002). The majority of whom had another pathogen detected. So, the exact role of *Cryptosporidium* in the respiratory symptoms is not clear.

Dunand et al reported on 5 of their own cases and reviewed 14 other cases of parasitic sinusitis in HIV-positive patients from the literature (Dunand et al, 1997). Symptoms often included fever and chills in addition to local tenderness and discharge. Although the prognosis was frequently poor, this was due to other complications of HIV infection.

5. Diagnosis

For intestinal cryptosporidiosis, a parasitological examination of the stools is not only readily accessible and repeatable, but also non invasive for the patient. Oocysts are eliminated at intermittent intervals so stool tests should be repeated three times at three-day intervals (Weber et al, 1991; John & Petri, 2006).

Because of the small size of the *Cryptosporidium* oocysts, they are difficult to identify in fresh samples without specific coloration.

Oocysts may be examined under phase-contrast microscopy after concentration by different techniques. Oocysts may be concentrated by the modified zinc sulfate centrifugal flotation technique or by Sheather's sugar flotation.

Another concentration technique involves formalin-ethyl acetate sedimentation followed by layering and flotation over hypertonic sodium chloride solution to separate oocysts from stool debris (Weber et al, 1991). Oocysts appear as highly refractile spherical bodies (4 to 6 µm).

Several staining techniques can be used, applied to the swabs realized after concentration.

Modified Ziehl Neelsen stain is the best staining technique. The oocysts appear as rose spherical elements and contain four sporozoites (fig 1). The background is stained blue or green depending on the counter-stain used (Fast Green, malachite green or aniline blue) (Weber et al, 1991; Sunnotel et al, 2006).

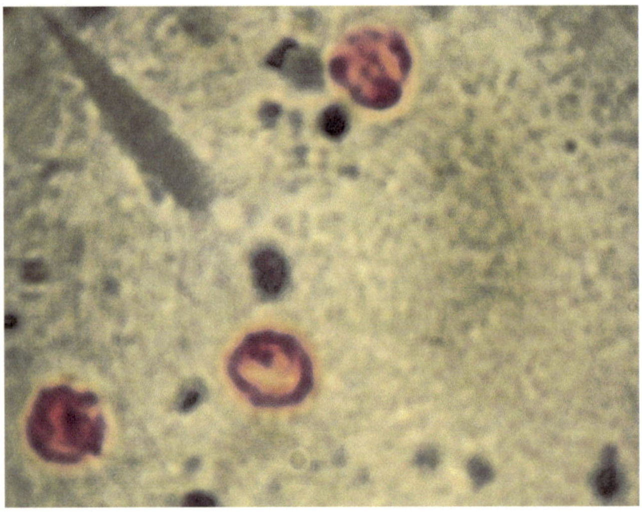

Fig. 1. Oocysts of *Cryptosporidium* sp stained by Modified Ziehl Neelsen stain

Cryptosporidium can also be detected by staining air-dried, methanol-fixed fecal smears with Giemsa's stain.

More recently, detection of oocysts is made by the use of copro-antigen detection kits, such as immunofluorescent antibody stains for microscopy, enzyme linked immunosorbent assays (ELISA) or immunochromatographic tests (Johnston et al, 2003).

Cryptosporidium oocysts also have been detected in fecal specimens by fluorescent stain like auramine-rhodamine.

The analytical sensitivity of these methods is generally in excess of 10^4 oocysts per gram faeces, depending on faecal consistency (Anusz et *al*, 1990; Weber et *al*, 1991), although immunofluorescence microscopy offers improved sensitivity (Arrowood, 1997).

Cryptosporidiosis can be diagnosed by identifying organisms (meronts containing merozoites and gamonts containing micro- and macrogametes) in intestinal biopsy material. Organisms stain lightly with hematoxylin and eosin and appear as small round bodies on the mucosal surface of biopsy specimens. With Masson's stain, a small red nucleus and blue cytoplasm can be distinguished in many of the organisms.

Species identification is an important element of outbreak investigations particularly where the source is not clear, and it is important that this is underpinned by routine species identification to establish the background epidemiology (Chalmers, 2008).

Even though oocysts of many *Cryptosporidium* spp are morphologically similar, morphometric measurement of oocysts can play a vital role in the differentiation of some *Cryptosporidium* spp. For example, the established species (interval) in birds and reptiles can easily be differentiated on the basis of the size and shape of oocysts. (Xiao et al, 2004).

However, laboratory techniques are unable to discriminate between the two main species involved in human disease, *C. hominis* and *C. parvum*. Species identification can be achieved with molecular methods which provide a precious tool for detecting *Cryptosporidium* and differentiating species in biological samples of infected patients (Chalmers, 2008).

However, *Cryptosporidium* presents two main problems for the isolation of DNA; the robust nature of the oocysts, requiring a disruption step prior to DNA extraction and the richness of PCR inhibitors in the sample matrix, requiring separation during DNA extraction.

Currently, there is no international consensus of typing methods and many rely on DNA sequence analysis which can be time-consuming and costly (Chalmers, 2008).

In 1991, Mark Laxer was the first to apply PCR to the detection of *Cryptosporidium* oocysts (Laxer et al, 1991).

Among molecular methods, PCR combined with restriction fragment length polymorphism (PCR-RFLP), which was first applied to *Cryptosporidium* typing by Awad-El-Kariem (Awad-El-Kariem et al, 1994) is the most used. PCR-RFLP assay detecting an RsaI polymorphism in the *Cryptosporidium* oocyst wall protein (COWP) gene (Spano et al, 1997), and a species-specific assay targeting the small-subunit rRNA gene (Xiao et al, 1999) are the most popular. Papers describing such assays or their application to *Cryptosporidium* typing are too numerous to cite here. Other methods such as random amplification methods (Morgan et al, 1995), sequencing (Lopez-Velez et al, 1995), length polymorphisms of repetitive sequences (Feng et al, 2000) and conformational polymorphism detection methods (Gasser et al, 2001) should also be mentioned in this context. However, the relatively high cost of molecular methods at present has limited their application in developed and developing countries.

The methodologies used in the detection of *Cryptosporidium*-specific antibodies vary widely, which complicates comparison of results. The use of the recombinant CP 41 antigen in a standardized serodiagnostic assay could provide a reliable and cost-effective method for assessing human exposure to *Cryptosporidium* in developing countries (Kjos et al, 2005).

6. Treatment

Despite the importance of cryptosporidiosis in mondial health, there has been any effective therapeutic specifically against *Cryptosporidium* infection, probably because of the unique intracellular extracytoplasmic location of *Cryptosporidium* and the poorly understood host-parasite interface. In addition, difficulties in laboratory propagation, including the absence of an ideal cell culture method, have limited high-throughput drug screening. Hundreds of drugs have been tested in the laboratory, and putative reports suggest that several,

including paromomycin, macrolides (e.g., azithromycin and spiramycin) and albendazole, are partially effective (Mor & Tzipori, 2008; Tzipori, 1998).
Clinical evaluations of these drugs have been disappointing, largely because they failed to clear the parasite from patients with HIV/AIDS.
To date, the broad-spectrum, anti-infective nitazoxanide (NTZ) has shown the most promise against *Cryptosporidium* (Mor & Tzipori, 2008).
It is used in many areas of the world because it appears to be well tolerated, it has a relatively low incidence of adverse effects, and it displays no significant known drug-to-drug interactions (Bobak, 2006). However, it is not effective against cryptosporidiosis in immunocompromised persons.
A meta-analysis of randomized, placebo-controlled trial of NTZ (of which there are only 2) among immunocompromised patients concluded that NTZ was no more effective than placebo in resolving diarrhea and achieving parasitological clearance in HIV-positive persons (Abubakar, 2007).
It has been speculated that HIV-positive persons may benefit from longer-duration regimens or higher doses of NTZ. However, a sustained clinical response was observed in only 59% of patients with HIV/AIDS who received off-label NTZ in a compassionate-use program (Rossignol, 2006).
This study indicate that the drug should be administered 500 mg b.d. until clinical symptoms resolve and oocysts are eliminated from the stool. Doses may be escalated to 1000 mg b.d. to accelerate or improve parasitological response. Fourteen days of treatment are generally sufficient in patients with CD4 counts above 50 cells/mm^3 while at least 8 weeks of treatment are likely required in patients with CD4 counts below 50 cells/mm^3.
Although refinement of the dosing regimen may improve clinical efficacy of NTZ, a prolonged therapeutic course will be impracticable in developing countries because of the expense and likely patient noncompliance.
ColoPlus is a product which may be an important alternative or additional treatment in HIV-associated diarrhoea. It is a product based on bovine colostrums witch is the first milk the suckling calf receives from the cow. It is rich in immunoglobulins, growth factors, antibacterial peptides and nutrients. It supplies the calf with a passive immunity before its own active immunity is established. As well as having a high nutritional value, it is designed for slow passage through the gastrointestinal tract.
Floren et al conducted a study on thirty patients with HIV-associated diarrhoea. The patients were treated with ColoPlus for 4 weeks in an open-labelled non-randomised study, after an observational period of one week. After a post-treatment period of another two weeks, treatment with anti-HIV drugs was started, if deemed appropriate. The effects on the frequency of stool evacuations per day, on body-weight, fatigue, haemoglobin, levels and CD4 + counts before and after treatment with ColoPlus were measured. There was a dramatic decrease in stool evacuations per day, a substantial decrease in body-weight and an increase in CD4 count by 125 % (Floren et al, 2006).
In part because of the failure of other therapeutic approaches, there have been several attempts at passive antibody-based immunotherapy for cryptosporidial infections (Crabb, 1998). These have also had limited success.
One therapeutic intervention that has a dramatic effect on cryptosporidiosis in AIDS patients is antiretroviral therapy leading to recovery of the CD4 count. (Foudraine, 1998; Maggi et al, 2000; Miao et al, 2000; Morpeth & Thielman, 2006). The authors noted that resolution of the diarrhea seemed to be related to an increased CD4 - cell count rather than

to the viral load. These findings give further support to the observation that it is cellular immunity that is of paramount importance in clearing *Cryptosporidium* infection.

7. Prophylaxis

Because of the risk of acquiring a life-threatening disease, people with AIDS should take the following specific measures to help reduce the risk of waternborne cryptosporidiosis: boil drinking water for 1 minute, or filter drinking water with devices that remove particles 1 μm and larger, or use bottled drinking water, especially water obtained from underground sources (eg. springs or wells), which are less likely to be contamined by *Cryptosporidium* oocysts. However, the boiling of water is the most certain method of killing *Cryptosporidium* oocysts. They should take additional precautions, including avoiding contact with young pets, and avoiding swallowing water while swimming (John & Petri, 2006).

The realization that *Cryptosporidium* oocysts are resistant to many chemical disinfectants (Tzipori & Giovanni, 2008; Rochelle et al, 2005) led to a search for methods that can inactivate oocysts without generating harmful by products. Much attention has focused on UV irradiation and ozone as alternative methods capable of inactivating waterborne oocysts (Tzipori & Giovanni, 2008; Lloyd & Drury, 2002). However, control of surface-water contamination is being emphasized as a first measure to reduce the occurrence of waterborne oocysts. Regulations aimed at reducing the risk of exposure to waterborne oocysts have been put in place; for example, the Long Term 2 Enhanced Surface Water Treatment Rule in the USA and regulations in the UK requiring continuous monitoring for *Cryptosporidium* oocysts in drinking water. A treatment-based standard of one oocyst in 10 l has been adopted (Sidhu et al, 1994).

8. Conclusion

We would conclude that research over the last three decades has dramatically increased our knowledge on cryptosporidiosis, but key questions still remain unclear.

With the new interest in *Cryptosporidium* generated by the emergence of the latter as the cause of human disease, much research is ongoing and will provide continuing information concerning cryptosporidiosis in the future.

Future developments need to include harmonisation of rapid and more cost effective methods.

Effective therapies are likely to become available in the near future. Access to endogenous forms and immortalization of strains in culture or by cryopreservation remain major challenges, which will require new ideas and new approaches.

Identification of *Cryptosporidium* isolates to species level and of subtyping is indispensable for appropriate control measures during outbreaks.

9. References

Abubakar, I., Aliyu, SH, Arumugam, C, Usman, NK & Hunter, PR. (2007). Treatment of cryptosporidiosis in immunocompromised individuals: systematic review and meta-analysis. *Br J Clin Pharmacol*, Vol.63, No.4, (April 2007), pp. 387-393.

Alvarez-Pellitero, P. & Sitja-Bobadilla, A. (2002). *Cryptosporidium molnari* n. sp. (Apicomplexa: Cryptosporidiidae) infecting two marine fish species, *Sparus aurata* L. and *Dicentrarchus labrax*. *Int J Parasitol*, Vol.32, No.8, (July 2002), pp. 1007-21.

Awad-el-Kariem, FM., Warhurst, DC & McDonald, V. (1994).Detection and species identification of *Cryptosporidium* oocysts using a system based on PCR and endonuclease restriction. *Parasitology*, Vol.109, No.1, (July 1994), pp. 19-22.

Barker, IK. & Carbonell, PL. (1974). *Cryptosporidium agni* sp.n. from lambs, and *Cryptosporidium bovis* sp.n. from a calf, with observations on the oocyst. *Z Parasitenkd*, Vol.44, No.4, (1974), pp. 289-98

Beaugerie, L., Carbonnel, F, Carrat, F, Rached, AA, Maslo, C, Gendre, JP, Rozenbaum, W & Cosnes, J.(1998). Factors of weight loss in patients with HIV and chronic diarrhea. *J Acquired Immune Defic Syndr*, Vol.19, No.1, (September 1998); pp. 34-9.

Bern, C., Hernandez, B, Lopez, MB, Arrowood, MJ, De Merida, AM. & Klein, R. E. (2000). The contrasting epidemiology of *Cyclospora* and *Cryptosporidium* among outpatients in Guatemala. *Am J trop Med Hyg*, Vol.63, No.(5-6), (Nov-Dec 2000), pp.231-5.

Bhattacharya, MK., Teka, T, Faruque, AS. & Fuchs, GJ.(1997). *Cryptosporidium* infection in children in urban Bangladesh. *J Trop Pediatr*, Vol.43, No.5, (October 1997), pp. 282-6.

Blanshard, C., Jackson, AM, Shanson, DC, Francis, N. & B. G. Gazzard.(1992). Cryptosporidiosis in HIV-seropositive patients. *Q J Med*, Vol.85, No. (307-308), (Nov-Dec 1992), pp. 813-23.

Bobak, DA.(2006). Use of nitazoxanide for gastrointestinal tract infections: treatment of protozoan parasitic infection and beyond. *Curr Infect Dis Rep*, Vol.8, No.2, (March 2006), pp. 91-5.

Calzetti, C., Magnani, G, Confalonieri, D, Capelli, A, Moneta, S, Scognamiglio, P. & Fiaccadori, F.(1997). Pancreatite da *Cryptosporidium parvum* in pazienti con grave deficit immunitario correlato ad infezione da HIV. *Ann Ital Med Int*, Vol.12, No.2, (Apr-Jun 1997), pp. 63-6.

Chalmers RM. (2008). *Cryptosporidium*: from laboratory diagnosis to surveillance and outbreaks. *Parasite*, Vol.15, No. 3, (September 2008), pp. 372-8.

Chen, X-M., Keithly, JS, Paya, CV. & LaRusso, NF. (2002). Cryptosporidiosis. *N Engl J Med*, Vol.346, No.22, (May, 2002), pp. 1723-31.

Clark, DP. (1999). New insights into human cryptosporidiosis. *Clin Microbiol Rev*, Vol.12, No.4, (October 1999), pp. 554-63.

Clavel, A., Arnal, AC, Sanchez, EC, Cuesta, J, Letona, S, Amiguet, JA, Castillo, FJ, Varea, M. & Gomez-Lus, R.(1996). Respiratory cryptosporidiosis: case series and review of the literature. *Infection*, Vol.24, No.5, (Sep-Oct 1996), pp. 341-6.

Crabb, JH. (1998). Antibody-based immunotherapy of cryptosporidiosis. *Adv. Parasitol*, Vol.40, (1998), pp. 121-49.

Dann, SM., Wang, H-C, Robinson, P, Castellanos-Gonzalez, A, Lewis, DE & Clinton White, A. (2008). Intestinal Immune Response to Human *Cryptosporidium* sp. infection *Infection and immunity*, Vol.76, No.1, (January 2008), pp. 23-9.

Dunand, VA., Hammer, SM, Rossi, R, Poulin, M, Albrecht, MA, Doweiko, JP, DeGirolami, PC, Coakley, E, Piessens, E. & Wanke, CA.(1997). Parasitic sinusitis and otitis in patients infected with human immunodeficiency virus: report of five cases and review. *Clin Infect Dis*, Vol.25, No.2, (August 1997), pp. 267-72.

Fayer, R., Trout, JM, Xiao, L, Morgan, UM, Lai, AA. & Dubey, JP. (2001). *Cryptosporidium canis* n. sp. from domestic dogs. *J Parasitol*, Vol.87, No.6, (December 2001), pp. 1415-22.

Feng, X., Rich , SM, Akiyosh, D, Tumwine, JK, Kekitiinwa, A, Nabukeera, N, Tzipori, S & Widmer, G.(2000). Extensive polymorphism in *Cryptosporidium parvum* identified by multilocus microsatellite analysis. *Appl Environ Microbiol*, Vol.66, No.8, (August 2000), pp. 3344-9.

Floren, CH., Chinenye, S, Elfstrand, L, Hagman, C & Ihse, I. (2006); ColoPlus, a new product based on bovine colostrum, alleviates HIV-associated diarrhoea. *Scand J Gatsroenterol*, Vol.41, No.6, (June 2006), pp. 682-6.

Forbes, A., Blanshard, C & Gazzard, B. (1993). Natural history of AIDS related sclerosing cholangitis: a study of 20 cases. *Gut*, Vol.34, No.1, (January 1993), pp. 116-21.

Foudraine, NA., Weverling, GJ, van Gool, T, Roos, MT, de Wolf, F, Koopmans, PP, van den Broek, PJ, Meenhorst, PL, Leeuwen, Rvan, Lange JM & Reiss, P.(1998). Improvement of chronic diarrhoea in patients with advanced HIV-1 infection during potent antiretroviral therapy. *AIDS*, Vol.12, No.1, (January 1998), pp. 35-41

Gasser, RB., Zhu, X, Caccio, S, Chalmers, R, Widmer, G, Morgan, UM, Thompson, RC, Pozio, E & Browning, GF.(2001).Genotyping *Cryptosporidium parvum* by single-strand conformation polymorphism analysis of ribosomal and heat shock gene regions. *Electrophoresis*, Vol.22, No.3, (February 2001), pp. 433-7.

Gatei, W., Wamae, CN, Mbae, C, Waruru, A, Mulinge, E, Waithera, T, Gatika, SM, Kamwati, SK, Revathi, G & Hart, CA. (2006). Cryptosporidiosis: prevalence, genotype analysis, and symptoms associated with infections in children in Kenya. *Am J Trop Med Hyg*, Vol.75, No.1, (July 2006), pp. 78-82.

Godwin, TA. (1991). Cryptosporidiosis in the acquired immunodeficiency syndrome: a study of 15 autopsy cases. *Hum Pathol*, Vol.22, No.12, (December 1991), pp. 1215-24.

Griffiths, JK.(1998). Human cryptosporidiosis: epidemiology, transmission, clinical disease, treatment, and diagnosis. *Adv Parasitol*, Vol.40, (1998), pp. 37–85.

Houpt, ER., Bushen, OY, Sam, NE, Kohli, A, Asgharpour, A, Ng, CT, Calfee, DP, Guerrant, RL, Maro, V, Ole-Nguyaine, S & Shao, JF.(2005).Short report: asymptomatic *Cryptosporidium hominis* infection among human immunodeficiency virus–infected patients in Tanzania. *Am J Trop Med Hyg*, Vol.73, No.3, (September 2005), pp. 520-2.

Hunter, PR., Nichols G.(2002). Epidemiology and clinical features of *Cryptosporidium* infection in immunocompromised patients. *Clin Microbiol Rev*, Vol.15, No.1, (January 2002), pp. 145-54.

Iribarren, JA., Castiella, A, Lobo, C, Lopez, P, Wichmann, M A von, Arrizabalaga, JF, Rodriguez-Arrondo, J. & Alzate, LF.(1997). AIDS associated cryptosporidiosis with antral narrowing. A new case. *J Clin Gastroenterol*, Vol.25, No.4, (December 1997), pp. 693-4.

John, DT Petri WA. (2006). Lumen-Dwelling Protozoa. In Medical Parasitology, Saunders Elsevier, pp.(68-71).

Johnston, sp., Ballar, MM, Beach, MJ, Causer, L. & Wilkins, PP. (2003). Evaluation of three commercial assays for fecal speciments. *J Clin Microbiol*, Vol.41, No.2, (February 2003), pp. 623-6.

Kazlow, PG., Shah, K, Benkov, KJ, Dische, R. & LeLeiko, NS. (1986). Esophageal cryptosporidiosis in a child with acquired immune deficiency syndrome. *Gastroenterology*, Vol.91, No.5, (November 1986), pp. 1301-3.

Kjos, SA., Jenkins, M, Okhuysen, PC. & Chappell, CL. (2005). Evaluation of recombinant oocyst protein CP 41 for detection of *Cryptosporidium*-specific antibodies. *Clin Diag Lab Immunol*, Vol.12, No.2, (February 2005), pp. 268-72.

Laxer, MA., Timblin, BK & Patel, RJ. (1991). DNA sequences for the specific detection of *Cryptosporidium parvum* by the polymerase chain reaction. *Am J Trop Med Hyg*, Vol.45, No.6, (December 1991), pp. 688-94.

Levine, ND.(1984). Taxonomy and review of the coccidian genus *Cryptosporidium* (protozoa, apicomplexa). *J Protozool*, Vol. 31, No.1, (February 1984), pp.94-98.

Lindsay, DS., Upton, SJ, Owens, DS, Morgan, UM, Mead, JR. & Blagburn, BL.(2000). *Cryptosporidium andersoni* n. sp. (Apicomplexa: *Cryptosporiidae*) from cattle, Bos taurus. *J Eukaryot Microbiol*, Vol. 47, No.1, (Jan-Feb 2000), pp. 91-5.

Lloyd, A & Drury, D.(2002). Continuous monitoring for *Cryptosporidium*–a novel approach to public health protection. *Water Sci Technol*, Vol.46, No. (11-12), (2002), pp. 297-301.

Lopez-Velez, R., Tarazona, R, Garcia Camacho, A, Gomez-Mampaso, E, Guerrero, A, Moreira, V & Villanueva, R.(1995). Intestinal and extraintestinal cryptosporidiosis in AIDS patients. *Eur J Clin Microbiol Infect Dis*, Vol.14, No.8, (August 1995), pp. 677-81.

Ma, P. & Soave, R. (1983). Three-step stool examination for cryptosporidiosis in 10 homosexual men with protracted watery diarrhea. *J Infect Dis*, Vol.147, No.5, (1983) pp.824-8.

Ma P. (1984). *Cryptosporidium* and the enteropathy of immune deficiency. *J Pediatr Gastroenterol Nutr*, Vol.3, No.4, (September 1984), pp. 488-90.

Mac Kenzie., WR, Hoxie, NJ, Proctor, ME, Gradus, MS, Blair, KA, Peterson, DE, Kazmierczak, JJ, Addiss, DG, Fox, KR, Rose, JB. & al.(1994). A massive outbreak in Milwaukee of *Cryptosporidium* infection transmitted through the public water supply. *N Engl J Med;* Vol.331, No.3, (July 1994), pp. 161-7.

MacKenzie, WR., Hoxie, NJ, Proctor, ME, Gradus, MS, Blair, KA, Peterson, DE, Kazmierczak, J J, Addiss, DG, Fox, K R, Rose, JB & al.(1994). A massive outbreak in Milwaukee of *Cryptosporidium* infection transmitted through the public water supply. *N Engl J Med*, Vol.331, No.3, (July 1994), pp. 161-7.

Maggi, P., Larocca, AM, Quarto, M, Serio, G, Brandonisio, O, Angarano, G & Pastore, G. (2000). Effect of antiretroviral therapy on cryptosporidiosis and microsporidiosis in patients infected with human immunodeficiency virus type 1. *Eur J Clin Microbiol Infect Dis*, Vol.19, No.3, (March 2000), pp. 213-7.

Manabe, YC., Clark, DP, Moore, R D, Lumadue, JA, Dahlman, H R. Belitsos, PC, Chaisson RE. & Sears. C. L. (1998). Cryptosporidiosis in patients with AIDS: correlates of disease and survival. *Clin Infect Dis*, Vol.27, No.3, (September 1998), pp. 536-42.

Mc Gowan, I., Hawkins, AS & Weller, IV.(1993).The natural history of cryptosporidial diarrhoea in HIV-infected patients. *AIDS*, Vol.7, No.3, (March 1993), pp. 349-54.

Meisel, JL., Perera, DR, Meligro, C & Rubin, CE.(1976). Overwhelming watery diarrhoea associated with a *Cryptosporidium* in an immunosuppressed patient. *Gastroenterology*, Vol.70, No.6, (June 1976), pp. 1156-60.

Mersha, D & Tiruneh, M.(1992). Frequency of isolation of *Cryptosporidium* oocysts in Ethiopian children with acute diarrhoeal disease. *East Afr Med J*, Vol.69, No.6, (June 1992), pp. 314-5.

Miao, YM., Awad-El-Kariem, FM, Franzen, C, Ellis, DS, Muller, A, Counihan, HM, Hayes, PJ. & Gazzard, BG.(2000). Eradication of *Cryptosporidia* and *Microsporidia* following successful antiretroviral therapy. *J Acquired Immune Defic Syndr*, Vol.25, No.2, (October 2000), pp. 124-9.

Miron, D., Kenes, J & Dagan, R.(1991). Calves as a source of an outbreak of cryptosporidiosis among young children in an agricultural closed community. *Pediatr Infect Dis J*, Vol.10, No.6, (June 1991), pp. 438-41.

Moon, A., Spivak, W. & Brandt,L. J.(1999).*Cryptosporidium*-induced gastric obstruction in a child with congenital HIV infection: case report and review of the literature. *J Pediatr Gastroenterol Nutr*, Vol.28, No.1, (January 1999), pp. 108-11.

Mor, MS., & Tzipori, S. (2008). Cryptosporidiosis in Children in Sub-Saharan Africa: A Lingering. *Clin Infect Dis*, Vol.47, No.7, (October 2008), pp. 15-21.

Morgan, UM, Constantine, CC, O'Donoghue, P, Meloni, BP, O'Brien, PA & Thompson ,RC.(1995). Molecular characterization of *Cryptosporidium* isolates from humans and other animals using random amplified polymorphic DNA analysis. *Am J Trop Med Hyg*, Vol.52, No.6, (June 1995), pp. 559-64.

Morgan-Ryan, UM., Fall, A, Ward, LA, Hijjawi, N, Sulaiman, I, Fayer, R, Thompson, RC, Olson, M, Lal,A. & Xiao, L.(2002). *Cryptosporidium hominis* n. sp. (Apicomplexa: Cryptosporidiidae) from Homo sapiens. *J Eukaryot Microbiol*, Vol.49, No.6, (November 2002), pp. 433-40.

Morpeth, SC, Thielman, NM. (2006).Diarrhea in patients with AIDS. *Curr Treat Options Gastroenterol*, Vol.9, No.1, (February 2006), pp. 23-37.

Muthusamy,D, Rao, SS, Ramani, S, Monica, B, Banerjee, I, Abraham, OC, Mathai, DC, Primrose, B, Muliyil, J, Wanke, CA, Ward, HD & Kang, G.(2006). Multilocus genotyping of *Cryptosporidium* sp. Isolates from human immunodeficiency virus-infected individuals in south india. *J Clin Microbiol*, Vol.44, No.2, (February 2006), pp. 632-4.

Navin, TR., Weber, R, Vugia, DJ, Rimland, DJ, Roberts, M, Addiss, DG, Visvesvara, GS, Wahlquist, SP, Hogan, SE, Gallagher, L E, Juranek, DD, Schwartz, DA, Wilcox, CM, Wilcox, JM, Stewart, SE, Thompson, r & Bryan, RT.(1999). Declining CD4 T-lymphocyte count is associated with increased risk of enteric parasitosis and chronic diarrhea: results of a 3-year longitudinal study. *J Acquir Immune Defic Synd*, Vol.20, No.2, (February 1999), pp. 154-9.

Neill, MA., Rice, SK, Ahmad, NV & Flanigan, T. P.(1996). Cryptosporidiosis: an unrecognized cause of diarrhea in elderly hospitalized patients. *Clin Infect Dis*, Vol.22, No.1, (January 1996), pp. 168-70.

Newman, RD., Sears, CL, Moore, SR, Nataro, JP, Wuhib, TD, Agnew, A, Guerrant R L. & Lima, AAM. (1999). Longitudinal study of *Cryptosporidium* infection in children in northeastern Brazil. *J Infect Dis*, Vol.180, No.1, (July 1999), pp. 167-75

Nime, FA., Burek, JD, Page, DL, Holscher, MA. & Yardley, JH.(1976). Acute enterocolitis in a human being infected with the protozoan *Cryptosporidium. Gastroenterology*, Vol.70, No.4, (April 1976), pp. 592-8.

Nina, JM, McDonald, V, Deer, RM, Wright, SE, Dyson, DA, Chiodini, PL & McAdam, KP. 1992. Comparative study of the antigenic composition of oocyst isolates of *Cryptosporidium parvum* from different hosts. *Parasite Immunol*, Vol.14, No.2, (March 1992), pp. 227-32.

Oberhuber, G., Lauer, E, Stolte, M & Borchard, F.(1991). Cryptosporidiosis of the appendix vermiformis: a case report. *Z Gastroenterol*, Vol.29, No.11, (November 1991), pp. 606-8.

Ogunkolade, BW, Robinson, HA, McDonald, V, Webster, K & Evans, DA.(1993). Isoenzyme variation within the genus *Cryptosporidium. Parasitol Res*, Vol.79, No.5, (1993), pp. 385-8.

Ortega, YR., Sheehy, RR, Cama, VA, Oishi KK & Sterling CR. (1991). Restriction fragment length polymorphism analysis of *Cryptosporidium parvum* isolates of bovine and human origin. *J Protozool*, Vol.38, No.6, (Nov-Dec 1991), pp.(40S-41S).

Pedersen, C., Danner, S, Lazzarin, A, Glauser, M. P, Weber, R, Katlama, C, Barton, S. E & Lundgren, J. D.(1996). Epidemiology of cryptosporidiosis among European AIDS patients. *Genitourin Med*, Vol. 72, No.2, (April 1996) pp.128–131.

Pozio, E., Rezza, G, Boschini, A, Pezzotti, P, Tamburrini, A, Rossi, P, Di Fine, M, Smacchia, C, Schiesari, A, Gattei, E, Zucconi, R. & Ballarini, P. (1997). Clinical cryptosporidiosis and human immunodeficiency virus (HIV)-induced immunosuppression: findings from a longitudinal study of HIV-positive and HIV-negative former injection drug users. *J Infec Dis*, Vol.176, No.4, (October 1997), pp.969-75.

Richardson, AJ., Frankenberg, RA, Buck, AC, Selkon, JB, Colbourne, JS, Parsons, JW & Mayon-White, RT.(1991).An outbreak of waterborne cryptosporidiosis in Swindon and Oxfordshire. *Epidemiol Infect*, Vol.107, No.3, (December 1991), pp. (485-95).

Rochelle, PA., Upton, SJ, Montelone, BA & Woods, K.(2005). The response of *Cryptosporidium parvum* to UV light. *Trends Parasitol*, Vol.21, No.2, (February 2005), pp.81-7.

Rossignol, JF.(2006). Nitazoxanide in the treatment of acquired immune deficiency syndrome-related cryptosporidiosis: results of the United States compassionate use program in 365 patients. *Aliment Pharmacol Ther*, Vol.24, No.5, (September 2006), pp.887-94.

Samson, VE. & Brown, W. R. (1996). Pneumatosis cystoides intestinalis in AIDS-associated cryptosporidiosis. More than an incidental finding? *J Clin Gastroenterol*, Vol.22, No.4, (June 1996), pp.311-2.

Tzipori, S & Widmer, G.(2008).A hundred-year retrospective on cryptosporidiosis.*Trends Parasitol*, Vol.24, No.4, (April 2008), pp.184-9.

Sidhu, S., Flamm, S & Chopra, S. (1994). Pneumatosis cystoides intestinalis: an incidental finding in a patient with AIDS and cryptosporidial diarrhea. *Am. J. Gastroenterol*, Vol.89, No.9, (September 1994), pp. 578-9.

Sorvillo, F., Beall, G, Turner, PA, Beer, VL, Kovacs, AA, Kraus, P, Masters, D. & Kerndt, PR.(1998). Seasonality and factors associated with cryptosporidiosis among individuals with HIV infection. *Epidemiol Infect*, Vol.21, No.1, (August 1998), pp.197-204.

Spano, F., Putignani, L, Crisanti, A, Sallicandro, P, Morgan, UM, Le Blancq, SM, Tchack, L, Tzipori, S & Widmer, G.(1998). Multilocus genotypic analysis of *Cryptosporidium parvum* isolates from different hosts and geographical origins. *J Clin Microbiol*, Vol.36, No.11, (November 1998), pp.3255-9.

Spano, F., Putignani, L, McLauchlin, J, Casemore, DP & Crisanti, A.(1997). PCR-RFLP analysis of the *Cryptosporidium* oocyst wall protein (COWP) gene discriminates between *C. wrairi* and *C. parvum*, and between *C. parvum* isolates of human and animal origin. *FEMS Microbiol Lett*, Vol.150, No.2, (May 1997), pp.209-17.

Strong, WB., Gut, J & Nelson, RG.(2000). Cloning and sequence analysis of a highly polymorphic *Cryptosporidium parvum* gene encoding a 60-kilodalton glycoprotein and characterization of its 15- and 45-kilodalton zoite surface antigen products. *Infect Immun*, Vol.68, No.7, (July 2000), pp. 4117-34.

Sunnotel, O., Lowery, CJ, Moore, JE, Dooley, JS, Xiao, L, Millar, BC, Rooney, PJ & Snelling, WJ. (2006). *Cryptosporidium*. *Lett Appll Microbiol*, Vol.43, No.1, (July 2006), pp. 7-16.

Tangermann, RH., Gordon, S, Wiesner, P & Kreckman L.(1991). An outbreak of cryptosporidiosis in a day-care center in Georgia. *Am J Epidemiol*, Vol.133, No.5, (March 1991), pp. 471-6.

Tyzzer, E.E.(1907). A sporozoon found in the peptic glands of the common mouse. *Proc Soc Exp Biol Med*, Vol.5, (1907), pp.12–13.

Tyzzer, E.(1910). An extracelluar coccidium, *Cryptosporidium muris* (gen. & sp. nov.), of the gastric glands of the common mouse. *J Med Res*, Vol.18, (1910), pp.487–509.

Tyzzer, E. (1912). *Cryptosporidium parvum* (sp. nov.), a coccidium found in the small intestine of the common mouse. *Arch Protisenkd*, Vol.26, (1912), pp.394–412.

Tzipori, S. (1998). Cryptosporidiosis: laboratory investigations and chemotherapy. *Adv. Parasitol*, Vol.40, (1998), pp.187–221.

Weber, R., Bryuan, RT, Bishop, HS, Walquist, SP, Sullivan, JJ, & Juranek, D,D. (1991). Threshold of detection of *Cryptosporidium* oocysts in human stool specimens: evidence for low sensitivity of current methods. *Journal of Clinical Microbiology*, Vol.29, No.7, (July 1991), pp.1323-7.

Weinstein, P., Macaitis, M, Walker, C & Cameron, S. (1993). Cryptosporidial diarrhoea in South Australia. An exploratory case-control study of risk factors for transmission. *Med J Aust*, Vol.158, No.2, (January 1993), pp.117-9.

Xiao, L., Escalante, L, Yang, C, Sulaiman, I, Escalante, AA, Montali, RJ, Fayer, R & Lal, AA.(1999). Phylogenetic analysis of *Cryptosporidium* parasites based on the small-subunit Rrna gene locus. *Appl Environ Microbiol*, Vol.65, No.4, (April 1999), pp.1578-83.

Xiao, L., Fayer, R, Ryan, U & Steve, J. (2004). *Cryptosporidium* Taxonomy: Recent Advances and Implications for Public Health. *Clinical Microbial Reviews*, Vol.17, No.1, (January 2004), pp.72-97.

Xiao, L. & Ryan, UM.(2004). Cryptosporidiosis: an update in molecular epidemiology. *Curr Opin Infect Dis*, Vol.17, No.5, (October 2004), pp.483-90.

Xiao, L. (2010). Molecular epidemiology of cryptosporidiosis: An update. *Experimental Parasitology*, Vol.124, No.1, (January 2010), pp.80-9.

15

Toxoplasmosis in HIV/AIDS Patients - A Living Legacy

Veeranoot Nissapatorn
University of Malaya
Malaysia

1. Introduction

The coccidian *Toxoplasma gondii* (*T. gondii*) is a ubiquitous, intracellular, protozoan parasite that causes toxoplasmosis, a cosmopolitan zoonotic disease. *Toxoplasma* infections are reported in approximately half of the world's population but most are asymptomatic. *T. gondii* may serve as one factor that can enhance the immunodeficiency found after HIV-1 infections. Co-infection with other pathogens in humans infected with HIV-1 may enhance the progression of the disease to AIDS (Lin & Bowman, 1992). In concurrence with HIV infection, cerebral toxoplasmosis (CT) occurs primarily due to reactivation of latent *Toxoplasma* infection and is one of the most frequent opportunistic infections, particularly in patients with full-blown AIDS. CT is the most common clinical presentation of toxoplasmosis (Luft & Remington, 1992), and is one of the most frequent causes of focal intracerebral lesions that complicates AIDS (Nissapatorn et al, 2004). CT is undoubtedly a serious life-threatening disease but it is treatable when there is a timely diagnosis and prompt treatment, and there are no other concurrent co-infections. When HIV-infected patients develop CT this poses many diagnostic and therapeutic challenges for clinicians (Israelski & Remington, 1992), particularly in developing countries where the infrastructure is limited but the number of patients infected with HIV is increasing. This chapter focuses on the clinico-epidemiological aspects of toxoplasmosis in HIV/AIDS patients at the time of transition to treatment with highly active anti-retroviral therapy (HAART). The course of toxoplasmosis in HIV/AIDS patients should be able to provide us with a better understanding of the clinical scenario and future management of this so-called "enigmatic parasite" of the tropics.

2. Pathogenesis - from source to host defense mechanism

2.1 Morphology

T. gondii is a coccidian, that is ubiquitous and an obligate intracellular parasite with a complex life cycle and felids are the definitive hosts. There are three infectious stages of *T. gondii* in the environment. Tachyzoites (or endozoites), crescent to oval in shape, are seen in an active infection. They can be transmitted through the placenta from mother to fetus, by blood transfusion, or by organ transplantation. Tissue cysts, containing thousands of bradyzoites, the terminal life cycle stage, are transmitted by eating infected meat or organs, and may persist life-long in an intermediate host. In this stage, they are associated with latent infections, but reactivation occurs in persons who lose their immunity. Bradyzoites (or cystozoites) are less susceptible to chemotherapy and the presence of this infective stage in host tissues is of clinical significance, particularly in immunosuppressed individuals. The oocyst stage, is excreted in the cat's feces, and this most tolerant form of *T. gondii*, is ubiquitous in nature, is highly resistant to disinfectants and environmental influences, as well as playing a key role in transmission through the fecal-oral route.

2.1.1 Life cycle and transmission

The life cycle of *T. gondii* was described in 1970, before it was determined that members of the family Felidae, including domestic cats, were the definitive hosts and warm-blooded animals including most livestock and humans serve as intermediate hosts (Figure 1). In contrast to other protozoans, *T. gondii* is a parasite that can parasitize all mammals. *T. gondii* has a large host range; this parasite can be found throughout the world. *T. gondii* is a common infection in humans; it becomes more important in the field of veterinary and medical infectious diseases. *T. gondii* is a potential organism causing a serious public health hazard due to infected meat-producing animals and a severe economic loss to the livestock owners. *T. gondii* can be transmitted (Figure 2) through one of the following routes (Tenter et al, 2000; Derouin et al, 2008).

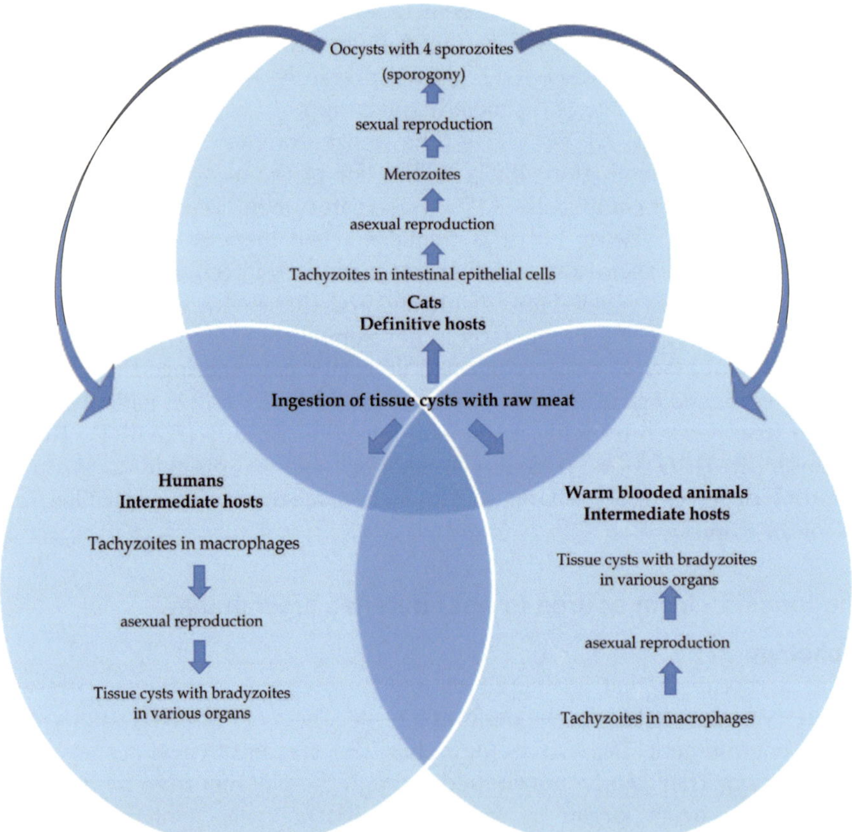

Fig. 1. The life cycle of *T. gondii*.

In the definitive hosts, infection with *T. gondii* occurs following not only ingestion of tissue cysts in under-cooked meat but also after ingesting the rapidly-multiplying tachyzoite forms or the oocysts shed in feces. The cyst wall of *T. gondii* is dissolved by the proteolytic enzymes of both stomach and small intestine, releasing the slowly-multiplying bradyzoite form. The asexual cycle begins after the invasion of *T. gondii* into the epithelial cells of the small intestine. While, the sexual cycle is very specific and occurs only in the gut epithelial cells of feline species. The oocyst forms are produced by gamete fusion and are then shed in the feces of the definitive hosts. These oocysts are highly infective to other definitive and intermediate hosts once they are in contact with a susceptible environment (Frenkel, 1973). The oocysts of *T. gondii* are less infective and pathogenic in the definitive host (cat) as compared with intermediate hosts (mice, pigs, humans) (Dubey, 1998).

In intermediate hosts, *T. gondii* undergoes two phases of asexual development. The infective stages (sporozoites or bradyzoites) transform into tachyzoites following *Toxoplasma* infection of the intestinal epithelial cells. In the first phase, tachyzoites multiply rapidly by repeated endodyogeny in an intracellular parasitophorous vacuole in many different types of host cells. The second phase develops from the tachyzoites of the last generation and results in tissue cysts (Tenter et al, 2000). Within the tissue cyst, bradyzoites multiply slowly by endodyogeny. Tissue cysts have a high affinity for neural and muscular tissues and are located mainly in the central nervous system (CNS), eye, skeletal and cardiac muscles as well as other visceral organs (Dubey et al, 1998). Tissue cysts break down periodically, with bradyzoites transforming into tachyzoites that reinvade host cells and again transform to bradyzoites within new tissue cysts (Dubey, 1998).

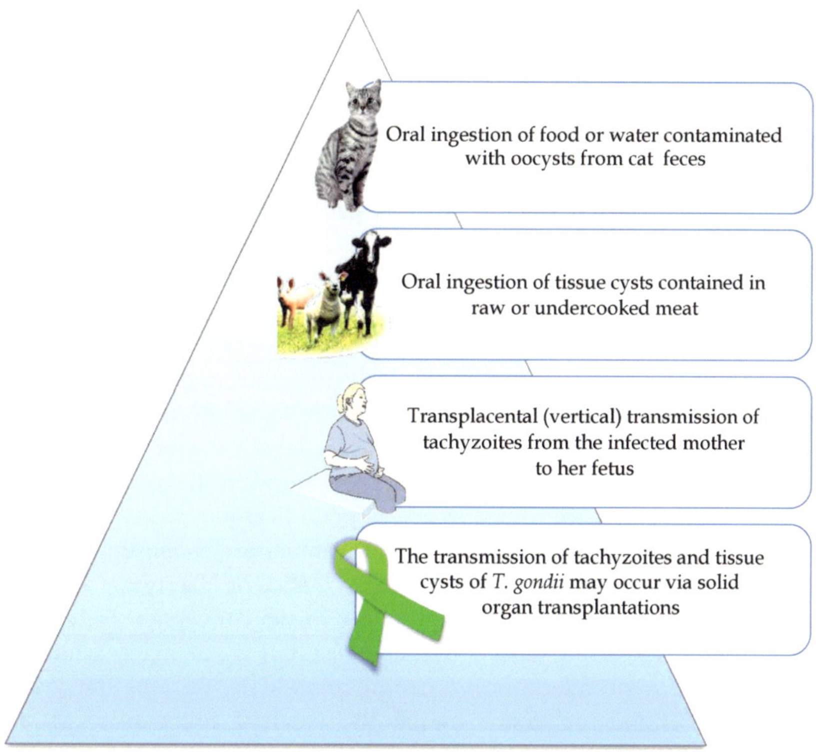

Fig. 2. The different routes of *T. gondii* transmission.

2.1.2 *T. gondii* antigens, host defense mechanisms and cerebral toxoplasmosis

In patients with AIDS, tissue cysts rupture and the released bradyzoites may multiply locally and spread to other organs. Infected patients may have serious complications or even death from symptomatic toxoplasmosis. The pathology of *Toxoplasma* infection is due to the invasion process initiating the lytic cycle that consequently leads to cell and tissue destruction. In the host cell cytoplasm, *T. gondii* induces the formation of a parasitophorous vacuole that contains secretions of both parasite and host proteins that normally promote phagosome maturation, , and thereby prevent lysosome fusion (Dubey et al, 1998; Carruthers, 2002). Despite this rapid, dynamic and significant process, there are very few secretory proteins that have so far been discovered (Zhou et al, 2005). These proteins (antigens) are essential components for low-grade stimulation that boosts the immune system. These antigens have been shown to stimulate antibody production as well as a T-cell response (Carruthers, 2002).

T. gondii excretory/secretory antigens (ESAs) represent the majority of the circulating antigens in host sera of patients with acute toxoplasmosis (Pereira-Chioccola et al, 2009). ESAs include the tachyzoite, sporozoite and encysted bradyzoite stages (Tilley et al, 1997). The secretions by the bradyzoite cysts maintain a long-lasting immunity to *T. gondii* (Cesbron-Delauw & Capron, 1993). The ESAs released by tachyzoites are highly immunogenic (Prigione et al, 2000; Carruthers, 2002) and may induce either antibody dependent or cell mediated immunity (Costa-Silva et al, 2008). Anti-ESA antibodies develop in high titers when circulating blood tachyzoites are present in AIDS-associated CT patients (Meira et al, 2008). *Toxoplasma* infection results in pathological changes such as inflammation and is usually followed by necrosis. This parasitic infection also induces strong type 1 polarized innate and adaptive immune responses. It is known that the host defense mechanism to infection with *T. gondii* is mediated by production of pro-inflammatory cytokines, including IL-12, IFN-γ and TNF-α (Suzuki et al, 1989). The important sources of IFN-γ in response to *Toxoplasma* infection are CD4-T lymphocytes, CD8-T lymphocytes, natural killer cells and T cells responding to IL-12 (Yap et al, 2000). These major mechanisms prevent rapid replication of tachyzoites and subsequent pathological changes (Denkers, 2003). Of these, T lymphocytes are a crucial source of IFN-γ during the first 2-3 weeks after infection, as demonstrated in antibody-mediated T-cell depletion experiments that resulted in reactivation of *Toxoplasma* infection (Denkers, 2003). In the chronic phase, the tissue cysts can persist indefinitely in the brain and muscle, developing lifelong protective immunity against re-infection (Dubey, 1998; Montoya & Liesenfeld, 2004). There are re-infections in some cases because slightly different genotypes of *T. gondii* strains have been found in the same patients (Ferreira et al, 2008). In the clinical phase, tissue cysts are periodically ruptured, but the bradyzoites released are normally destroyed by the host immune response. At the time when asymptomatic individuals become immune deficient, secondary reactivation of latent/chronic infection may occur, culminating in the conversion of bradyzoites to the active and rapidly replicating tachyzoites, as a result of tissue injury which is often fatal. As the cysts have a predilection for neural, muscle tissue and the eye, most cases reactivate chorioretinitis or, more frequently, cerebral toxoplasmosis, which is the predominant manifestation in patients with AIDS. Apart from these mechanisms, the development of cerebral toxoplasmosis has recently been studied and shown to have a significant correlation with the HLA genes (class I and class II) in HIV-infected patients. The MHC is one of the most polymorphic genetic systems in humans and controls the adaptive immune response by class I (HLA-A, HLA-B, HLA-Cw) and class II (HLA-DRB1, HLA-DQB1, HLA-DPB1) against both intra-and extracellular microorganisms as well as it being correlated with infection susceptibility or resistance. Class I HLA-B35 antigen was associated with retinochoroiditis (Veronese Rodrigues et al, 2004). Class I HLA-B8 and class II HLA-DRB1*17 antigens were associated with cerebral toxoplasmosis (Castro Figueiredo et al, 2000). The presence of class II HLA-DQB1*0402 and DRB1*08 alleles (Habegger de Sorrentino et al, 2005) and the HLA-DR52 haplotype represent risk factors to the development of cerebral toxoplasmosis, whereas the HLA-DR53 haplotype was associated with resistance to *Toxoplasma* infection (Pereira-Chioccola et al, 2009).

Among patients with AIDS, CT is a multifocal process that occurs spontaneously. The use of the highly sensitive technique of magnetic resonance imaging (MRI) reveals that >80% of patients will have multiple lesions (Ciricillo & Rosenblum, 1990). With this technique, the percentages are probably an underestimation of the multifocal pathological process that may be occurring as they will be below its resolution. The spontaneous and simultaneous development of multifocal brain lesions strongly indicates that although CT arises because of reactivation of a latent infection, the multiple areas of the brain that are involved are likely a result of the hematogenous spread of the parasite, and involvement of the brain is due to the particular proclivity of *T. gondii* for causing disease in the CNS (Luft & Remington, 1992). The latter is likely due to the fact that the brain is an immunologically original site rather than an actual site of the organism. This supposition is further supported by the observation that patients who relapse after receiving an adequate course of therapy often develop new lesions in areas of the brain previously free of infection (Leport et al, 1989).

3. Epidemiology - from source to gene

The high rates of latent *Toxoplasma* infection (41.9–72%) were reported in South America and in approximately half of the studies (≥ 40%) from the Asian continent. In North America, however, the rate of *Toxoplasma* infection was low. Surprisingly, only 8 of the 50 studies were conducted on HIV-infected pregnant women and 2 of those studies, interestingly, reported a very high seroprevalence of toxoplasmosis of 53.7% in Thailand and 72% in Brazil. Latent toxoplasmosis is still prevalent as an infection that coexists with HIV infection. The level of anti-*Toxoplasma* (IgG) antibodies was, interestingly, unaffected by either antiretroviral drugs or therapeutic regimes/prophylaxis used for toxoplasmosis in these patients (Machala et al, 2009). Supporting these epidemiological studies, screening for *Toxoplasma* infection should be included in routine investigations in order to monitor primary infections even though it is not very common in such patients. It may also prevent secondary reactivation of latent infections, especially in HIV-infected patients with limited resource settings where the majority are unable to access primary chemoprophylaxis and/or antiretroviral therapy.

How do the plausible risk factors play their roles in association with *Toxoplasma* infection in HIV-infected patients? Age and race/ethnicity, among other demographic characteristics, were shown to have a positive interaction with this parasite. A study from the United States demonstrated that *Toxoplasma* prevalence rates reported in HIV-infected women aged ≥ 50 years were significantly higher compared to those who were younger (Falusi et al, 2002). This was dissimilar to a study from Malaysia which reported that HIV-infected patients in the younger age group had higher *Toxoplasma* seroprevalence rates than the older age group although it was not statistically significant (Nissapatorn et al, 2001). Based on these findings, *Toxoplasma* infection is acquired irrespective of age, and preventive measures are needed to curb the prevalence rate especially in areas where the parasite is highly endemic. The study by Falusi and colleagues in 2001 further pointed out that those women born outside the U.S. were more likely to have higher rates of latent toxoplasmosis although race did not affect *Toxoplasma* seroprevalence between black and white women in that country (Falusi et al, 2002). In a country like Malaysia, a higher rate of *Toxoplasma* infection was more likely to be found among Malays, the predominant ethnic group in this region compared to others including Chinese and Indian (Nissapatorn et al, 2007). Traditionally, Malays keep cats as pets, which could explain this association. Based on these studies, demographic characteristics certainly make significant contributions to the epidemiological surveillance of *Toxoplasma* infection in a given population, such as HIV/AIDS patients.

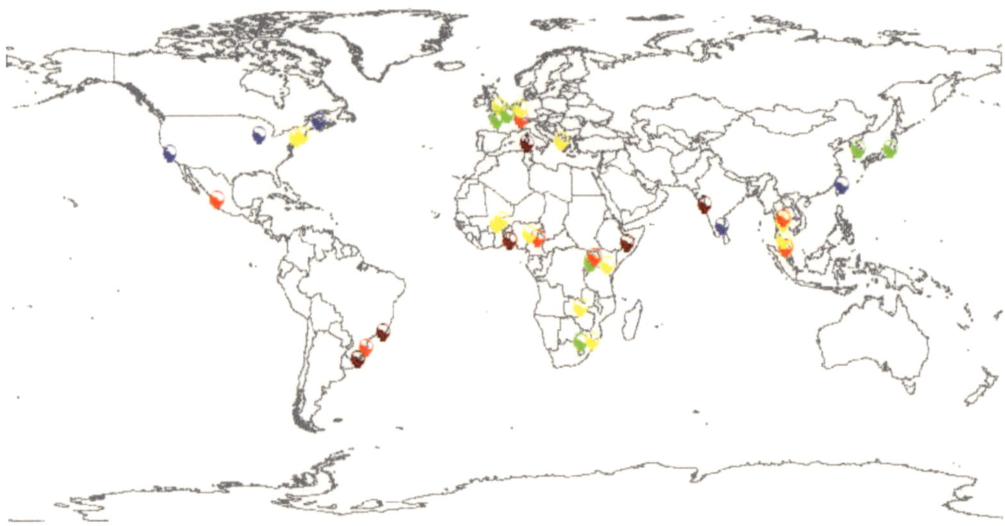

Fig. 3. Global status of latent *Toxoplasma* infection in HIV-infected patients.

Dark red equals prevalence above 60%, light red equals 40-60%, yellow 20-40%, blue 10-20% and green equals prevalence <10%. White equals absence of data. (Courtesy of Dr. Rattanasinchaiboon O and Dr Phumkokrux S, Bangkok, Thailand.)

There are not many studies on how the T-cell response could affect *Toxoplasma*-seropositive patients. It has been recognized that T-helper (CD4) cells, among several types of T-cell responses, are involved in *Toxoplasma* infection by stimulating T-cytotoxic cells which are then able to lyse tachyzoites directly and participate in the activation of B-cells which then go on to produce antibodies against *Toxoplasma* (Ho-Yen, 1992.). An earlier study showed that there is a greater likelihood of problems with *Toxoplasma* infection in situations in which there is a reduction of T-cell function (Pendry et al, 1990). Supporting this literature, a U.S.

study demonstrated a significant association between CD4 counts of 200-499 cells/mm^3 and *Toxoplasma*-seropositivity in patients (Falusi et al, 2002). The authors were unable to provide an explanation for this association except that patients with low CD4 counts were more likely to be foreign born. So far, similar findings have not been reported from previous studies (Nissapatorn et al, 2001; Nissapatorn et al, 2002). Looking at other possible risk factors such as a history of close contact with cats, consumption of contaminated meat, and receiving blood transfusions from *Toxoplasma*-seropositive patients, there was however no significant association found from studies reported earlier (Wallace et al, 1993; Nissapatorn et al, 2001; Nissapatorn et al, 2002). This possibly explains that these patients had been constantly exposed to *Toxoplasma* infections (with no definite time frame) before acquiring HIV infection. The other reason is that patients acquired *Toxoplasma* infection from other sources such as eating raw vegetables or drinking contaminated water, risk factors that were not included in these studies. However, primary behavioral practice such as avoiding close contact with cats, consumption of clean and properly cooked foods is necessary and advisable for HIV-infected patients regardless of *Toxoplasma* serostatus. Interestingly, patients with *Toxoplasma*-seropositivity were more likely to develop CT and tended to be patients receiving HAART (Nissapatorn et al, 2007). From this observation, primary chemoprophylaxis or antiretroviral drugs including HAART (if available) should be instituted to these patients after clinical evaluation.

Apart from the host immune status, the genotype of the infecting parasites may influence the course of disease (Lindström et al, 2006). Genetic analyses have shown that the vast majority of all *T. gondii*-strains typed to date fall into one of three clonal lineages, type I, II, and III (Howe & Sibley, 1995), which differ in virulence but do not show clear host or geographic boundaries (Lindström et al, 2006). Studies from different parts of the world have produced similar findings in which the genotyping of the SAG2-locus revealed that the type II allele was the most disease-causing strain (reactivation of chronic infections) found in immunocompromised individuals (Dardé et al, 1992; Howe and Sibley, 1995; Howe et al, 1997; Fuentes et al, 2001; Lindström et al, 2006; Ajzenberg et al, 2009).

This high prevalence of type II strains in human toxoplasmosis may simply reflect the source of the strains that led to human infections (Howe et al, 1997). Also, the low level of gamma interferon and other factors related to the immune system in these patients might increase the possibility of reactivation of the infective forms of the parasite by developing bradyzoites and increasing the formation of cysts in the brain (Gross et al, 1997). During this same period, a few studies have reported on uncommon type I strains (Khan et al, 2005), type I/III (Genot et al, 2007), and a high rate of genetic polymorphism (Ferreira et al, 2008) in *T. gondii* strains isolated from immunocompromised patients. Despite these differences, genotyping studies could serve as an important mile-stone for improving the diagnosis and management of human toxoplasmosis, in addition, for the development of novel drugs and vaccines. Surprisingly, genotyping studies on *T. gondii* strains have not been reported from HIV-infected patients in the Asian continent even though there are a number of these patients, in endemic areas for latent *Toxoplasma* infections (Subsai et al, 2006; Nissapatorn et al, 2007), and cases of clinical toxoplasmosis detected in AIDS patients (Subsai et al, 2006; Lian et al, 2007). Future studies are recommended to elucidate the distribution of genotypes and to establish any correlations between genotyping of *T. gondii* strains and human toxoplasmosis in Asian HIV patients.

Based on these findings, it certainly poses a question as to whether there is an association between genotyping of *T. gondii* strains and human toxoplasmosis. One study interestingly indicates that the type of infecting parasitic strain does not predominantly influence the pathogenesis of toxoplasmosis in immunocompromised patients and fully support the need for specific prophylaxis in patients infected by *T. gondii*, regardless of the strain genotype (Honoré et al, 2000). In addition, other host factors are more involved than parasite factors in patients' resistance or susceptibility to toxoplasmosis in immunocompromised hosts (Ajzenberg et al, 2009).

A total of 50 studies have been reported from different parts of the world including Asia, Europe, North America, South America and Africa (Table 1). The varying seroprevalence of toxoplasmosis (latent/chronic infection) interestingly showed low to high rates of infection being >60% (9 studies), 40-60%, (12 studies), 20-40% (21 studies), 10-20% (3 studies), and <10% (5 studies).

Study (Ref)	City, Country	No. of HIV/AIDS patients	Seroprevalence in %
Asia			
Wongkamchai et al, 1995	Bangkok, Thailand	40	42.5
Meisheri et al, 1997	Bombay, India	89	67.8
Yoong and Cheong, 1997	Kuala Lumpur, Malaysia	49	59.0
Chintana et al, 1998	Bangkok, Thailand	253 (pregnancy)	21.1
Sukthana et al, 2000	Bangkok, Thailand	190	23.2
Oh et al, 1999	Seoul, South Korea	173	4.0
Nissapatorn et al, 2001	Bangkok, Thailand	183	22.4
Shivaprakash et al, 2001	Pondicherry, India	216	11.5 (IgM)
Wanachiwanawin et al, 2001	Bangkok, Thailand	838 (pregnancy)	53.7
Shamilah et al, 2001	Kuala Lumpur, Malaysia	729	31.3
Nissapatorn et al, 2002	Kuala Lumpur, Malaysia	100	21.0
Nissapatorn et al, 2003	Kuala Lumpur, Malaysia	406	51.2
Nissapatorn et al, 2004	Kuala Lumpur, Malaysia	505	44.8
Hung et al, 2005	Taipei, Taiwan	844	10.2
Nissapatorn et al, 2005	Kuala Lumpur, Malaysia	162	35.8 and 14.8 (IgM)
Naito et al, 2007	Tokyo, Japan	56	5.40
Nissapatorn et al, 2007	Kuala Lumpur, Malaysia	693	43.85
Nissapatorn et al, [In print]	Songkhla, Thailand	300	36.3
Europe			
Holliman, 1990	London, UK	500	26.6 and 1.4 (IgM)
Sykora et al, 1992	Prague, Czechoslovakia	67	29.8

Study (Ref)	City, Country	No. of HIV/AIDS patients	Seroprevalence in %
Zufferey et al, 1993	Lausanne, Switzerland	715	50.0
Oksenhendler et al, 1994	Villejuif, France	499	25.4
Raffi et al, 1997	Nantes cedex, France	186	97
Bossi et al, 1998	Paris, France	399	97
Letillois et al, 1995	Grenoble, France	37	64.9
Reiter-Owona et al, 1998	Bon, Germany	183	33.3 (in 1987) and 36.6 (in 1995)
Millogo et al, 2000	Burkina Faso, France	1,828	25.4
Machala et al, 2009	Prague, Czech Republic	626	33.2
North America			
Grant et al, 1990	New York, USA	411	32.0
Israelski et al, 1993	California, USA	1,073	11.0
Minkoff et al, 1997	Brooklyn, USA	138	20.2
Ruiz et al, 1997	Rhode Island, USA	169 (pregnancy)	22.0
Falusi et al, 2002	Chicago, USA	1,975	15.1
South America			
Wainstein et al, 1993	RS, Brazil	516	65 and 49 (CSF)
Galván Ramirez et al, 1997	Universidad de Guadalajara, Mexico	92	50.0 and 1.0 (IgM)
Cruz et al, 2007	RJ, Brazil	767 (pregnancy)	74.0
Lago et al, 2009	Rio Grande do Sul, Brazil	168 (pregnancy)	72.0
Africa			
Brindle et al, 1991	Kenya, Nairobi	94	22
Zumla et al, 1991	Zambia and Uganda	373 (186-Uganda and 187-Zambia)	34 (Ugandan) and 4 (Zambian)
Woldemichael et al, 1998	Addis Ababa, Ethiopia	127	74.2
Maïga et al, 2001	Bamako, Mali	?	22.6 and 60
Uneke et al, 2005	Jos, Nigeria	219	38.8
Lindström et al, 2006	Kampala, Uganda	130	54
Hari et al, 2007	Johannesburg, South Africa	307	8
Ouermi et al, 2009	Burkina faso, agadougou	138 (pregnancy)	31.9 and 3.6 (IgM)
Akanmu et al, 2010	Lagos, Nigeria	380	54
Sitoe et al, 2010	Maputo, Mozambique	58 (pregnancy)	31.3
Oshinaike et al, 2010	Lagos, Idi Araba, Nigeria	83	85.5

Table 1. Summary of studies on seroprevalence of toxoplasmosis in HIV-infected patients.

4. Toxoplasmosis - from epidemiology to clinical implication

4.1 Congenital toxoplasmosis

Seven of the 50 studies were conducted on HIV-infected pregnant women, 2 reported a high seroprevalence, 53.7% in Thailand (Wanachiwanawin et al, 2001) and 74% in Brazil (Cruz et al, 2007). Considering these epidemiological studies (Table 1), geographical location, environment, socio-economic, clinical and diagnostic methods are among the factors that can pin point the differences of *Toxoplasma* infections between these affected areas. Latent toxoplasmosis is still prevalent and coexists with HIV infections. The level of anti-*Toxoplasma* (IgG) antibodies does not appear to be affected by antiretroviral drugs or therapeutic regimes/prophylaxis used to treat toxoplasmosis in these patients (Machala et al, 2009). Given the results of these epidemiological studies, screening for *Toxoplasma* serostatus should be carried out among HIV-infected women in the prenatal period even though it is not a common practice. It may also prevent secondary reactivation of latent toxoplasmosis during pregnancy, especially among HIV-infected women in limited resource settings where the majority of these patients are unable to access primary chemoprophylaxis and/or antiretroviral therapy.

In HIV-infected pregnant women, a secondary reactivation of chronic *Toxoplasma* infection may occur during pregnancy particularly in those who are severely immunocompromised. There are cases of cerebral toxoplasmosis reported in HIV-infected pregnant women and congenital toxoplasmosis in the fetus of these infected mothers but it is found only at a low incidence (Dunn et al, 1997). A case of CT was earlier reported in an HIV-infected pregnant woman who responded well with a standard regimen of pyrimethamine and sulfadiazine, with a normal fetal outcome (Hedriana et al, 1993). Another case of CT was confirmed in an HIV-infected pregnant woman during the puerperium with her CD4 count being < 200 cells/cumm (Biedermann et al, 1995). A prophylactic treatment was recommended to prevent maternal reactivation and congenital transmission of toxoplasmosis in such a case. In recent years, an HIV-infected pregnant woman with CT who was at risk for transmitting HIV (low CD4 and high viral load) and *Toxoplasma* infections to her fetus; she responded well to anti-*Toxoplasma* therapy and HAART (Nogueira et al, 2002). In this case, the combined *Toxoplasma* therapy (pyrimethamine and sulfadiazine) and HAART were benefitial not only to the mother but also prevented transmission to the fetus. Despite this evidence of success in most cases, there have been reports of poor outcomes when an HIV-infected mother has CT during pregnancy, with vertical transmission of one or both infections to the fetus and an increase of morbidity and mortality in the mother (Mitchell et al, 1990; O'Riordan & Farkas, 1998; Fernandes et al, 2009). Maternal-fetal transmission of toxoplasmosis due to reactivation of chronic infection during pregnancy occurs in mothers with a very low CD4 cell counts (Minkoff et al, 1997) or in the presence of other immunological disorders (Montoya & Liesenfeld, 2004). A case of severe congenital toxoplasmosis was reported from an HIV-infected mother with moderate immunosuppression as a result of reactivation (Bachmeyer et al, 2006). This indicates that a routine screening for not only children from HIV-infected mothers should be used to detect congenital toxoplasmosis but also in pregnant women to confirm an early diagnosis of a reactivation of a chronic *Toxoplasma* infection. The first case of congenital toxoplasmosis was reported in Brazil, this was from an HIV-infected mother with a high titer of IgG but negative for IgM antibodies (Cruz et al, 2007). This highlights the special attention needed for analysis of maternal titers of anti-*Toxoplasma* antibody during HIV prenatal care. Two years later, a contrasting study reported a case of congenital toxoplasmosis in an HIV-infected pregnant woman with a low titer of IgG to *T. gondii* and a negative result for IgM antibodies (Lago et al, 2009). It is important to keep this in mind that a high titer for IgG antibody is fairly common in HIV-infected mothers. This phenomenon is not significantly associated with an increased risk of congenitally acquired toxoplasmosis during pregnancy. Compliance to antiretroviral therapy is a medical challenge which led to a rare case of congenital toxoplasmosis from a severely immunosuppressed HIV-infected woman as a result of reactivation (Fernandes et al, 2009). Under this circumstance, prophylaxis is required in addition for strict adherence to therapy in pregnant women infected with HIV. The most recent cases of congenital toxoplasmosis were reported from HIV-infected mothers who had a high titer for IgG and were negative for IgM antibodies (Azevedo et al, 2010). Due to the increasing number of HIV- infected women in childbearing age worldwide, the possibility of maternal-fetal transmission from mothers infected with chronic *Toxoplasma* infection is more likely to occur and may have a huge impact on public health perspectives, especially in those endemic areas with *Toxoplasma* infection. It is surprising that there has been no reported case of clinically confirmed congenital toxoplasmosis or CT in HIV-infected pregnant women from Asian countries. In fact, HIV infection is fast growing in this region compared to other parts of the world. This could be explained either because of the overall low prevalence of toxoplasmosis in HIV-infected women or those cases of toxoplasmosis are under-reporting. Therefore, clinicians should be more aware of this parasitic infection to establish an early diagnosis and better management in both qualities of care and treatment among HIV-infected pregnant women in this continent. To conclude, HIV and *Toxoplasma* infections are common in developing countries with resource limited settings, it is therefore imperative that drugs related to both infections are easily accessible particularly for pregnant women living in low-socio-economic conditions. Due to the effectiveness of anti-*Toxoplasma* therapy and increasing global availability of HAART in HIV-infected pregnant women, the incidence of congenital toxoplasmosis should decline or even disappear.

4.2 Cerebral toxoplasmosis

Neurological complications of AIDS patients are often due to opportunistic infections (OIs) in the central nervous system (CNS). Toxoplasmosis is one of the most common CNS-OIs and causes high rates of morbidity and mortality in patients with advanced HIV infection. With the advent of the HIV pandemic, epidemiological studies have shown CT to be one of the most common OIs in AIDS patients and the most commonly reported CNS-OIs on 5 continents: Asia (India, Malaysia and Thailand), Europe (France, United Kingdom and Germany), North America (USA), South America (Brazil and Mexico), and recently from South Africa (Amogne et al, 2006; Oshinaike et al, 2010). The incidence of CT varies according to geographical locations and the prevalence of *Toxoplasma* infections in the general population. Other factors such as the mode of transmission, gender, ethnicity, severe immunodeficiency, and differences in genotypes of *T. gondii* isolates are also found to influence the occurrence of CT (Richards et al, 1995; Khan et al, 2005). In the pre-HAART era, ~25% of AIDS patients from France had CT compared to ~10% in some cities from the USA (Dal Pan & McArthur, 1996). The rate of CT was found to vary from between 16-40%

in the USA and UK, ~60% in Spain, 50-80% in Brazil, 75-90% in France (Pereira-Chioccola et al, 2009), and <20% in Asian countries including India (Sharma et al, 2004), Malaysia (Nissapatorn et al, 2003-2007), or Thailand (Anekthananon et al, 2004; Subsai et al, 2004). CT is frequently diagnosed in adults but rarely occurs in children with AIDS; the infection accounted for 0.86% of AIDS-defining illnesses (Richards et al, 1995) or <1.0 per 100 person years (Dankner et al, 2001; Gupta et al, 2009). CT is the most common cause of focal intracerebral lesion(s) in patients with AIDS. More than 95% of CT is caused by the reactivation of latent (chronic) *Toxoplasma* infection as a result of the progressive loss of cellular immunity in AIDS patients (Luft & Remington, 1988). In clinical practice, the incidence of CT patients is related both to *Toxoplasma* IgG seropositivity and the CD4 cell count. The risk of developing CT among seropositive patients with AIDS was 27 times that of seronegative ones (Oksenhendler et al, 1994). AIDS patients who are *Toxoplasma* seropositive, have CD4 count of <100 cells/cumm, and failure to receive prophylaxis are among the identified risk of developing CT (Luft and Remington, 1992; Nascimento et al, 2001; Nissapatorn et al, 2004). The clinical presentations of CT depend on the number of lesions and location. Headache, hemiparesis and seizure (Nissapatorn et al, 2004; Vidal et al, 2005a) are among the most common neurological presentations found in CT patients. Other clinical manifestations include disarthria, movement disorders, memory and cognitive impairments and neuropsychiatric abnormalities. These neurological deficits remain in surviving patients even after good clinical response to therapy (Hoffmann et al, 2007). More than 50% of CT patients may have focal neurological findings. CT is a life-threatening but treatable condition provided there is early diagnosis and treatment. CT can be prevented by primary behavioral practices in avoiding acquisition of *Toxoplasma* infection such as consumption of well cooked meat, avoiding close contact with stray cats, contaminated soil and/or water, and receiving unscreened blood transfusions. Compliance to both therapeutic regimens for treatment and prophylaxis of toxoplasmosis is an imperative to prevent relapse of CT in areas where HAART is not fully accessible for people living with HIV/AIDS. This ultimately reduces the number of hospital admissions as well as the mounting medical care cost of AIDS-associated CT patients, particularly in limited resource settings.

There are atypical/unusual clinical manifestations reported in AIDS-associated CT patients. Ventriculitis and obstructive hydrocephalus, characteristics of congenital toxoplasmosis, are rarely seen in adult AIDS-associated CT. Ventriculitis has so far been reported in nine adult AIDS patients (Cota et al, 2008), accompanied by hydrocephalus, occurred as the primary manifestations of toxoplasmosis or as complications of a preexisting, recognized cerebral toxoplasmosis. In addition, hydrocephalus without mass lesions was the only abnormal finding from a computed tomography (CAT) scan in an adult AIDS patient (Nolla-Salas et al, 1987). It is very rare for patients with CT to present as a neuropsychiatric illness with an acute psychosis followed by a rapid mental and somatic decline, however one case has been reported in a patient with AIDS (Ilniczky et al, 2006). Extrapyramidal movement disorders are one of the atypical clinical manifestations reported in AIDS patients. Toxoplasmosis is one of the main underlying opportunistic infections and causes movement disorders in AIDS patients. These movement disorders are becoming well known and increasingly recognized as a potential neurological complication in AIDS patients (Tse et al, 2004). In hyperkinetic movements, holmes (also known as rubral or midbrain tremor) tremor is the earliest reported symptom of CT and might present with other focal neurological signs that indicates a midbrain localization (Koppel & Daws, 1980). The appearance of hemichorea-hemiballism is considered as a pathognomonic of CT and is most commonly associated with a subthalamic abscess (Navia et al, 1986; Maggi et al, 1996). The presence of hemichorea-hemiballism in CT patients is low (7.4% of cases) compared to the pathological studies which show 50% of *Toxoplasma* abscesses occur in the basal ganglia (Navia et al, 1986; Maggi et al, 1996). Generalized chorea may occur as a result of bilateral abscesses of toxoplasmosis (Gallo et al, 1996). Myoclonus, is generalized and elicited by sudden auditory stimuli that resembles a startled response, has also been described in AIDS-associated CT patients (Maher et al, 1997). A case of focal dystonia of the left arm and hand has been reported in an AIDS patient due to the right lenticular nucleus and thalamic abscesses of toxoplasmosis (Tolge & Factor, 1991). A few cases with parkinsonian features, hypokinetic movement disorders, due to toxoplasmosis were also described in patients with AIDS (Carrazana et al, 1989; Murakami et al, 2000). Movement disorders in AIDS patients and particularly in countries with a high prevalence of toxoplasmosis, should indicate the possibility of CT (Noël et al, 1992). In AIDS patients, opportunistic infections may affect endocrine organs. Diabetes insipidus (DI) is uncommon but has also been reported in relation to CT. Imaging studies may demonstrate pathological situations and assist in the diagnosis (Brändle et al, 1995). A case of CT with massive intracerebral hemorrhage leading to a fatal vehicular crash was also reported in a patient with AIDS (Gyori & Hyma, 1998). Cerebellar toxoplasmosis is another infrequent complication of HIV/AIDS that should prompt a high index of clinical suspicion and early institution for presumptive therapy in poor resource settings (Emeka et al, 2010). These unusual neurological presentations of AIDS patients associated toxoplasmosis have rarely been reported in Asia (Chaddha et al, 1999; Nissapatorn et al, 2004; Subsai et al, 2006; Nissapatorn et al, 2007).

4.3 Extracerebral toxoplasmosis

Overall, the prevalence of extracerebral toxoplasmosis (ECT) in patients with AIDS is estimated to be 1.5%-2% (Rabaud et al, 1994) which is far less common than CNS toxoplasmosis. Ocular toxoplasmosis (OT) is the most common form of ECT associated with CT, being detected in 50% of ECT in AIDS patients and has the best prognosis (Rabaud et al, 1994; Zajdenweber et al, 2005). OT, in contrast to intracranial disease, is uncommon in patients with AIDS (Lamichhane et al, 2010). However, OT is a serious eye problem in HIV-infected patients, especially in developing countries (Chakraborty, 1999). OT is an important disorder and may be the first manifestation of life-threatening intracranial or disseminated *T. gondii* infections. Accurate diagnosis may allow early referral to a neurologist and infectious diseases specialist (Holland et al, 1988). Generally, OT tends to cause retinochoroidal scars with less retinal pigment epithelium hyperplasia (Arevalo et al, 1997). It has no association between the ocular findings and a positive titer of toxoplasmosis (Mansour, 1990.). However, the presence of IgM antibodies may support this diagnosis, although antibody levels in AIDS patients may not reflect the magnitude of the disease (Gagliuso et al, 1990). OT was first reported in 2 of 34 AIDS patients with a 'cotton wool' spot as one of the most common retinal manifestations (Schuman & Friedman, 1983). It is also characterized by several features, including single or multifocal retinal lesions in one or both eyes or massive areas of retinal necrosis. These lesions that are not associated with a pre-existing retinochoroidal scar indicate a manifestation of acquired rather than congenital disease (Gagliuso et al, 1990). A unique pattern of bilateral retinitis due to OT was observed in a patient in the late stages of AIDS in which the recognition of this pattern is important for providing the appropriate treatment of an immunosuppressed patient (Berger et al, 1993). Toxoplasmosis should therefore be considered in the differential diagnosis in an AIDS patient with necrotizing retinitis (Moorthy et al, 1993). There have been few studies reported on toxoplasmosis as being one of the most common causes of neuro-ophthalmological disorders in neurologically symptomatic HIV-infected patients such as palsy involving the sixth and third cranial nerves (Mwanza et al, 2004). Thus, clinicians should be more aware of this pathogen to avoid consequences, such as damaging visual pathways leading to visual impairment or blindness in these patients. With more affordable and accessibility of HAART, the prevalence of ocular toxoplasmosis will decline over time.

Toxoplasmosis is known to cause widely disseminated and extracerebral disease which is less common and more difficult to diagnose in AIDS patients. *Toxoplasma*-induced cystitis or pseudoneoplastic bullous cystitis is rarely detected in these patients. The diagnosis may be difficult because this condition is associated with misleading radiologic and endoscopic findings (Welker et al, 1994). With these studies, the diagnosis was eventually confirmed by the presence of *Toxoplasma* cysts on histopathological examination of bladder biopsies (Hofman et al, 1993). Therefore, disseminated toxoplasmosis should be considered in the differential diagnosis of AIDS patients with culture-negative cystitis (Welker et al, 1994). For unclear reasons, gastrointestinal involvement is exceedingly rare and occurs only in the context of severe immunosuppression and disseminated disease (Merzianu et al, 2005). Gastric toxoplasmosis has been reported in AIDS patients. It presents as diarrheoa and other nonspecific GI symptoms. Biopsy shows the presence of *Toxoplasma* trophozoites in the forms of tachyzoites, bradyzoites, and pseudocysts which are mandatory for definite diagnosis. It responds well to anti-*Toxoplasma* therapy (Alpert et al, 1996; Merzianu et al, 2005). It is of interest, that disseminated toxoplasmosis with sepsis has also been found in AIDS patients and should be considered in patients with sepsis of unknown origin (Artigas et al, 1994). ECT has also been diagnosed in the heart (Guerot et al, 1995; Chimenti et al, 2007), lung (Touboul et al, 1986; Kovari et al, 2010), liver (Mastroianni et al, 1996), and spinal cord (Harris et al, 1990; Kung et al, 2011). ECT has a low incidence in AIDS patients. Many HIV-infected patients lack access to primary chemoprophylaxis and antiretroviral therapy, in limited resource settings hence, more cases are reported in this group.

5. Neuropathology of toxoplasmosis: from pre to HAART era

Toxoplasmosis is an important opportunistic infection, causing short-term and chronic mortality (Neuen-Jacob et al, 1993; Kumarasamy et al, 2010). Multifocal necrotizing encephalitis is the predominant neuropathological finding of CT in AIDS patients. Localization of multiple with ring enhancing lesions on neuroimaging in basal ganglia, frontoparietal cortex and thalamus suggests haematogenous spread. The predilection of *T. gondii* in the basal ganglia can result in a variety of movement disorders (Nath et al, 1993). The cerebral edema, encephalitic process and tissue destruction are significant and responsible for majority of neurological morbidity in HIV-infected patients presenting with focal brain lesion (Ammassari et al, 2000). Rupture of tissue cysts in AIDS- associated CT patients result in multiplication of bradyzoites into tachyzoites, which causes severe inflammatory reaction. Three morphological patterns of brain lesions in patients with CT are produced based on the stage of infection and degree of tissue reaction (Shankar et al, 2005): (i) In the acute stage (less than a few weeks duration): appearance of a necrotizing abscess or encephalitis seen as poorly circumscribed necrotic foci with variable degrees of haemorrhage, perifocal edema, acute and chronic inflammation, macrophage infiltration, with numerous *T. gondii* tachyzoites and encysted bradyzoites along the periphery. Also common are vascular thrombosis/fibrinoid necrosis of vessel walls, with polymorph infiltration, hypertrophy and the presence of tachyzoites in the hypertrophie arterial wall. (ii) A chronic lesion (weeks to months) : organized abscesses are found in CT cases treated for ≥ 2 weeks and seen as well circumscribed foci of central necrosis with a rim of congestion. In contrast to the acute phase, the central foci of an acellular necrosis is surrounded by a granulomatous reaction, with macrophages containing tightly packed lipid and haemosiderin, prominent hypertrophic occlusive arteritis with dense lymphocytic cuffing, and only a few organisms. (iii) Patients treated for ≥ 1 month show chronic abscesses in CT appear as small cystic cavities or linear orange-yellow scars and macrophages containing lipid and haemosiderin surrounded by a dense gliotic reaction. Calcification of vessels occurs and organisms are rarely found. In addition, a CAT scan can present as a diffuse, non-necrotizing, rapidly progressive encephalitis. The histological appearance seen as nodules of micrioglial cells with encysted bradyzoites and dispersed tachyzoites within the nodules.

Autopsy findings confirm the presence of the parasite and demonstration of *Toxoplasma* cysts is diagnostic of disseminated toxoplasmosis in AIDS patients (Holch et al, 1993). Despite the effectiveness of HAART, involvement of the brain in patients with AIDS remains a frequent autopsy finding (Masliah et al, 2000). AIDS-associated CT continues to be the major cause of mortality in the era of HAART (Rajagopalan et al, 2009; Kumarasamy et al, 2010). The expansion of earlier access to HAART could substantially reduce mortality, particularly in limited resource settings (Mzileni et al, 2008; Rajagopalan et al, 2009).

The seroprevalence of toxoplasmosis is generally high in HIV-infected patients and approximately 10% of CT is reported in AIDS patients. There has been no report of such neuropathological findings related to toxoplasmosis found in AIDS patients from Malaysia and its neighboring countries in the Southeast Asian region such as Thailand. This may be due to the fact it is not a common practice to conduct an autopsy in HIV/AIDS patients that could give the actual prevalence of AIDS-associated CT being underestimated. CT is one of the most common opportunistic infections of the CNS (Wadia et al, 2001; Nobre et al, 2003) as reported in an autopsy series conducted in India (Lanjewar et al, 1998a; Lanjewar et al, 1998b) and in other clinical settings (Petito et al, 1986; Souza et al, 2008). The majority of AIDS-related diseases diagnosed at autopsy had not been clinically diagnosed or suspected antemortem (Eza et al, 2006). The importance of an autopsy in evaluating clinical management and diagnosis (Eza et al, 2006) should be periodically done; particular in areas of high endemic toxoplasmosis where antiretroviral drugs, such as HAART, cannot be fully accessed.

There is scanty data about AIDS-associated neuropathological findings during the HAART era in Asia and Sub-Sahara Africa. This is mainly due to delayed introduction of these agents to these regions. It is expected that more autopsy studies will be carried out in this part of the world in the near future. The incidence of toxoplasmosis in autopsy studies has declined since the introduction of HAART in various countries, such as the USA (Langford et al, 2003) and France (Vallat-Decouvelaere et al, 2003). These studies show that autopsy findings can be a valuable means for determining the range and relative frequency of infectious diseases in these patients (Lucas et al, 1993). In addition, this can potentially have an immediate impact on patient care by enabling appropriate interventions, based on the results obtained (Lucas et al, 1993).

6. Diagnostic approaches - from conventional to advanced technology

Among patients with AIDS, cerebral involvement is more common and more serious than extracerebral toxoplasmosis. The definitive diagnosis is crucial for CT patients by directly demonstrating the presence of the tachyzoite form of *T. gondii* in the cerebral tissues. The presumptive diagnosis for CT, including the clinical presentations, radio-imaging findings, molecular and sero-diagnosis for *Toxoplasma* infection, and good response to anti-*Toxoplasma* therapy are widely accepted in clinical practice. The favorable outcome of CT is the improvement of clinical and radiological features after 2 to 3 weeks of initiated empirical therapy. The clinical diagnosis is a dilemma due to CT mimics with other brain diseases making it difficult to diagnose. Differential diagnosis of AIDS-associated CT is extremely important and the local neuroepidemiology and the degree of immunosuppression in the host are two key factors involved (Vidal et al, 2008). Primary CNS lymphoma is the main differential diagnosis of CT reported from developed countries (Manzardo et al, 2005). While, focal forms of cerebral tuberculosis (tuberculoma and, less likely tuberculous brain abscess) allow for differential diagnosis of CT mainly in developing countries (Trujillo et al, 2005). Primary CNS lymphoma usually presents with a CD4 count of less than 50 cells/cumm, CT occurs below 100 cells/cumm, and cerebral TB is more frequently present with a CD4 count above 200 cells/cumm (Vidal et al, 2004a; Vidal et al, 2005a; Vidal et al, 2005b). In addition to these more common neurological diseases, the differential diagnosis of CT includes other opportunistic infections such as progressive multifocal leucoencephalopathy, herpes simplex encephalitis, and cryptococcal meningitis; AIDS-and non-AIDS-associated tumors such as metastases of disseminated lymphoma and glioblastoma multiforme, respectively; and vascular diseases. Overall, a rapid and accurate diagnosis of CT is necessary, as the earlier the treatment the better the clinical outcome and survival rate of these patients.

6.1 Radiological diagnosis

Radio-imaging findings, either by computed tomography (CAT scan) or magnetic resonance imaging (MRI), are useful tools for the presumptive or empirical diagnosis of CT. CT usually causes unifocal, and more frequently multifocal lesions, and less likely diffuse encephalitis. These findings are however not pathognomonic of CT. Radiological diagnosis (Vidal et al, 2005a) can be classified as typical findings of hypodense lesions with ring-enhancing and perilesional edema, are observed in ~80% of CT cases. A typical pattern of hypodense lesions found without contrast enhancing and with an expansive effect, CT patients without focal lesions and MRI demonstrating focal lesions, and diffuse cerebral encephalitis without visible focal lesions, are shown in ~20% of these cases. An unusual but highly suggestive image of patients with CT is the 'eccentric target sign', which is a small asymmetric nodule along the wall of the enhancing ring (Pereira-Chioccola et al, 2009). Figure 2 shows the main radiological features of AIDS-associated CT patients. A CAT scan seems to be a sensitive diagnostic method for patients with focal neurological deficits; however it may underestimate the minimal inflammatory responses seen during early disease (Gill et al, 1986).

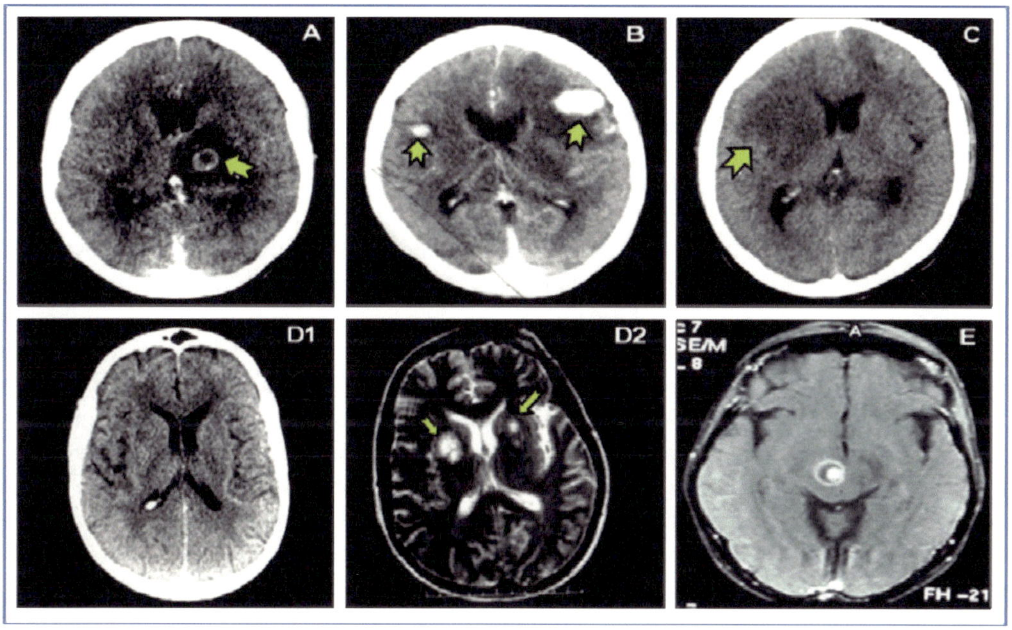

Fig. 4. Computed tomography images showing the spectrum of radiological findings of cerebral toxoplasmosis in HIV-infected patients.

Hypodense lesion with ring-enhancing and perilesional edema **(A)**; nodular enhancing and perilesional edema **(B)**; without contrast enhancing and with expansive effect **(C)**. A CAT scan with contrast enhancement showed no abnormalities **(D1)** and corresponding T2-weighted MRI showed multiple basal ganglia focal lesions, with high-intensity signals **(D2)**. T1-weighted MRI showed a ring-enhancing lesion with a small, enhancing asymmetric nodule along the wall of the lesion **(E)** ('the eccentric target sign'). The arrows show the abnormalities. (Courtesy of Dr. Pereira-Chioccola VL and Dr. Vidal JE, São Paulo, Brazil.)

MRI is recommended to be performed in patients with; neurological symptoms and positive serology to anti-*Toxoplasma* antibodies whose CAT scans show no or only a single abnormality, or persistent or worsening focal neurological deficits of disease if results of the initial procedure were negative (Luft & Remington, 1992). A CAT scan or MRI is useful for assessment of patients who had responded to initial empirical treatment. There may be a worsening of radiographic appearance in patients with a clinically improved condition before 3 weeks, and complete resolution of cerebral lesions seen on a CAT scan may vary from 3 week to 6 months after initiation of therapy (Luft & Remington, 1992). An evidence of either clinical or radiographic improvement within 3 weeks of initial therapy provides a confirmed diagnosis of patients with CT.

6.2 Serological diagnosis

Cerebral toxoplasmosis poses a diagnostic problem that relies on classical serological methods to detect anti-*Toxoplasma* immunoglobulins because clinical blood samples from patients with immunodeficiency can fail to produce sufficient titers of specific antibodies. Sero-evidence of *Toxoplasma* infection, independent of antibody levels, is generally seen in all patients before developing CT (Carme et al, 1988). Most CT patients have high titers of anti-*Toxoplasma* IgG antibodies with high IgG avidity that provides serological evidence of infection (Raffi et al, 1997; Vidal et al, 2005a), and this also supports a conclusion that this is the result of a secondary reaction of latent or chronic *Toxoplasma* infection (Dardé, 1996). Therefore, it is important to determine the *Toxoplasma* serostatus in all HIV-infected patients in order to define the population at risk for CT. At the onset of CT, significant rises in anti-*Toxoplasma* antibody titers are found in only a minority of these patients (Carme et al, 1988). The level of rising titers may occur before the onset of CT and it does not seem to predict the occurrence of CT. Anti-*Toxoplasma* IgM antibody, as measured by the indirect fluorescent or ELISA tests, is rarely found in CT patients (Luft & Remington, 1992). In cases of CT, a negative or low titer of serological results or even the absence of anti-*Toxoplasma* antibodies does not exclude positive diagnosis and the initiation of anti-*Toxoplasma* therapy should be immediately started without delay if clinical and radiological presentations are consistent with CT (Luft & Remington, 1992; Nissapatorn et al, 2004). A positive serology result seems to be even less useful in areas where there is a high prevalence of toxoplasmosis in the general population (Pereira-Chioccola et al, 2009). While, a negative result does have a high negative predictive value (Vidal et al, 2008) Determination of an increase of intrathecal anti-*Toxoplasma* IgG antibody production is normally characterized by the presence of *T. gondii* oligoclonal bands (OCBs) of IgG antibody in CT patients (Potasman et al, 1988). Immunological diagnosis using other clinical samples such as cerebrospinal fluid (CSF) is of limited use because of the sensitivity and specificity being only about 60-70% (Collazos, 2003). *T. gondii* excretory/secretory antigens (ESAs) are an excellent serological marker for the diagnosis of CT in AIDS patients (Pereira-Chioccola et al, 2009). ESAs are produced by *T. gondii* tachyzoites, the form responsible for disease dissemination, which plays an important role in stimulating humoral and cellular immunities in order to control *Toxoplasma* infection (Carruthers & Sibley, 1997; Cérède et al, 2005). Anti-ESA IgG antibodies are also present in CSF sample of AIDS patients with CT which can be determined by ESA-ELISA and immunoblot techniques and these samples are clearly distinguishable from AIDS patients who are *Toxoplasma* seropositive but with other brain diseases (Pereira-Chioccola et al, 2009).

6.3 Molecular diagnosis

Since the serological status is solely useful to recognize whether the patient is at risk for reactivation, the direct detection of *T. gondii* DNA in biological specimens by polymerase chain reaction (PCR) has provided a major breakthrough for the diagnosis of toxoplasmosis (Reischl et al, 2003). Over a period of two decades, these molecular methods based on PCR and specific genetic markers have been developed for routine use in assisting serology for the diagnosis of CT patients. PCR techniques are suitable for patients with AIDS because these methods do not depend on the host immune responses and allow for direct detection of *T. gondii* DNA from a variety of clinical samples. In addition, these methods are rapid, sensitive, specific, less time consuming, and can be used to replace invasive procedures such as stereotactic brain biopsy. The sensitivity and specificity of the PCR reactions depends on the types of reagents, protocols for DNA extraction, storage of clinical samples, and the timing between the start of a specific therapy and collection of clinical samples, which can make the interpretation of results difficult (Pereira-Chioccola et al, 2009). Among clinical/biological samples, blood and CSF are the most frequently used for the detection of *T. gondii* DNA in patients with CT. To yield a better result, clinical samples should be collected before or up until the first 3 days of anti-*Toxoplasma* therapy because the diagnostic sensitivity will be reduced after the first week of this specific treatment (Vidal et al, 2004b). In CSF samples, the varying sensitivity of the PCR technique ranges from 11.5% to 100% but a high specificity (96-100%) has been reported using CSF specimens (Novati et al, 1994; Dupon et al, 1995; Vidal et al, 2004b). The collection of CSF sample is invasive and is not recommended for patients with multiple brain lesions (Pereira-Chioccola et al, 2009). PCR in blood samples, as an alternative approach, has been reported with a wide range of sensitivities of between 16% and 86% (Dupouy-Camet et al, 1993; Dupon et al, 1995). A quantitative real-time PCR (qrtPCR), is a recent development among molecular methods, and accelerates the detection of *T. gondii* DNA in most positive samples and allows for amplification and simultaneous detection of DNA in 1 hour (Hierl et al, 2004). Its advantages over conventional and nested PCR include rapid, improved sensitivity, a broad dynamic range of targets, DNA quantitation and reduction of contamination. Despite these advantages, in some patients with low parasite load particularly in CSF samples; there is still the need for comparative results of both conventional nested and real-time quantitative PCR methods (Bretagne, 2003; Hierl et al, 2004; Apfalter et al, 2005). Future prospect on the diagnosis of patients with CT is more likely to rely on the development of molecular methods based on qrtPCR which provides quantitative results and is less time-consuming in preparation. However, this technique needs to have improved specificity and more importantly a reduction of the high cost of the necessary equipment.

6.4 Other diagnostic methods

There is a need for more specific or invasive approaches that will assist confirmation of the diagnosis of CT. Brain biopsy is generally reserved for those patients who present with a diagnostic dilemma or do not fulfill the criteria for presumptive treatment and for those patients who fail to improve clinically or radiologically over the succeeding 10-14 days after being empirically treated for toxoplasmosis initially so they do warrant a stereotactic brain biopsy (SBB) in order to institute specific and appropriate therapy (Luft & Remington, 1992). For patients with expansive brain lesions who fail to respond to empirical treatment initiated for CT within 14 days, SBB should be seriously considered relatively early in the course of treatment, with or without change in therapy (Pereira-Chioccola et al, 2009). Surprisingly, SBB is not commonly used for the diagnosis of CT or CT-associated other opportunistic CNS diseases in Asian countries (Yeo et al, 2000) compared to other settings where CT cases have been reported in patients with AIDS. Brain biopsies do not influence survival of CT patients (Sadler et al, 1998). SBB is an efficient, safe and important diagnostic procedure. In selected patients even expensive investigations should be undertaken before considering specific therapy and cost effective homecare (Armbruster et al, 1998). This procedure should be performed early during the patient's evolution in order to achieve a prompt and accurate diagnosis and to guide the therapeutic scheme for AIDS patients with FBL (Corti et al, 2008).

Recently, genotyping analysis of *T. gondii* strains isolated from clinical samples has been conducted in HIV-infected patients from different settings. However, it remains doubtful on how to ascertain the association between *T. gondii* strains and human toxoplasmosis since the majority of infected individuals are chronic and without any clinical symptoms, and it is difficult to isolate *T. gondii* strains from these patients. Therefore, a larger sample size should be carried out in human patients to identify specific *T. gondii* strains using high resolution typing methods such as multiplex nested PCR-RFLP which can genotype some DNA samples extracted directly from infected tissues. Serotyping of *T. gondii* strains has proved to be a promising tool using serum samples to overcome the diagnostic challenge (Kong et al, 2003; Peyron et al, 2006; Morisset et al, 2008; Sousa et al, 2008; Sousa et al, 2009). However, due to the limitation of serotyping it is not possible to differentiate type II from non-type II strains particularly in South America where there is a high diversity of *T. gondii* strain types. At present, this requires further developments of typing analyses to facilitate and be incorporated into the routine diagnosis of patients with CT.

7. Therapeutic approaches: from specific treatment to HAART

7.1 Anti-*Toxoplasma* therapy

One of the keys after diagnoses is how patients respond to the different therapeutic regimens used for treating this opportunistic disease. Most patients with CT respond well to anti-*Toxoplasma* agents as demonstrated by findings from studies in various settings. However, about 10% of CT cases died despite what was thought to be adequate treatment (Vidal et al, 2005a). There are few options other than anti-*Toxoplasma* regimens used as first-choice initial therapy; 6 weeks with sufadiazine (1.0-1.5 g per oral [PO] every 6 h) with pyrimethamine (100-200 mg PO loading dose, then 50 mg PO daily) and folinic acid (10-20 mg PO daily) that can reduce the hemato-toxicities related to pyrimethamine (Portegies et al, 2004). This standard combination has been successfully used in treating CT but has been associated with high toxicities such as Lyell's syndrome or Steven-Johnson syndrome (Katlama et al, 1996a; Torre et al, 1998). The other regimen is trimethoprim/sulfamethoxazole (Co-trimoxazole, 5/25 mg/kg PO or intravenous (IV) every 12 h for 4-6 weeks) (Canessa et al, 1992). This therapeutic regimen has been confirmed for its efficacy and safety in a single available randomized clinical trial (Canessa et al, 1992; Torre et al, 1998; Dedicoat & Livesley, 2006; Béraud et al, 2009). Several alternative therapies, principally used in patients who are intolerant to this combination, have been reported to be effective, including clindamycin and pyrimethamine or sulfadiazine (Katlama et al, 1996a; Tsai et al, 2002), clarithromycin and pyrimethamine (Fernandez-Martin et al, 1991), clindamycin and 5-fluoro-uracil (Dhiver et al, 1993), azithromycin and pyrimethamine (Saba et al, 1993; Jacobson et al, 2001), clindamycin and fansidar (Nissapatorn et al, 2004), sulfadoxine and pyrimethamine (Amogne et al, 2006), and atovaquone (Torres et al, 1997). There was no superior regimen among the three following combinations: pyrimethamine plus sulfadiazine, pyrimethamine plus clindamycin (Katlama et al, 1996a), and pyrimethamine plus sulfadiazine with Co-trimoxazole (Torre et al, 1998) that were reported in a recent review of comparative studies (Dedicoat & Livesley, 2006).

There is one case of toxoplasmosis resistant to standard combination therapy (pyrimethamine and sulfadiazine) that was improved with clindamycin and pyrimethamine (Huber et al, 1995). The other case was an AIDS patient with toxoplasmic myelopathy and myopathy

resistant to standard anti-*Toxoplasma* therapy due to the possibility of immune reconstitution of the inflammatory syndrome, was reported (Kung et al, 2011). Another study suggested atovaquone as being effective in AIDS cases with resistant toxoplasmosis (Lafeuillade et al, 1993). This helps to identify drugs that are effective and may act synergistically (McFadden et al, 2001). Relapses of CT are frequently observed in AIDS patients non-compliant to therapy or prophylaxis, and in those who develop adverse drug effects (Luft & Remington, 1992; Nissapatorn et al, 2004; Béraud et al, 2009). There has been no evidence of treatment-induced resistance so far reported that have contributing to a relapse of CT. Few studies have arrived at a solution of how to prevent relapses. Pyrimethamine and sulfadoxine twice a week appears to give promising results for prevention of CT. Allergic reactions are usually mild and disappear on continuation, but may limit the value of this regimen (Ruf et al, 1993). Daily doses of pyrimethamine and sulfadiazine are more effective as maintenance therapy for preventing relapses of CT (4.4 compared to 19.5 per 100 patient-years; incidence rate ration, 4.36; $p=0.024$) than twice weekly administration (Podzamczer et al, 1995). Pyrimethamine and clindamycin has been shown to be a valuable alternative for treatment but is less effective, particularly for the long term prevention of relapses (Katlama et al, 1996a). Azithromycin and pyrimethamine have been used as alternative therapy, but maintenance with this combination or oral azithromycin alone is associated with relapses (Jacobson et al, 2001).
Atovaquone is a unique naphthoquinone with broad-spectrum antiprotozoal activity. It has been found to be effective against tachyzoites in vitro and may kill bradyzoites within cysts at a higher concentration. Atovaquone is frequently used in combination with other agents in treating CT. Experimental studies have shown that the efficacy of atovaquone was enhanced when other agents were added, such as pyrimethamine, sulfadiazine, clindamycin, or clarithromycin (Guelar et al, 1994). An intravenous preparation is highly effective in murine models with reactivated toxoplasmosis (Schöler et al, 2001; Dunay et al, 2004). In AIDS patients, the only study to report failure with atovaquone during treatment found that a high temperature may induce inactivation of the product in the absence of food intake (Duran et al, 1995). Atovaquone has consistently been found to be a promising therapeutic for salvage therapy in CT patients who were intolerant to or who failed standard regimens (Guelar et al, 1994; Katlama et al, 1996a; Torres et al, 1997; Chirgwin et al, 2002). However, the role of atovaquone in the treatment and prophylaxis of CT in AIDS patients is not well defined and more studies are required before a firm recommendation can be made (Baggish & Hill, 2002). The treatment of choice is often directed by the available therapy, particularly in resource-poor settings. An important question is whether the incidence of secondary reactivation or relapse cases of CT may begin to rise in the future. This depends on how the efficacy of the current treatment regimens and new novel drugs, especially those that can destroy cyst/bradyzoite forms of the *Toxoplasma* parasite. Another important factor is increasing resistance to antiretroviral drugs in HIV-positive patients and the subsequent decline in CD4 cell counts (Kuritzkes et al, 2000) which has been reported in the recent years.

7.2 Primary and secondary chemoprophylaxis

Toxoplasmosis is one of the leading CNS-OIs, that causes morbidity and mortality in advanced stages of HIV-infected patients. Effective primary and secondary prophylaxis has been formulated to prevent the occurrence of CT (Katlama et al, 1996a; Bucher et al, 1997). Before the era of HAART, co-trimoxazole played an important role as a primary prophylactic agent in preventing the reactivation of toxoplasmosis in HIV-positive patients (van Oosterhout et al, 2005). CT was still reported in HIV-infected patients with or without prophylaxis (Nissapatorn et al, 2004; Nissapatorn et al, 2007). To be consistent with previous reports and present situations in most resource limited settings, a current guideline recommends the use of a daily dose of a double-strength tablet of co-trimoxazole in *Toxoplasma*-seropositive patients who have a CD4 cell count below100 cells/cumm (CDC, 2009). For AIDS patients who survive their first episode of CT, the risk of relapse is between 30% and 50% if lifelong suppressive therapy is not provided (Leport et al, 1988; de Gans et al, 1992). Discontinuation of maintenance therapy (secondary/ suppressive therapy) for established CT patients is not recommended (USPHS/IDSA Prevention of opportunistic infections working group, 1997). In the pre HAART era, relapse rates of CT after discontinuation of maintenance therapy was approximately 50% (Katlama et al, 1996b). There are few regimens that have been used for secondary prophylaxis for CT patients; the combination of pyrimethamine (25-50 mg/day) plus sulfadiazine (500 mg every 6 h) plus leucovorin (10-20 mg/day) is a highly effective treatment. The use of this combined thrice-weekly regimen (Podzamczer et al, 1995) or the same doses of sulfadiazine twice a day (Jordan et al, 2004) is an alternative option among non-compliance patients. The recommendation is for pyrimethamine plus clindamycin (600 mg clinidamycin every 8 h) for patients who are intolerant to sulfa drugs (CDC, 2009). Co-trimoxazole (960 mg twice daily) is another potential drug used in secondary prophylaxis for patients with CT (Duval et al, 2004). This agent (2.5/12.5 mg/kg PO every 12 h) is considered as safe, cheap and effective and can be an alternative choice (Pereira-Chioccola et al, 2009) to increase drug adherence in areas where other maintenance therapies are not available.

7.3 Highly active anti-retroviral therapy (HAART)

For more than two decades now, the use of HAART in HIV-infected patients has resulted in an improved quality of life and an increase in the length of time that patients remain free from opportunistic infections (Mocroft et al, 1998; Palella et al, 1998). A higher CNS Penetration-Effectiveness (CPE) score of antiretroviral drugs is increasing the survival rate of CT patients (Lanoy et al, 2011). In CT cases, there is no recommendation for the timing of HAART when CT is present in antiretroviral-naïve patients. However, HAART should be started at least 2 weeks after an anti-*Toxoplasma* regimen was initiated in these patients (Manzardo et al, 2005; Pereira-Chioccola et al, 2009). In HIV-infected patients receiving HAART, primary prophylaxis for CT can be safely discontinued in patients whose CD4 cell counts increase to >200 cells/mm^3 (CDC, 2009). It is a medical challenge to decide whether secondary prophylaxis should be continued while HIV-infected patients are receiving HAART. If maintenance therapy is stopped, recurrence of toxoplasmosis may allow for permanent damage to cerebral and visual functions which is potentially harmful to an affected person (Stout et al, 2002). While maintenance therapy is still essential, evaluation of *T. gondii*-specific immune responses might be the other important step for improving estimates of the individual risk of CT and CT relapse (Hoffmann et al, 2007). Otherwise, secondary prophylaxis can be safely discontinued in CT patients receiving HAART with CD4 cell count of > 200 cells/cumm after 6 months (Pereira-Chioccola et al, 2009). This same prophylaxis should be reintroduced in patients with CD4 cell count of < 200 cells/cumm (CDC, 2009). While, primary and secondary prophylaxis against CT can also be safely discontinued after the CD4 cell count has increased to ≥ 200 cells/cumm for more than 3 months in HIV-infected patients receiving HAART (Miro et al, 2006). These strategies can help in reducing the toxicity, pill overload, and expense associated with complicated therapeutic regimens. Considering that CT patients have a high chance of early death, HAART should be immediately initiated after CT diagnosis and prophylaxis should be maintained in these patients who fail to respond to antiretroviral therapy.

8. Immune Reconstitution Inflammatory Syndrome (IRIS) - from past to future concerns

Anti-retroviral therapy partially restores the immune function of HIV-infected patients, thereby remarkably reducing morbidity and mortality of opportunistic infections in general and CT in particular. The incidence of opportunistic infections, including CT and ECT has decreased, particularly in areas where antiretroviral therapy, including HAART, is accessible (Kaplan et al, 2000; Subsai et al, 2006; Lian et al, 2007). HAART has reduced relapse in cases of toxoplasmosis and has improved survival in these HIV-infected patients. This may be due to the successful suppression of virus replications followed by an increase in CD4+ lymphocytes, a partial recovery of T-cell specific immune responses and decreased susceptibility to both local and systemic opportunistic pathogens (Silva & Araújo, 2005). HIV-associated IRIS is the clinical worsening of opportunistic infections that result from enhancement of pathogen-specific immune responses among patients responding to antiretroviral treatment (Lawn & Wilkinson, 2006). IRIS has been widely recognized in CT patients following initiation of HAART and development of a paradoxical clinical deterioration despite an increased CD4 cell count and decreased HIV viral load which leads to the rapid restoration of the immune system (Gray et al, 2005). So far, more than 20 cases of IRIS-associated CT have been reported in the literature (Table 2). A low CD4 cell count has been identified as a significant risk factor in AIDS patients with CT (Tsambiras et al, 2001; de Boer et al, 2003; Sendi et al, 2006; Chen et al, 2009; Caby et al, 2010; Kung et al, 2011) due to impaired proliferative response to *Toxoplasma* antigen (Belanger et al, 1999), a decreased production of interferon γ (Ullum et al, 1997), and it is found to be more common that IRIS develops in HIV-infected patients (Jevtović et al, 2005). Therefore, monitoring of CD4/CD8 T cells in patients on HAART might serve as a better marker for the restoration of *T. gondii*-specific immune responses than the total number of CD4 cells count (Furco et al, 2008). Immune reconstitution under HAART has been associated with a restoration of immune responses against *T. gondii* (Fournier et al, 2001). In the case where IRIS is suspected in CT patient, close observation for 7-15 days, a higher steroid dose to control IRIS (Venkataramana et al, 2006), uninterrupted HAART, and continued treatment for toxoplasmosis can resolve this problem without biopsy (Tremont-Lukats et al, 2009). Based on reported cases of CT-associated IRIS from different studies, this could verify its association that it can develop in a substantial numbers of HIV-infected patients receiving HAART. No case of IRIS-related toxoplasmosis has ever been reported among AIDS patients in Malaysia even though CT was one of the most common systemic opportunistic infections in AIDS patients (Nissapatorn et al, 2004; Lian et al, 2007). Toxoplasmosis is a common neurological opportunistic infection in industrialized countries for which HAART is often initiated fairly early compared to developing or resource-limited settings. As for the increasing use of HAART worldwide, the care for patients receiving HAART will need to incorporate monitoring for and treating complications of IRIS (Agmon-Levin et al, 2008), including impaired CD4-cell immune reconstitution upon HIV therapy in patients with CT

Reference	Country	No. of cases	Clinical presentation	Baseline CD4 cell count/µL
Rodríguez-Rosado et al, 1998	Spain	3	Cerebral toxoplasmosis	-
González-Castillo et al, 2001	Spain	1	Cerebral toxoplasmosis	456
Tsambiras et al, 2001	USA	1	Cerebral toxoplasmosis	83
de Boer et al, 2003	The Netherlands	1	Cerebral toxoplasmosis	43
Jevtović et al, 2005	Serbia & Montenegro	1	Cerebral toxoplasmosis	<100
Sendi et al, 2006	Switzerland	1	Immune recovery vitritis with isolated toxoplasmic retinochoroiditis	11
Subsai et al, 2006	Thailand	2	Cerebral toxoplasmosis	-
Huruy et al, 2008	Ethiopia	2	Cerebral toxoplasmosis	-
Chen et al, 2009	USA	1	Cerebral toxoplasmosis	29
Klotz et al, 2009	Ethiopia	7	Cerebral toxoplasmosis	50-100
McCombe et al, 2009	Canada	1	Cerebral toxoplasmosis	2
Tremont-Lukats et al, 2009	USA	1	Cerebral toxoplasmosis	14
Cabral et al, 2010	Brazil	1	Cerebral toxoplasmosis	276
Caby et al, 2010	France	1	Placental IRIS	7 (pregnancy)
Martin-Blondel et al, 2010	France	3	Cerebral toxoplasmosis	9, 25, 23
Kung et al, 2011	USA	1	Toxoplasmic myelopathy and myopathy	67
Shah, 2011	India	1 (child)	Cerebral toxoplasmosis	-

Table 2. Summary on reported cases of immune reconstitution inflammatory syndrome (IRIS) associated toxoplasmosis in HIV-infected patients.

(Kastenbauer et al, 2009). As the number of AIDS-associated CT cases treated with HAART increases, the complications of IRIS-CT may become more common and easily recognizable, particularly in areas where toxoplasmosis is endemic. Therefore, increased awareness of IRIS is importance to clinicians along with early diagnosis and appropriate treatment in managing AIDS patients.

9. Conclusion

Despite a decline in both morbidity and mortality in HIV-infected patients in developed countries including the United States and Europe, toxoplasmosis remains an important disease and is unlikely to be eradicated. Toxoplasmosis still occurs in those not diagnosed with HIV and not receiving medical care, those not receiving prophylaxis, and those not taking or not responding to HAART. There are very few reports regarding resistance to the drugs used for toxoplasmosis. Resistance in HIV cases and the action of anti-retroviral therapy with or without IRIS may contribute to an increase in the incidence of CT. In developing countries where anti-retroviral therapy is still lacking, HIV-infected patients are at high risk for CT, these regions include China, India, South America, Southeast Asia and most importantly sub-Saharan Africa. A better understanding of the clinico-epidemiology of toxoplasmosis, and improved efforts in prevention, diagnosis and treatment, are needed. The role of infections with this parasite requires further study, including as to whether infections, such as CT have an impact on HIV/AIDS patients.

10. Acknowledgement

I express my sincere thanks to Assoc. Prof. Dr. Nongyao Sawangjaroen, Department of Microbiology, Faculty of Science, Prince of Songkhla University, Hat Yai, Songkhla, Thailand and Dr. Sucheep Phiriyasamith, Master of Public Administration Program, Graduate School, Kasem Bundit University, Bangkok, Thailand for their assistance during preparation of this chapter. Also, I would like to thank the University of Malaya Research Grant (UMRG094/09HTM) for financial support.

11. References

Agmon-Levin, N., Elbirt, D. & Sthoeger, Z.M. (2008). Immune reconstitution inflammatory syndrome in human immunodeficiency (HIV) infected patients. *Harefuah*, Vol.147, No.5, pp. 439-444, 476, 477, ISSN 0017-7768.

Ajzenberg, D., Year, H., Marty, P., Paris, L., Dalle, F., Menotti, J., Aubert, D., Franck, J., Bessières, M.H., Quinio, D., Pelloux, H., Delhaes, L., Desbois, N., Thulliez, P., Robert-Gangneux, F., Kauffmann-Lacroix, C., Pujol, S., Rabodonirina, M., Bougnoux, M.E., Cuisenier, B., Duhamel, C., Duong ,T.H., Filisetti, D., Flori, P., Gay-Andrieu, F., Pratlong, F., Nevez, G., Totet, A., Carme, B., Bonnabau, H., Dardé, M.L. & Villena, I. (2009). Genotype of 88 *Toxoplasma gondii* isolates associated with toxoplasmosis in immunocompromised patients and correlation with clinical findings. *Journal of Infectious Diseases*, Vol.199, No.8, pp. 1155-1167, ISSN 0022-1899.

Akanmu, A.S., Osunkalu, V.O., Ofomah, J.N. & Olowoselu, F.O. (2010). Pattern of demographic risk factors in the seroprevalence of anti-*Toxoplasma gondii* antibodies in HIV infected patients at the Lagos University Teaching Hospital. *Nigerian Quarterly Journal of Hospital Medicine*, Vol.20, No.1, pp.1-4, ISSN 0189 - 2657.

Alpert, L., Miller, M., Alpert, E., Satin, R., Lamoureux, E. & Trudel, L. (1996). Gastric toxoplasmosis in acquired immunodeficiency syndrome: antemortem diagnosis with histopathologic characterization. *Gastroenterology*, Vol.110, No.1, pp. 258-264, ISSN 0016-5085.

Alves, J.M., Magalhães, V. & Matos, M.A. (2010). Toxoplasmic retinochoroiditis in patients with AIDS and neurotoxoplasmosis. *Arquivos Brasileiros de Oftalmologia*, Vol.73, No.2, pp.150-154, ISSN 0004-2749.

Ammassari, A., Cingolani, A., Pezzotti, P., De Luca, D.A., Murri, R., Giancola, M.L., Larocca, L.M. & Antinori, A. (2000). AIDS-related focal brain lesions in the era of highly active antiretroviral therapy. *Neurology*, Vol.55, No.8, pp. 1194-1200, ISSN 0028-3878.

Amogne, W., Teshager, G. & Zenebe, G. (2006). Central nervous system toxoplasmosis in adult Ethiopians. *Ethiopian Medical Journal*, Vol.44, No.2, pp.113-120, ISSN 0014-1755.

Anekthananon, T., Ratanasuwan, W., Techasathit, W., Rongrungruang, Y. & Suwanagool, S. (2004). HIV infection/acquired immunodeficiency syndrome at Siriraj Hospital, 2002: time for secondary prevention. *Journal of the Medical Association of Thailand*, Vol.87, No.2, pp. 173-179, ISSN 0125-2208.

Apfalter, P., Reischl, U. & Hammerschlag, M.R. (2005). In-house nucleic acid amplification assays in research: how much quality control is needed before one can rely upon the results? *Journal of Clinical Microbiology*, Vol.43, No.12, pp. 5835-5841, ISSN 0095-1137.

Arevalo, J.F., Quiceno, J.I., García, R.F., McCutchan, J.A., Munguia, D., Nelson, J.A. & Freeman, W.R. (1997). Retinal findings and characteristics in AIDS patients with systemic *Mycobacterium avium-intracellulare complex* and toxoplasmic encephalitis. *Ophthalmic Surgery & Lasers*, Vol.28, No.1, pp. 50-54, ISSN 1082-3069.

Armbruster, C., Alesch, F., Budka, H. & Kriwanek, S. (1998). Stereotactic brain biopsy in AIDS patients: a necessary patient-oriented and cost-effective diagnostic measure? *Acta Medica Austriaca*, Vol.25, No.3, pp. 91-95, ISSN 0303-8173.

Arshad, S., Skiest, D. & Granowitz, E.V. (2009). Subacute onset of paralysis in a person with AIDS. *The AIDS Reader*, Vol.19, No.1, pp. 32-35, ISSN 1053-0894.

Artigas, J., Grosse, G., Niedobitek, F., Kassner, M., Risch, W. & Heise, W. (1994). Severe toxoplasmic ventriculomeningoencephalomyelitis in two AIDS patients following treatment of cerebral toxoplasmic granuloma. *Clinical Neuropathology*, Vol.13, No.3, pp. 120-126, ISSN 0722-5091.

Azevedo, K.M., Setúbal, S., Lopes, V.G., Camacho, L.A. & Oliveira, S.A. (2010). Congenital toxoplasmosis transmitted by human immunodeficiency-virus infected women. *The Brazilian Journal of Infectious Diseases*, Vol.14, No.2, pp. 186-189, ISSN 1413-8670.

Bachmeyer, C., Mouchnino, G., Thulliez, P. & Blum, L. (2006). Congenital toxoplasmosis from an HIV-infected woman as a result of reactivation. *Journal of Infection*, Vol.52, No.2, pp. e55-e57, ISSN 0163-4453.

Baggish, A.L. & Hill, D.R. (2002). Antiparasitic agent atovaquone. *Antimicrobial Agents and Chemotherapy*, Vol.46, No.5, pp. 1163-1173, ISSN 0066-4804.

Belanger, F., Derouin, F., Grangeot-Keros, L. & Meyer, L. (1999). Incidence and risk factors of toxoplasmosis in a cohort of human immunodeficiency virus-infected patients: 1988-1995. HEMOCO and SEROCO Study Groups. *Clinical Infectious Diseases*, Vol.28, No.3, pp. 575-581, ISSN 1058-4838.

Berger, B.B., Egwuagu, C.E., Freeman, W.R. & Wiley, C.A. (1993). Miliary toxoplasmic retinitis in acquired immunodeficiency syndrome. *Archives of Ophthalmology*, Vol.111, No.3, pp. 373-376, ISSN 0003-9950.

Béraud, G., Pierre-François, S., Foltzer, A., Abel, S., Liautaud, B., Smadja, D. & Cabié, A. (2009). Cotrimoxazole for treatment of cerebral toxoplasmosis: an observational cohort study during 1994-2006. *The American Journal of Tropical Medicine and Hygiene*, Vol.80, No.4, pp. 583-587, ISSN 0002-9637.

Biedermann, K., Flepp, M., Fierz, W., Joller-Jemelka, H. & Kleihues, P. (1995). Pregnancy, immunosuppression and reactivation of latent toxoplasmosis. *Journal of Perinatal Medicine*, Vol.23, No.3, pp. 191-203, ISSN 0300-5577.

Bossi, P., Caumes, E., Astagneau, P., Li, T.S., Paris, L., Mengual, X., Katlama, C. & Bricaire, F. (1998). Epidemiologic characteristics of cerebral toxoplasmosis in 399 HIV-infected patients followed between 1983 and 1994. *La Revue de Medecine Interne*, Vol.19, No.5, pp. 313-317, ISSN 0248-8663.

Brändle, M., Vernazza, P.L., Oesterle, M. & Galeazzi, R.L. (1995). Cerebral toxoplasmosis with central diabetes insipidus and panhypopituitarism in a patient with AIDS. *Schweizerische medizinische Wochenschrift*, Vol.125, No.14, pp. 684-687, ISSN 0036-7672.

Bretagne, S. (2003). Molecular diagnostics in clinical parasitology and mycology: limits of the current polymerase chain reaction (PCR) assays and interest of the real-time PCR assays. *Clinical Microbiology and Infection*, Vol.9, No.6, pp. 505-511, ISSN 1198-743X.

Brindle, R., Holliman, R., Gilks, C. & Waiyaki, P. (1991). *Toxoplasma* antibodies in HIV-positive patients from Nairobi. *Transactions of the Royal Society of Tropical Medicine and Hygiene*, Vol.85, No.6, pp. 750-751, ISSN 0035-9203.

Brion, J.P., Pelloux, H., Le Marc'hadour, F., Stahl, J.P., Vilde, J.L. & Micoud, M. (1992). Acute toxoplasmic hepatitis in a patient with AIDS. *Clinical Infectious Diseases*, Vol.15, No.1, pp. 183-184, ISSN 1058-4838.

Bucher, H.C., Griffith, L., Guyatt, G.H. & Opravil, M. (1997). Meta-analysis of prophylactic treatments against *Pneumocystis carinii* pneumonia and toxoplasma encephalitis in HIV-infected patients. *Journal of Acquired Immune Deficiency Syndromes and Human Retrovirology*, Vol.15, No.2, pp. 104-114, ISSN 1077-9450.

Cabral, R.F., Valle Bahia, P.R., Gasparetto, E.L. & Chimelli, L. (2010). Immune reconstitution inflammatory syndrome and cerebral toxoplasmosis. *American Journal of Neuroradiology*, Vol.31, No.7, pp.E65-E66, ISSN 0195-6108.

Caby, F., Lemercier, D., Coulomb, A., Grigorescu, R., Paris, L., Touafek, F., Carcelain, G., Canestri, A., Pauchard, M., Katlama, C., Dommergues, M. & Tubiana, R. (2010). Fetal death as a result of placental immune reconstitution inflammatory syndrome. *The Journal of Infection*, Vol.61, No.2, pp. 185-188, ISSN 0163-4453.

Canessa, A., Del Bono, V., De Leo, P., Piersantelli, N. & Terragna, A. (1992). Cotrimoxazole therapy of *Toxoplasma gondii* encephalitis in AIDS patients. *European Journal of Clinical Microbiology & Infectious Diseases*, Vol.11, No.2, pp. 125-130, ISSN 0934-9723.

Cantos, G.A., Prando, M.D., Siqueira, M.V. & Teixeira, R.M. (2000). Toxoplasmosis: occurrence of antibodies anti- *Toxoplasma gondii* and diagnosis. *Revista da Associacao Medica Brasileira* (Sao Paulo), Vol.46, No.4, pp. 335-341, ISSN 0104-4230

Carme, B., M'Pele, P., Mbitsi, A., Kissila, A.M., Aya, G.M., Mouanga-Yidika, G., Mboussa, J. & Itoua-Ngaporo, A. (1988). Opportunistic parasitic diseases and mycoses in AIDS. Their frequencies in Brazzaville (Congo). *Bulletin de la Société de Pathologie Exotique et de ses Filiales*, Vol.81, No.3, pp. 311-316, ISSN 0037-9085.

Carrazana, E.J., Rossitch, E., Jr. & Samuels, M.A. (1989). Parkinsonian symptoms in a patient with AIDS and cerebral toxoplasmosis. *Journal of Neurology, Neurosurgery, and Psychiatry*, Vol.52, No.12, pp. 1445-1447, ISSN 0022-3050.

Carruthers, V.B. (2002). Host cell invasion by the opportunistic pathogen *Toxoplasma gondii*. *Acta Tropica*, Vol.81, No.2, pp.111-122, ISSN 0001-706X.

Carruthers, V.B. & Sibley, L.D. (1997). Sequential protein secretion from three distinct organelles of *Toxoplasma gondii* accompanies invasion of human fibroblasts. *European Journal of Cell Biology*, Vol.73, No.2, pp. 114-123, ISSN 0171-9335.

Castro Figueiredo, J.F., de Lourdes Veronese, R.M., Costa Passos, A.D. Saloum Deghaide, N., Romeo, E., Tokunaga, N.C. & Donadi, E.A. (2000). HLA typing in patients with AIDS and neurotoxoplasmosis. Presented at XIII International AIDS Conference, 9-14 July, Durban, South Africa, (Abstract MoPeB2141).

CDC. (2009). Guidelines for prevention and treatment of opportunistic infection in HIV-infected adults and adolescents. Recommendations from CDC, the National Institutes of Health, and the HIV Medicine Association of the Infectious Diseases Society of America. *MMWR. Morbidity and Mortality Weekly Report*, Vol.58, No.RR-4, pp. 1-207, ISSN 0149-2195.

Cérède, O., Dubremetz, J.F., Soêten, M., Deslée, D., Vial, H., Bout, D. & Lebrun, M. (2005). Synergistic role of micronemal proteins in *Toxoplasma gondii* virulence. *The Journal of Experimental Medicine*, Vol.201, No.3, pp. 453-463, ISSN 0022-1007.

Cesbron-Delauw, M.F. & Capron, A. (1993). Excreted/secreted antigens of *Toxoplasma gondii*--their origin and role in the host-parasite interaction. *Research in Immunology*, Vol.144, No.1, pp.41-44, ISSN 0923-2494.

Chaddha, D.S., Kalra, S.P., Singh, A.P., Gupta, R.M. & Sanchetee, P.C. (1999). Toxoplasmic encephalitis in acquired immunodeficiency syndrome. *The Journal of the Association of Physicians of India*, Vol.47, No.7, pp. 680-684, ISSN 0004-5772.

Chakraborty, J. (1999). HIV/AIDS and ocular manifestations. *Journal of the Indian Medical Association*, Vol.97, No.8, pp. 299-304, ISSN 14743655.

Chen, K.C., Chen, J.Y. & Tung, G.A. (2009). Case 149: Immune reconstitution inflammatory syndrome. *Radiology*, Vol.252, No.3, pp. 924-928, ISSN 0033-8419.

Chimenti, C., Del Nonno, F., Topino, S., Abbate, I., Licci, S., Paglia, M.G., Capobianchi, M.R., Petrosillo, N. & Frustaci, A. (2007). Fatal myocardial co-infection by *Toxoplasma gondii* and Parvovirus B19 in an HIV patient. *AIDS*, Vol.21, No.10, pp. 1386-1388, ISSN 1473-5571.

Chintana, T., Sukthana, Y., Bunyakai, B. & Lekkla, A. (1998). *Toxoplasma gondii* antibody in pregnant women with and without HIV infection. *Southeast Asian Journal of Tropical Medicine and Public Health*, Vol.29, No.2, pp. 383-386, ISSN 0125-1562.

Chirgwin, K., Hafner, R., Leport, C. Remington, J., Andersen, J., Bosler, E.M., Roque, C., Rajicic, N., McAuliffe, V., Morlat, P., Jayaweera, D.T., Vilde, J.L. & Luft, B.J. (2002). Randomized phase II trial of atovaquone with pyrimethamine or sulfadiazine for treatment of toxoplasmic encephalitis in patients with acquired immunodeficiency syndrome: ACTG 237/ANRS 039 Study. AIDS Clinical Trials Group 237/Agence Nationale de Recherche sur le SIDA, Essai 039. *Clinical Infectious Diseases*, Vol.34, No.9, pp. 1243-1250, ISSN 1058-4838.

Ciricillo, S.F. & Rosenblum, M.L. (1990). Use of CT and MR imaging to distinguish intracranial lesions and to define the need for biopsy in AIDS patients. *Journal of Neurosurgery*, Vol.73, No.5, pp.720-724, ISSN 0022-3085.

Collazos, J. (2003). Opportunistic infections of the CNS in patients with AIDS: diagnosis and management. *CNS Drugs*, Vol.17, No.12, pp. 869-887, ISSN 1172-7047.

Corti, M., Metta, H., Villafañe, M.F., Yampolsky, C., Schtirbu, R., Sevlever, G. & Garrido, D. (2008). Stereotactic brain biopsy in the diagnosis of focal brain lesions in AIDS. *Medicina*, Vol.68, No.4, pp. 285-290, ISSN 0025-7680.

Costa-Silva, T.A., Meira, C.S., Ferreira, I.M., Hiramoto, R.M. & Pereira-Chioccola, V.L. (2008). Evaluation of immunization with tachyzoite excreted-secreted proteins in a novel susceptible mouse model (A/Sn) for *Toxoplasma gondii*. *Experimental Parasitology*, Vol.120, No.3, pp.227-234, ISSN 0014-4894.

Cota, G.F., Assad, E.C., Christo, P.P., Giannetti, A.V., Santos Filho, J.A. & Xavier, M.A. (2008). Ventriculitis: a rare case of primary cerebral toxoplasmosis in AIDS patient and literature review. *The Brazilian Journal of Infectious Diseases*, Vol.12, No.1, pp. 101-104, ISSN 1413-8670.

Cruz, M.L., Cardoso, C.A., Saavedra, M.C., Santos, E.D. & Melino, T. (2007). Congenital toxoplasmosis infection in an infant born to an HIV-1-infected mother. *Brazilian Journal of Infectious Diseases*, Vol.11, No. 6, pp. 610-611, ISSN 1413-8670.

Dal Pan, G.J. & McArthur, J.C. (1996). Neuroepidemiology of HIV infection. *Neurologic Clinics*, Vol.14, No.2, pp. 359-382, ISSN 0733-8619.

Dankner, W.M., Lindsey, J.C., Levin, M.J., Pediatric AIDS Clinical Trials Group Protocol Teams 051, 128, 138, 144, 152, 179, 190, 220, 240, 245, 254, 300 and 327. (2001). Correlates of opportunistic infections in children infected with the human immunodeficiency virus managed before highly active antiretroviral therapy. *The Pediatric Infectious Disease Journal*, Vol.20, No.1, pp. 40-48, ISSN 0891-3668.

Dardé, M.L. (1996). Biodiversity in *Toxoplasma gondii*. *Current Topics in Microbiology and Immunology*, Vol.219, pp. 27-41, ISSN 0070-217X.

Dardé, M.L., Bouteille, B. & Pestre-Alexandre, M. (1992). Isoenzyme analysis of 35 *Toxoplasma gondii* isolates and the biological and epidemiological implications. *Journal of Parasitology*, Vol.78, No.5, pp. 786-794, ISSN 0022-3395.

de Boer, M.G., Kroon, F.P., Kauffmann, R.H., Vriesendorp, R., Zwinderman, K. & van Dissel, J.T. (2003). Immune restoration disease in HIV-infected individuals receiving highly active antiretroviral therapy: clinical and immunological characteristics. *The Netherlands Journal of Medicine*, Vol.61, No.12, pp. 408-412, ISSN 0300-2977.

Dedicoat, M. & Livesley, N. (2006). Management of toxoplasmic encephalitis in HIV-infected adults (with an emphasis on resource-poor settings). *Cochrane Database of systematic reviews*, Vol.3, pp. CD005420, ISSN 1613-4125

de Gans, J., Portegies, P., Reiss, P., Troost, D., van Gool, T. & Lange, J.M. (1992). Pyrimethamine alone as maintenance therapy for central nervous system toxoplasmosis in 38 patients with AIDS. *Journal of Acquired Immune Deficiency Syndromes*, Vol.5, No.2, pp. 137-142, ISSN 0894-9255.

Denkers, E.Y. (2003) From cells to signaling cascades: manipulation of innate immunity by *Toxoplasma gondii*. *FEMS Immunology & Medical Microbiology*, Vol.39, No.3, pp.193-203, ISSN: 1574-695X.

Derouin, F., Pelloux, H. & ESCMID Study Group on Clinical Parasitology. (2008). Prevention of toxoplasmosis in transplant patients. *Clinical Microbiology & Infection*, Vol.14, No.12, pp.1089-1101, ISSN 1198-743X.

Dhiver, C., Milandre, C., Poizot-Martin, I., Drogoul, M.P., Gastaut, J.L. & Gastaut, J.A. (1993). 5-Fluoro-uracil-clindamycin for treatment of cerebral toxoplasmosis. *AIDS*, Vol.7, No.1, pp. 143-144, ISSN 1473-5571.

Dubey, J.P. (1998). Advances in the life cycle of *Toxoplasma gondii*. *International Journal of Parasitology*, Vol.28, No.7, pp.1019-1024, ISSN 0020-7519.

Dubey, J.P., Lindsay, D.S. & Speer, C.A. (1998). Structures of *Toxoplasma gondii* tachyzoites, bradyzoites, and sporozoites and biology and development of tissue cysts. *Clinical Microbiology Review*, Vol.11, No.2, pp.267-299, ISSN 0893-8512.

Dunay, I.R., Heimesaat, M.M., Bushrab, F.N., Müller, R.H., Stocker, H., Arasteh, K., Kurowski, M., Fitzner, R., Borner, K. & Liesenfeld, O. (2004). Atovaquone maintenance therapy prevents reactivation of toxoplasmic encephalitis in a murine model of reactivated toxoplasmosis. *Antimicrobial Agents and Chemotherapy*, Vol.48, No.12, pp. 4848-4854, ISSN 0066-4804.

Dunn, D., Newell, M.L. & Gilbert, R. (1997). Low risk of congenital toxoplasmosis in children born to women infected with human immunodeficiency virus. *The Pediatric Infectious Disease Journal*, Vol.16, No.1, pp. 84, ISSN 0891-3668.

Dupon, M., Cazenave, J., Pellegrin, J.L., Ragnaud, J.M., Cheyrou, A., Fischer, I., Leng, B. & Lacut, J.Y. (1995). Detection of *Toxoplasma gondii* by PCR and tissue culture in cerebrospinal fluid and blood of human immunodeficiency virus-seropositive patients. *Journal of Clinical Microbiology*, Vol.33, No.9, pp. 2421-2426, ISSN 0095-1137.

Dupouy-Camet, J., de Souza, S.L., Maslo, C., Paugam, A., Saimot, A.G., Benarous, R., Tourte-Schaefer, C. & Derouin, F. (1993). Detection of *Toxoplasma gondii* in venous blood from AIDS patients by polymerase chain reaction. *Journal of Clinical Microbiology*, Vol.31, No.7, pp. 1866-1869, ISSN 0095-1137.

Duran, J.M., Cretel, E., Bagneres, D., Guillemot, E., Kaplanski, G. & Soubeyrand, J. (1995). Failure of atovaquone in the treatment of cerebral toxoplasmosis. *AIDS*, Vol.9, No.7, pp. 812-813, ISSN 1473-5571.

Duval, X., Pajot, O., Le Moing, V., Longuet, P., Ecobichon, J.L., Mentre, F., Leport, C. & Vilde, J.L. (2004). Maintenance therapy with cotrimoxazole for toxoplasmic encephalitis in the era of highly active antiretroviral therapy. *AIDS*, Vol.18, No.9, pp. 1342-1344, ISSN 1473-5571.

Emeka, E.U., Ogunrin, A.O. & Olubunmi, A. (2010). Cerebellar toxoplasmosis in HIV/AIDS: a case report. *West African Journal of Medicine*, Vol.29, No.2, pp. 123-126, ISSN 0189-160X.

Eza, D., Cerrillo, G., Moore, D.A. Castro, C., Ticona, E., Morales, D., Cabanillas, J., Barrantes, F., Alfaro, A., Benavides, A., Rafael, A., Valladares, G., Arevalo, F., Evans, C.A. & Gilman, RH. (2006). Postmortem findings and opportunistic infections in HIV-positive patients from a public hospital in Peru. *Pathology Research and Practice*, Vol.202, No.11, pp. 767-775, ISSN 0344-0338.

Falusi O, French AL, Seaberg EC, Tien, P.C., Watts, D.H., Minkoff, H., Piessens ,E., Kovacs, A., Anastos, K. & Cohen, M.H. (2002). Prevalence and predictors of *Toxoplasma* seropositivity in women with and at risk for human immunodeficiency virus infection. *Clinical Infectious Diseases*, Vol.35, No.11, pp. 1414-1417, ISSN 1058-4838.

Fernandes, R.C., Vasconcellos, V.P., Araújo, L.C. & Medina-Acosta, E. (2009). Vertical transmission of HIV and *Toxoplasma* by reactivation in a chronically infected woman. *The Brazilian Journal of Infectious Diseases*, Vol.13, No.1, pp. 70-71, ISSN 1413-8670.

Fernandez-Martin, J., Leport, C., Morlat, P., Meyohas, M.C., Chauvin, J.P. & Vilde, J.L. (1991). Pyrimethamine-clarithromycin combination for therapy of acute *Toxoplasma* encephalitis in patients with AIDS. *Antimicrobial Agents and Chemotherapy*, Vol.35, No.10, pp. 2049-2052, ISSN 0066-4804.

Ferreira, I.M., Vidal, J.E., Costa-Silva, T.A., Meira, C.S., Hiramoto, R.M., Penalva de Oliveira, A.C. & Pereira-Chioccola, V.L. (2008). *Toxoplasma gondii*: genotyping of strains from Brazilian AIDS patients with cerebral toxoplasmosis by multilocus PCR-RFLP markers. *Experimental Parasitology*, Vol.118, No. 2, pp.221-227, ISSN 0014-4894.

Fournier, S., Rabian, C., Alberti, C., Carmagnat, M.V., Garin, J.F., Charron, D., Derouin, F. & Molina, J.M. (2001). Immune recovery under highly active antiretroviral therapy is associated with restoration of lymphocyte proliferation and interferon-gamma production in the presence of *Toxoplasma gondii* antigens. *The Journal of Infectious Diseases*, Vol.183, No.11, pp. 1586-1591, ISSN 0022-1899.

Frenkel, J.K. (1973). *Toxoplasma* in and around us. *Journal of Biological Sciences*, Vol.23, pp.343-352, ISSN 1727-3048.

Fuentes, I., Rubio, J.M., Ramírez, C. & Alvar, J. (2001). Genotypic characterization of *Toxoplasma gondii* strains associated with human toxoplasmosis in Spain: direct analysis from clinical samples. *Journal of Clinical Microbiology*, Vol.39, No.4, pp. 1566-1570, ISSN 0095-1137.

Furco, A., Carmagnat, M., Chevret, S., Garin, Y.J., Pavie, J., De Castro, N., Charron, D., Derouin, F., Rabian, C. & Molina, J.M. (2008). Restoration of *Toxoplasma gondii*-specific immune responses in patients with AIDS starting HAART. *AIDS*, Vol.22, No.16, pp. 2087-2096, ISSN 1473-5571.

Gagliuso, D.J., Teich, S.A., Friedman, A.H. & Orellana, J. (1990). Ocular toxoplasmosis in AIDS patients. *Transactions of the American Ophthalmological Society*, Vol.90, pp. 63-86, discussion 86-88, ISSN 0065-9533.

Gallo, B.V., Shulman, L.M., Weiner, W.J., Petito, C.K. & Berger, J.R. (1996). HIV encephalitis presenting with severe generalized chorea. *Neurology*, Vol.46, No.4, pp. 1163-1165, ISSN 0028-3878.

Galván Ramírez, M.L., Valdez Alvarado, V., Vargas Gutierrez, G., Jiménez González, O., García Cosio, C. & Vielma Sandoval, M. (1997). Prevalence of IgG and IgM anti-*Toxoplasma* antibodies in patients with HIV and acquired immunodeficiency syndrome (AIDS). *Revista da Sociedade Brasileira de Medicina Tropical*, Vol.30, No.6, pp. 465-467, ISSN 0037-8682.

Genot, S., Franck, J., Forel, J.M., Rebaudet, S., Ajzenberg, D., de Paula, A.M., Dardé, M.L., Stein, A. & Ranque, S. (2007). Severe *Toxoplasma gondii* I/III recombinant-genotype encephalitis in a human immunodeficiency virus patient. *Journal of Clinical Microbiology*, Vol.45, No.9, pp. 3138-3140, ISSN 0095-1137.

Gill, P.S., Graham, R.A., Boswell, W., Meyer, P., Krailo, M. & Levine, A.M. (1986). A comparison of imaging, clinical, and pathologic aspects of space-occupying lesions within the brain in patients with acquired immune deficiency syndrome. *American Journal of Physiologic Imaging*, Vol.1, No.3, pp. 134-141, ISSN 0885-8276.

González-Castillo, J., Blanco, F., Soriano, V., Barreiro, P., Concepción Bravo, M., Jiménez-Nácher, I. & González-Lahoz, J. (2001). Opportunistic episodes in patients infected with the human immunodeficiency virus during the first 6 months of HAART. *Medicina Clinica*, Vol.17, No.3, pp. 81-84, ISSN 0025-7753.

Grant, I.H., Gold, J.W., Rosenblum, M., Niedzwiecki, D. & Armstrong, D. (1990). *Toxoplasma gondii* serology in HIV-infected patients: the development of central nervous system toxoplasmosis in AIDS. *AIDS*, Vol.4, No.6, pp. 519-521, ISSN 0269-9370.

Gray, F., Bazille, C., Adle-Biassette, H., Mikol, J., Moulignier, A. & Scaravilli, F. (2005). Central nervous system immune reconstitution disease in acquired immunodeficiency syndrome patients receiving highly active antiretroviral treatment. *Journal of Neurovirology*, Vol.11, No.Suppl 3, pp. 16-22, ISSN 1355-0284.

Gross, U., Kempf, M.C., Seeber, F., Lüder, C.G., Lugert, R. & Bohne, W. (1997). Reactivation of chronic toxoplasmosis: is there a link to strain-specific differences in the parasite? *Behring Institute Mitteilungen*, Vol.99, pp. 97-106, ISSN 0955-8810.

Guelar, A., Miró, J.M., Mallolas, J., Zamora, L., Cardenal, C., Gatell, J.M. & Soriano, E. (1994). Therapeutic alternatives for cases of cerebral toxoplasmosis in patients with AIDS: clarithromycin and atovaquone. *Enfermedades Infecciosas y Microbiologia Clinica*, Vol.12, No.3, pp. 137-140, ISSN 0213-005X.

Guerot, E., Aissa, F., Kayal, S., Leselbaum, A., Grenier, O., Guerot, C. & Labrousse, J. (1995). *Toxoplasma* pericarditis in acquired immunodeficiency syndrome. *Intensive Care Medicine*, Vol.21, No.3, pp.229-230, ISSN 0342-4642.

Guex, A.C., Radziwill, A.J. & Bucher, H.C. (2000). Discontinuation of secondary prophylaxis for toxoplasmic encephalitis in human immunodeficiency virus infection after immune restoration with highly active antiretroviral therapy. *Clinical Infectious Diseases*, Vol.30, No.3, pp. 602-603, ISSN 1058-4838.

Gupta, S., Shah, D.M. & Shah, I. (2009). Neurological disorders in HIV-infected children in India. *Annals of Tropical Paediatrics*, Vol.29, No.3, pp. 177-181, ISSN 0272-4936.

Gyori, E. & Hyma, B.A. (1998). Fatal automobile crash caused by cerebral toxoplasmosis. *The American Journal of Forensic Medicine and Pathology*, Vol.19, No.2, pp. 178-180, ISSN 0195-7910.

Habegger de Sorrentino, A., López, R., Motta, P., Marinic, K., Sorrentino, A., Iliovich, E., Rubio, A.E., Quarleri, J. & Salomón, H. (2005). HLA class II involvement in HIV-associated toxoplasmic encephalitis development. *Clinical Immunology*, Vol.115, No.2, pp.133-137, ISSN 1521-6616.

Hari, K.R., Modi, M.R., Mochan, A.H. & Modi, G. (2007). Reduced risk of *Toxoplasma* encephalitis in HIV-infected patients--a prospective study from Gauteng, South Africa. *International Journal of STD & AIDS*, Vol.18, No.8, pp. 555-558, ISSN 0956-4624.

Harris, T.M., Smith, R.R., Bognanno, J.R. & Edwards, M.K. (1990). Toxoplasmic myelitis in AIDS: gadolinium-enhanced MR. *Journal of Computer Assisted Tomography*, Vol. 14, No.5, pp. 809-811, ISSN 0363-8715.

Hedriana, H.L., Mitchell, J.L., Brown, G.M. & Williams, S.B. (1993). Normal fetal outcome in a pregnancy with central nervous system with toxoplasmosis and human immunodeficiency virus infection. A case report. *The Journal of Reproductive Medicine*, Vol.38, No.9, pp.747-750, ISSN 0024-7758.

Hierl, T., Reischl, U., Lang, P., Hebart, H., Stark, M., Kyme, P. & Autenrieth, I.B. (2004). Preliminary evaluation of one conventional nested and two real-time PCR assays for the detection of *Toxoplasma gondii* in immunocompromised patients. *Journal of Medical Microbiology*, Vol.53, No.7, pp. 629-632, ISSN 0022-2615.

Hirose, G. (2000). Parkinsonism in a patient with AIDS. *Internal Medicine*, Vol.39, No.12, pp. 1006-1007, ISSN 0918-2918.

Hoffmann, C., Ernst, M., Meyer, P., Wolf, E., Rosenkranz, T., Plettenberg, A., Stoehr, A., Horst, H.A., Marienfeld, K. & Lange, C. (2007). Evolving characteristics of toxoplasmosis in patients infected with human immunodeficiency virus-1: clinical course and *Toxoplasma gondii*-specific immune responses. *Clinical Microbiology and Infection*, Vol.13, No.5, pp. 510-515, ISSN 1198-743X.

Hofman, P., Quintens, H., Michiels, J.F., Taillan, B., Thyss, A., (1993). *Toxoplasma* cystitis associated with acquired immunodeficiency syndrome. *Urology*, Vol.42, No.5, pp.589-592, ISSN 0090-4295.

Holch, A., Opravil, M., Moradpour, D., Siegenthaler, W., Schneider, J. & Lüthy, R. (1993). Disseminated toxoplasmosis in AIDS. *Deutsche Medizinische Wochenschrift*, Vol.118, No.22, pp. 814-819, ISSN 0012-0472.

Holland, G.N., Engstrom, R.E. Jr., Glasgow, B.J., Berger, B.B., Daniels, S.A., Sidikaro, Y., Harmon, J.A., Fischer, D.H., Boyer, D.S. & Rao, N.A. (1988). Ocular toxoplasmosis in patients with the acquired immunodeficiency syndrome. *American Journal of Ophthalmology*, Vol.106, No.6, pp.653-667, ISSN 0002-9394.

Holliman, R.E. (1990). Serological study of the prevalence of toxoplasmosis in asymptomatic patients infected with human immunodeficiency virus. *Epidemiology and Infection*, Vol.105, No.2, pp. 415-418, ISSN 1469-4409.

Honoré, S., Couvelard, A., Garin, Y.J., Bedel, C., Hénin, D., Dardé, M.L. & Derouin, F. (2000). Genotyping of *Toxoplasma gondii* strains from immunocompromised patients. *Pathologie Biologie*, Vol.48, No.6, pp. 541-547, ISSN 0369-8114.

Howe, D.K., Honoré, S., Derouin, F. & Sibley, L.D. (1997). Determination of genotypes of *Toxoplasma gondii* strains isolated from patients with toxoplasmosis. *Journal of Clinical Microbiology*, Vol.35, No.6, pp.1411-1414, ISSN 0095-1137.

Howe, D.K. & Sibley, L.D. (1995). *Toxoplasma gondii* comprises three clonal lineages: correlation of parasite genotype with human disease. *Journal of Infectious Diseases*, Vol.172, No.6, pp.1561-1566, ISSN 0022-1899.

Ho-Yen, D.O. (1992). Immunocompromised patients, In: *Human Toxoplasmosis*, D.O. Ho-Yen, & A.W.L. Joss, (Eds.), 184-213, Oxford University Press, ISBN 0198547501, New York, USA.

Huber, W., Bautz, W., Classen, M. & Schepp, W. (1995). Pyrimethamine-sulfadiazine resistant cerebral toxoplasmosis in AIDS. *Deutsche Medizinische Wochenschrift*, Vol.120, No.3, pp. 60-64, ISSN 0012-0472.

Hung, C.C., Chen, M.Y., Hsieh, S.M., Hsiao, C.F., Sheng, W.H. & Chang, S.C. (2005). Prevalence of *Toxoplasma gondii* infection and incidence of *Toxoplasma* encephalitis in non-haemophiliac HIV-1-infected adults in Taiwan. *International Journal of STD & AIDS*, Vol.16, No.4, pp. 302-6, ISSN 0956-4624.

Huruy, K., Mulu, A., Mengistu, G., Shewa-Amare, A., Akalu, A., Kassu, A., Andargie, G., Elias, D. & Torben, W. (2008). Immune reconstitution inflammatory syndrome among HIV/AIDS patients during highly active antiretroviral therapy in Addis Ababa, Ethiopia. *Japanese Journal of Infectious Diseases*, Vol.61, No.3, pp. 205-209, ISSN 1344-6304.

Ilniczky, S., Debreczeni, R., Kovács, T., Várkonyi, V., Barsi, P. & Szirmai, I. (2006). [Aids-related *Toxoplasma*-encephalitis presenting with acute psychotic episode]. *Ideggyógyászati Szemle*, Vol.59, No.7-8, pp. 289-293, ISSN 0019-1442.

Israelski, D.M., Chmiel, J.S., Poggensee, L., Phair, J.P. & Remington, J.S. (1993). Prevalence of *Toxoplasma* infection in a cohort of homosexual men at risk of AIDS and toxoplasmic encephalitis. *Journal of Acquired Immune Deficiency Syndrome*, Vol.6, No.4, pp. 414-418, ISSN 0894-9255.

Israelski, D.M. & Remington, J.S. (1992). AIDS-associated toxoplasmosis. In: *The medical management of AIDS*, M.A. Sande, & P.A. Volberding (Eds.), 319-345, WB Saunders, ISBN 0721637310, Philadelphia, USA.

Jacobson, J.M., Hafner, R., Remington, J. Farthing, C., Holden-Wiltse, J., Bosler, E. M., Harris, C., Jayaweera, D.T., Roque, C., Luft, B.J. & Members of the ACTG 156 Study Team.

(2001). Dose-escalation, phase I/II study of azithromycin and pyrimethamine for the treatment of toxoplasmic encephalitis in AIDS. *AIDS*, Vol.15, No.5, pp. 583-589, ISSN 1473-5571.

Jevtović, D.J., Salemović, D., Ranin, J., Pesić, I., Zerjav, S. & Djurković-Djaković, O. (2005). The prevalence and risk of immune restoration disease in HIV-infected patients treated with highly active antiretroviral therapy. *HIV Medicine*, Vol.6, No.2, pp. 140-143, ISSN 1464 -2662.

Jordan, M.K., Burstein, A.H., Rock-Kress, D., Alfaro, R.M., Pau, A.K., Kovacs, J.A. & Piscitelli, S.C. (2004). Plasma pharmacokinetics of sulfadiazine administered twice daily versus four times daily are similar in human immunodeficiency virus-infected patients. *Antimicrobial Agents and Chemotherapy*, Vol.48, No.2, pp. 635-637, ISSN 0066-4804.

Jubault, V., Pacanowski, J., Rabian, C. & Viard, J.P. (2002). Interruption of prophylaxis for major opportunistic infections in HIV-infected patients receiving triple combination antiretroviral therapy. *Annales de Médecine Interne*, Vol.151, No.3, pp. 163-168, ISSN 0003-410X.

Kaplan, J.E., Hanson, D., Dworkin, M.S., Frederick, T., Bertolli, J., Lindegren, M.L., Holmberg, S. & Jones, J.L. (2000). Epidemiology of human immunodeficiency virus-associated opportunistic infections in the United States in the era of highly active antiretroviral therapy. *Clinical Infectious Diseases*, Vol.30, No.Suppl 1, pp. S5-S14, ISSN 1058-4838.

Kastenbauer, U., Wolf, E., Kollan, C., Hamouda, O., Bogner, J.R. & ClinSurv Study Group. (2009). Impaired CD4-cell immune reconstitution upon HIV therapy in patients with toxoplasmic encephalitis compared to patients with pneumocystis pneumonia as AIDS indicating disease. *European Journal of Medical Research*, Vol.14, No.6, pp. 244-249, ISSN 0949-2321.

Katlama, C., De Wit, S., O'Doherty, E., Van Glabeke, M. & Clumeck, N. (1996a). Pyrimethamine-clindamycin vs. pyrimethamine-sulfadiazine as acute and long-term therapy for toxoplasmic encephalitis in patients with AIDS. *Clinical Infectious Diseases*, Vol.22, No.2, pp. 268-275, ISSN 1058-4838.

Katlama, C., Mouthon, B., Gourdon, D., Lapierre, D. & Rousseau, F. (1996b). Atovaquone as long-term suppressive therapy for toxoplasmic encephalitis in patients with AIDS and multiple drug intolerance. Atovaquone Expanded Access Group. *AIDS*, Vol.10, No.10, pp. 1107-1112, ISSN 1473-5571.

Khan, A., Su, C., German, M., Storch, G.A., Clifford, D.B. & Sibley, L.D. (2005). Genotyping of *Toxoplasma gondii* strains from immunocompromised patients reveals high prevalence of type I strains. *Journal of Clinical Microbiology*, Vol.43, No.12, pp. 5881-5887, ISSN 0095-1137.

Klotz, S.A., Aziz Mohammed, A., Girmai Woldemichael, M., Worku Mitku, M., Handrich, M. (2009). Immune reconstitution inflammatory syndrome in a resource-poor setting. *Journal of the International association of Physicians in AIDS Care*, Vol.8, No.2, pp. 122-127, ISSN 1545-1097.

Kong, J.T., Grigg, M.E., Uyetake, L., Parmley, S. & Boothroyd, J.C. (2003). Serotyping of *Toxoplasma gondii* infections in humans using synthetic peptides. *The Journal of Infectious Diseases*, Vol.187, No.9, pp. 1484-1495, ISSN 0022-1899.

Kongsaengdao, S. (2009). Neurologic immune reconstitution inflammatory syndrome in HIV/AIDS: outcome and epidemiology. *Neurology*, Vol.73, No.23, pp. 2046-2047, ISSN 0028-3878.

Koppel, B.S. & Daws, M. (1990). Rubral tremor due to midbrain toxoplasmosis abscess. *Movement Disorders*, Vol.5, No.3, pp. 254-256, ISSN 0885-3185.

Kovari, H., Ebnöther, C., Schweiger, A., Berther, N., Kuster, H. & Günthard, H.F. (2010). Pulmonary toxoplasmosis, a rare but severe manifestation of a common opportunistic infection in late HIV presenters: report of two cases. *Infection*, Vol.38, No.2, pp.141-144, ISSN 0300-8126.

Kumarasamy, N., Venkatesh, K.K., Devaleenol, B., Poongulali, S., Yephthomi, T., Pradeep, A., Saghayam, S., Flanigan, T., Mayer, K.H. & Solomon, S. (2010). Factors associated with mortality among HIV-infected patients in the era of highly active antiretroviral therapy in southern India. *Internal Journal of Infectious Diseases*, Vol.4, No.2, pp. e127-e131, ISSN 1201-9712.

Kung, D.H., Hubenthal, E.A., Kwan, J.Y., Shelburne, S.A., Goodman, J.C. & Kass, J.S. (2011). Toxoplasmosis myelopathy and myopathy in an AIDS patient: a case of immune reconstitution inflammatory syndrome? *The Neurologist*, Vol.17, No.1, pp. 49-51, ISSN 1074-7931.

Kuritzkes, D.R., Shugarts, D., Bakhtiari, M., Poticha, D., Johnson, J., Rubin, M., Gingeras, T.R., Kennedy, M., & Eron, J.J. (2000). Emergence of dual resistance to zidovudine and lamivudine in HIV-1-infected patients treated with zidovudine plus lamivudine as initial therapy. *Journal of Acquired Immune Deficiency Syndromes*, Vol.23, No.1, pp. 26-34, ISSN 0894-9255.

Lafeuillade, A., Pellegrino, P., Poggi, C., Profizi, N., Quilichini, R., Chouette, I. & Navarreté, M.S. (1993). Efficacy of atovaquone in resistant toxoplasmosis in AIDS. *Presse médicale*, Vol.22, No.33, pp.1708, ISSN 0755-4982.

Lago, E.G., Conrado, G.S., Piccoli, C.S., Carvalho, R.L. & Bender, A.L. (2009). *Toxoplasma gondii* antibody profile in HIV-infected pregnant women and the risk of congenital toxoplasmosis. *European Journal of Clinical Microbiology & Infectious Diseases*, Vol.28, No.4, pp. 345-351, ISSN 0934-9723.

Lamichhane, G., Shah, D.N., Sharma, S. & Chaudhary, M. (2010). Ocular manifestations in HIV/AIDS cases in Nepal. *Nepalese Journal of Ophthalmology*, Vol.2, No.1, pp. 45-50, ISSN 2072-6805.

Langford, T.D., Letendre, S.L., Larrea, G.J. & Masliah, E. (2003). Changing patterns in the neuropathogenesis of HIV during the HAART era. *Brain Pathology*, Vol.13, No.2, pp. 195-210, ISSN 1015-6305.

Lanjewar, D.N., Jain, P.P. & Shetty, C.R. (1998a). Profile of central nervous system pathology in patients with AIDS: an autopsy study from India. *AIDS*, Vol.12, No.3, pp. 309-313, ISSN 1473-5571.

Lanjewar, D.N., Surve, K.V., Maheshwari, M.B., Shenoy, B.P. & Hira, S.K. (1998b). Toxoplasmosis of the central nervous system in the acquired immunodeficiency syndrome. *Indian Journal of Pathology & Microbiology*, Vol.41, No.2, pp.147-151, ISSN 0377-4929.

Lanoy, E., Guiguet, M., Bentata, M., Rouveix, E., Dhiver, C., Poizot-Martin, I., Costagliola, D., Gasnault, J. & FHDH-ANRS CO4. (2011). Survival after neuroAIDS: Association with antiretroviral CNS Penetration-Effectiveness score. *Neurology*, Vol.76, No.7, pp. 644-651, ISSN 0028-3878.

Lawn, S.D. & Wilkinson, R.J. (2006). Immune reconstitution disease associated with parasitic infections following antiretroviral treatment. *Parasite Immunology*, Vol.28, No.11, pp. 625-633, ISSN 0141-9838.

Leport, C., Bastuji-Garin, S., Perronne, C., Salmon, D., Marche, C., Briçaire, F. & Vilde, J.L. (1989). An open study of the pyrimethamine-clindamycin combination in AIDS patients with brain toxoplasmosis. *Journal of Infectious Diseases*, Vol.160, No.3, pp.557-558, ISSN 0022-1899.

Leport, C., Raffi, F., Matheron, S., Katlama, C., Regnier, B., Saimot, A.G., Marche, C., Vedrenne, C. & Vilde, J.L. (1988). Treatment of central nervous system toxoplasmosis with pyrimethamine/sulfadiazine combination in 35 patients with the acquired immunodeficiency syndrome. Efficacy of long-term continuous therapy. *The American Journal of Medicine*, Vol.84, No.1, pp. 94-100, ISSN 0002-9343.

Letillois, M.F., Laigle, V., Santoro, F., Micoud, M. & Chumpitazi, B.F. (1995). *Toxoplasma gondii* surface antigen-1 in sera of HIV-infected patients as an indicator of reactivated toxoplasmosis. *European Journal of Clinical Microbiology & Infectious Diseases*, Vol.14, No.10, pp. 899-903, ISSN 0934-9723.

Lian, Y.L., Heng, B.S., Nissapatorn, V. & Lee, C. (2007). AIDS-defining illnesses: a comparison between before and after commencement of highly active antiretroviral therapy (HAART). *Current HIV Research*, Vol.5, No.5, pp. 484-489, ISSN 1570-162X.

Lin, D.S. & Bowman, D.D. (1992). *Toxoplasma gondii*: an AIDS enhancing cofactor. *Medical Hypotheses*, Vol.39, No.2, pp. 140-142, ISSN 0306-9877.

Lindström, I., Kaddu-Mulindwa, D.H., Kironde, F. & Lindh, J. (2006). Prevalence of latent and reactivated *Toxoplasma gondii* parasites in HIV-patients from Uganda. *Acta Tropica*, Vol.100, No.3, pp. 218-222, ISSN 0001-706X.

Lucas, S.B., Hounnou, A., Peacock, C., Beaumel, A., Djomand, G., N'Gbichi, J.M., Yeboue, K., Hondé, M., Diomande, M., Giordano, C., Doorly, R., Brattegaard, K., Kestens, L., Smithwick, R., Kadio, A., Ezani, N., Yapi, A. & De Cock, K.M. (1993). The mortality and pathology of HIV infection in a West Africa city. *AIDS*, Vol.7, No.12, pp.1569-1579, ISSN 1473-5571.

Luft, B.J. & Remington, J.S. (1985). Toxoplasmosis of the central nervous system. In: *Current clinical topics in infectious diseases*, J.S. Remington, M.N. Swartz, (Eds.), 315-358, McGraw-Hill, ISBN 0070518556, New York. USA.

Luft, B.J. & RemIngton, J.S. (1988). AIDS Commentary. Toxoplasmic encephalitis. *Journal of Infectious Diseases*, Vol. 157, No.1, pp.1-6. ISSN 0022-1899.

Luft, B.J. & Remington, J.S. (1992). Toxoplasmic encephalitis in AIDS. *Clinical Infectious Diseases*, Vol.15, No.2, pp. 211-222, ISSN 1058-4838.

Machala, L., Malý, M., Hrdá, S., Rozsypal, H., Stanková, M. & Kodym, P. (2009). Antibody response of HIV-infected patients to latent, cerebral and recently acquired toxoplasmosis. *European Journal of Clinical Microbiology & Infectious Diseases*, Vol.28, No.2, pp. 179-182, ISSN 0934-9723.

Maggi, P., de Mari, M., De Blasi, R., Armenise, S., Romanelli, C., Andreula, C., Zimatore, G. & Angarano, G. (1996). Choreoathetosis in acquired immune deficiency syndrome patients with cerebral toxoplasmosis. *Movement Disorders*, Vol.11, No.4, pp. 434-436, ISSN 0885-3185.

Maher, J., Choudhri, S., Halliday, W., Power, C. & Nath, A. (1997). AIDS dementia complex with generalized myoclonus. *Movement Disorders*, Vol.12, No.4, pp. 593-597, ISSN 0885-3185.

Maïga, I., Kiemtoré, P. & Tounkara, A. (2001). Prevalence of antitoxoplasma antibodies in patients with Acquired immunodeficiency syndrome and blood donors in Bamako. *Bulletin de la Société de pathologie exotique*, Vol.94, No.3, pp. 268-270, ISSN 0002-9637.

Mansour, A.M. (1990). Neuro-ophthalmic findings in acquired immunodeficiency syndrome. *Journal of Clinical Neuro-Ophthalmology*, Vol.10, No.3, pp. 167-174, ISSN 0272-846X.

Manzardo, C., Del Mar Ortega, M., Sued, O., García, F., Moreno, A. & Miró, J.M. (2005). Central nervous system opportunistic infections in developed countries in the highly active antiretroviral therapy era. *Journal of Neurovirology*, Vol.11, No.Suppl 3, pp. 72-82, ISSN 1355-0284.

Martin-Blondel, G., Alvarez, M., Delobel, P., Uro-Coste, E., Cuzin, L., Cuvinciuc, V., Fillaux J., Massip, P. & Marchou, B. (2010). Toxoplasmic encephalitis IRIS in HIV-infected patients: a case series and review of the literature. *Journal of Neurology, Neurosurgery, and Psychiatry*, 10.1136/JNNP.2009.199919, ISSN 0022-3050.

Masliah, E., DeTeresa, R.M., Mallory, M.E. & Hansen, L.A. (2000). Changes in pathological findings at autopsy in AIDS cases for the last 15 years. *AIDS*, Vol.14, No.1, pp. 69-74, ISSN 1473-5571.

Mastroianni, A., Coronado, O., Scarani, P., Manfredi, R. & Chiodo, F. (1996). Liver toxoplasmosis and acquired immunodeficiency syndrome. *Recenti Progressi in Medicina*, Vol.87, No.7-8, pp.353-355, ISSN 0034-1193.

McCombe, J.A., Auer, R.N., Maingat, F.G., Houston, S., Gill, M.J. & Power, C. (2009). Neurologic immune reconstitution inflammatory syndrome in HIV/AIDS: outcome and epidemiology. *Neurology*, Vol.72, No.9, pp. 835-841, ISSN 0028-3878.

McFadden, D.C., Camps, M. & Boothroyd, J.C. (2001). Resistance as a tool in the study of old and new drug targets in *Toxoplasma*. *Drug Resistance Updates*, Vol.4, No.2, pp. 79-84, ISSN 1368-7646.

Meira, C.S., Costa-Silva, T.A., Vidal, J.E., Ferreira, I.M., Hiramoto, R.M. & Pereira-Chioccola, V.L. (2008). Use of the serum reactivity against *Toxoplasma gondii* excreted-secreted antigens in cerebral toxoplasmosis diagnosis in human immunodeficiency virus-infected patients. *Journal of Medical Microbiology*, Vol.57, No.Pt 7, pp. 845-850, ISSN 0022-2615.

Meisheri, Y.V., Mehta, S. & Patel, U. (1997). A prospective study of seroprevalence of Toxoplasmosis in general population, and in HIV/AIDS patients in Bombay, India. *Journal of Postgraduate Medicine*, Vol.43, No.4, pp. 93-97, ISSN 0022-3859.

Merzianu, M., Gorelick, S.M., Paje, V., Kotler, D.P. & Sian, C. (2005). Gastric toxoplasmosis as the presentation of acquired immunodeficiency syndrome. *Archives of Pathology & Laboratory Medicine*, Vol.129, No.4, pp.e87-e90, ISSN 0003-9985.

Millogo, A., Ki-Zerbo, G.A., Traoré, W., Sawadogo, A.B., Ouédraogo, I. & Péghini, M. (2000). *Toxoplasma* serology in HIV infected patients and suspected cerebral toxoplasmosis at the Central Hospital of Bobo-Dioulasso (Burkina Faso). *Bulletin de la Société de pathologie exotique*, Vol.93, No.1, pp. 17-19, ISSN 0002-9637.

Minkoff, H., Remington, J.S., Holman, S., Ramirez, R., Goodwin, S. & Landesman, S. (1997). Vertical transmission of toxoplasma by human immunodeficiency virus-infected women. *American Journal of Obstetrics and Gynecology*, Vol.176, No.3, pp. 555-559, ISSN 0002-9378.

Miro, J.M., Lopez, J.C., Podzamczer, D., Peña, J.M., Alberdi, J.C., Martínez, E., Domingo, P., Cosin, J., Claramonte, X., Arribas, J.R., Santín, M., Ribera, E. & GESIDA 04/98 Study Group. (2006). Discontinuation of primary and secondary *Toxoplasma gondii* prophylaxis is safe in HIV-infected patients after immunological restoration with highly active antiretroviral therapy: results of an open, randomized, multicenter clinical trial. *Clinical Infectious Diseases*, Vol.43, No.1, pp. 79-89, ISSN 1058-4838.

Mitchell, C.D., Erlich, S.S., Mastrucci, M.T., Hutto, S.C., Parks, W.P. & Scott, G.B., (1990). Congenital toxoplasmosis occurring in infants perinatally infected with human immunodeficiency virus 1. *The Pediatric Infectious Disease Journal*, Vol.9, No.7, pp. 512-518, ISSN 0891-3668.

Mocroft, A., Vella, S., Benfield, T.L., Chiesi, A., Miller, V., Gargalianos, P., d'Arminio Monforte, A., Yust, I., Bruun, J.N., Phillips, A.N. & Lundgren, J.D., (1998). Changing patterns of mortality across Europe in patients infected with HIV-1. EuroSIDA Study Group. *The Lancet*, Vol.352, No.9142, pp. 1725-1730, ISSN 0140-6736.

Montoya, J.G. & Liesenfeld, O. (2004). Toxoplasmosis. *The Lancet*, Vol.363, No.9425, pp.1965-1976, ISSN 0140-6736.

Moorthy, R.S., Smith, R.E. & Rao, N.A. (1993). Progressive ocular toxoplasmosis in patients with acquired immunodeficiency syndrome. *American Journal of Ophthalmollogy*, Vol.115, No.6, pp. 742-747, ISSN 1549-4713.

Morisset, S., Peyron, F., Lobry, J.R., Garweg, J., Ferrandiz, J., Musset, K., Gomez-Marin, J.E., de la Torre, A., Demar, M., Carme, B., Mercier, C., Garin, J.F. & Cesbron-Delauw, M.F. (2008). Serotyping of *Toxoplasma gondii*: striking homogeneous pattern between symptomatic and asymptomatic infections within Europe and South America. *Microbes and Infections*, Vol.10, No.7, pp. 742-747, ISSN 1286-4579.

Murakami, T., Nakajima, M., Nakamura, T., Hara, A., Uyama, E., Mita, S., Matsushita, S., Uchino, M.. (2000). Parkinsonian symptoms as an initial manifestation in a Japanese patient with acquired immunodeficiency syndrome and *Toxoplasma* infection. *Internal Medicine*, Vol.39, No.12, pp. 1111-1114, ISSN 0918-2918.

Mwanza, J.C., Nyamabo, L.K., Tylleskär, T. & Plant, G.T. (2004). Neuro-ophthalmological disorders in HIV infected subjects with neurological manifestations. *The British Journal of Ophthalmology*, Vol.88, No.11, pp. 1455-1459, ISSN 0007-1161.

Mzileni, M.O., Longo-Mbenza, B. & Chephe, T.J. (2008). Mortality and causes of death in HIV-positive patients receiving antiretroviral therapy at Tshepang Clinic in Doctor George Mukhari Hospital. *Polskie Archiwum Medycyny Wewnętrznej*, Vol.118, No.10, pp. 548-554, ISSN 0032-3772.

Naito, T., Inui, A., Kudo, N., Matsumoto, N., Fukuda, H., Isonuma, H., Sekigawa, I., Dambara, T. & Hayashida, Y. (2007). Seroprevalence of IgG anti-*Toxoplasma* antibodies in asymptomatic patients infected with human immunodeficiency virus in Japan. *Internal Medicine*, Vol.46, No. 14, pp. 1149-1150.

Nascimento, L.V., Stollar, F., Tavares, L.B., Cavasini, C.E., Maia, I.L., Cordeiro, J.A. & Ferreira, M.U. (2001). Risk factors for toxoplasmic encephalitis in HIV-infected patients: a case-control study in Brazil. *Annals of Tropical Medicine and Parasitology*, Vol.95, No.6, pp. 587-593, ISSN 0003-4983.

Nath, A., Hobson, D.E. & Russell, A. (1993). Movement disorders with cerebral toxoplasmosis and AIDS. *Movement Disorders*, Vol.8, No.1, pp. 107-112, ISSN 0885-3185.

Navia, B.A., Petito, C.K., Gold, J.W., Cho, E.S., Jordan, B.D. & Price, R.W. (1986). Cerebral toxoplasmosis complicating the acquired immune deficiency syndrome: clinical and neuropathological findings in 27 patients. *Annals of Neurology*, Vol.19, No.3, pp. 224-238, ISSN 0364-5134.

Neuen-Jacob, E., Figge, C., Arendt, G., Wendtland, B., Jacob, B. & Wechsler, W. (1993). Neuropathological studies in the brains of AIDS patients with opportunistic diseases. *International Journal of Legal Medicine*, Vol.105, No.6, pp. 339-350, ISSN 0937-9827.

Nissapatorn, V., Wattanagoon, Y., Pungpak, S., Supanaranond, W., Bowonwatnuwong, C., Sukthana, Y., Desakorn, V., Khamboonruang, C., Thang, D.Q. & Kumar, S.M. (2001). Seroprevalence of toxoplasmosis in HIV infected patients in Chonburi regional hospital, Chonburi, Thailand. *Tropical Biomedicine*, Vol.18, No.2, pp. 123-129, ISSN 0127-5720.

Nissapatorn, V., Kamarulzaman, A., Init, I., Tan, L.H., Rohela, M., Norliza, A., Chan, L.L., Latt, H.M., Anuar, A.K. & Quek, K.F. (2002). Seroepidemiology of toxoplasmosis among HIV-infected patients and healthy blood donors. *Medical Journal of Malaysia*, Vol.57, No.3, pp. 304-310, ISSN 0300-5283.

Nissapatorn, V., Lee, C.K. & Khairul, A.A. (2003). Seroprevalence of toxoplasmosis among AIDS patients in Hospital Kuala Lumpur, 2001. *Singapore Medical Journal*, Vol.44, No.4, pp. 194-196, ISSN 0037 - 5675.

Nissapatorn V, Lee C, Quek KF, Leong CL, Mahmud R, Abdullah KA. (2004). Toxoplasmosis in HIV/AIDS patients: a current situation. *Japanese Journal of Infectious Diseases*, Vol.57, No.4, pp. 160-165, ISSN 1344-6304.

Nissapatorn, V., Lim, Y.A., Jamaiah, I., Agnes, L.S., Amyliana, K., Wen, C.C., Nurul, H., Nizam, S., Quake, C.T., Valartmathi, C., Woei, C.Y. & Anuar, A.K. (2005). Parasitic infections in Malaysia: changing and challenges. *Southeast Asian Journal of Tropical Medicine and Public Health*, Vol.36, No.suppl4, pp. 50-59, ISSN 01251562.

Nissapatorn, V., Lee, C.K.C., Lim, Y.A.L., Tan, K.S., Jamaiah, I., Rohela, M., Sim, B.L.H., Ahmad, A., Hadita, S., Lott, P.W., Ng, K.T., Poh, M.E., Zuliana, J. & Khairul Anuar, A. (2007). Toxoplasmosis: a silent opportunistic disease in HIV/AIDS patients. *Research Journal of Parasitology* Vol.2, No.1, pp. 23-31, ISSN 1816-4943.

Nissapatorn, V., Sawangjaroen, N., Hortiwakul, T., Jareonmark, B., Andiappan, H. & Siripaitoon P. Prevalence of latent and reactivated *Toxoplasma gondii* infection in HIV-infected patients from Southern Thailand. (In press).

Nobre, V., Braga, E., Rayes, A., Serufo, J.C., Godoy, P., Nunes, N., Antunes, C.M. & Lambertucci, J.R. (2003). Opportunistic infections in patients with AIDS admitted to an university hospital of the Southeast of Brazil. *Revista do Instituto de Medicina Tropical de São Paulo*, Vol.45, No.2, pp. 69-74, ISSN 0036-4665.

Noël, S., Guillaume, M.P., Telerman-Toppet, N. & Cogan, E. (1992). Movement disorders due to cerebral *Toxoplasma gondii* infection in patients with the acquired immunodeficiency syndrome (AIDS). *Acta neurologica Belgica*, Vol.92, No.3, pp. 148-156, ISSN 0300-9009.

Nogueira, S.A., Guedes, A.L., Machado, E.S., Matos, J.A., Costa, T.P., Cortes, E.M. & Lambert, J.S. (2002). Toxoplasmic encephalitis in an HIV infected pregnant woman: successful outcome for both mother and child. *The Brazilian Journal of Infectious Diseases*, Vol.6, No.4, pp. 201-205, ISSN 1413-8670.

Nolla-Salas, J., Ricart, C., D'Olhaberriague, L., Galí, F. & Lamarca, J. (1987). Hydrocephalus: an unusual CT presentation of cerebral toxoplasmosis in a patient with acquired immunodeficiency syndrome. *European Neurology*, Vol.27, No.2, pp. 130-132, ISSN 0014-3022.

Novati, R., Castagna, A., Morsica, G., Vago, L., Tambussi, G., Ghezzi, S., Gervasoni, C., Bisson, C., d'Arminio Monforte, A. & Lazzarin, A. (1994). Polymerase chain reaction for *Toxoplasma gondii* DNA in the cerebrospinal fluid of AIDS patients with focal brain lesions. *AIDS*, Vol.8, No.12, pp. 1691-1694, ISSN 1473-5571.

Oh, M.D., Park, S.W., Kim, H.B., Kim, U.S., Kim, N.J., Choi, H.J., Shin, D.H., Lee, J.S. & Choe, K.(1999). Spectrum of opportunistic infections and malignancies in patients with human immunodeficiency virus infection in South Korea. *Clinical Infectious Diseases* 1999; Vol.29, No.6, pp. 1524-1528, ISSN 1058-4838.

Oksenhendler, E., Charreau, I., Tournerie, C., Azihary, M., Carbon, C. & Aboulker, J.P. (1994). *Toxoplasma gondii* infection in advanced HIV infection. *AIDS*, Vol. 8, No.4, pp. 483-487, ISSN 0269-9370.

O'Riordan, S.E. & Farkas, A.G. (1998). Maternal death due to cerebral toxoplasmosis. *British Journal of Obstetrics and Gynaecology*, Vol.105, No.5, pp. 565-566, ISSN 0306-5456.

Oshinaike, O.O., Okubadejo, N.U., Ojini, F.I. & Danesi, M.A. (2010). A preliminary study of the frequency of focal neurological deficits in HIV/AIDS patients seropositive for *Toxoplasma gondii* IgG in Lagos, Nigeria. *Nigerian Quarterly Journal of Hospital Medicine*, Vol.20, No.3, pp.104-107, ISSN 0189-2657.

Ouermi, D., Simpore, J., Belem, A.M., Sanou, D.S., Karou, D.S., Ilboudo, D., Bisseye, C., Onadja, S.M., Pietra, V., Pignatelli, S., Gnoula, C., Nikiema, J.B. & Kabre, G.B. (2009). Co-infection of *Toxoplasma gondii* with HBV in HIV-infected and uninfected pregnant women in Burkina Faso. *Pakistan Journal of Biological Sciences*, Vol.12, No.17, pp. 1188-1193, ISSN 1028-8880.

Palella, F.J, Jr., Delaney, K.M., Moorman, A.C., Loveless, M.O., Fuhrer, J., Satten, G.A., Aschman, D.J. & Holmberg, S.D. (1998). Declining morbidity and mortality among patients with advanced human immunodeficiency virus infection. HIV Outpatient Study Investigators. *The New England Journal of Medicine*, Vol.338, No.13, pp. 853-860, ISSN 0028-4793.

Pendry, K., Tait, R.C., McLay, A., Yen, D.H., Baird, D. & Burnett, AK. (1990). Toxoplasmosis after BMT for CML. *Bone Marrow Transplantation*, Vol.5, No.1, pp.65-66, ISSN 0268-3369.

Pereira-Chioccola, V.L., Vidal, J.E. & Su, C. (2009). *Toxoplasma gondii* infection and cerebral toxoplasmosis in HIV-infected patients. *Future Microbiology*, Vol.4, No.10, pp. 1363-1379, ISSN 1746-0913.

Pestre, P., Milandre, L., Farnarier, P. & Gallais, H. (1991). Hemichorea in acquired immunodeficiency syndrome. Toxoplasmosis abscess in the striatum. *Revue Neurologique*, Vol.147, No.12, pp. 833-837, ISSN 0035-3787.

Petito, C.K., Cho, E.S., Lemann, W., Navia, B.A. & Price, R.W. (1986). Neuropathology of acquired immunodeficiency syndrome (AIDS): an autopsy review. *Journal of*

Neuropathology and Experimental Neurology, Vol.45, No.6, pp. 635-646, ISSN 0022-3069.

Peyron, F., Lobry, J.R., Musset, K., Ferrandiz, J., Gomez-Marin, J.E., Petersen, E., Meroni, V., Rausher, B., Mercier, C., Picot, S. & Cesbron-Delauw, M.F. (2006). Serotyping of *Toxoplasma gondii* in chronically infected pregnant women: predominance of type II in Europe and types I and III in Colombia (South America). *Microbes and Infections*, Vol.8, No.9-10, pp. 2333-2340, ISSN 1286-4579.

Pfeffer, G., Prout, A., Hooge, J. & Maguire, J. (2009). Biopsy-proven immune reconstitution syndrome in a patient with AIDS and cerebral toxoplasmosis. *Neurology*, Vol.73, No.4, pp. 321-322, ISSN 0028-3878.

Podzamczer, D., Miró, J.M., Bolao, F., Gatell, J.M., Cosin, J., Sirera, G., Domingo, P., Laguna, F., Santamaria, J., Verdejo, J. & The Spanish Toxoplasmosis Study Group. (1995). Twice-weekly maintenance therapy with sulfadiazine-pyrimethamine to prevent recurrent toxoplasmic encephalitis in patients with AIDS. Spanish Toxoplasmosis Study Group. *Annals of Internal Medicine*, Vol.123, No.3, pp. 175-180, ISSN 0003-4819.

Portegies, P., Solod, L., Cinque, P., Chaudhuri, A., Begovac, J., Everall, I., Weber, T., Bojar, M., Martinez-Martin, P. & Kennedy, P.G. (2004). Guidelines for the diagnosis and management of neurological complications of HIV infection. *European Journal of Neurology*, Vol.11, No.5, pp. 297-304, ISSN 1351-5101.

Potasman, I., Resnick, L., Luft, B.J. & Remington, J.S. (1988). Intrathecal production of antibodies against *Toxoplasma gondii* in patients with toxoplasmic encephalitis and the acquired immunodeficiency syndrome (AIDS). *Annnals of Internal Medicine*, Vol.108, No.1, pp. 49-51, ISSN 0003-4819.

Prigione, I., Facchetti, P., Lecordier, L., Deslée, D., Chiesa, S., Cesbron-Delauw, M.F. & Pistoia, V. (2000). T cell clones raised from chronically infected healthy humans by stimulation with *Toxoplasma gondii* excretory-secretory antigens cross-react with live tachyzoites: characterization of the fine antigenic specificity of the clones and implications for vaccine development. *Journal of Immunology*, Vol.164, No.7, pp.3741-3748, ISSN 0022-1767.

Rabaud, C., May, T., Amiel, C., Katlama, C., Leport, C., Ambroise-Thomas, P. & Canton, P. (1994). Extracerebral toxoplasmosis in patients infected with HIV. A French National Survey. *Medicine*, Vol.73, No.6, pp.306-314, ISSN 0025-7974.

Raffi, F., Aboulker, J.P., Michelet, C., Reliquet, V., Pelloux, H., Huart, A., Poizot-Martin, I., Morlat, P., Dupas, B., Mussini, JM. & Leport, C. (1997). A prospective study of criteria for the diagnosis of toxoplasmic encephalitis in 186 AIDS patients. The BIOTOXO Study Group. *AIDS*, Vol.11, No.2, pp. 177-184, ISSN 0269-9370.

Rajagopalan, N., Suchitra, JB., Shet, A., Khan, ZK., Martin-Garcia, J., Nonnemacher, M.R., Jacobson, J.M. & Wigdahl, B. (2009). Mortality among HIV-Infected Patients in Resource Limited Settings: A case controlled analysis of inpatients at a community care center. *American Journal of Infectious Diseases*, Vol.5, No.3, pp. 219-224, ISSN 1553-6203.

Reischl, U., Bretagne, S., Krüger, D., Ernault, P. & Costa, J.M. (2003). Comparison of two DNA targets for the diagnosis of Toxoplasmosis by real-time PCR using fluorescence resonance energy transfer hybridization probes. *BMC Infectious Diseases*, Vol.3, pp. 7, ISSN 1471-2334.

Reiter-Owona, I., Bialek, R., Rockstroh, J.K. & Seitz, H.M. (1998). The probability of acquiring primary *Toxoplasma* infection in HIV-infected patients: results of an 8-year retrospective study. *Infection*, Vol.26, No.1, pp. 20-25, ISSN 0300-8126.

Richards, F.O Jr., Kovacs, J.A. & Luft, B.J. (1995). Preventing toxoplasmic encephalitis in persons infected with human immunodeficiency virus. *Clinical Infectious Diseases*, Vol.21, No.Suppl 1, pp. S49-S56, ISSN 1058-4838.

Rodríguez-Rosado, R., Soriano, V., Dona, C. & González-Lahoz, J. (1998). Opportunistic infections shortly after beginning highly active antiretroviral therapy. *Antiviral Therapy*, Vol.3, No.4, pp. 229-231, ISSN 1359-6535.

Ruf, B., Schürmann, D., Bergmann, F., Schüler-Maué, W., Grünewald, T., Gottschalk, H. J., Witt, H. & Pohle, H.D. (1993). Efficacy of pyrimethamine/sulfadoxine in the prevention of toxoplasmic encephalitis relapses and *Pneumocystis carinii* pneumonia in HIV-infected patients. *European Journal of Clinical Microbiology & Infectious Diseases*, Vol.12, No.5, pp. 325-329, ISSN 0934-9723.

Ruiz, R., Cu-Uvin, S., Fiore, T. & Flanigan, T.P. (1997). Toxoplasmosis in HIV-positive women: seroprevalence and the role of prophylaxis in preventing disease. *AIDS*, Vol.11, No.1, pp. 119-120, ISSN 0269-9370.

Saba, J., Morlat, P., Raffi, F., Hazebroucq, V., Joly, V., Leport, C. & Vildé J. L. (1993). Pyrimethamine plus azithromycin for treatment of acute toxoplasmic encephalitis in patients with AIDS. *European Journal of Clinical Microbiology & Infectious Diseases*, Vol.12, No.11, pp. 853-856, ISSN 0934-9723.

Sadler, M., Brink, N.S. & Gazzard, B.G. (1998). Management of intracerebral lesions in patients with HIV: a retrospective study with discussion of diagnostic problems. *QJM: Monthly Journal of the Association of Physicians*, Vol.91, No.3, pp. 205-217, ISSN 1460-2725.

Schöler, N., Krause, K., Kayser, O., Müller, R.H., Borner, K., Hahn, H. & Liesenfeld, O. (2001). Atovaquone nanosuspensions show excellent therapeutic effect in a new murine model of reactivated toxoplasmosis. *Antimicrobial Agents and Chemotherapy*, Vol.45, No.6, pp. 1771-1779, ISSN 0066-4804.

Schuman, J.S. & Friedman, A.H. (1983). Retinal manifestations of the acquired immune deficiency syndrome (AIDS): cytomegalovirus, *Candida albicans*, cryptococcus, toxoplasmosis and *Pneumocystis carinii*. *Transactions of the Ophthalmological Societies of the United Kingdom*, Vol.103, No.Pt2, pp. 177-190, ISSN 0078-5334.

Sendi, P., Sachers, F., Drechsler, H. & Graber, P. (2006). Immune recovery vitritis in an HIV patient with isolated toxoplasmic retinochoroiditis. AIDS, Vol.20, No.17, pp. 2237-2238, ISSN 0269-9370.

Shah, I. (2011). Immune Reconstitution Syndrome in HIV-1 Infected Children-A Study from India. *Indian Journal of Pediatrics*, Vol.78, No.5, pp. 540-543, ISSN 0019-5456.

Shamilah, H., Hakim, L., Noor Azian, S., Malkith, K.M.Y. & Yisri, M.Y. (2001). Seroprevalence of *Toxoplasma gondii* antibodies in HIV positive and negative patients using the immunofluorescence antibody test (IFAT) methods. *Tropical Biomedicine*, Vol.18, No.2, pp. 137-141, ISSN 0127-5720.

Shankar, S.K., Mahadevan, A., Satishchandra, P., Kumar, R.U., Yasha, T.C., Santosh, V., Chandramuki, A., Ravi, V. & Nath, A. (2005). Neuropathology of HIV/AIDS with an overview of the Indian scene. *The Indian Journal of Medical Research*, Vol.121, No.4, pp. 468-488, ISSN 0971-5916.

Sharma, S.K., Kadhiravan, T., Banga, A., Goyal, T., Bhatia, I. & Saha, P.K. (2004). Spectrum of clinical disease in a series of 135 hospitalised HIV-infected patients from north India. *BMC Infectious Diseases*, Vol.22, No.4, pp. 52. ISSN 1471-2334.

Shivaprakash, M.R., Parija, S.C. & Sujatha, S. (2001). Seroprevalence of toxoplasmosis in HIV infected patients in Pondicherry. *Journal of Communicable Diseases*, Vol.33, No.3, pp. 221-223, ISSN 0019-5138.

Silva, M.T. & Araújo, A. (2005). Highly active antiretroviral therapy access and neurological complications of human immunodeficiency virus infection: impact versus resources in Brazil. *Journal of Neurovirology*, Vol.11, No.Suppl 3, pp. 11-15, ISSN 1355-0284.

Sitoe, S.P., Rafael, B., Meireles, L.R., Andrade, H.F. Jr. & Thompson, R. (2010). Preliminary report of HIV and *Toxoplasma gondii* occurrence in pregnant women from Mozambique. *Revista do Instituto de Medicina Tropical de São Paulo*, Vol.52, No.6, pp. 291-295, ISSN 0036-4665.

Sousa, S., Ajzenberg, D., Vilanova, M., Costa, J. & Dardé, M.L. (2008). Use of GRA6-derived synthetic polymorphic peptides in an immunoenzymatic assay to serotype *Toxoplasma gondii* in human serum samples collected from three continents. *Clinical and Vaccine Immunology*, Vol.15, No.9, pp. 1380-1386, ISSN 1556-6811.

Sousa, S., Ajzenberg, D., Marle, M., Aubert, D., Villena, I., da Costa, J.C. & Dardé, M.L. (2009). Selection of polymorphic peptides from GRA6 and GRA7 sequences of *Toxoplasma gondii* strains to be used in serotyping. *Clinical and Vaccine Immunology*, Vol.16, No.8, pp. 1158-1169, ISSN 1556-6811.

Stout, J.E., Lai, J.C., Giner, J. & Hamilton, C.D. (2002). Reactivation of retinal toxoplasmosis despite evidence of immune response to highly active antiretroviral therapy. *Clinical Infectious Diseases*, Vol.35, No.4, pp. e37-e39, ISSN 1058-4838.

Subsai, K., Kanoksri, S., Siwaporn, C. & Helen, L. (2004). Neurological complications in AIDS patients: the 1-year retrospective study in Chiang Mai University, Thailand. *European Journal of Neurology*, Vol.11, No.11, pp. 755-759, ISSN 1351-5101.

Subsai, K., Kanoksri, S., Siwaporn, C., Helen, L., Kanokporn, O. & Wantana, P. (2006). Neurological complications in AIDS patients receiving HAART: a 2-year retrospective study. *European Journal of Neurology*, Vol.13, No.3, pp. 233-239, ISSN 1351-5101.

Sukthana, Y., Chintana, T. & Lekkla, A. (2000). *Toxoplasma gondii* antibody in HIV-infected persons. *Journal of the Medical Association of Thailand*, Vol.83, No.6, pp. 681-684, ISSN 0125-2208.

Suzuki, Y., Conley, F.K. & Remington, J.S. (1989). Importance of endogenous IFN-gamma for prevention of toxoplasmic encephalitis in mice. *Journal of Immunology*, Vol.143, No.6, pp. 2045-2050, ISSN 0022-1767.

Sýkora, J., Zástěra, M. & Stanková, M. (1992). Toxoplasmic antibodies in sera of HIV-infected persons. *Folia Parasitologica*, Vol.39, No.2, pp. 177-180, ISSN 0015-5683.

Tenter, A.M., Heckeroth, A.R. & Weiss, L.M. (2000). *Toxoplasma gondii*: from animals to humans. *International Journal of Parasitology*, Vol.30, No.12-13, pp.1217-1258, ISSN 0020-7519.

Tilley, M., Fichera, M.E., Jerome, M.E., Roos, D.S. & White, M.W. (1997). *Toxoplasma gondii* sporozoites form a transient parasitophorous vacuole that is impermeable and contains only a subset of dense-granule proteins. *Infection and Immunity*, Vol.65, No.11, pp.4598-605, ISSN 1098-5522.

Tolge, C.F. & Factor, S.A. (1991). Focal dystonia secondary to cerebral toxoplasmosis in a patient with acquired immune deficiency syndrome. *Movement Disorders*, Vol.6, No.1, pp. 69-72, ISSN 0885-3185.

Torre, D., Speranza, F., Martegani, R., Zeroli, C., Banfi, M. & Airoldi, M. (1998). A retrospective study of treatment of cerebral toxoplasmosis in AIDS patients with trimethoprim-sulphamethoxazole. *The Journal of Infection*, Vol.37, No.1, pp. 15-18, ISSN 3163-4453.

Torres, R.A., Weinberg, W., Stansell, J., Leoung, G., Kovacs, J., Rogers, M. & Scott, J. (1997). Atovaquone for salvage treatment and suppression of toxoplasmic encephalitis in patients with AIDS. Atovaquone/Toxoplasmic Encephalitis Study Group. *Clinical Infectious Diseases*, Vol.24, No.3, pp. 422-429, ISSN 1058-4838.

Touboul, J.L., Salmon, D., Lancastre, F., Mayaud, C., Fermand, J.P., Fouret, P. & Akoun, G. (1986). *Toxoplasma gondii* pneumopathy in a patient with the acquired immunodeficiency syndrome: demonstration of the parasite by bronchioloalveolar lavage. *Revue de Pneumologie Clinique*, Vol.42, No.3, pp. 150-152, ISSN 0761-8417.

Tremont-Lukats, I.W., Garciarena, P., Juarbe, R. & El-Abassi, R.N. (2009). The immune inflammatory reconstitution syndrome and central nervous system toxoplasmosis. *Annals of Internal Medicine*, Vol.150, No.9, pp. 656-657, ISSN 0003-4819.

Trujillo, J.R., Jaramillo-Rangel, G., Ortega-Martinez, M., Penalva de Oliveira, A.C., Vidal, J.E., Bryant, J. & Gallo, R.C. (2005). International NeuroAIDS: prospects of HIV-1 associated neurological complications. *Cell Research*, Vol.15, No.11-12, pp. 962-969, ISSN 1001-0602.

Tsai, H.C., Lee, S.S., Lin, H.H., Lin, W.R., Chen, Y.S., Huang, C.K., Liu, Y.C. & Chen, E.R. (2002). Treatment of *Toxoplasma* brain abscess with clindamycin and sulfadiazine in an AIDS patient with concurrent atypical *Pneumocystis carinii pneumonia*. *Journal of the Formosan Medical Association*, Vol.101, No.9, pp. 646-649, ISSN 0929-6646.

Tsambiras, P.E., Larkin, J.A. & Houston, S.H. (2001). Case report. *Toxoplasma* encephalitis after initiation of HAART. *The AIDS Reader®*, Vol.11, No.12, pp. 608-610, 615-616, ISSN 1053-0894.

Tse, W., Cersosimo, M.G., Gracies, J.M., Morgello, S., Olanow, C.W. & Koller, W. (2004). Movement disorders and AIDS: a review. *Parkinsonism Related Disorders*, Vol.10, No.6, pp. 323-334, ISSN 1353-8020.

Ullum, H., Cozzi Lepri, A., Bendtzen, K., Victor, J., Gøtzsche, P.C., Phillips, A.N., Skinhøj, P. & Klarlund Pedersen, B. (1997). Low production of interferon gamma is related to disease progression in HIV infection: evidence from a cohort of 347 HIV-infected individuals. *AIDS Research and Human Retroviruses*, Vol.13, No.12, pp. 1039-1046, ISSN 0889-2229.

Uneke, C.J., Duhlinska, D.D., Njoku, M.O. & Ngwu, B.A. (2005). Seroprevalence of acquired toxoplasmosis in HIV-infected and apparently healthy individuals in Jos, Nigeria. *Parassitologia*, Vol.47, No.2, pp. 233-236, ISSN 0048-2951.

USPHS/IDSA Prevention of opportunistic infections working group. (1997). USPHS/IDSA guidelines for the prevention of opportunistic infections in persons infected with human immunodeficiency virus. *MMWR. Morbidity and Mortality Weekly Report*, Vol.46, No.RR-12, pp. 1-46, ISSN 0149-2195.

Vallat-Decouvelaere, A.V., Chrétien, F., Lorin, de la Grandmaison, G., Carlier, R., Force, G. & Gray, F. (2003). The neuropathology of HIV infection in the era of highly active antiretroviral therapy. *Annales de Pathologie*, Vol.23, No.5, pp. 408-423, ISSN 0242-6498.

van Oosterhout, J.J., Laufer, M.K., Graham, S.M., Thumba, F., Perez, M.A., Chimbiya, N., Wilson, L., Chagomerana, M., Molyneux, M.E., Zijlstra, E.E., Taylor, T.E. & Plowe, C.V. (2005). A community-based study of the incidence of trimethoprim-sulfamethoxazole-preventable infections in Malawian adults living with HIV. *Journal of Acquired Immune Deficiency Syndromes*, Vol.39, No.5, pp. 626-631, ISSN 0894-9255.

van Vaerenbergh, K., Debaisieux, L., De Cabooter, N., Declercq, C., Desmet, K., Fransen, K., Maes, B., Marissens, D., Miller, K., Muyldermans, G., Sprecher, S., Stuyver, L., Vaira, D., Verhofstede, C., Zissis, G., Van Ranst, M., De Clercq, E., Desmyter, J. & Vandamme, A.M. (2001). Prevalence of genotypic resistance among antiretroviral drug-naive HIV-1-infected patients in Belgium. *Antiviral Therapy*, Vol.6, No.1, pp. 63-70, ISSN 1359-6535.

Venkataramana, A., Pardo, C.A., McArthur, J.C., Kerr, D.A., Irani, D.N., Griffin, J.W., Burger, P., Reich, D.S., Calabresi, P.A. & Nath, A. (2006). Immune reconstitution inflammatory syndrome in the CNS of HIV-infected patients. *Neurology*, Vol.67, No.3, pp. 383-388, ISSN 0028-3878.

Veronese Rodrigues, M., Demarco, A.L.G., Donadi, E.A., Demarco, L.A., Deghaide, N.H.S., Romão, E. & Figueiredo, J.F.C. (2004). HLA class I profile in patients with AIDS and *Toxoplasma gondii* chorioretinitis. *Investigative Ophthalmology & Visual Science*, Vol.45, pp.E-1672, ISSN 0146-0404.

Vidal, J.E., Hernández, A.V., Oliveira, A.C., de Souza, A.L., Madalosso, G., Silva, P.R. & Dauar, R. (2004a). Cerebral tuberculomas in AIDS patients: a forgotten diagnosis? *Arquivos de Neuro-Psiquiatria*, Vol.62, No.3B, pp. 793-796, ISSN 0004-282X.

Vidal, J.E., Colombo, F.A., de Oliveira, A.C., Focaccia, R. & Pereira-Chioccola, V.L. (2004b). PCR assay using cerebrospinal fluid for diagnosis of cerebral toxoplasmosis in Brazilian AIDS patients. *Journal of Clinical Microbiology*, Vol.42, No.10, pp. 4765-4768, ISSN 0095-1137.

Vidal, J.E., Hernandez, A.V., de Oliveira, A.C., Dauar, R.F., Barbosa, S.P.Jr. & Focaccia, R. (2005a). Cerebral toxoplasmosis in HIV-positive patients in Brazil: clinical features and predictors of treatment response in the HAART era. *AIDS Patient Care and STDs*, Vol.19, No.10, pp. 626-634, ISSN 1087-2914.

Vidal, J.E., Penalva, de Oliveira, A.C., Bonasser Filho, F., Schiavon Nogueira, R., Dauar, R.F., Leite, A.G., Lins, D.L. & Coelho, J.F. (2005b). Tuberculous brain abscess in AIDS patients: report of three cases and literature review. *Internal Journal of Infectious Diseases*, Vol.9, No.4, pp. 201-207, ISSN 1201-9712.

Vidal, J.E., Dauar, R.F. & de Oliveira, A.C. (2008). Utility of brain biopsy in patients with acquired immunodeficiency syndrome before and after introduction of highly active antiretroviral therapy. *Neurosurgery*, Vol.63, No.6, pp. E1209, ISSN 0148-396X.

Wadia, R.S., Pujari, S.N., Kothari, S., Udhar, M., Kulkarni, S., Bhagat, S.& Nanivadekar, A. (2001). Neurological manifestations of HIV disease. *The Journal of the Association of Physicians of India*, Vol.49, pp. 343-348, ISSN 0004-5772.

Wainstein, M.V., Wolffenbuttel, L., Lopes, D.K., González, H.E., Golbspan, L., Ferreira, L., Sprinz, E., Kronfeld, M. & Edelweiss, M.I. (1993). The sensitivity and specificity of the clinical, serological and tomographic diagnosis of *Toxoplasma gondii* encephalitis in the acquired immunodeficiency syndrome (AIDS). *Revista da Sociedade Brasileira de Medicina Tropical*, Vol.26, No.2, pp. 71-75, ISSN 0037-8682.

Wallace, M.R., Rossetti, R.J. & Olson, P.E. (1993). Cats and toxoplasmosis risk in HIV-infected adults. *The Journal of the American Medical Association*, Vol.269, No.1, pp. 76-77, ISSN 0098-7484.

Wanachiwanawin, D., Sutthent, R., Chokephaibulkit, K., Mahakittikun, V., Ongrotchanakun, J. & Monkong, N. (2001). *Toxoplasma gondii* antibodies in HIV and non-HIV infected Thai pregnant women. *Asian Pacific Journal of Allergy and Immunology*, Vol.19, No.4, pp. 291-293, ISSN 0125-877X.

Welker, Y., Geissmann, F., Benali, A., Bron, J., Molina, J.M. & Decazes, J.M. (1994). *Toxoplasma*-induced cystitis in a patient with AIDS. *Clinical Infectious Diseases*, Vol.18, No.3, pp.453-454, ISSN 1058-4838.

Woldemichael, T., Fontanet, A.L., Sahlu, T., Gilis, H., Messele, T., Rinke de Wit, T.F., Yeneneh, H., Coutinho, R.A. & Van Gool, T. (1998). Evaluation of the Eiken latex agglutination test for anti-*Toxoplasma* antibodies and seroprevalence of *Toxoplasma* infection among factory workers in Addis Ababa, Ethiopia. *Transactions of the Royal Society of Tropical Medicine and Hygiene*, Vol.92, No.4, pp. 401-403, ISSN 0035-9203.

Wongkamchai, S., Rungpitaransi, B., Wongbunnate, S. & Sittapairochana, C. (1995). *Toxoplasma* infection in healthy persons and in patients with HIV or ocular disease. *Southeast Asian Journal of Tropical Medicine and Public Health*, Vol.26, No.4, pp. 655-658, ISSN 0125-1562.

Yap, G., Pesin, M. & Sher, A. (2000). Cutting edge: IL-12 is required for the maintenance of IFN-gamma production in T cells mediating chronic resistance to the intracellular pathogen, *Toxoplasma gondii*. *Journal of Immunology*, Vol.165, No.2, pp.628-631, ISSN 0022-1767.

Yeo, K.K., Yeo, T.T., Chan, C.Y., Sitoh, Y.Y., Teo, J. & Wong, S.Y. (2000). Stereotactic brain biopsies in AIDS patients--early local experience. *Singapore Medical Journal*, Vol.41, No.4, pp. 161-166, ISSN 0037-5675.

Yoong, K.Y. & Cheong, I. (1997). A study of Malaysian drug addicts with human immunodeficiency virus infection. *International Journal of STD & AIDS*, Vol.8, No.2, pp. 118-123, ISSN 0956-4624.

Zajdenweber, M., Muccioli, C. & Belfort, R. Jr. (2005). Ocular involvement in AIDS patients with central nervous system toxoplasmosis: before and after HAART. *Arquivos Brasileiros de Oftalmologia*, Vol.68, No.6, pp. 773-775, ISSN 0004-2749.

Zhou, X.W., Kafsack, B.F., Cole, R.N., Beckett, P., Shen, R.F. & Carruthers, V.B. (2005). The opportunistic pathogen *Toxoplasma gondii* deploys a diverse legion of invasion and survival proteins. *The Journal of Biological Chemistry*, Vol.280, No.40, pp. 34233-44, ISSN 0021-9258.

Zufferey, J., Sugar, A., Rudaz, P., Bille, J., Glauser, M.P. & Chave, J.P. (1993). Prevalence of latent toxoplasmosis and serological diagnosis of active infection in HIV-positive patients. *European Journal of Clinical Microbiology & Infectious Diseases*, Vol.12, No.8, pp. 591-595, ISSN 0934-9723.

Zumla, A., Savva, D., Wheeler, R.B., Hira, S.K., Luo, N.P., Kaleebu, P., Sempala, S.K., Johnson, J.D. & Holliman, R. (1991). *Toxoplasma* serology in Zambian and Ugandan patients infected with the human immunodeficiency virus. *Transactions of the Royal Society of Tropical Medicine and Hygiene*, Vol.85, No.2, pp. 227-229, ISSN 0035-9203.

16

Use of Polymerase Chain Reaction for the Determination of About 2.5 kb fpvA and fpvB Gene Sequences in *Pseudomonas aeruginosa* Strains

Julie Osaretin Osayande
Department of Molecular and Cellular Interactions (MINT)
Vrije Universiteit Brussels
Belgium

1. Introduction

Pseudomonas aeruginosa produces three different pyoverdines, types I-III (Cornelis *et al.*, 1989), which are able to chelate iron and form ferripyoverdine complexes that are recognized and transported by different ferripyoverdine receptors present on the outer membrane. The ferripyoverdine receptor gene, *fpvA* of *P. aeruginosa* (PAO1) has been characterized previously (Poole *et al.*, 1993). In addition, the other iron-repressible outer membrane receptor proteins for types II and III ferripyoverdine complexes were recently identified and characterized by cloning (De Chial *et al.*, 2003). Following the observation that an *fpvA* mutant could demonstrate low ferripyoverdine uptake compared with wild type (Poole *et al.*, 1991; Gensberg *et al.*, 1992), an alternative ferripyoverdine receptor gene *fpvB* was identified and a fragment (562 bp) was amplified by polymerase chain reaction (Ghysels *et al.* 2004). In addition, the growth of several *P. aeruginosa* pyoverdine-negative mutants, found to inhabit the lungs of cystic fibrosis patients, were stimulated by existing pyoverdine types, providing additional confirmation for the existence of an alternative route for ferripyoverdine uptake (De Vos *et al.*, 2001; Ghysels *et al.*, 2004).
PCR was developed in 1983 by Kary Mullis (Karry Mullis Nobel Lecture, December 8, 1993) and involves the selective amplification of specific regions of DNA for extensive use in molecular biology (Sambrook and Russell, 2001). Using primers designed in this study, the complete sequence of the ferripyoverdine receptor genes (*fpvA* and *fpvB*) from several *P. aeruginosa* clinical and environmental isolates were amplified and sequenced, allowing the identification of variant forms of these receptor genes.

2. Experimental procedures

Bacterial strains used in this study. The strains used in this study included reference and test strains and are as listed in Table 1.
Primers. Several internal and external primers were designed from the *fpvA* (I-III) gene sequences of reference strains (PAO1, PA 14, ATCC 27853, 7NSK2, and 59.20) present in the

Strain	***fpvA* type**	***fpvB* gene (562 bp)**	**Source**
PAO1	I	Positive	Stover *et al.*, 2000
ATCC 27853	IIb	Negative	Spencer *et al.*, 2003
7NSK2	IIa	Positive	De Chial *et al.*, 2003
59.20	III	Positive	De Chial *et al.*, 2003
W15 Aug 16	III	Positive	Woluwe River water
W15 Dec 9	III	Positive	Woluwe River water
W15 Dec 10	III	Positive	Woluwe River water
W15 Aug 15	IIa	Positive	Woluwe River water
W15 Dec 11	IIb	Positive	Woluwe River water
W15 Dec 1	I	Positive	Woluwe River water
W15 Dec 6	I	Positive	Woluwe River water
W15 Aug 21	I	Positive	Woluwe River water
Br678	II	Positive	Burn wound (Pirnay *et al.*, 2005)

Table 1. List of strains used in this study

database for the purpose of amplification and sequencing of the ferripyoverdine receptor (*fpvA* and *fpvB*) genes in the strains under study. The primer sequences are shown in Table 2.

DNA preparation method. DNA was extracted from bacterial samples either by boiling in filter-sterilized water or using a PCR template preparation kit (Roche) according to the manufacturer's instructions.

Sequencing of PCR products. All sequencing was performed at the VIB sequencing facility. Using the CAP2 software program (*www.infobiogen.com*), the resulting external forward and reverse sequences, in addition to the internal sequences for all test strains, were aligned, and the resulting consensus sequence was approximately 2.5 kb.

PCR conditions. The various PCR mixes and cycling conditions are shown in Tables 3A-D.

3. Amplification of the *fpvB* gene (2.5 kb) in *P. aeruginosa* strains

List of bacterial strains used is shown in Table 1.

DNA preparation method. Sterile colonies from 13 bacterial samples were grown on LB media overnight at 37°C and then boiled in 400 μL water at 95°C for 10 min. The resulting templates were used for PCR.

	Primer name	Sequences 5' → 3'
External primers for *fpvA* type I gene amplification	1A-PF	ATGCCAGCACCACACGGTC
	1A-PR	GCGAGTGCTGAACATCAGGT
Internal primers for sequencing the *fpvA* type I gene	Int1-AF1	CCTGATCCGCAAGAAACCT
	Int1-AR1	GGCCGCTGACGTCCAGTT
	Int1-BF1	GTGACCGATGACCTGAACC
	Int1-BR1	CGGACTCGCGAATGGTCGG
External primers for *fpvA* type IIa gene amplification	2A-PF	CAGCACTCCGCACACTCC
	2A-PR	GTCAAGTCGGAGGTGATGG
Internal primers for sequencing the *fpvA* type IIa and IIb genes	EFT-2A	TCCAGTTCGACATCGGCGC
	Int2-AF2	CAAGCGCAGCGGTACCGGC
	Int2-AR2	AACCGCGCGCCTTGATCTC
	Int2-BF2	CGACCGCGACCAGTTCGT
	Int2-BR2	TGCCGAA(G/C)(A/G/C)CTTTGTTGGT
	2A-int2AF	AATCAATCGGCCGCCATGC
External primers for *fpvA* type IIb gene amplification	ExtF-2A	GCGCAACACCCTGACG(C/T)TGC
	ExtR-2A	TTACCAGTTGTAGGTCAG(G/A)TCG
External primers *fpvA* type III gene amplification	EFT-IIIA	ATGTCCAGGCTTGGCCTGGC
	ERT-IIIA	GTAGTCGACCCAGGAGCG
	ExFN-IIIA	GAGCGCCCAGGCGGTCGC
Internal primers for sequencing the *fpvA* type III gene	Int3AF3	TGCGCAAGCGACCGACGG
	Int3AR3	GCCGGCCTTGGCAGTCAG
	Int3BF3	ACGCTTCGATCCAGAAAGGC
	Int3BR3	ACTCCTTGGCCACCGCCTTC
	Int3-BF3	
	FpVAint3F	AACCTGCTGCGTTACCAGG
	FpVA-3PR	AGCACGTTGCGCGGATCG
External primers for *fpvB* gene amplification	PA4168F	CCATCCAGGAACTGCAGAT
	PA4168R	GGATCAGAGCGATACTTCA
Internal primers for sequencing the *fpvB* gene	FpvbF1	AGGCAGCGTCGGCACCTG
	FpvbF2	AAACGTCGGCCTCGCTGC
	FpvbR1	CTGAAAGTGATCCTCGGCG
	FpvbR2	CTTGTACCAGTCCAGGCG
Degenerate primers for amplification and sequencing the *fpvA* type II gene*	FpVAF1	AGA CCG A (T/C) A CCC CGC TCA AG
	FpVAF2	(C/A)G(C/G)(C/G)(T/C)(G/A)(G/A)(T/C) (C/A)(C/A)(T/G)(G/A)(A/G)C(T/A)(T/C)C(A/G)(C/ A)G
	FpVAR1	CTT GGT GTA CTT GA (T/C) GTC GTT (T/G)
	FpVAR2	G (T/A) G GGT (A/G)T A G(C/G)C (A/G) GC (C/A)T(G/A) (A/T)ACC

* Degenerate primer used to amplify and sequence *fpvA* gene in *P. aeruginosa* strain Br678.

Table 2. List of external and internal primers designed and used in this study.

Reagents	Volume (µL)
Water	774.0
Buffer	120.0
Q-solution	240.0
Primers (100 µM)	6.0 each
dNTP mix (10 mM)	24
Enzyme (*Taq* polymerase)	6.0
DNA	2

Table 3A. PCR mix for *fpvB* gene amplification using primers PA4168F and PA4168R (Ghysels *et al.*, 2004)

	Temperature (°C)	Time	
Initial denaturation	94	3-5 min	
Denaturation	94	30 s	
Annealing	55	30 s	35 cycles
Extension	72	2.30 min	
Final extension	72	10 min	

Table 3B. PCR cycling conditions

Reagents	Volume (µL)
Water	258
Buffer	40
Q-solution	80
$MgCl_2$	12
Primers (100 µM)	2 each
dNTP mix (10 mM)	8
Enzyme (*Taq* polymerase)	2
DNA	2

Table 3C. PCR mix for *fpvA* type I gene amplification using primers 1A-PF and 1A-PR

Reagents	Volume (µL)
Water	516
Buffer	80
Q-solution	160
$MgCl_2$	20
Primers (100 µM)	4 each
dNTP mix (10 mM)	16
Enzyme (Taq polymerase)	4
DNA	2

Table 3D. PCR mix for *fpvA* gene amplification using primers FpVAF1, FpVAF2, FpVAR1, and FpVAR2

Gel electrophoresis. Amplified PCR products were run on an agarose gel (0.8%) at 100 V for 70 min. Subsequently, the gel was stained in ethidium bromide for 12 min. Stained gels were visualized and illuminated under UV light (260 nm).

Sequencing of PCR products. Amplified DNA was purified using a Sigma Gen-Elute PCR clean up kit, and 100 ng/µl of purified DNA was sent for sequencing with 5 µM of each primer; these primers were used to sequence the external portions of the *fpvB* gene of nine *P. aeruginosa* strains as shown below:

Strain	***fpvA* type**	**Source**
W15 Aug 21	I	Woluwe River water
W15 Dec 1	I	Woluwe River water
W15 Dec 6	I	Woluwe River water
W15 Aug 15	IIa	Woluwe River water
W15 Dec 11	IIb	Woluwe River water
59.20	III	*De Chial et al.*, 2003
W15 Aug 16	III	Woluwe River water
W15 Dec 9	III	Woluwe River water
W15 Dec 10	III	Woluwe River water

Table 4. Primers used to sequence the external portions of the *fpvB* gene of nine *P. aeruginosa* strains

The resulting sequences were aligned with the sequence of the PAO1 *fpvB* gene using DNA-manager software. The alignment was performed for the PAO1 *fpvB* sequence plus all resulting forward sequences (for nine sequenced strains) and the PAO1 *fpvB* sequence plus all resulting reverse sequence (for nine sequenced strains).

The purpose of this alignment was to facilitate the design of internal primers for the sequencing of the internal portion of the *fpvB* gene, and two sets of internal primers were designed for this purpose as shown below:

- FpVBF1 (forward) from position (803-820) of aligned forward sequences;
- FpVBF2 (reverse) from position (833-850) of aligned forward sequences;
- FpVBR1 (forward) from position (1609-1628) of aligned reverse sequences; and
- FpVBR2 (reverse) from position (1631-1648) of aligned reverse sequences.

100 ng/µl of purified DNA plus 5 µM of each primer was used for sequencing the internal portion of the gene.

2.5 kb *fpvB* gene sequence for nine strains. Using the CAP2 software program, the resulting external forward and reverse sequences, in addition to four internal sequences for each of the nine strains, were aligned; the resulting consensus sequence was approximately 2.5 kb.

Amplification of the *fpvA* gene (2.5 kb) in *P. aeruginosa* strains. Amplification of the *fpvA* types I, IIa, IIb, and III genes in eight *P. aeruginosa* strains in which about 2.5 kb *fpvB* gene was previously amplified was performed using primers designed in this study (Table 2: List of primers)

DNA preparation method. Sterile colonies of 12 bacterial samples (eight Woluwe River water strains that included *fpvA* types I-III plus four positive controls) were grown and templates were prepared for PCR as described above.

Strain	**Source**	***fpvB* (2.5 kb)** This study
(PAO1 (+)	Stover *et al.*, 2000	Positive
ATCC 27853(+)	Spencer *et al.*, 2003	Negative
7NSK2 (+)	De Chial *et al.*, 2003	Positive
59.2O (+)	De Chial *et al.*, 2003	Positive
W15 Aug 16	Woluwe	Positive
W15 Dec 9	Woluwe	Positive
W15 Dec 10	Woluwe	Positive
W15 Aug 15	Woluwe	Positive
W15 Dec 11	Woluwe	Positive
W15 Dec 1	Woluwe	Positive
W15 Dec 6	Woluwe	Positive
W15 Aug 21	Woluwe	Positive
Other Reference strains		***fpvA* type**
PA 14		I
10-15	Smith *et al.*, 2005	I
MSH	Smith *et al.*, 2005	II
1-60	Spencer *et al.*, 2003	II
2-164	Spencer *et al.*, 2003	II
ATCC013	Smith *et al.*, 2005	III
206-12	Smith *et al.*, 2005	III

Table 5. Additional information for strains used in this study.

Gel electrophoresis. Amplified PCR products were run and processed as described above.
Sequencing of PCR products. Amplified DNA was purified as described above and 100 ng/µl of purified DNA was sequenced with 5 µM of each primer; these primers were used to sequence the external portions of the *fpvA* gene of three *P. aeruginosa* strains as shown below:

Strain	*fpvA* type	Source
W15 Aug 21	I	Woluwe River water
W15 Dec 1	I	Woluwe River water
W15 Dec 6	I	Woluwe River water

Table 6. Three *P. aeruginosa* strains

The resulting sequences were aligned with the complete sequence of the *fpvA* gene of three reference strains (PAO1, PA14, and 10-15) as described above. The alignment was done for the *fpvA* sequences of three reference strains plus all resulting forward sequences (for three sequenced strains) and the *fpvA* sequences of three reference strains plus all resulting reverse sequences (for three sequenced strains).
The purpose of this alignment was to facilitate the design of internal primers for the sequencing of the internal portion of the *fpvA* gene, and two sets of internal primers were designed for this purpose as shown below:

- Int1AF1 (forward) from position (800-818) of aligned forward sequences;
- Int1AR1 (Reverse) from position (860-879) of aligned forward sequences;
- Int1BF1 (forward) from position (1632-1650) of aligned reverse sequences; and
- Int1BR1 (Reverse) from position (1718-1736) of aligned reverse sequences.

100 ng/µl of purified DNA plus 5 µM of each internal primer was used to sequence the internal portion of the *fpvA* gene.
***fpvA* gene (2.5 kb) sequence for three strains.** Using the CAP2 software program, the resulting external forward and reverse sequences, in addition to four internal sequences for each of the three strains, were aligned, and the resulting consensus sequence was approximately 2.5 kb.
PCR mix for *fpvA* type IIa gene amplification using primers 2A-PF and 2A-PR was as in Table 3C, except that no $MgCl_2$ was used.
PCR cycling conditions were as in Table 3B.
Gel electrophoresis was performed as described above.
Sequencing of PCR products. Amplified DNA was purified as described above and100 ng/µl of purified DNA was sequenced with 3 µM of each primer and these primers were used to sequence the external portions of the *fpvA* gene of *P. aeruginosa* strain W15 Aug 15 as shown below:

Strain	*fpvA* type	Source
W15 Aug 15	IIa	Woluwe River water

Table 7. *P. aeruginosa* strain W15 Aug 15

The resulting sequence was aligned with the sequence of the *fpvA* gene of five reference strains (7NSK2, ATCC 27853, MSH, 2-164, and 1-60) as described above. The alignment was done for the *fpvA* gene sequences of five reference strains plus resulting forward sequences (for 1 sequenced strain) and the *fpvA* gene sequences of five reference strains plus resulting reverse sequences (for one sequenced strain).
The purpose of this alignment was to facilitate the design of internal primers to enable the sequencing of the internal portion of the *fpvA* gene; the internal primers designed are shown below:

- EFT-2A (forward) from position (500-519) of aligned forward sequences;
- Int2AF2 (forward) from position (801-819) of aligned forward sequences;
- Int2AR2 (Reverse) from position (880-898) of aligned forward sequences;
- Int2BF2 (forward) from position (1537-1554) of aligned reverse sequences;
- Int2BR2 (Reverse) from position (1736-1754) of aligned reverse sequences;
- 2A-Int2AF (forward) from position (2344-2362**)** of aligned reverse sequences; and ERT-2A (Reverse) from position (2400-2419) of aligned reverse sequences.

100 ng/µl of purified DNA plus 5µM each of internal primers were used for sequencing the internal portion of the gene. The same procedure was followed for type 11b except for the external primers that differed (ExtF-2A and ExtR-2A) and only internal primers shown in bold above were used.
***fpvA* gene (2.5 kb) sequence for two strains.** Using the CAP2 software program, the resulting external forward and reverse sequences in addition to the four internal sequences for each of the two strains (seven internal sequences in the case of W15Aug15) were aligned and the resulting consensus sequence was approximately 2.5 kb.
PCR mix for *fpvA* type III gene amplification using primers EFT-II1A and ERT-II1A is as shown in Table 3C.
PCR cycling conditions are as shown in Table 3B.
Gel electrophoresis was performed as described above.
Sequencing of PCR products. Amplified DNA was purified as described above and 100 ng/µl of purified DNA was sequenced with 3 µM of each primer; these primers were used to sequence the external portions of the *fpvA* gene of three *P. aeruginosa* strains as shown below:

Strain	*fpvA* type	Source
W15 Aug 16	III	Woluwe River water
W15 Dec 10	III	Woluwe River water
W15 Dec 9	III	Woluwe River water

Table 8. Three *P. aeruginosa* strains.

The resulting sequences were aligned with the sequence of the *fpvA* gene of three reference strains (59.2O, ATCC 013, and 206-12) as described above. The alignment was done for the *fpvA* sequences of three reference strains plus all resulting forward sequences (for three sequenced strains) and the *fpvA* sequences of three reference strains plus all resulting reverse sequences (for three sequenced strains).

The purpose of this alignment was to facilitate the design of internal primers for the sequencing of the internal portion of the *fpvA* gene; the internal primers (in bold) are shown below:

- **Int3AF3** (forward) from position (940-958) of aligned forward sequences;
- **Int3AR3** (Reverse) from position (975-992) of aligned forward sequences;
- **Int3BF3** (forward) from position (1690-1709) of aligned reverse sequences;
- Int3-BF3 (forward) from position (1604-1622) of aligned forward sequences;
- **Int3BR3** (Reverse) from position (1820-1839) of aligned reverse sequences;
- **FpVAint3F** (forward) from position (2219-2237); and
- FpVA-3PR (Reverse) from position (2542-2559).

100 ng/µl of purified DNA plus 3 µM (5µM in the case of int3AF3 and int3BR3) each of internal primers were used for sequencing the internal portion of the gene. Also, a new PCR amplification using primers int3-BF3 and FpVA-3PR was performed to enable sequencing of the end portion of the *fpvA* gene.

***fpvA* gene (2.5kb) sequence for 3 strains.** Using the CAP2 software program, the resulting external forward and reverse sequences, in addition to five internal sequences for each of the three strains, were aligned; the resulting consensus sequence was approximately 2.5 kb.

Strain	**Source**	**Pvd siderotype** (Pirnay *et al.*, 2005)	***fpvB* (562 bp)** Primers (Ghysels *et al.*, 2004)	***fpvB* (2.5 kb)**
Br678	Burn	II	Positive (+)	NA, not analyzed

Table 9. PCR amplification of *fpvA* gene (1.5 kb) in *Pseudomonas* strain Br678

Strains	***fpv type***
PAO1, PA14, 10-15	I
7NKS2, ATCC27853, MSH, 1-60, 2-164	II
59.20, ATCC013, 206-12	III

Primers	**Position**	**Tm (°C)**
FpVAF1	836-855	67.4
FpVAF2	836-855	53.8
FpVAR1	2501-2522	60.5
FpVAR2	2501-2522	60.4

Table 10. ClustalX alignment of *fpvA* sequences

Design of primers. Two sets of degenerate primers were designed in this study following a ClustalX alignment of the *fpvA* sequences of 11 *P. aeruginosa* strains as shown above.
DNA was purified and prepared for PCR as described above.
PCR cycling conditions were as described above except that the annealing temperature was increased to 57°C.
Gel electrophoresis. Gel electrophoresis of amplified DNA involved an application of 8 μL amplified PCR product and 2 μL loading dye on a 0.8% agarose gel in 1× TAE buffer and performed at 100 V for 65 min. Subsequently, the gel was stained in ethidium bromide for 12 min and illuminated under UV light.
Sequencing of PCR products. Amplified DNA was purified and sequenced as described above with 5μM each of primer; these primers were used to sequence the amplified purified PCR product of strain Br678.
***fpvA* gene (1.5 kb) sequence for strain Br678.** Using the CAP2 software program, the resulting forward and reverse sequences were aligned, and the resulting consensus sequence was approximately 1.5 kb.
The 1.5-kb *fpvA* sequence of Br678 was 96% identical and 97% similar to *fpvA* type II of *P. aeruginosa* isolate 2-164 at nucleotide and amino acid levels, respectively.

4. Amplification of *fpvB* gene (2.5 kb) in *P. aeruginosa* strain Br678

DNA was purified and prepared for PCR as described above.
PCR cycling conditions were as described above in Table 3B.
Gel electrophoresis was as described above.
Sequencing of PCR products. Amplified DNA was purified and sequenced as described above with 5 μM of each primer (PA4168F and PA4168R as above); these primers were used to sequence the external portions of the *fpvB* gene of strain Br678.
In addition, the two sets of internal primers previously designed for the sequencing of the internal portion of the *fpvB* gene were used to sequence the internal portion of the *fpvB* gene in this strain as shown below:

- FpVBF1 (forward) from position (803-820) of aligned forward sequences;
- FpVBF2 (Reverse) from position (833-850) of aligned forward sequences;
- FpVBR1 (forward) from position (1609-1628) of aligned reverse sequences; and
- FpVBR2 (Reverse) from position (1631-1648) of aligned reverse sequences.

100 ng/μl of purified DNA of filter sterilized water plus 5μM of each internal primer was used to sequence the internal portion of the gene.

5. *fpvB* gene (2.5 kb) sequence for strain Br678

Using the CAP3 software program, the resulting external forward and reverse sequences, in addition to four internal sequences for strain Br678, were aligned, and the resulting consensus sequence was approximately 2.5 kb.

6. Results

The nucleotide sequences of both *FpvA* and *FpvB* determined in this study have been deposited in the GenBank database (Bodilis *et al.*, 2009).

Primer name	*fpvA* type	*fpvA* (bp)	Primer name
1A-PF	I	~2500	PA4168F
1A-PR			PA4168R
Int1-AF1			FpvbF1
Int1-AR1			FpvbF2
Int1-BF1			FpvbR1
Int1-BR1			FpvbR2
2A-PF	II a	~2500	PA4168F
2A-PR			PA4168R
EFT-2A			FpvbF1
Int2-AF2			FpvbF2
Int2-AR2			FpvbR1
Int2-BF2			FpvbR2
Int2-BR2			
2A-int2AF			
ExtF-2A	II b	~2500	PA4168F
ExtR-2A			PA4168R
Int2-AF2			FpvbF1
Int2-AR2			FpvbF2
Int2-BF2			FpvbR1
Int2-BR2			FpvbR2
EFT -IIIA	III	~2500	PA4168F
ERT-IIIA	III		PA4168R
ExFIIIAN	III		FpvbF1
FpVA-3PR			FpvbF2
Int3AF3			FpvbR1
Int3BF3			FpvbR2
int3BF3			
Int3-BF3			
Int3BR3			
FpVAint3F			
FpVAF1	II	1500	PA4168F
FpVAF2			PA4168R
FpvAR1			FpvbF1
FpvAR2			FpvbF2

Table 11. External and internal primers used in this study.

fpvB (bp) ~2500 bp for the primers used

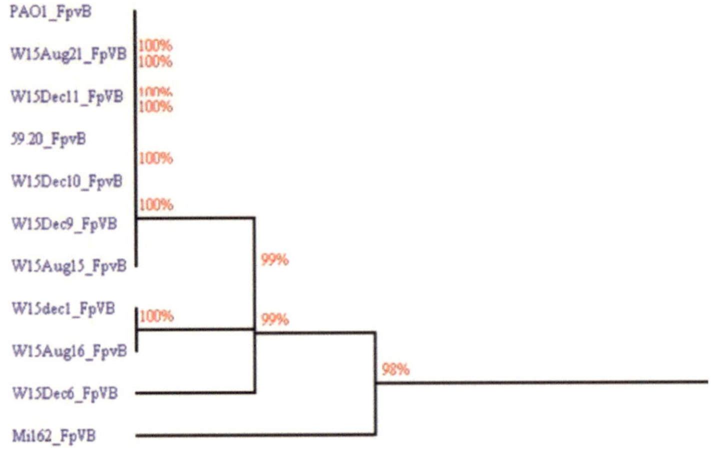

Homology tree a

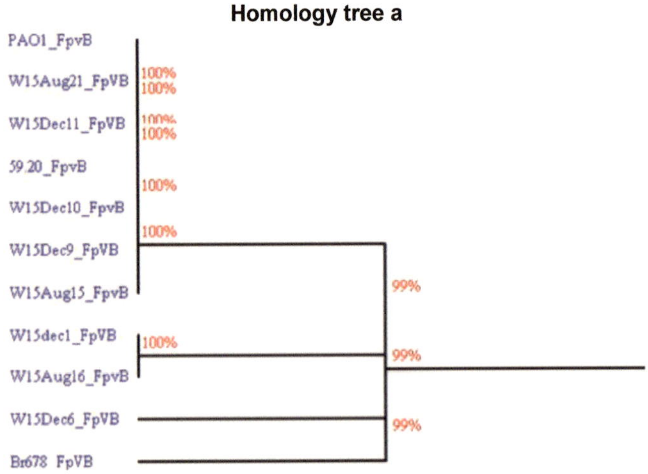

Homology tree b

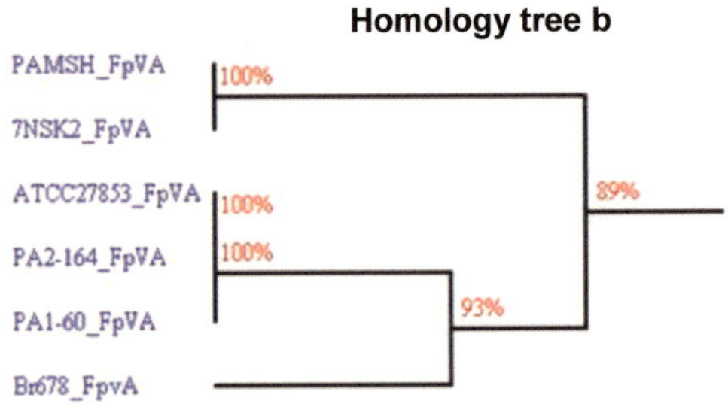

Homology tree c

Fig. 1. Homology trees (a-c) show the percent relatedness of the *fpvA* and *fpvB* genes in *P. aeruginosa* strains *Br678* and *Mi162* (*fpvA* gene sequence of strain Mi162; homology tree is shown in another manuscript in preparation) and other test strains to those of reference strains MSH (Smith *et al.*, 2005), ATCC 27853, 1-60, 2-164 (Spencer *et al.*, 2003), 7NSK2 (De Chial *et al.*, 2003), and PAO1 (Stover *et al.*, 2000). Trees were constructed using the DNA manager software following the alignment of all the nucleotide (*fpvA* and *fpvB*) sequences for the individual *P. aeruginosa* test and reference strains.

7. Gel images of *fpvA* and *fpvB* gene amplification in *P. aeruginosa* strains

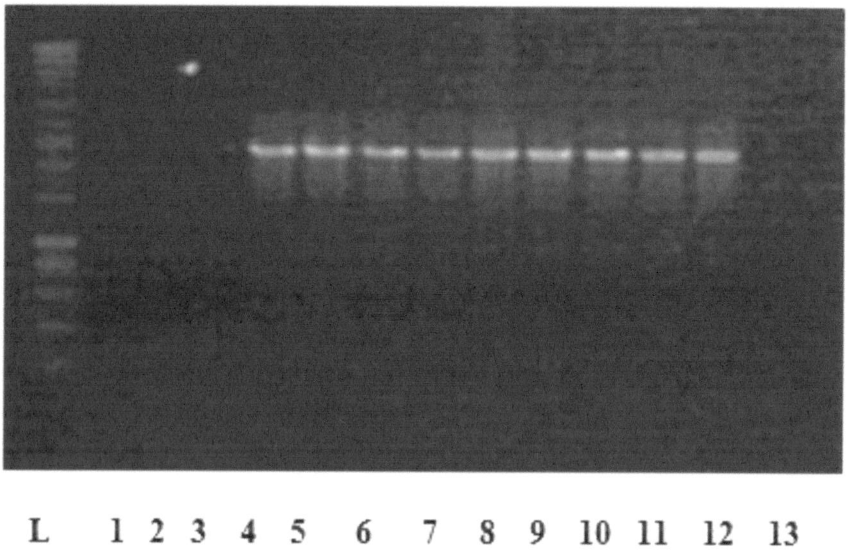

Fig. 2. Gel image of *fpvB* (2.5 kb) gene amplification in *P. aeruginosa* strains. Lanes 1-13: PAOI (positive control), ATCC 27853, 7NSK2, 59.20, W15 Aug 21,

W15 Aug 16, W15 Aug 15, W15 Dec 11, W15 Dec 10, W15 Dec 9, W15 Dec 6, W15 Dec 1, and negative control (200-bp ladder).

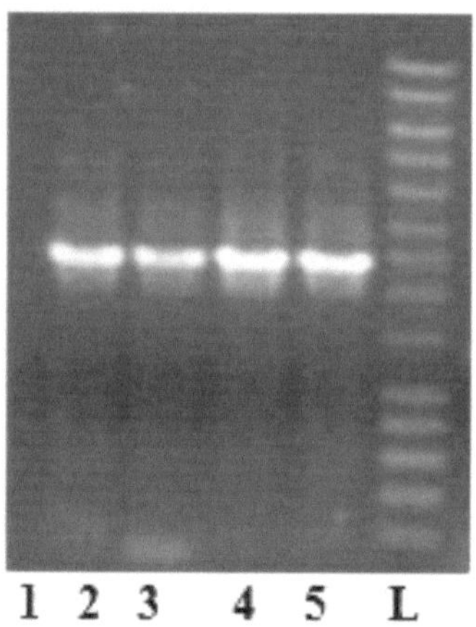

Fig. 3. Gel image of *fpvA* (2.5 kb) gene amplification in *fpvA* type I *P. aeruginosa* strains. Lanes 2-5: PAOI (positive control), W15 Aug 21, W15 Dec 6, W15 Dec 1; negative control (lane L, 200-bp ladder).

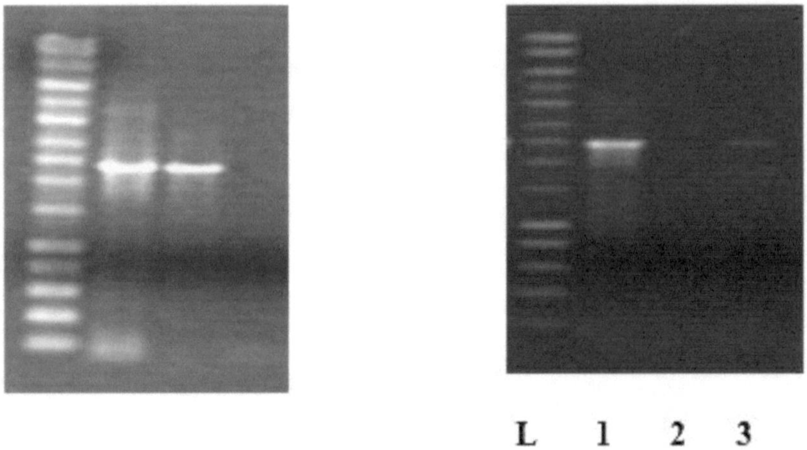

(a) (b)

Fig. 4. Gel image of *fpvA* (2.5 kb) gene amplification in *fpvA* type IIa *P. aeruginosa* strains (a). Lanes 1-3: 7NSK2 (positive control), W15 Aug 15, and negative control; L, 200-bp ladder. Gel image of *fpvA* (2.5 kb) gene amplification in *fpvA* type IIb *P. aeruginosa* strains (b). Lanes 1-3: ATCC 27853 (positive control), negative control, W15 Dec 11; L, 200-bp ladder).

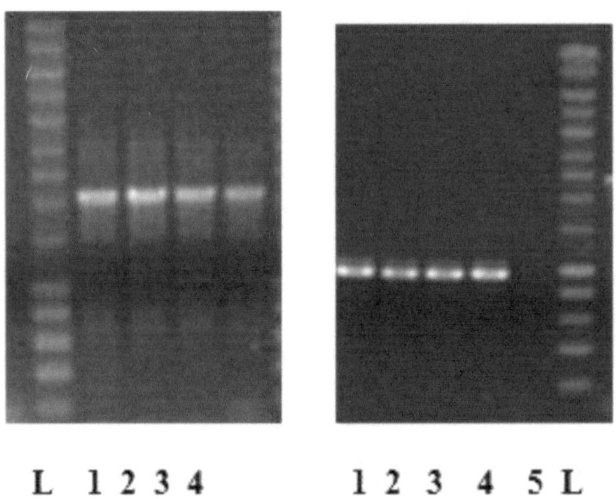

(a) (b)

Fig. 5. Gel images of *fpvA* (2.0 and 1.0 kb) gene amplification in *fpvA* type III *P. aeruginosa* strains. Lanes 1-5 (a, Lanes 1-4): 59.2O (positive control), W15 Dec 9, W15 Dec 10, W15 Aug 16, and negative control (b); L, 200-bp ladder.

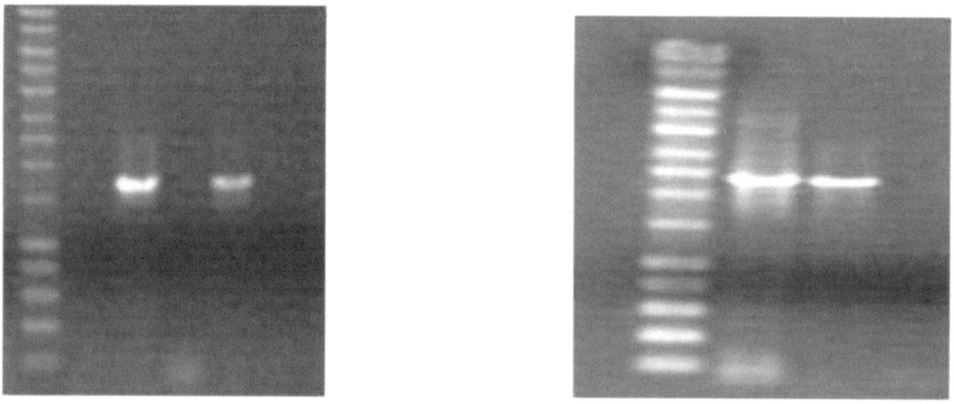

(a) (b)

Fig. 6. Gel images of *fpvA* and *fpvB* (2.5 kb) gene amplification in *P. aeruginosa* strain *Br678*. Bands correspond to *fpvA* and *fpvB* genes in test strain (*Br678*) and positive control (PAO1), respectively.

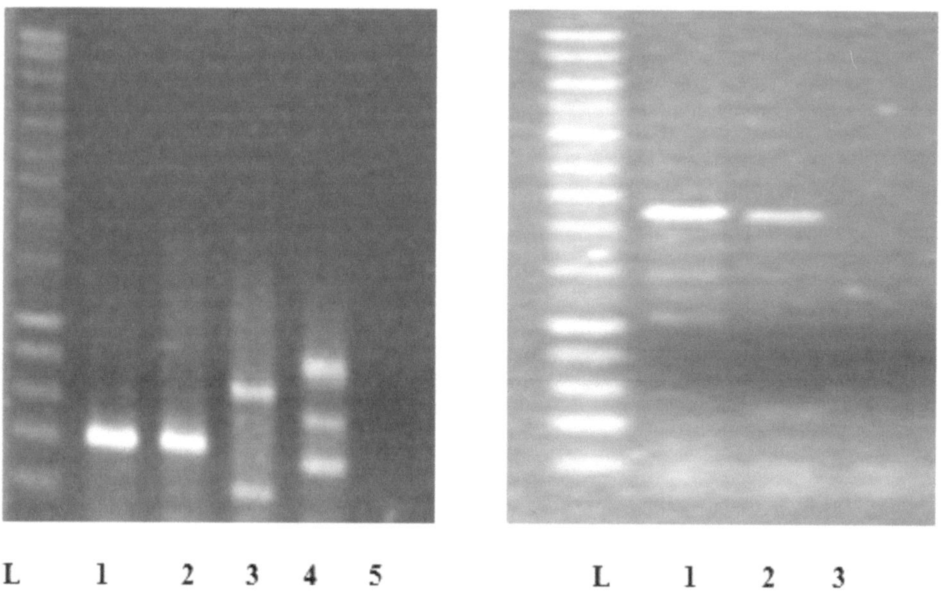

(a) (b)

Fig. 7. Gel images of *fpvA* (500 bp) and *fpvB* (2.5 kb) gene amplification in *P. aeruginosa* strain *Mi162*. Bands correspond to *fpvA* (Lane 1; a, and *fpvB* (Lane 1 b) gene amplification in test strain (*Mi162*) and positive controls (*PAO1* for *fpvB* (Lanes 2, Figure 7b) and ATCC 27853 for *fpvA*) (Lane 2, a).

8. Percent identity and similarity of *fpvA* and *fpvB* at the nucleotide and amino acid levels (BLAST search against the NCBI database)

	Strain	Pvd type	Source	*fpvA*: % identity (nucleotide level)	*fpvB*: % identity (nucleotide level)
1	59.20	III	De Chial *et al.*, 2003		99% identical to *fpvB* of PAO1
2	W15 Aug 21	I	Woluwe	99% identical to *fpvA* of PAO1	99% identical to *fpvB* of PAO1
3	W15 Dec 1	I	Woluwe	99% identical to *fpvA* of PAO1	99% identical to *fpvB* of PAO1
4	W15 Dec 6	I	Woluwe	99% identical to *fpvA* of PAO1	99% identical to *fpvB* of PAO1
5	W15 Aug 15	11a	Woluwe	99% identical to *fpvA* of 7NSK2	99% identical to *fpvB* of PAO1
6	W15 Dec 11	11b	Woluwe	95% identical to *fpvA* of ATCC27853	99% identical to *fpvB* of PAO1
7	W15 Aug 16	III	Woluwe	100% identical to *fpvA* of ATCCO13	99% identical to *fpvB* of PAO1
8	W15 Dec 9	III	Woluwe	100% identical to *fpvA* of ATCCO13	99% identical to *fpvB* of PAO1
9	W15 Dec 10	III	Woluwe	100% identical to *fpvA* of ATCCO13	99% identical to *fpvB* of PAO1
10	Br678	II	Burn	97% identical to ferrichrome iron receptor PA7	99% identical to *fpvB* of PAO1
11	Mi162	II	Burn	99% identical to PA strain MSH type II pyoverdine region	98% identical to *fpvB* of PA14

Table 12. Percent identity at the nucleotide level for each individual test strain in relation to the reference strains.

	Strain	Pvd type	Source	*fpvA*: % similarity (amino acid level)	*fpvB*: % similarity (amino acid level)
1	59.20	III	De Chial *et al.*, 2003		100% similar to ferric coprogen and ferric rhodoturolic acid of PA 2192
2	W15 Aug 21	I	Woluwe	96% similar to *fpvA* of UCBPP-PA14	100% similar to ferric coprogen and ferric rhodoturolic acid of PA 2192
3	W15 Dec 1	I	Woluwe	99% similar to *fpvA* of PAO1	99% similar to ferric coprogen and ferric rhodoturolic acid of PA UCBPP-PA14
4	W15 Dec 6	I	Woluwe	100% similar to *fpvA* of PAO1	99% similar to *fpvB* PAO1
5	W15 Aug 15	11a	Woluwe	99% similar to *fpvA* of PA C3719	99% similar to ferric coprogen and ferric rhodoturolic acid of PA 2192
6	W15 Dec 11	11b	Woluwe	99% similar to *fpvA* of PA MSH	99% similar to *fpvB* of PAO1
7	W15 Aug 16	III	Woluwe	100% similar to *fpvA* of PA206-12	99% similar to ferric coprogen and ferric rhodoturolic acid of PA UCBPP-PA14
8	W15 Dec 9	III	Woluwe	100% similar to *fpvA* of ATCCO13	99% similar to ferric coprogen and ferric rhodoturolic acid of PA 2192
9	W15 Dec 10	III	Woluwe	100% similar to *fpvA* of ATCCO13	99% similar to *fpvB* PAO1
10	Br678	II	Burn	98% similar to *fpvA* of PA C3719	99% similar to ferric coprogen and ferric rhodoturolic acid of PA 2192
11	Mi162	II	Burn	100% similar to *fpvA* II *Pseudomonas aeruginosa*	99% similar to *fpvB* second ferripyoverdine receptor of PA UCBPP-PA14

Table 13. Percent similarity of *fpvA* and *fpvB* at the nucleotide and amino acid levels (BLAST search against the NCBI database)

9. Discussion

Under iron limiting conditions, pyoverdine is produced by *Pseudomonas aeruginosa*, a human opportunistic pathogen, several studies track its occurrence as a noscomial pathogen indicating that antibiotic resistance is increasing in clinical isolates (**which may be true for the strains I worked with**). Pyoverdine is a metal chelating compound, *P. aeruginosa*, in the past has been studied to acquire plasmid (Mercer and Loutit, 1979), several transporting mechanisms have been extensively studied in this organism of which is the pyoverdine transport. Based on the different pyoverdine types, three siderovars which exists within the *P. aeruginosa* group have been detected by siderotyping, (Fuchs *et al.*, 2001; Meyer *et al.*, 1997; 2002); this technique, however, is limited. The existence of pyoverdine-negative isolates of *P. aeruginosa* (De Vos *et al.*, 2001) has prompted the need for accurate and enhanced genotyping procedures based on the determination of the gene sequence of ferripyoverdine receptor *fpvA* of *P. aeruginosa*. Cloning techniques have been used to characterize iron-regulated genes in *P. aeruginosa* (Poole *et al.*, 1993; Visca *et al.*, 1994; Cunliffe *et al.*, 1995, McMorran *et al.*, 1996; Ochsner *et al.*, 2002; Ochsner and Vasil, 1996), and several simple and inexpensive methods exist for the typing of *P. aeruginosa* isolates (AL-Samarrai *et al.*, 2000). Several studies have involved the use of PCR-based techniques in the identification and characterization of Gram-negative bacteria (Bej *et al.*, 1991; De Vos *et al.*, 1997; Fricker and Fricker, 1994; Mcintosh *et al.*, 1992; Laguerre *et al.*, 1994; Kasai *et al.*, 1998; Anzai *et al.*, 2000; Qin *et al.*, 2003) using PCR-specific primers designed for the amplification of genes in these organisms. PCR is not limited by pyoverdine production as is siderotyping and, as such, is considered reliable and less time-intensive than cloning. Since PCR-specific primers are designed to carry out amplification procedures, the problems with false positives may not likely arise, although this has not always been the case. *P. aeruginosa* secretes pyocyanin which has been documented to strip iron from transferrin (Cox, C. 1986), it also produces pyoverdine, which strips iron and contributes to the virulence of this organism, thus pyoverdine production is accompanied by virulence factor secretion (Meyer, 1996; Clarke *et al.*, 2001; Beare *et al.*, 2003). Pyoverdine growth stimulation assays have also been used to type *P. aeruginosa*, but situations have arisen whereby the observable growth had been stimulated by more than one pyoverdine (Pirnay *et al.*, 2002; Meyer, 1992; Meyer *et al.*, 1999; Stintzi *et al.*, 2000). The outcome of such assays may only be predictions, and, therefore, not of use for molecular diagnosis (Pirnay *et al.* 2005). The *fpvA* gene sequence has been proposed to be diverse (Thupvong *et al.*, 1999; Smith *et al.*, 2005); with such diversity, it may be difficult to perform PCR on such a gene without problems of non-specific amplification. However, in this study, single bands arising as a result of *fpvA* or *fpvB* gene amplification were either purified directly or excised and purified from the gel. Results of sequencing following a BLAST search against the NCBI database revealed that these sequences were approximately 95-100% identical and similar at both the nucleotide and amino acid levels to those of reference strains used in this study. Homology trees showing percent relatedness of the *fpvA* and *fpvB* genes in *P. aeruginosa* test and reference strains were also constructed using the DNA manager software following an alignment of all nucleotide sequences for the individual test and reference strains.

The purpose of this study was to use PCR for the determination of about 2.5 kb gene sequence of the ferripyoverdine receptor genes (*fpvA* types *I*, *IIa*, *IIb*, and *III*, and *fpvB*) in *P. aeruginosa* clinical and environmental strains, and this goal was achieved using a series of external and internal primers designed for both amplification and sequencing. This study has provided for the first time a means to determine the *fpvA* and *fpvB* gene sequences (~2.5 kb) in *P. aeruginosa* clinical and environmental isolates using experimental PCR.

10. Future perspective

Pseudomonas aeruginosa affects immunocompromised individuals like the AIDS patients undergoing antiretroviral therapy, in these individuals, it has been documented that *P. aeruginosa* causes a range of infections amongst which are urinary tract infections, respiratory infections, gastrointestinal infections, bone and joint infections and bacteremia, the case fatality rate in these patients is near 50% (Todar, K. 2004).

Pyoverdine the siderophore secreted by *P. aeruginosa* is very important to it and siderophore biosynthesis has been documented to represent an attractive antibiotic target (Quadri, 2000). *fpvA* has also been proposed to drive diversity at the pyoverdine locus (Smith *et al.*, 2005), looking at the strains I worked with, especially the clinical isolates (Isolated from burn wound), the primers used for amplification were different from those used for the existing *fpvA* type II pyoverdine isolates and following amplification and sequencing, a variant form (different from the already existing ferripyoverdine receptor gene types) of the ferripyoverdine receptor genes is presented (strain Br678, *fpvA* 93% identical to the *fpvA* gene of other strains in the homology tree (see homology tree c); comparison based on the sequenced 1.5 kb sized *fpvA* gene, strain Mi162 *fpvB* 98% identical to the *fpvB* gene of other strains in the homology tree (see homology tree a); comparison based on the sequenced 2.5 kb sized *fpvB* gene), this may then justify a correlation between amino acid sequence diversity of immunogenic bacterial proteins and evasion of host immune defense mechanisms (Tummler and Cornelis, 2005).

It would be interesting to study these strains in the future to pave way for the full understanding of underlying mechanism of antibiotic resistance. More research would be done in this regard hopefully.

11. Citation

J. Osayande : Use of Polymerase Chain Reaction for the Determination of about 2.5 kb fpvA and fpvB Gene Sequences in *Pseudomonas aeruginosa* Strains. *The Internet Journal of Microbiology.* 2009 Volume 7 Number 2

12. Acknowledgement

I am grateful to Professor P. Cornelis and the Vrije Universiteit Brussels (VUB) for the provision of Academic Scholarship.

13. References

[1] Al-Samarrai, T.H, Zhang, N., Lamont, I.L., Martin, Lois, Kolbe, J., Wilsher, M., Morris, A.J., and Schmid, J. 2000. Simple and inexpensive but highly discriminating method for computer-assisted DNA fingerprinting of *Pseudomonas aeruginosa*. J. Clin. Microbiol. 38(12): 4445-4452.

[2] Anzai, Y., Kim, H., Park, J.Y., Wakabayashi, H., and Oyaizu, H. 2000. Phylogenetic affiliation of the pseudomonads based on 16S rRNA sequence. Int. J. Syst. Evol. Microbiol. 50: 1563-1589.

[3] Beare, P.A., For, R.J., Martin, L.W., and Lamont I.L. 2003. Siderophore-mediated cell signaling in *Pseudomonas aeruginosa*: divergent pathways regulate virulence factor production and siderophore receptor synthesis. Mol. Microbiol. 47 (1): 195-207

[4] Bej, A.K., McCarty, S.C., and Atlas, R.M. 1991. Detection of coliform bacteria and Eschericia coli by multiplex polymerase chain reaction: Comparison with defined substrate and plating methods for water quality monitoring. Appl. Environ. Microbiol. 57(8): 2429-2432.

[5] Bodilis, J., Ghysels, B., Osayande, J., Matthijs, S., Pirnay, J.P., Denayer, S., De Vos, D., and Cornelis, P. 2009. Distribution and evolution of ferripyoverdine. April 21 [Epup ahead of print].

[6] Clarke, T.E., Tari, L.W., and Vogel, H.J. 2001. Structural biology of bacterial iron uptake systems. Curr. Top. Med. Chem. 1:7-30.

[7] Cornelis, P., Hohnadel, D., and Meyer, J.M. 1989. Evidence for different pyoverdine-mediated iron uptake systems among *Pseudomonas aeruginosa* strains. Infect. Immun. 57:3491-3497.

[8] Cox, C.D. 1986. Role of Pyocyanin in the acquisition of iron from transferrin. Infect. Immun. 52(1): 263-270.

[9] Cunliffe, H.E., Merriman, T.R., and Lamont, I.L. 1995. Cloning and characterisation of pvdS, a gene required for pyoverdine synthesis in *Pseudomonas aeruginosa*: PvdS is probably an alternative sigma factor. J. Bacteriol. 177: 2744-2750.

[10] De Chial, M., Ghysels, B., Beatson, S., Geoffroy, V., Meyer, J. M., Pattery, T., Baysse, C., Chablain, P., Parsons, Y.N., Winstanley, C., Cordwell, S., and Cornelis, P. 2003. Identification of type II and type III pyoverdine receptors from *Pseudomonas aeruginosa*. Microbiology 149: 821-831.

[11] De Vos, D., Lim, J. A., Pirnay, J.P., Struelens, M., Vandenvelde, C., Duinslaeger, L., Vanderkelen, A., and Cornelis, P. 1997. Direct detection and identification of *Pseudomonas aeruginosa* in clinical samples such as skin biopsy specimens and expectorations by multiplex PCR Based on two outer membrane lipoprotein Genes, OprI and OprL.J. Clin. Microbiol. 35(6): 1295-1299.

[12] De Vos, D., De Chial, M., Cochez, C., Jansen, S., Tummler, B., Meyer, J.M., and Cornelis, P. 2001. Study of pyoverdine type and production by *Pseudomonas aeruginosa* isolated from cystic fibrosis patients: prevalence of type II pyoverdine isolates and accumulation of pyoverdine –negative mutations. Arch. Microbiol. 175:384-388.

[13] Fricker, E.J., and Fricker, C.R. 1994. Application of the polymerase chain reaction to the identification of Escherichia coli and coliforms in water. Lett. Appl. Microbiol. 19: 44-46.

[14] Fuchs, R., Schafer, M., Geoffroy V., and Meyer, J.M. 2001. Siderotyping - A powerful tool for the characterization of pyoverdines. Curr. Top. Med. Chem. 1:31-57.

[15] Gensberg, K., Hughes, K., and Smith, A.W. 1992. Siderophore-specific induction of iron uptake in *Pseudomonas aeruginosa*. J. Gen. Microbiol. 138:2381-2387.

[16] Ghysels, B., Dieu, B.T., Beatson, S.A., Pirnay, J.P., Ochsner, U.A., Vasil, M.L., and Cornelis, P. 2004. FpvB, an alternative type I ferripyoverdine receptor of *Pseudomonas aeruginosa*. Microbiology 150: 1671-1680.

[17] Guerinot, M.L. 1994. Microbial iron transport. Annu. Rev. Microbiol. 48: 743-72.
[18] Karry Mullis Nobel Lecture, December 8, 1993.
[19] Kasai, H., Watanabe, K., Gasteiger, E., Bairoch, A., Isono, K., Yamamoto, S., and Harayama, S. 1998. Construction of the gyrB database for the identification and classification of bacteria. Genome Inform. 9:13-21.
[20] Laguerre, G., Gois-Rigottier, L., and Lemanceau, P. 1994. Fluorescent Pseudomonas species categorized by using polymerase chain reaction (PCR)/ restriction fragment analysis of 16S rDNA. Mol. Ecol., 3: 479-487.
[21] Mcintosh, I., Govan, J.R.W., and Brock, D.J.H. 1992. Detection of *Pseudomonas aeruginosa* in sputum from cystic fibrosis patients by the polymerase chain reaction. Mol. Cell. Probes 6: 299-304.
[22] McMorran, B.J., Merriman, M.E., Rombel, I.T., and Lamont, I.L. 1996. Characterization of the pvdE gene which is required for pyoverdine synthesis in *Pseudomonas aeruginosa*. Gene 176: 55-59.
[23] Mercer, A.A and Loutit , J.S. 1979. Transformation and transfection of *Pseudomonas aeruginosa*: Effects of Metal Ions. J. Bacteriol. 140 (1) 37-42.
[24] Meyer, J.M. 1992. Exogenous siderophore-mediated iron uptake in *Pseudomonas aeruginosa*: possible involvement of porin OprF in iron translocation. J. Gen. Microbiol. 138:951-958.
[25] Meyer, J.M., Geoffroy, V.A., Baida, N., Gardan, L., Izard, D., Lemanceau, P., Achouk, W., and Palleroni, N. 2002. Siderophore typing, a powerful tool for the identification of fluorescent and non-fluorescent pseudomonads. Appl. Environ. Microbiol. 68: 2745-2753.
[26] Meyer, J.M., Neely, A., Stintzi, A., Georges, C., and Holder, I.A. 1996. Pyoverdine is essential for virulence of Pseudomonas aeruginosa. Infect. Immun. 64: 518-523.
[27] Meyer, J.M., Stintzi, A., and Poole, K. 1999. The ferripyoverdine receptor FpvA of *Pseudomonas aeruginosa* PAO1 recognizes the ferripyoverdines of P. aeruginosa and P. fluorescens ATCC 13525. FEMS Microbiol. Lett. 170: 145-150.
[28] Pirnay, J.P., De Vos, D., Cochez, C., Bilcoq, F., Vanderkelen, A., Zizi, M., Ghysels, B., and Cornelis, P. 2002. *Pseudomonas aeruginosa* displays an epidemic population structure. Environ. Microbiol. 4: 898-911.
[29] Pirnay, J.P., Matthijs, S., Colak, H., Chablain, P., Bilocq, F., Van Eldere, J., De Vos, D., Zizi, M., Triest L., and Cornelis, P. 2005. Global *Pseudomonas aeruginosa* biodiversity as reflected in a Belgian river. Environ. Microbiol. 7(7): 969-980.
[30] Poole, K., Neshat, S., and Heinrichs, D. 1991. Pyoverdine-mediated iron transport in *Pseudomonas aeruginosa*: involvement of a high -molecular -mass outer membrane protein. FEMS Microbiol. Lett. 78: 1-6.
[31] Poole, K., Neshat, S., Krebes, K., and Heinrichs, D.E. 1993. Cloning and nucleotide sequence analysis of the ferripyoverdine receptor fpvA of *Pseudomonas aeruginosa.* J. Bacteriol. 175: 4597-4604.
[32] Qin, X., Emerson, J., Stapp, J., Stapp, L., Abe, P., and Burns, J.L. 2003. Use of real-time PCR with multiple targets to identify *Pseudomonas aeruginosa* and other nonfermenting Gram-negative Bacilli from patients with cystic fibrosis. J. Clin. Microbiol. 41: 4312-4317.
[33] Quadri, L.E.N. 2000. Assembly of aryl-capped siderophores by modular peptide synthetases and polyketide synthases. Mol. Microbiol. 37(1): 1-12.

[34] Smith, E.E., Sims, E.H., Spencer, D.H., Kaul, R., and Olson, M.V. 2005. Evidence for diversifying selection at the pyoverdine locus of *Pseudomonas aeruginosa*. J. Bacteriol. 187(6): 2138-2147.

[35] Spencer, D. H., Kas, A., Smith, E. E., Raymond, C. K., Sims, E. H., Hastings, M., Burns, J. L., Kaul, R., and Olson, M. V. 2003. Whole-genome sequence variation among multiple isolates of *Pseudomonas aeruginosa*. J. Bacteriol. 185, 1316–1325.

[36] Stinzi, A., Barnes, C., Xu, J., and Raymond, K.N. 2000. Microbial iron transport via a siderophore shuttle: a membrane ion transport paradigm. Proc. Natl. Acad. Sci. USA, 97: 10691-10696.

[37] Stover, C.K., Pham, X.Q., Erwin, A.L., Mizoguchi, S.D., Warrener, P., Hickey, M.J., Brinkman, F.S., Hufnagle, W.O., Kowalik, D.J., Lagrou, M., Garber, R.L., Goltry, L., Tolentino E, Westbrock-Wadman, S., Yuan, Y., Brody, L.L., Coulter, S.N., Folger, K.R., Kas, A., Larbig, K., Lim, R., Smith, K., Spencer, D., Wong, G.K., Wu, Z., Paulsen, I.T., Reizer, J., Saier, M.H., Hancock, R.E., Lory, S., Olson, M.V. 2000. Complete genome sequence of *Pseudomonas aeruginosa* PA01, an opportunistic pathogen. Nature 406(6799):959-64.

[38] Thupvong, T., Wiideman, A., Dunn, D., Oreschalk, K., Jankowicz, B., Doering, J., and Castignetti, D. 1999. Sequence heterogeneity of the ferripyoverdine uptake (fpvA), but not the ferric uptake regultaor (fur), genes among strains of the fluorescent pseudomonads *Pseudomonas aeruginosa, Pseudomonas aureofaciens, Pseudomonas fluorescens and Pseudomonas putida*. Biometals 12: 265-274.

[39] Todar, K. 2004.The Good, the Bad and the Deadly. Science Magazine, 304: Pg. 1421

[40] Tummler, B., and Cornelis, P. 2005. Pyoverdine Receptor: a case of Darwinian selection in *Pseudomonas aeruginosa*. J. Bacteriol. 187(10): 3289-3292.

[41] Visca, P., Ciervo, A., and Orsi, N. 1994. Cloning and nucleotide sequence of the pvdA gene encoding the pyoverdine biosynthetic enzyme L-ornithine N5-oxygenase in *Pseudomonas aeruginosa*. J. Bacteriol. 176(4): 1128-1140.

17

The Role of Bacteria and Yeasts in AIDS

Vladimír Zajac[1,2], Zuzana Adamcikova[1], Vladimir Holec[2], Katarina Hainova[1], Viola Stevurkova[1] and Lenka Wachsmannova[1]

[1]*The Cancer Reasearch Institute, Department of Cancer Genetics, SAS, Bratislava,*
[2]*Comenius University, Medical Faculty, Bratislava,*
Slovak Republic

1. Introduction

Human immunodeficiency virus type I (HIV-1) is widely accepted as the cause of AIDS. It is also believed that HIV-1 itself is sufficient to cause immunodeficiency and to destroy parenchyma cells inducing widespread organ failure. Despite the unquestionable success in diagnosis and therapy of this disease, there are many unanswered questions. The substantial argument of this predication is the fact that it is still not possible to stop the worldwide pervasion of AIDS, especially in Africa and Asia. Without giving answers to all these questions a more successful treatment of patients cannot be expected. The fight against this disease is challenging and should be realized in a more complex manner, overcoming all the taboos and dogmas surrounding the disease. It is necessary to deliberate other potential factors, not only HIV, which may take part in this disease.

Plasma HIV RNA is dramatically reduced in HIV/AIDS patients treated with highly active antiretroviral therapy (HAART), but residual viral replication is detected after suppression of plasma viraemia (Chun et al., 2000; Cusisni et al., 2004). It has also been expressly proven that various forms of HIV reservoirs persist in practically all patients receiving HAART (Finzi et al., 1997; Siliciano et al., 2003). The range of viral reservoirs in the human body is probably very much wider, as claimed in recent studies. Reservoirs were detected in macrophages and other cells of the blood system, in which even very effective HAART was not able to eliminate the virus. HIV persists in peripheral blood mononuclear cells despite sustained, undetectable plasma viraemia resulting from long-term antiretroviral therapy (Veazey et al., 1998; Brenchley et al., 2004). The source of persistent HIV in these infected persons remains however unclear.

Over the last period of time AIDS research has been focused on the gut and other mucosal tissue, and not blood, as the major site of HIV infection and CD4+ T cells loss (Veazey et al., 2005). Mattapallil and Li both showed that the major focus of destruction of memory CD4+ T cells by simian immunodeficiency virus (SIV) is in mucosal cells, where most T cells expressing CD4 and CCR5 with a "memory" phenotype reside (Mattapallil et al., 2005; Li et al., 2005). The loss of $CD4^+$ T cells in the intestine coincided with productive infection of large numbers of mononuclear cells at this site (Veazey et al., 1990). These recent findings support the idea that the mucosal and intestine immune system is the major site of viral replication, persistence and CD4+ T cells loss in HIV-1 infected persons (Guadalupe et al., 2006; Dandekar et al., 2007; Ling et al., 2007, 2010; Lackner et al., 2009; Hatziioannou et al., 2009). HIV-1 has been also detected in bowel crypt cells and the lamina propria from patients with gastrointestinal symptoms (Nelson et al., 1988). The pathogenesis of HIV infection is presumably centered on these mucosal viral "target" cells. Since these cells are in close vicinity to intestinal bacteria, the idea has been raised that bacteria may also be involved in AIDS pathogenesis.

This interest in investigating bacteria and mycoplasma was also supported by Montagnier's finding, confirmed by Shyh-Ching Lo, that mycoplasma is a very important "co-factor" which accelerates the progression of HIV infection in AIDS patients (Montagnier, 1986; Lo et al., 1991). And finally, Cantwell and Broxmeyer pointed out that there is a very close relationship between bacteria and cancer, resp. AIDS (Cantwell, 1983, 1993; Broxmeyer & Cantwell, 2008).

2. Molecular biology analysis of bacteria and yeasts of HIV positive patients

2.1 Dot blot DNA hybridization.

To verify this idea, bacterial DNA isolated from the gastrointestinal tract and blood DNA of 51 AIDS patients and 10 healthy subjects were tested for the presence of HIV-1 sequences by colony and dot blot hybridization (Zajac et al., 2005, 2006, 2007, 2011). In dot blot hybridization, the lymphocyte/bacterial DNA of American and Slovak HIV/AIDS patients were in most cases positive (Figure 1). Of 27 patient samples, 23 lymphocyte DNA and 20 bacterial were positive, with respective 85% and 74%. Yet positivity of all the 41 patients tested was approximately the same. The selected patients 23, 33, 44, 78, 30, P1 and P15 are localized as follows: patient 23 in line 2 - position 1,2; patient 33 in line 1 - 5,6; patient 44 in line 4 - 3,4; patient 78 in line 6 - 1,2; patient 30 in line 7 - 1,2; patient P1 in line 7 -3,4 and patient P15 in line 7 - 5,6. The intensity of the hybridization signal was in correlation with the origin of the probes used, the signal of human samples was more intensive with the applied human probes and vice versa for bacterial probes (data not shown). These findings suggest some differences in sequences between the two sources of material. The hybridization signals of samples from patients 96, 83, 62 (line 3, position 5, 6; line 4, position 1, 2; line 2, position 5, 6) were not intensive either in lymphocyte or bacterial DNA. These patients were classified as A1 stage of their CDC clinical category with $CD4^+$ around 400/µl. The obtained results are in correlation with the common usage of 68; 69 primers in AIDS diagnostics. The hybridization signal was not detected in samples of control subjects, with the exception of samples from one subject (line 12, position 5,6).

Bacteria and yeasts from the respiratory tract (nose, pharyngeal swabs) were isolated from 39 Cambodian and 28 Kenyan HIV-positive children. The majority of microbes were characterized as *Staphylococcus aureus, Klebsiella pneumoniae* and *Candida albicans.* In some cases, *E. coli, Streptococcus pyogenes, Proteus mirabilis* and *Candida tropicalis* were identified. Bacteria and yeasts of 16 Cambodian (41%) and 8 Kenyan (31%) children were found to be positive in colony and dot-blot DNA hybridization (17). Bacteria and yeasts from the respiratory tract of 41% of Cambodian (Figure 2) and 31% of Kenyan HIV-positive children bear HIV-like sequences.

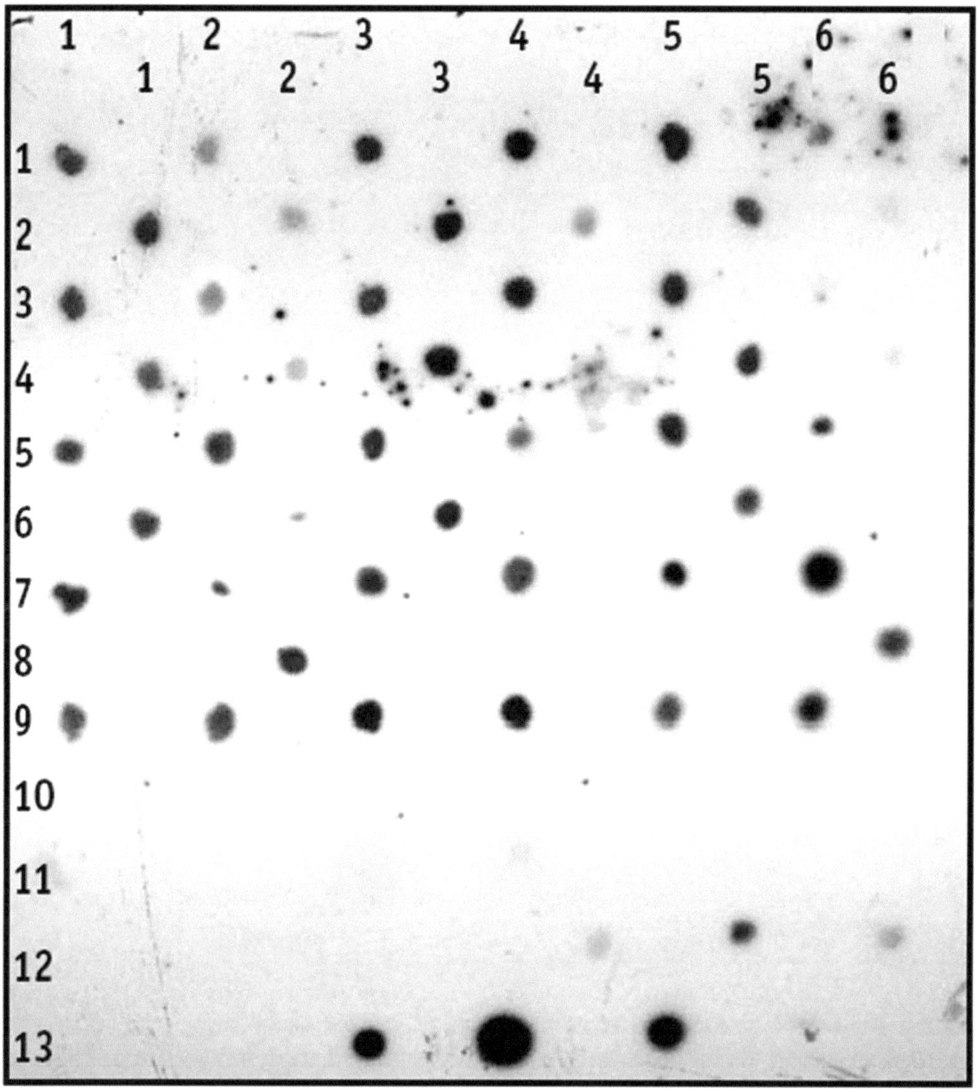

Fig. 1. Dot blot hybridization. DNA of lymphocyte/bacterial DNA (0.2 µg) from 27 HIV positive patients are on lines 1-9 and from 9 healthy subjects are on lines 10-12. The PCR products 38;39, 68;69 and mixture, synthesized on the template of patient 30's DNA were used as probes. They are on line 13 in position 3, 4, 5 diluted 1:100.

The PCR specific for HIV sequences was carried out using HIV-1-specific primers. The analysis was performed by colony and dot-blot hybridization using HIV-1-specific primers, which represent *gag, pol* and *env* genes of the virus.

2.2 PCR and sequencing

Subsequently, bacterial DNA of positive isolates was amplified by the PCR using two sets of primers. The PCR products of 142 bp (primers 68;69, *env* gene of HIV-1) were detected in all

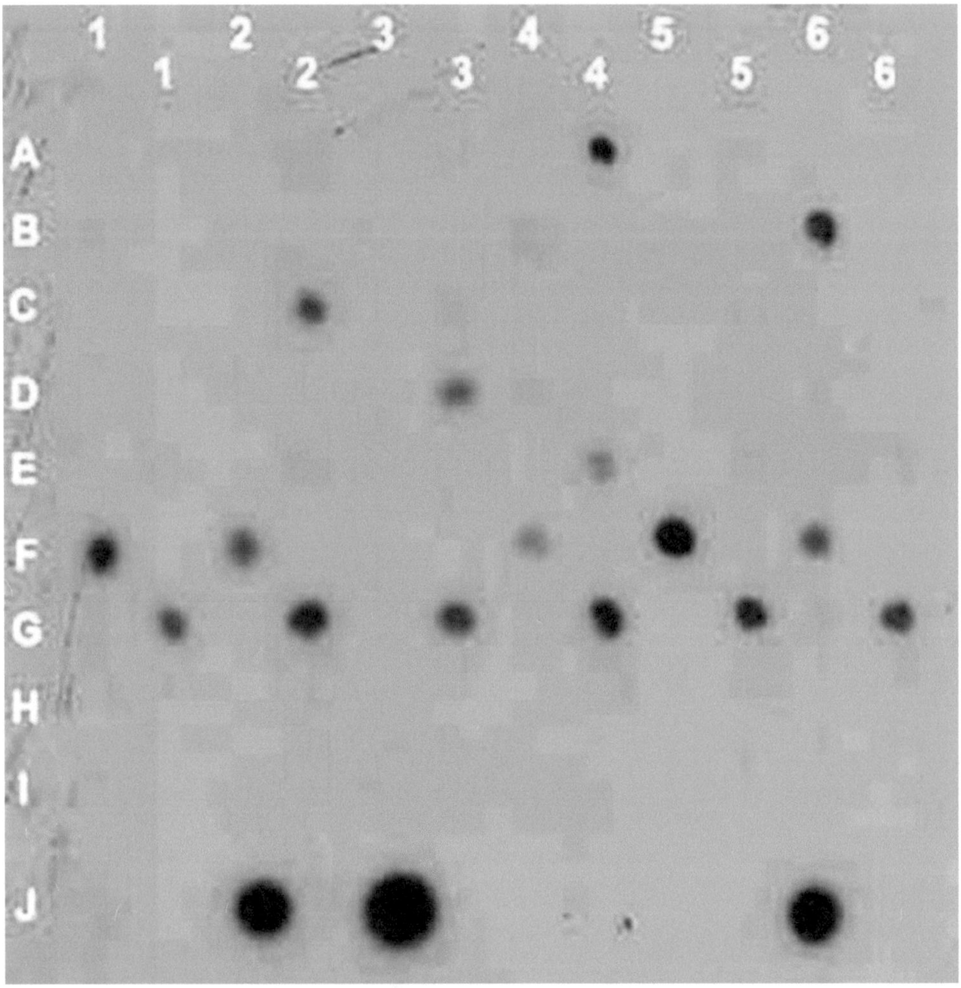

Fig. 2. Dot-blot hybridization of bacterial DNA from Cambodian and Kenyan HIV positive children. Lines A-G: samples of 42 patients; lines H-I: samples of 8 healthy subjects; line J: in position 6 is DNA of AIDS child and in position 2, 3 are probes diluted 1:100 and 1:50.

bacterial samples tested. The longest PCR products of 1484 bp determined by primers P10: CATTTGGAAAGGACCAGCAAAACTACT (HIV-1 *pol* gene position 4430); E1:TCATATGCTTTAGCATCTGATGCACAA (HIV-1 *env* gene position 5914) were detected in 70% of the patient bacterial DNA: M11, P1, P3, P6, P15, P9, M1, M2, M15, M12, M22 (Figure 3).

The PCR products synthesized on the template of bacterial DNA analyzed and on the template of patient's DNA using primers from *gag*, *pol* and *env* genes were sequenced. By sequencing PCR products synthesized on the template of the patients' bacterial DNA using primers 68;69 *env* HIV-1 gene, 68for: AGCAGCAGGAAGCACTATGG, 69rev: CCAGACTGTGAGTTGCAACAG) homology greater than 90% with HIV-1 isolate HXB2 (HIVHXB2CG) was revealed. Sequences of intestinal bacteria of patients revealed at least 90% homology with three crucial HIV-1 genes (*gag, pol, env*). Amplified fragments longer than 120 bp were directly sequenced on the ABI 373 DNA Sequencer.

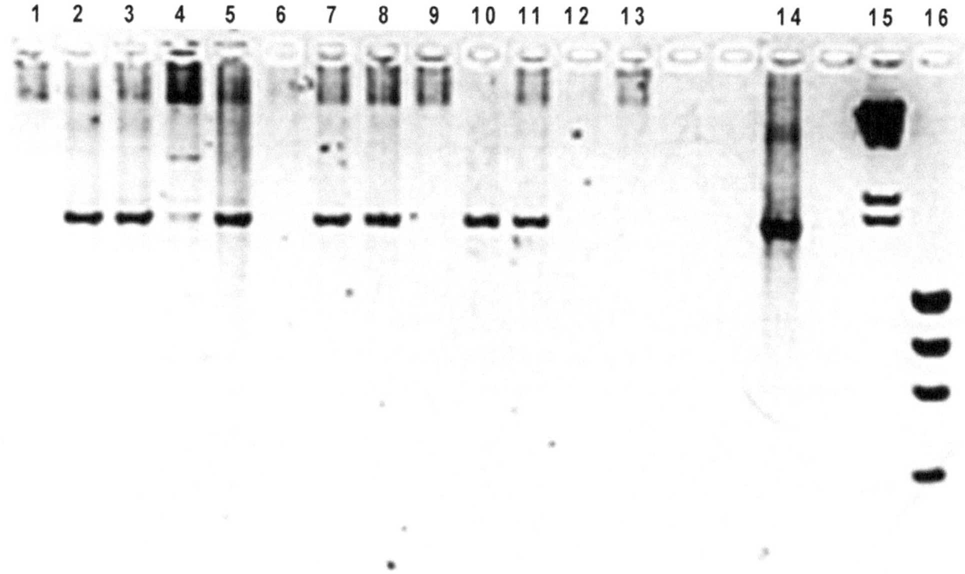

Fig. 3. The PCR products of 1484 bp determined by primers P10for ; E1rev synthesized on the template of bacterial DNA. Lines 1 - 11: AIDS patients; line 12 – PCR without DNA; line 13 - negative control; line 14 - pBH10; line 15 – marker λDNA×HindIII; line 16 - marker ϕX174×HaeIII.

```
               (1) 1        10        20        30        40        50        60        70        80        90             105
  23h 68;69    (1) AGCAGCAGGAAGCACTATGGGCGCAGCGTCAATGACGCTGACGGTACAGGCCAGACAGTTATTGTCTGGTATAGTGCACCAGCAGAACAATTTGCTGAGGGCTAT
  23b 68;69    (1) AGCAGCAGGAAGCACTATGGGCGCAGCGTCAATGACGCTGACGGTACAGGCCAGACAGTTATTGTCTGGTATAGTGCACCAGCAGAACAATTTGCTGAGGGCTAT
  33h 68;69    (1) AGCAGCAGGAAGCACTATGGGCGCAGCGTCAATGACGCTGACGGTACAGGCCAGACAGTTATTGTCTGGTATAGTGCACCAGCAGAACAATTTGCTGAGGGCTAT
  33b 68;69    (1) AGCAGCAGGAAGCACTATGGGCGCAGCGTCAATGACGYTGACGGTACAGGCCAGACAGTTATTGTCTGGTATAGTGCACCAGCAGAACAATTTGCTGAGGGCTAT
  44h 68;69    (1) AGCAGCAGGAAGCACTATGGGCGCAGCGTCAATGACGCTGACGGTACAGGCCAGACAGTTATTGTCTGGTATAGTGCACCAGCAGAACAATTTGCTGAGGGCTAT
  44b 68;69    (1) AGCAGCAGGAAGCACTATGGGCGCAGCGTCAATGACGYTGACGGTACAGGCCAGACAGTTATTGTCTGGTATAGTGCACCAGCAGAACAATTTGCTGAGGGCTAT
  78h 68;69    (1) AGCAGCAGGAAGCACTATGGGCGCAGCGTCAATGACGCTGACGGTACAGGCCAGACAGTTATTGTCTGGTATAGTGCACCAGCAGAACAATTTGCTGAGGGCTAT
  78b 68;69    (1) AGCAGCAGGAAGCACTATGGGCGCAGCGTCAATGACGYTGACGGTACAGGCCAGACAGTTATTGTCTGGTATAGTGCACCAGCAGAACAATTTGCTGAGGGCTAT
  30h 68;69    (1) AGCAGCAGGAAGCACTATGGGCGCAGCGTCAATGACGCTGACGGTACAGGCCAGACAGTTATTGTCTGGTATAGTGCACCAGCAGAACAATTTGCTGAGGGCTAT
  30b 68;69    (1) AGCAGCAGGAAGCACTATGGGCGCAGCGTCAATGACGSTGACGGTACAGGCCAGACAGTTATTGTCTGGTATAGTGCACCAGCAGAACAATTTGCTGAGGGCTAT
  P1h 68;69    (1) AGCAGCAGGAAGCACTATGGGCGCAGCGTCAATGACGTTGACGGTACAGGCCAGACAGTTATTGTCTGGTATAGTGCACCAGCAGAACAATTTGCTGAGGGCTAT
  P15h 68;69   (1) AGCAGCAGGAAGCACTATGGGCGCAGCGTCAATGACGYTGACGGTACAGGCCAGACAGTTATTGTCTGGTATAGTGCACCAGCAGAACAATTTGCTGAGGGCTAT
  P1b 68;69    (1) AGCAGCAGGAAGCACTATGGGCGCAGCGTCAATGACGCTGACGGTACAGGCCAGACAATTATTGTCTGGTATAGTGCACCAGCAGAACAATTTGCTGAGGGCTAT
  P15b 68;69   (1) AGCAGCAGGAAGCACTATGGGCGCAGCGTCAATGACGMTGACGGTACAGGCCAGACAATTATTGTCTGGTATAGTGCACCAGCAGAACAATTTGCTGAGGGCTAT
  pBH10 68-69  (1) AGCAGCAGGAAGCACTATGGGCGCAGGCTCAATAACGCTAACGGTACAGGCCAGACACTTATTGTCTGGTATAGTGCAACAGCAAAACAATTTGCTGAGGGCTAT
  Consensus    (1) AGCAGCAGGAAGCACTATGGGCGCAGCGTCAATGACGCTGACGGTACAGGCCAGACAGTTATTGTCTGGTATAGTGCACCAGCAGAACAATTTGCTGAGGGCTAT

             (106) 106          120       130    142
  23h 68;69  (106) WGAGGCGCAACAGCATCTGTTGCAACTCACAGTCTGG
  23b 68;69  (106) AGAGGCGCAACAGCATCTGTTGCAACTCACAGTCTGG
  33h 68;69  (106) TGAGGCGCAACAGCATCTGTTGCAACTCACAGTCTGG
  33b 68;69  (106) WGAGGCGCAACAGCATCTGTTGCAACTCACAGTCTGG
  44h 68;69  (106) WGAGGCGCAACAGCATCTGTTGCAACTCACAGTCTGG
  44b 68;69  (106) TGAGGCGCAACAGCATCTGTTGCAACTCACAGTCTGG
  78h 68;69  (106) WGAGGCGCAACAGCATCTGTTGCAACTCACAGTCTGG
  78b 68;69  (106) WGAGGCGCAACAGCATCTGTTGCAACTCACAGTCTGG
  30h 68;69  (106) WGAGGCGCAACAGCATCTGTTGCAACTCACAGTCTGG
  30b 68;69  (106) AGAGGCGCAACAGCATCTGTTGCAACTCACAGTCTGG
  P1h 68;69  (106) TGAGGCGCAACAGCATCTGTTGCAACTCACAGTCTGG
  P15h 68;69 (106) TGAGGCGCAACAGCATCTGTTGCAACTCACAGTCTGG
  P1b 68;69  (106) TGAGGCGCAACAGCATCTGTTGCAACTCACAGTCTGG
  P15b 68;69 (106) WGAGGCGCAACAGCATCTGTTGCAACTCACAGTCTGG
  pBH10 68-69(106) TGAGGCGCAACAGCATCTGTTGCAACTCACGGTCTGG
  Consensus  (106)  GAGGCGCAACAGCATCTGTTGCAACTCACAGTCTGG
```

Fig. 4. Comparison of the sequences of 142 bp PCR products synthesized on the template of patients' lymphocyte (h) and bacterial (b) DNA, determined by primers 68; 69, of selected patients 23, 33, 44, 78, 30, P1 and P15. Abbreviations: Y - C or T, M - A or C, S – G or C, W - A or T.

The sequences of 142 bp PCR products synthesized on the template of patients' lymphocyte (h) and bacterial (b) DNA, determined by primers 68; 69, were remarkably similar, with some differences occurring between isolates (Figure 4). These minor differences in the isolates strongly suggest that the DNA has a common recent ancestry in HIV-1. Important is the finding of rather marked differences between bacterial sequences and sequences of pBH10 in all fragments tested. On the basis of these results, the possibility of contamination of our samples by pBH10 plasmid DNA is practically excluded.

2.3 Protein analysis of patient's bacteria and yeasts

The expression of HIV-1 antigens in bacteria and yeasts of HIV positive patients was detected by using specific monoclonal antibodies against HIV-1 antigens p17, p24, p55, gp41 and gp120 (Abcam, UK). 55 kDa protein was detected using MAbs against HIV-1 p24 approximately in 30-35% bacterial extracts of HIV positive Cambodian (Km) and Kenyan (Ke) tested patients: 14Km, 31Km, 3'Km, 32'Km, 21Ke, 17'Ke, 14'Ke. (Figure 5).
Using MAbs against gp41 the protein of 41 kDa was identified in 30-35% of bacterial extracts of Cambodian and Kenyan and of American and Slovak patients: P79, PEC, P14, P5, P15, P1. (Figure 6).

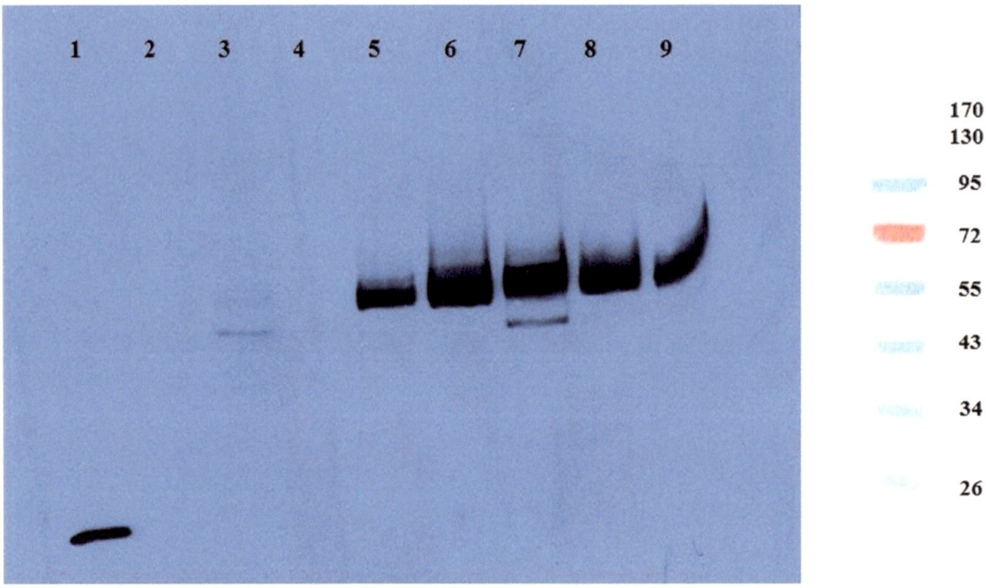

Fig. 5. Western blotting of proteins isolated from bacteria and yeasts of the respiratory tract (nose, pharyngeal swabs) of Cambodian (Km) and Kenyan (Ke) HIV positive children. Detection was performed using monoclonal antibodies against HIV-1 p24. Line 1: p24 diluted 1:500; line 2: control bacteria Muta 104-0; lines 3-9 tested samples.

55 kDa protein was also detected in bacteria and yeasts from bacteria and yeasts of the respiratory tract (nose, pharyngeal swabs) of Cambodian (Km) and Kenyan (Ke) HIV positive children: 14Km, 17'Ke, 21Ke, 32'Km, 3'Km, 31Km, 14'Ke, using by MAbs against HIV1 p17, p55 (Figure 7).

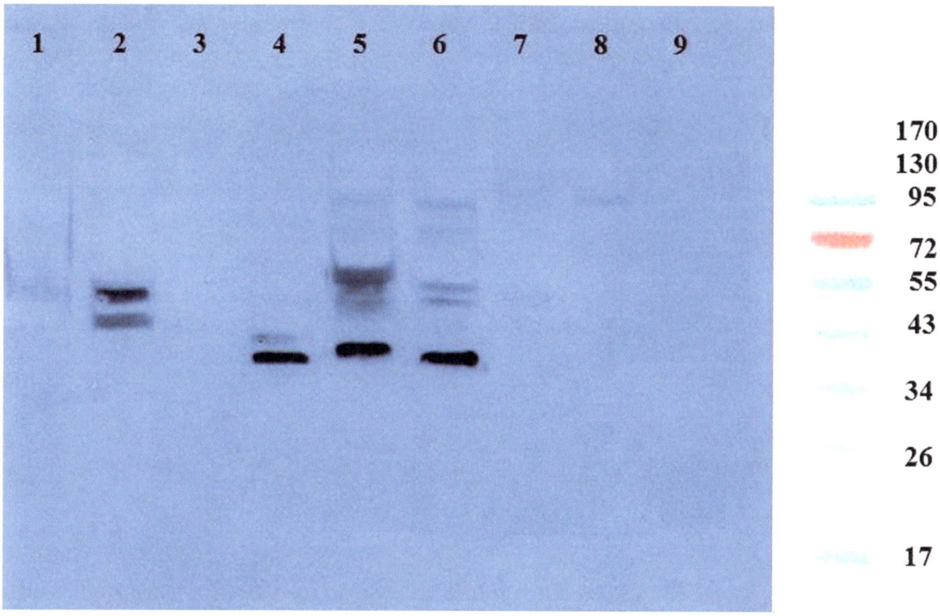

Fig. 6. Western blotting of proteins isolated from intestinal bacteria of Slovak and American HIV positive patients. For detection monoclonal antibodies against HIV-1 gp41 diluted 1:750 were used. Line 1: negative control; line 2: serum of AIDS patient; line 3: control HB101; lines 4-9 tested patients.

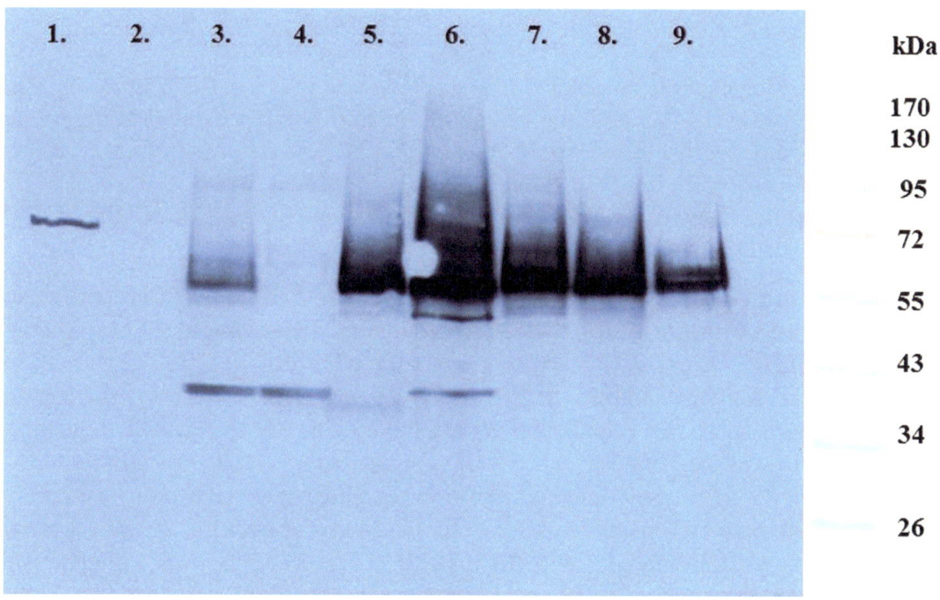

Fig. 7. Western blotting of proteins isolated from bacteria and yeasts of the respiratory tract (nose, pharyngeal swabs) of Cambodian (Km) and Kenyan (Ke) HIV positive children. Detection was performed using monoclonal antibodies against HIV-1 p17, p55 diluted 1:750. Line 1: serum of AIDS patient diluted 1:100; line 2: negative control; lines 3-9 tested samples.

Using monoclonal antibodies against HIV-1 gp120 (1:750), proteins of 75-80 kDa were detected in protein extracts from bacteria and yeasts of the respiratory tract (nose, pharyngeal swabs) of Cambodian (Km) and Kenyan (Ke) HIV positive children: 14Km, 17'Ke, 21Ke, 32'Km, 3'Km, 31Km, 14'Ke (Figure 8).

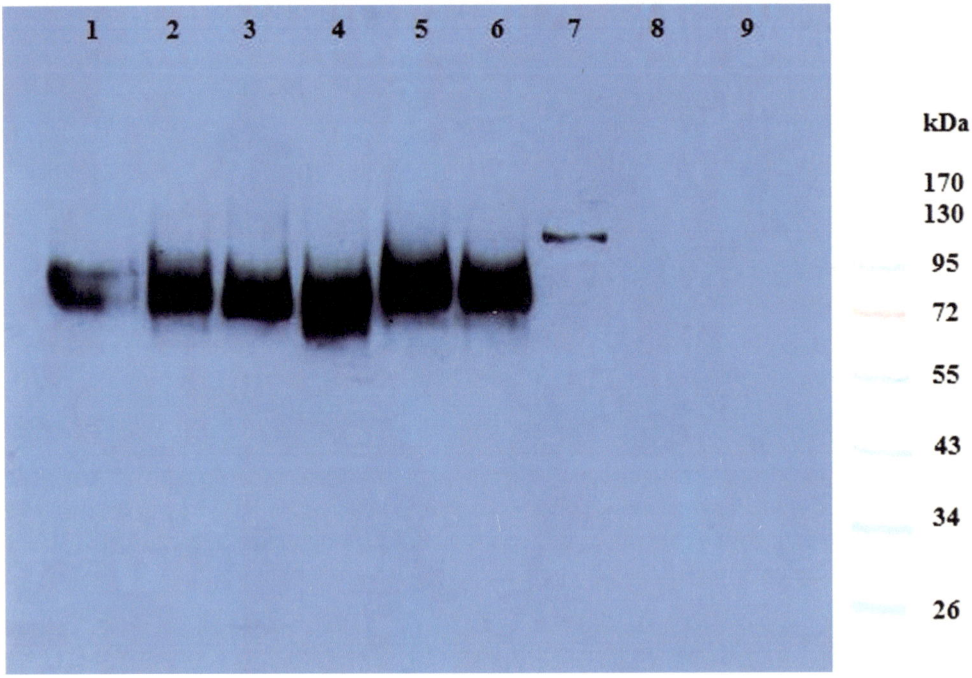

Fig. 8. Western blotting of proteins isolated from bacteria and yeasts of the respiratory tract (nose, pharyngeal swabs) of Cambodian (Km) and Kenyan (Ke) HIV positive children. Used monoclonal antibodies against HIV-1 gp120 (1:750). lines 1-6 tested samples. Line 7: serum of AIDS patient diluted 1:100; line 9: negative control bacteria Muta 104-0.
In samples of Slovak and American HIV positive patients using MAbs against HIV p17, p55 proteins of about 30 kDa was found.

In addition, the protein of molecular weight 55 kDa was detected in Cambodian and Kenyan samples by MAbs anti HIV-1 p17 and p55. Its molecular weight is comparable to *gag*-encoded Pr55Gag precursor. By MAbs against HIV p24, protein of 55 kDa was found in Cambodian and Kenyan samples. Surprisingly, no proteins were found in bacterial extract of 10 American and 24 Slovak AIDS patients by this MAbs. Protein detected by Mabs against gp41 was identified in 30-35% of samples from all cohorts of patients. The protein of about 85 kDa was detected only in *Candida* species protein extracts of Cambodian and Kenyan HIV positive children by the MAbs against gp120. In Slovak and American samples, protein reacting with MAbs anti gp120 was not found. These results suggest that there are specific differences between bacterial proteins of Slovak and American HIV positive patients on one side and Cambodian and Kenyan on the other. These differences suggest a diverse bacterial evolution in various geographical areas. Microbes of Slovak and American HIV/AIDS patients were most often identified as *Klebsiella pneumoniae, Escherichia coli, Proteus mirabilis, Citrobacter freundii* and *Enterobacter aerogenes.* Microbes from respiratory tract of Cambodian and Kenyan HIV/AIDS patients were most often identified as *Staphylococcus aureus, Klebsiella pneumoniae, Candida albicans, Candida tropicalis, Enterobacter aerogenes,* but also as *Escherichia coli* and *Proteus mirabilis.*

2.4 Tests for internalization capacity of patient's bacteria

The obtained results raise the question, what is the role of intestinal bacteria bearing HIV sequences in the AIDS process (Simon & Gorbach, 1984). Analogous to the finding of Swidsinski (Swidsinski et al., 1998, 2002) and our previous works (Mego et al., 2005, 2006) that bacteria isolated from biopsies of polyps, adenomas, and carcinomas are able to internalize epithelial cells, we tested bacteria purified from the intestinal tract of Slovak and American HIV/AIDS patients for their capacity to be internalized by cells of HL-60 cell line and normal human lymphocytes. In the present study, the specific characteristic was found to be their vigorous ability to be internalized by HL-60 cells and human lymphocytes, as confirmed by a gentamicin protection assay. In comparison with intramucosal bacteria isolated from patients with colorectal cancer, their capacity to be internalized by normal human lymphocytes was 5-10 times higher and in most cases the cells were lysed. Bacteria 725/5 were classified as *Enterobacter cloacae* and all other clones tested were characterized as *Escherichia coli.* Internalization frequently resulted in partial (bacteria of patients M1, M22) or complete lysis (patients K1, M12) of HL-60 cells. Partial (patients P3, M22) and complete lysis (patients P1, K1, M1, M12) was detected also after infection of normal human lymphocytes.

What is the fate of bacteria after internalization? As we demonstrate, about 50-60% of the bacteria of tested AIDS patients are competent to lyse HL-60 and lymphocytes of host cells. The remaining part of intracellular bacteria survived in the host cells for a further 7-10 days, as shown by GPA. After this time the GPA test was negative. It can be assumed that in nature some pathogenic bacteria which penetrated into the blood system may infect or lyse lymphatic cells.

Patient/bacterial clone	Number of bacterial colonies
	HIV positive patients
P15/7	2264
P1/4	1340
P3/3	1680
725/5	1140
M1/6	481/partial lyses of HL-60 cells
M22/5	27/partial lyses of HL-60 cells
M12/5	complete lyses of HL-60 cells
K1/1	complete lyses of HL-60 cells
	Colon cancer patients
TuSG/1	71
883 S/3	104
MZRa/3	44
negative controls (healthy subjects)	<5

Table 1. Gentamicin protection assay. The number of colonies represents the number of intracellular bacteria in HL-60 cells. Number of cells used for assay: HL-60 $5x10^6$; bacteria $1x10^8$

Patient/bacterial clone	Number of bacterial colonies
	HIV positive patients
P15/7	1121
P3/3	320/partial lysis of human lymphocytes
725/5	1140
M22/5	423/partial lyses of human lymphocytes
P1/4	complete lyses of human lymphocytes
K1/1	complete lyses of human lymphocytes
M1/6	complete lyses of human lymphocytes
M12/5	complete lyses of human lymphocytes
	Colon cancer patients
TuSG/1	1
883 S/3	0
MZRa/3	4
negative controls (healthy subjects)	<5

Table 2. Gentamicin protection assay. The number of colonies represents the number of intracellular bacteria in normal human lymphocytes. Number of used cells: normal human lymphocytes $1,5x10^7$; bacteria $1x10^8$.

To analyze the role of bacteria in immunodeficiency, reduction of their amount in the intestinal tract of 20 AIDS patients was performed by oral administration of probiotic bacteria *Escherichia coli* strain Nissle 1917. After three months of probiotics treatment the viral load decreased or remained on the detection limit (<400 c/ml) in 55.5% of the patients tested. According to these findings, it is assumed that not only one biological component plays the most important role in the AIDS process, but that there are two – HIV and the bacterial host. These bacteria bearing rich extrachromosomal genetic information are able to penetrate from the GIT into the human body and attack strongly the human immune system.

3. Etiology and possible evolution of disease

The fundamental, still unanswered question is the origin of HIV (Gallo et al., 1985; Baltimore, 1985; Duesberg, 1987; Temin, 1988, 1989; Varmus, 1989; Sharp et al., 2001; Zhu et al., 1998; Apetrei & Marx, 2005). Is HIV a unique relative of other retroviruses? When looking at retroviruses, the rule applies that practically every species in the animal kingdom has its own retrovirus – mouse, rat, chicken, goat, sheep, cow, horse, monkey, chimpanzee, etc. Some of them are very contiguous, due to their phylogenetic relationship - mouse and rat, monkey and chimpanzee. Similarly, retroviruses of monkeys, chimpanzee and humans are evolutionarily collateral. Yet there is no substantial evidence about transmission of retroviruses between different species in nature. On the basis of these facts and our achieved results, it is possible to conclude - all retroviruses have been an integral part of a particular host organism since the beginning of their existence as species and they are passed on from generation to generation. The hosts – including humans - inherited them from their ancestors. In accordance with this idea, it is assumed that transfer of the HIV from apes to humans in Africa, as a consequence of their accidental contacts, is not the cause of AIDS pandemics.

But there is a very serious objection - if HIV were in our bacteria from our beginning, why did they emerge only about 25-35 years ago? Were they hidden without any implication all the time, for many thousands of years, in our bodies? To answer this question, we should go back into the ancient history of humankind. In the past, major epidemics frequently occurred when there were new patterns of communication and transportation between separately populated areas and/or new patterns of settlement. The first recorded great plague occurred in Athens during the Peloponnesian war in 430 BC. In the middle of the sixth century AD (542), there was a great outbreak of bubonic plague (Justinianus) in the Mediterranean countries, where 40 to 50% of the population died. The biggest cataclysm of bubonic plague epidemic started in 1346 in Europe and the population was finally decimated by 50 to 60%. Plague subsequently spread to Asia and at least 60 million people died just only in China alone. This plague continued up to the seventeenth and partially to the eighteenth century. In the sixteenth century, after Europeans reached America, new devastating epidemics started among the native peoples resulting in a 90% population loss among American Indians within 120 years.

Who were in particular the victims of these plagues? Mostly people who were malnourished, sick, with a debilitated immune system. As discussed above, bacteria carrying the rich extra-chromosomal genetic information, as plasmids, phages, transposomes, viruses and virus-like particles (HIV included), are mostly pathogenic for the host organism and continually attack the immune system after penetration. This attack depends on the amount of the microbes which penetrate into the blood. Thus the immune system of people with low amounts of these bacteria was stronger and their carriers had a chance to overwhelm any plague. One of the most important results of the set of plagues that occurred in the history of humankind, mainly in Europe, North Africa, North America and partially in Asia, was natural selection, resulting in sanitation of the human population. Hand in hand in this tremendous evolution process was the selection of people with a low level of bacteria carrying pathogenic, mainly extra-chromosomal genetic information, able to penetrate into the human body and attack the immune system. The outcome of this complex evolutional proceeding, which finished towards the end of the nineteenth century, was a great reduction of pathogenic bacteria in the human population and eventually the establishment of a balance between non-pathogenic and pathogenic ("good" and "bad") microbes in the microflora of surviving individuals. The effect of this process was limitation of bacteria bearing HIV sequences and the selection of people carrying CCR-5 receptor deficiency on white blood cells.

A consequence of many plagues in the history of mankind was the establishment of a balance between prokaryotic and eukaryotic kingdoms in our body, which led to a positive selection of people with a low amount of viral and retroviral genetic information in their intestinal bacteria. This tremendous process, whose victims were many millions of humans, was very intensive particularly in Europe. The stability, acquired over many centuries, between eukaryotic and prokaryotic kingdoms was interrupted in the middle of the twentieth century due to the use of antibiotics, narcotic drugs and changes in life style (homo and anal sex).

It is generally accepted that due to ATB practically all primary bacterial pathogens were liquidated throughout two-three decades. The success of antibiotics in elimination of many diseases induced by microbes was such expressive that in the mid-1950s US Surgeon General Steward effusively proclaimed that the era of bacterial diseases finished. This trend of ATB glorification was spread very quickly from USA to Europe and microbiology got to the scientific periphery. In 1969, only a few people heard the voice of the English scientist J. A. Reaburn who said that in the future years it would be shown that antibiotics could bring us unforeseen vicious tricks.

In this way resistant, potentially pathogenic microbes, bearing rich extra-chromosomal genetic information as plasmids, phages, transposomes, virus-like particles (VLP) or viruses (including HIV), went from minority to majority and attacked the human immune system. Microbes employed their ability to change their shape - cell wall deficient (CWD) to survive in these hard conditions or were internalized into host cells (Swidsinski et al., 1998, 2002; Martin et al., 2004; Beachey, 1981; Benjamin et al., Cohen & Laux, 1995). Some of these microbes are able to overcome insurmountable barriers existing between microbial DNA and DNA of more highly organized beings. The result of this process are health troubles and one of them, induced by HIV bacteria with strong affinity to T lymphocytes, is immunodeficiency.

This proceeding started between Afro-American drug users because they had not been going through plague selection and sanitation, as had other American inhabitants. Disease spread mainly in big American cities as Los Angeles, San Fransisco, New York, Chicago, and others. Microbes which might be harmless in a healthy body became deadly in conjunction with drugs. This hypothesis was put forward in an editorial of the New England Journal of Medicine by David Durack: Some new factors may have distorted the host-parasite relation. So-called "recreational" drugs are one possibility. They were widely used in the large cities where the most of these cases have occurred, and the only patients in the series reported with this issue who were not homosexual were drug users. Perhaps one of these recreational drugs is an immunosuppressive agent (Durack and Phil, 1981). The leading candidates were nitrites, which were commonly inhaled in the years 1960 to 1977 to intensify orgasm. Butyl nitrite very probably plays an important role in induction of Kaposi's sarcoma in AIDS (Mirwish & Hawerkos, 1987). Mice exposed to isobutyl nitrite showed dose-related immune system damage and became highly susceptible to disease and death caused by mycobacterial infection (Neefe et al., 1983).

The "classical" drugs have a similar but more intensive effect on the immune system and micro-flora of drug users. The elimination of "good" intestinal bacteria by continually used drugs opened the space for amplification of microbes, which had existed before in the minority. The result of this process is that the immune system is not able to react to the massive attack and many diseases are induced, as: pneumonia, tuberculosis, toxoplasmosis, Cryptococcus, hepatitis B, herpes simplex, cytomegalovirus, bacterial, yeast and fungal infections, lymph gland infections and immunodeficiency. Amplified pathogenic microbes are equipped with antibiotic resistance and some of them are bearing viral and retroviral genetic information. Many of these infections are chronic or recurring, often unrecognized at first, and difficult to treat. Consequent antibiotic treatment forwards the spiral process of natural micro-flora destruction. And finally, ingestion of antiretroviral drugs as AZT completed this distortion. The result of such continual, step by step attack of intestinal microbes is their unification, reduction of their heterogeneity and loss of their basic function for the host. In the intestinal tract of two American AIDS patients in the final phase we found only one type of bacteria bearing HIV-1 sequences - multi-resistant *Escherichia coli* with plasmids of about 50 kbp.

4. Conclusion

Hypothetically, bacteria are probably hosts not only for HIV but also for other retroviruses. The presence of HIV sequences in commensurate bacteria of the patients may be explained as follows: 1) intestinal bacteria were infected by HIV or virus-like particles (VLP) previously produced by human cells, in particular by macrophages and lymphocytes; 2) intestinal bacteria of AIDS patients are a natural host of HIV sequences in the form of a virus or VLP.

Effective vaccines for human immunodeficiency virus type 1 (HIV-1) will have to stimulate protective immunity in the intestinal mucosa, where HIV-1 infection causes severe $CD4^+$ T-cell depletion (Bealshe et al., 1994; Bartlett et al., 2003). While replication-competent recombinant adenovirus (rAd) vectors can stimulate adenovirus-specific mucosal immunity after replication, oral delivery of replication-defective rAd vectors encoding specific immunogens has proven challenging (Wang et al., 2009).

Recent studies suggest that induction of primary immune responses by recombinant bacterial vectors leads to gut immunization and subsequent systemic boosting elicits potent antigen-specific gut mucosal responses. Genetically modified bacteria have been experimentally used as recombinant probiotics also in gastrointestinal disorders, but clinical usage is currently not the case. Nevertheless, in the future a greater use of this kind of approach is expected. The expression of HIV-1 antigens in specific probiotic strains may be suitable for clinical use as a potential vaccine.

5. Acknowledgement

We would like to thank Danica Stanekova and all the people working at HIV/AIDS Reference Centre, Slovak Medical University, Bratislava, to Milos Mokras from Department of Infectious Diseases and Geographic Medicine, Derer's Hospital, Bratislava and to Vladimir Krcmery from St. Elizabeth University, Bratislava for patient's samples.

This work was supported by the grant VEGA 2/5025/27, 2/0081/08 and the grant APVV-0404-07.

6. References

Apetrei, C., and Marx, P.A. (2005). African lentiviruses related to HIV. *J. Neurovirol.* 11: 33-49.

Baltimore, D. (1985). Retroviruses and retrotransposos: The role of reverse transcription in shaping the eukaryotic genome. *Cell* 40: 481-482,

Bartlett, J.G., Carlos, del Rio, DeMaria, A., Sepkowitz K.A. (2003). Smallpox Vaccination and the HIV-Infected Patient: A Roundtable. *AIDS Clinical Care*, 15: 61-63.

Belshe, R.B., Bolognesi, D.P., Clements, M.L., Corey, L., Dolin, R., Mestecky, J., Mulligan, M., Stablein, D., Wright, P. (1994). HIV infection in vaccinated volunteers. *JAMA*, 10: 431.

Beachey, E.H. (1981). Bacterial adherence: adhesin-receptor interactions mediating the attachment of bacteria to mucosal surface. *J. Infect. Dis.*, 143: 325-345.

Benjamin, P., Federman, M., and Wanke, Ch.A. (1995). Characterization of an invasive phenotype associated with enteroaggregative *Escherichia coli*. *Infection and Immunity*, 63: 3417-342.

Brenchley, J.M., Schacker, T. W., Ruff, L.E., Price, D.A., Taylor, J.H., Beilman, G.J., Nguyen, P.L., Khoruts, A., Larson, M., Haase, A.T., Douek, D. (2004). CCD4+T Cell Depletion during all Stages of HIV Disease Occurs Predominantly in the Gastrointestinal Tract. *Journal of Experimental Medicine*, 200: 749-759.

Broxmeyer, L., and Cantwell, A. (2008). AIDS: "It's the bacteria, stupid!" *Medical Hypotheses*, 71, 741–748.

Cantwell Jr AR. (1983). Kaposi's sarcoma and variably acid-fast bacteria in vivo in two homosexual men. *Cutis*, 32(1): 58–61.

Cantwell Jr AR. (1993). Necroscopic findings of variably acid-fast bacteria in a fatal case of acquired immunodeficience syndrome and Kaposi's sarcoma. *Growth*, 47(2):129–34.

Cusini M., Salmaso F, Zerboni R, Carminati G, Vernaci C, Franchi C, Locatelli A, Alessi E. (2004). 5% Imiquimod cream for external anogenital warts in HIV infected patients under HAART therapy. *Int J STD AIDS*, 15: 17–20.

Cohen, P.S., and Laux, D.C.(1995). Bacterial adhesion to and penetration of intestinal Mucus *in vitro. Methods Enzymol.*, 253: 309-314.

Dandekar, S. (2007). Pathogenesis of HIV in the gastrointestinal tract. *Curr HIV/AIDS Rep.* 4 (1):10-15.

Duesberg, P.H.(1987). Retroviruses as Carcinogens and Pathogens: Expectations and Reality. *Cancer Research*, 47: 1199-1220.

Durack, D.T., Phil, M.B.D. (1981). Opportunistic Infections and Kaposi's Sarcoma in Homosexual Men. *New England Journal of Medicine,* 305:1465-1467.

Finzi, D., Hermankova, M., Pierson, T., Carruth, T.L., Buck, C., Chaisson, R.E., Quinn, T.C., Chadwick, K., Margolick, K.J., Brookmeyer, R., Gallant, J., Markowitz, M., Ho, D.D., Richman, D.D., Siliciano, R.F. (1997). Identification of a Reservoir for HIV-1 in Patients on Highly Active Antiretroviral Therapy. *Science*, 278: 1295–1300.

Gallo, R.C., and Wong-Staal, F. (1985). A human T-lymphotropic retrovirus (HTLV-III) as a the cause of the acquired immunodeficiency syndrome. *Ann.Intern. Med.*, 103:679-689.

Guadalupe, M., Sankaran, S., George, M.D., Reay, E., Verhoeven, D., Shacklett, B.L., Flamm, J., Wegelin, J., Prindiville, T., Dandekar, S. (2006). Viral suppression and immune restoration in the gastrointestinal mucosa of human immunodeficiency virus type1-infected patients initiating therapy during primary or chronic infection. *J. Virol.*, 80: 8236-47.

Hatziioannou, T., Ambrose, Z., Chung, N.P., Piatak, M. Jr, Yuan, F., Trubey, C.M., Coalter, V., Kiser, R., Schneider, D., Smedley, J., Pung, R., Gathuka, M., Estes, J.D., Veazey, R.S., KewalRamani, V.N., Lifson, J.D., Bieniasz, P.D. (2009). A macaque model of HIV-1 infection. *Proc Natl Acad Sci U S A.*, 17; 106 (11):4425-9.

Chun,T.W., Davey, R.T., Ostrowski, M., Shawn, J.J., Engel, D., Mullins, J.I., and Fauci, A.S. (2000). Relationship between pre-existing viral reservoirs and the re-emergence of plasma viremia after discontinuation of highly active anti-retroviral therapy. *Nature Medicine*, 6:757–61.

Lackner, A.A., Mohan, M., Veazey, R.S. (2009).The gastrointestinal tract and AIDS pathogenesis. *Gastroenterology,* 136(6):1965-78.

Li, Q.S., Duan, L.J., Estes, J.D., Ma, Z.M., Rourke, T., Wang, Y.CH., Reilly, C., Carlis, J., Miller, CH.J., Haase, A.T. (2005). Peak SIV replication in resting memory $CD4^{+}$ T cells depletes gut lamina propria CD4+ T cells. *Nature*; 434:1148–52.

Ling, B., Veazey, R.S., Hart, M., Lackner, A.A., Kuroda, M., Pahar, B., Marx, P. (2007). Early restoration of mucosal CD4 memory CCR5 T cells in the gut of SIV-infected rhesus predicts long term non-progression. *AIDS*, 21(18):2377-85.

Ling, B., Mohan, M., Lackner, A.A., Green, L.C., Marx, P.A., Doyle, L.A., Veazey, R.S. (2010). The large intestine as a major reservoir for simian immunodeficiency virus in macaques with long-term, nonprogressing infection. *J Infect Dis.*, 202(12): 1846-54.

Lo, S.-C., Tsai, S., Benish, J.R., Shih, J.W.-K., Wear, D.J., and Wong, D.M. (1991). Enhancement of HIV-1 cytocidal effects in CD_4^+ lymphocytes by the AIDS-associated mycoplasma. *Science*, 251: 1074-1076.

Martin, M.H., Campbell, B.J., Hart, C.A., Mpolfu, C., Nayar, M., Singh, R., Englyst, H., Williams, H.F., Rhodes, J.M. (2004). Enhanced Esherichia coli adherence and invasion in Crohn's disease and colon cancer. *Gastroenterology*,127: 80-93.

Mattapallil, J.J., Daniel, C., Douek, D.C., Hill, B., Nishimura, Y., Martin, M., Roederer, M. (2005). Massive infection and loss of memory $CD4^+$ T cells in multiple tissues during acute SIV infection. *Nature*, 434: 1093–7.

Mego, M., Majek, J., Koncekova, R., Ebringer, L., Ciernikova, S., Rauko, P., Kovac, M ., Trupl, J., Slezak, P., Zajac, V. (2005). Intramucosal bacteria in colon cancer and their elimination by probiotic strain *Enterococcus faecium* M-74 with organic selenium. *Folia Microbiologica*, 50: 443-447.

Mego,M., Koncekova, R., Mikusova, E., Ebringer, L., Demitrovicova, L., Nemova, I., Drgona, L., Trupl, J., Mardiak, J., Koza, I., Zajac, V. (2006). Prevention of febrile neutropenia in leukemic patients by probiotic strain *Enterococcus faecium* M-74. Phase II.study. *Support Care Cancer*, 14, 285-290.

Mirwish, S.S., Hawerkos, H.W.(1987). Butyl nitrite in induction of Kaposi sarcoma in AIDS.]. *New England Journal of Medicine*, 17: 1603.

Montagnier, L.: Vaincre le SIDA. (1986). Entretiens avec Pierre Bourget. Paris, Editations Cana.

Neefe, J.R., Ganjii, A., and Goedert, J.G. (1983) "Daily Amyl Nitrite Inhalation Decreases Mouse Splenocyte Response to Concanavalin A". (abstract 3850) *Federation Proceedings* 42 (4): 949, 5 March.

Nelson, J.A., Wiley, C.A., Reynolds-Kohler, C., Reese, C.E., Margaretten, M., Lecy, J.A. (1988). HIV detected in bowel epithelium from patients with gastrointestinal symptoms. *Lancet*, 6: 259-62.

Sharp, P.M., Bailes, E., Chaudhui, R.R., Rodenburg, C.M., Santiago, M.O., Hahn, B.H. (2001). The origin of acquired immune deficiency syndrome viruses: where and when? *Philos Trans R Soc Lond B Biol Sci.*, 29: 867-876.

Siliciano, J.D., Kajdas, J,, Finzi, D.C., Quinn, T.C., Chadwick, C., Margolick, J.B., Kovacs, C., Gange, S.J., and Siliciano, R.F. (2003). Long-term follow-up studies confirm the stability of the latent reservoir for HIV-1 in resting CD4+ T cells. *Nature Medicine*, 9: 727–8.

Simon, G.L., and Gorbach, S.L. (1984). Intestinal microflora in health and disease. *Gastroenterology*, 86: 174–193.

Swidsinski, A., Khilkin, M., Kerjaschki, D., Schreiber, S., Ortner, M., Weber, J., Lochs, H. (1998). Association between intraepthelial Escherichia coli and colorectal cancer. *Gastroenteology*, 115; 281-286.

Swidsinski, A., Ladhoff, A., Pernthaler, A., Swidsinski, S., Loening-Baucke, V., Orther, M., Weber, J., Hoffman, U., Schrei-Ber, S., Dietel, M., Lochs H. (2002). Mucosal flora in inflammatory bowel disease. *Gastroenterology* 122, 44–54.

Temin, H.M. (1988). Origin of retroviruses from cellular moveable genetic elements. *Cell*, 21: 599-600.

Temin, H.M. (1989). Retrons in bacteria. *Nature*, 39: 254-255.

Varmus, H.J. (1989). Reverse transcription in bacteria. *Cell* , 56: 721-724.

Veazey, R.S., DeMaria, M.A., Chalifoux, L.V., Shvetz, D.E., Pauley, D.R., Knight, H.L., Rosenzweig, M., Johnson, R.P., Desrosiers, R.C., Lackner, A.A. (1998). Gastrointestinal tract as a major site of CD4+ T cell depletion and viral replication in SIV infection. *Science*, 280: 427-31.

Veazey, R.S., Lackner, A.A. (2005). HIV swiftly guts the immune system. *Nature Medicine*, 11: 469 –70.

Wang, L.S., Cheng, Ch., Ko, S.Y., Kong, W-P., Kanekiyo, M., Einfeld, D., Schwartz, R.M., C. Richter King, R., Gall, J.G.D. and Nabel, G.J. Delivery of Human Immunodeficiency Virus Vaccine Vectors to the Intestine Induces Enhanced Mucosal Cellular Immunity. *J. Virol.* 2009: 83: 7166-7175.

Zajac, V., Kovac, M., Ciernikova, S., Mego, M., Rauko, P., Stevurkova, V., Stanekova, D., and Mokras, M. (2005). Detection of HIV sequences in colon bacteria of AIDS positive patients. ECCMID conference *Clin. Microbiol. Infec.* 11: 53, Copenhagen, April 2005.

Zajac, V., Stevurkova, V., Matelova, L., Ujhazy, E. (2007). Detection of HIV-1 sequences in intestinal bacteria of HIV/AIDS patients. *Neuroendocrinology Letters*, 28: 591- 595.

Zajac,V., Mego, M., Kovac, M., Stevurkova, V., Ciernikova, S., Ujhazy, E., Gajdosik, A., Gajdosikova A.(2006). Testing of bacteria isolated from HIV/AIDS patients in experimental models. *Neuroendocrinology Letters*, 27: 101-104.

Zajac, V., Matelova, L., Liskova, A., Mego, M., Holec, V., Adamcikova, Z., Stevurkova, V., Shahum, A., Krcmery, V. (2011). Confirmation of HIV-like sequences in respiratory tract bacteria of Cambodian and Kenyan HIV-positive pediatric patients. *Medical Science Monitor*, 17(3):154-158.

Zhu, T., Korber, B.T., Nahmias, A.J., Hooper, E., Sharp, P.M., Ho, D.D. (1998). An African HIV-1 sequence from 1959 and implications for the origin of the epidemic. *Nature*, 391: 594-7.